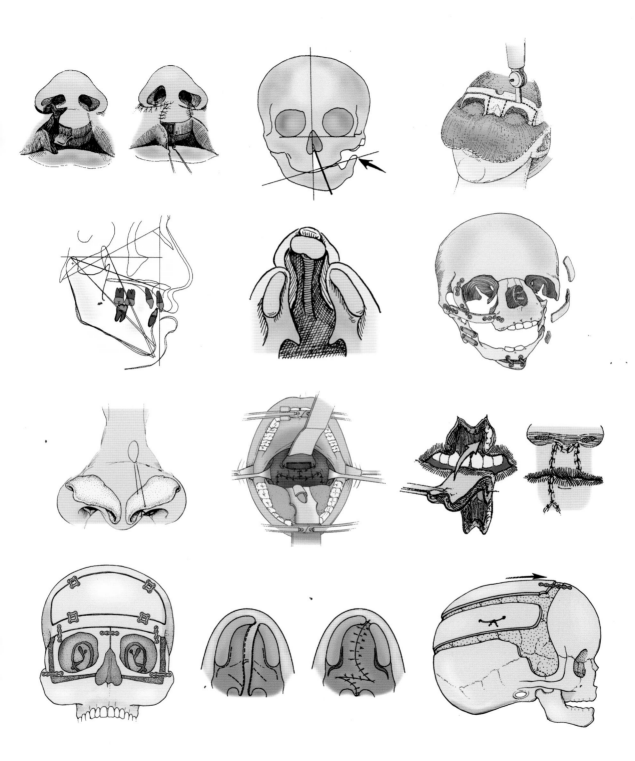

Plastic Surgery

Plastic Surgery

First Edition

Editor:
Joseph G. McCarthy, MD

Editors, Hand Surgery volumes:
James W. May, Jr., MD
J. William Littler, MD

Plastic Surgery

Second Edition

Editor
Stephen J. Mathes, MD
Professor of Surgery
Chief, Division of Plastic Surgery
University of California, San Francisco
School of Medicine
San Francisco, California

Editor, Hand Surgery Volumes
Vincent R. Hentz, MD
Professor of Surgery
Chief, Division of Plastic and Hand Surgery
Stanford University School of Medicine
Stanford, California

With illustrations by Kathy Hirsh and Scott Thorn Barrows, CMI, FAMI

Shireen L. Dunwoody, Editorial Coordinator

VOLUME *IV*

PEDIATRIC PLASTIC SURGERY

SAUNDERS

ELSEVIER

SAUNDERS
ELSEVIER

1600 John F. Kennedy Blvd.
Ste 1800
Philadelphia, PA 19103-2899

PLASTIC SURGERY, 2nd ed.

Volume I 0-7216-8812-8/978-0-7216-8812-1
Volume II 0-7216-8813-6/978-0-7216-8813-8
Volume III 0-7216-8814-4/978-0-7216-8814-5
Volume IV 0-7216-8815-2/978-0-7216-8815-2
Volume V 0-7216-8816-0/978-0-7216-8816-9
Volume VI 0-7216-8817-9/978-0-7216-8817-6
Volume VII 0-7216-8818-7/978-0-7216-8818-3
Volume VIII 0-7216-8819-5/978-0-7216-8819-0
8-Volume Set 0-7216-8811-X/978-0-7216-8811-4

Notice

Knowledge and best practice in this field are constantly changing. As new research and experience broaden our knowledge, changes in practice, treatment and drug therapy may become necessary or appropriate. Readers are advised to check the most current information provided (i) on procedures featured or (ii) by the manufacturer of each product to be administered, to verify the recommended dose or formula, the method and duration of administration, and contraindications. It is the responsibility of the practitioner, relying on his or her own experience and knowledge of the patient, to make diagnoses, to determine dosages and the best treatment for each individual patient, and to take all appropriate safety precautions. To the fullest extent of the law, neither the Publisher nor the Editors assume any liability for any injury and/or damage to persons or property arising out of or related to any use of the material contained in this book.

The Publisher

Previous edition copyrighted 1990.

Library of Congress Cataloging-in-Publication Data
Mathes, Stephen J.
     Plastic surgery / Stephen J. Mathes ; editor Vincent R. Hentz.—2nd ed.
       p.   cm.
     ISBN 0–7216–8811–X
     1. Surgery, Plastic.   I. Hentz, Vincent R.   II. Title.
RD118.M388 2006
617.9′5—dc21

2003041541

Acquisitions Editors: Sue Hodgson, Allan Ross, Joe Rusko, Judith Fletcher
Senior Developmental Editor: Ann Ruzycka Anderson
Publishing Services Manager: Tina Rebane
Senior Project Manager: Linda Van Pelt
Design Direction: Steven Stave
Cover Designer: Shireen Dunwoody

Printed in China

Last digit is the print number: 9   8   7   6   5   4   3   2   1

This text is dedicated to Mary H. McGrath, who is my inspiration and a source of joy in our daily life together, our adventures at home and away, and our shared enthusiasm and excitement as plastic surgeons.

✦ CONTRIBUTORS

STEPHEN B. BAKER, DDS, MD
Assistant Professor of Surgery
Division of Plastic Surgery
Georgetown University School of Medicine
Associate Residency Director and Section Chief
Craniomaxillofacial Surgery
Georgetown University Hospital
Washington, D.C.

SCOTT P. BARTLETT, MD, FACS
Associate Professor of Surgery (Plastic)
University of Pennsylvania School of Medicine
Director, Craniofacial Program
The Children's Hospital of Philadelphia
Philadelphia, Pennsylvania

JAMES P. BRADLEY, MD
Associate Professor of Surgery
Benard Sarnat Chair, Craniofacial Research
Division of Plastic Surgery
David Geffen School of Medicine at the University of
    California, Los Angeles
Chief, Pediatric Plastic Surgery
University of California, Los Angeles, Medical Center
Los Angeles, California

MICHAEL H. CARSTENS, MD, FACS
Associate Professor of Plastic Surgery
Saint Louis University School of Medicine
Director of Craniofacial Surgery
Cardinal Glennon Children's Hospital
St. Louis, Missouri

PHILIP KUO-TING CHEN, MD
Associate Professor of Surgery
Chang Gung University Medical College
Director, Craniofacial Center
Chang Gung Memorial Hospital
Kweishan, Taiwan

COURT BALDWIN CUTTING, MD
Associate Professor of Surgery (Plastic Surgery)
New York University School of Medicine
Attending Surgeon
New York University Medical Center
New York, New York

DAVID J. DAVID, MD, FRCS
Professor of Craniofacial Surgery
University of Adelaide Faculty of Medicine
Head, Australian Craniofacial Unit
Women's and Children's Hospital and Royal Adelaide
    Hospital
Adelaide, South Australia, Australia

ALVARO A. FIGUEROA, DDS, MS
Professor of Orthodontics
Department of Plastic Surgery
Rush Medical College
Co-Director, Rush Craniofacial Center
Chicago, Illinois

BARRY H. GRAYSON, DDS
Associate Professor of Clinical Surgery (Orthodontics)
New York University School of Medicine
Professor of Clinical Orthodontics
New York University College of Dentistry
Attending Surgeon
Institute of Reconstructive Plastic Surgery
New York University Medical Center
New York, New York

JUDITH M. GURLEY, MD
Staff Surgeon
Genesis Cosmetic Surgery and Medical Spa
St. Louis, Missouri

ROBERT A. HARDESTY, MD, FACS
Private Practice
Riverside, California
Former Professor of Surgery
Division of Plastic Surgery
Loma Linda University School of Medicine
Director, Plastic Surgery Training Program
Loma Linda University Medical Center
Loma Linda, California

ALEXES HAZEN, MD
Assistant Professor (Plastic Surgery)
New York University School of Medicine
Director
New York University
Aesthetic Plastic Surgery Center
Institute of Reconstructive and Plastic Surgery
Director
Division of Plastic Surgery
Manhattan Veterans Administration Medical Center
New York, New York

JILL A. HELMS, DDS, PhD
Associate Professor of Surgery
Stanford University School of Medicine
Stanford, California

WILLIAM Y. HOFFMAN, MD, FACS
Professor of Clinical Surgery
University of California, San Francisco, School of
    Medicine
Staff Surgeon
San Francisco General Hospital
San Francisco, California

LARRY H. HOLLIER, Jr., MD, FACS
Associate Professor of Surgery
Division of Plastic Surgery
Michael DeBakey Department of Surgery
Baylor College of Medicine
Co-Director, Craniofacial Clinic
Chief of Service, Plastic Surgery
Texas Children's Hospital and Ben Taub Hospital
Houston, Texas

RICHARD A. HOPPER, MD, FACS
Assistant Professor
Department of Surgery
University of Washington School of Medicine
Attending Surgeon
Children's Hospital and Regional Medical Center
Seattle, Washington

DENNIS J. HURWITZ, MD, FACS
Clinical Professor of Surgery (Plastic)
University of Pittsburgh School of Medicine
Attending Surgeon
Children's Hospital of Pittsburgh and Magee Women's
    Hospital
Pittsburgh, Pennsylvania

DAVID M. KAHN, MD
Assistant Professor of Surgery
Stanford University School of Medicine
Attending Surgeon
Lucile Packard Children's Hospital at Stanford
Stanford, California

ALEX A. KANE, MD, FACS
Assistant Professor of Surgery, Division of Plastic and
    Reconstructive Surgery
Washington University School of Medicine
Pediatric Plastic Surgeon
St. Louis Children's Hospital
St. Louis, Missouri

JOSEPH E. LOSEE, MD, FACS, FAAP
Assistant Professor of Surgery (Plastic) and Pediatrics
Program Director, Craniofacial Fellowship
University of Pittsburgh School of Medicine
Director, Pittsburgh Cleft and Craniofacial Center
Chief, Division of Pediatric Plastic Surgery
Children's Hospital of Pittsburgh
Pittsburgh, Pennsylvania

JEFFREY L. MARSH, MD, FACS
Clinical Professor in Surgery
Saint Louis University School of Medicine
Director, Cleft Lip/Palate and Craniofacial Deformities
    Center
St. John's Mercy Medical Center
St. Louis, Missouri

JOSEPH G. McCARTHY, MD, FACS
Lawrence D. Bell Professor of Plastic Surgery
New York University School of Medicine
Director, Institute of Reconstructive Plastic Surgery
New York University Medical Center
New York, New York

JOHN M. MENEZES, MD
Assistant Professor of Surgery
Division of Plastic and Reconstructive Surgery
University of Nevada School of Medicine
Head, Craniofacial Section
University Medical Center
Las Vegas, Nevada

DELORA L. MOUNT, MD, FACS
Assistant Professor of Surgery
Assistant Professor of Pediatrics
University of Wisconsin Medical School
Chief, Pediatric Plastic Surgery
University of Wisconsin Children's Hospital
Director
Craniofacial Anomalies Clinic
Madison, Wisconsin

RANDALL P. NACAMULI, MD, FACS
Resident in Surgery
University of California, San Francisco–East Bay Surgery
    Program
Alameda County Medical Center
Oakland, California
Postdoctoral Fellow
Children's Surgical Research Laboratory
Stanford University School of Medicine
Stanford, California

M. SAMUEL NOORDHOFF, MD
Professor of Surgery
Chang Gung University Medical College
Superintendent Emeritus and Chairman
Department of Plastic Surgery
Chang Gung Memorial Hospital
Taipei, Taiwan

JOHN W. POLLEY, MD
Professor and Chairman
Department of Plastic Surgery
Rush Medical College
Co-Director
Rush Craniofacial Center
Chicago, Illinois

ANIL P. PUNJABI, MD, DDS
Associate Professor of Surgery
Division of Plastic Surgery
Loma Linda University School of Medicine
Loma Linda, California
Chief
Division of Plastic Surgery
Riverside County Regional Medical Center
Moreno Valley, California

JAY RAPLEY, BS
Resident in Orthopaedic Surgery
University of Texas Medical Branch Health Care
Galueston, Texas

ALI SALIM, MD
Resident in Plastic Surgery
University of California, Davis, Medical Center
Sacramento, California
Postdoctoral Fellow
Children's Surgical Research Laboratory
Stanford University School of Medicine
Stanford, California

STEPHEN A. SCHENDEL, MD, DDS, FACS
Professor of Surgery
Division of Plastic Surgery
Stanford University School of Medicine
Director
Craniofacial Surgery Program
Lucile Packard Children's Hospital at Stanford
Stanford, California

YUN-YING SHI, BS
Medical Student/Research Fellow
Stanford University School of Medicine
Stanford, California

JOHN W. SIEBERT, MD
Associate Professor of Surgery
Division of Plastic Surgery
Department of Surgery
New York University School of Medicine
Staff
New York University Medical Center
New York, New York

GERALD M. SLOAN, MD, FACS
Ethel F. and James A. Valone Distinguished Professor
Chief (retired), Division of Plastic and Reconstructive
    Surgery
Department of Surgery
University of North Carolina School of Medicine
Medical Director (retired)
Craniofacial Center
University of North Carolina School of Dentistry
Chapel Hill, North Carolina

HOOMAN SOLTANIAN, MD
Attending Surgeon
St. Francis Care
Private Practice
Hartford, Connecticut

SAMUEL STAL, MD, FACS
Professor of Surgery, Division of Plastic Surgery
Michael DeBakey Department of Surgery
Baylor College of Medicine
Chief of Service, Department of Plastic Surgery
Director, Craniofacial Clinic
Texas Children's Hospital
Houston, Texas

CRAIG A. VANDER KOLK, MD, FACS
Professor of Surgery, Division of Plastic and
    Reconstructive Surgery
Johns Hopkins University School of Medicine
Director, Cleft and Craniofacial Center
Johns Hopkins Hospital
Baltimore, Maryland

PETER D. WITT, MD
Medical Director, Pediatric Plastic Surgery
Children's Hospital Central California
Madera, California

DAVID J. ZAJAC, PhD, CCC-SLP
Associate Professor of Dental Ecology
University of North Carolina School of Dentistry
Associate Professor of Speech and Hearing Sciences
University of North Carolina at Chapel Hill School of
    Medicine
Chapel Hill, North Carolina

✦ PREFACE

It is a great thing to start life with a small number of really good books which are your very own. Through the Magic Door (1908), Sir Arthur Conan Doyle

My meeting for lunch with Joseph McCarthy in Boston in 1998 during the annual meeting of the Society of Plastic Surgery was arranged to discuss the possibility of my becoming the editor of the new edition of *Plastic Surgery*. I was well aware of the responsibility of assuming this giant project. My admiration of the past editors, including Joseph McCarthy for the 1990 edition of *Plastic Surgery* and John Marquis Converse for the 1964 and 1977 editions of *Reconstructive Plastic Surgery*, was great since these texts in my estimation really defined our specialty of plastic surgery and provided the platform for future advances in treating congenital and acquired deformities. My memory of Converse's first edition started with my residency in plastic surgery on my first rotation at the private practice of William Schatten, John Hartley, and John Griffith in Atlanta, Georgia. There, in moments when I was not involved in patient care activities, I would enjoy reading the pages of clinical advice on all subjects related to plastic surgery in the five volumes of *Reconstructive Plastic Surgery*. Subsequently, in 1977, as a faculty member at Washington University, I was privileged to be able to purchase my own copy of the then six-volume edition of *Reconstructive Plastic Surgery*, again edited by Converse. This time, my reading of the exciting pages was less relaxed, since I was using the text as the reference in preparation for my plastic surgery board examinations.

By 1990, I was able to contribute a chapter to *Plastic Surgery*, edited by Joseph McCarthy, and I personally knew most of the contributors, having witnessed the evolution of many of the new advances and unique contributions contained within the then eight volumes. With this background, I was excited and honored to have been recommended as the next editor of this text, which has so well reflected the greatness of the specialty of plastic surgery. My meeting was punctuated by advice regarding the importance of the text and the selection of experts who would provide both guidance and stimulation to future readers on the many subjects important to physicians involved in plastic surgery. The complexity of orchestrating so many contributors in a timely fashion was also emphasized. I left this luncheon inspired to undertake this project, with the anticipation of capturing the best and most innovative surgeons as contributors to achieve an edition in keeping with the unique traditions of excellence of the past editions of *Plastic Surgery* and *Reconstructive Plastic Surgery*.

My first step was to find an academic hand surgeon to edit the two hand volumes. J. William Littler had served as the editor of the hand and upper extremity volume in Converse's two editions of *Reconstructive Plastic Surgery*. Littler was a master hand surgeon and one of the foremost innovators in hand surgery. McCarthy selected a unique combination of academic hand surgeons, James W. May and J. William Littler, to edit the two volumes dedicated to upper extremity and hand surgery in the 1990 edition of *Plastic Surgery*. With the many new techniques related to microvascular surgery, the space devoted to this important aspect of plastic surgery had been expanded into two volumes. Jim May, like Bill Littler, is a master hand surgeon, a gifted teacher, and an innovator in all aspects of plastic surgery and was able to include both his contributions and those of many other hand surgeons, who all took part in advancing this important discipline.

Fortunately, the decision regarding who should be the hand editor for this edition of *Plastic Surgery* was obvious. Vincent R. Hentz is a master hand surgeon and past president of the American Society of Surgery of the Hand. As an accomplished educator and chief of the division of plastic and hand surgery at Stanford, he is the ideal person to follow in the footsteps of Littler and May. In keeping with the many innovations and new techniques in upper extremity and hand surgery, this edition contains two volumes devoted to hand surgery. Of interest, we have shifted the editorial geography from the East Coast (New York City and Boston) to the West Coast (San Francisco and Palo Alto). Unfortunately, despite the improvement in weather characteristics of the western coastline of the United States, the commitment to continue the excellence of this text has kept the editors mostly indoors during the complex editing process necessary to complete these volumes.

The goal of this edition is to cover the scope of plastic surgery. The key was to select the best contributors to define the problems encountered in plastic surgery, to provide both the most current and the most successful solutions, and to deliver the challenge for future innovation in each area of plastic surgery. In this new edition, there are 219 chapters with 293 contributors. Each of the senior authors of the 219 chapters was carefully selected for his or her recognized expertise in the assigned subject of the chapter. Each author has personally contributed to the advancement in knowledge related to his or her area of expertise in our specialty.

The authors selected are inspirational leaders due to their many innovations toward improvement in the management of the plastic surgery patient. After the manuscripts were submitted, each chapter was carefully reviewed by the editors to ensure that all aspects of the authors' assigned topics were adequately covered and well illustrated so that the reader could readily incorporate the chapter content into the practice of plastic surgery.

In the eight volumes included in this edition, all subjects pertinent to the scope of plastic surgery are covered. Many new topics, 67 in all, have been developed or were enlarged from broader subjects and warranted a new individual chapter. Thirteen of these new chapter topics are included in Volume I: General Principles. The enlargement of the volume containing general principles reflects the continuing expansion of our specialty, the emphasis on experimental and clinical research, and the impact of research on the practice of plastic surgery. In the remaining volumes, devoted to specific clinical topics, two new types of chapter formats were added: 25 technique chapters and 7 secondary chapters. The technique chapters are added to complement the overview chapters and are designed to focus on particular techniques currently in use for a clinical problem. Likewise, the secondary chapters are again an extension of the overview chapters on particular subjects but focus on problems that persist despite the application of primary plastic surgery solutions. These secondary chapters are designed to demonstrate areas where operations may fail related to improper patient or technique selection or technique failures. They also discuss procedures to correct unsatisfactory outcomes following primary plastic surgery.

Volumes II through VII are divided into specific topographical areas of plastic surgery. Volume II: The Head and Neck (Part 1) is devoted to cosmetic procedures and contains six new topic chapters, seven new technique chapters, and three new secondary chapters. This volume now contains color illustrations, which will help the reader evaluate problems and results following cosmetic procedures. Many important subjects are expanded and introduced. For instance, there are now five chapters on the face lift, which provide the reader with the ability to compare techniques and focus on specific aspects of the procedure. Volume III: The Head and Neck (Part 2) is dedicated to reconstructive procedures and contains 10 new topics as well as the traditional subjects used in the previous edition. Volume IV: Pediatric Plastic Surgery contains five new topics and provides multispecialty approaches to children presenting with congenital facial anomalies. Volume V: Tumors of the Head, Neck, and Skin has seven new topics. Along with management principles of head and neck cancer, identification and treatment of melanoma and non-melanoma skin cancer have been added in new topic chapters. Volume VI: Trunk and Lower Extremity contains 34 added topics. For example, in the area of postmastectomy reconstruction, 12 new chapters have been added to provide specific diagnostic, management, and technical information on breast reconstruction issues. Similarly, four new chapter topics have been added on body contouring procedures. With emphasis on bariatric surgery and body contouring procedures, these chapters provide a complete array of information on techniques and outcomes. Volume VII: The Hand and Upper Limb (Part 1) contains introductory and general principles related to diagnosis and management of acquired disorders, both traumatic and nontraumatic. Volume VIII: The Hand and Upper Limb (Part 2) contains three parts: congenital anomalies, paralytic disorders, and rehabilitation. The two volumes on hand and upper extremity surgery contain an additional 22 chapters introducing new subjects to this edition of *Plastic Surgery*.

Education involves the process of observation as well as contact with teachers, mentors, colleagues, and students and the literature. Each component is essential to learning a specialty in medicine and maintaining competence in the specialty over the course of one's career. In plastic surgery, the abundance of master surgeons gives everyone the opportunity to observe excellence in technique, during residency and later through educational programs. Contact with teachers and colleagues must be maintained in order to keep abreast of the new innovations in medicine and to measure one's outcomes in the context of standard of care. Our professional society meetings and symposia, both locally and nationally, provide us with this opportunity. Contact with mentors and students is critical for innovation. The physician must seek out these sources of inspiration and stimulation to improve patient care. Collaboration with professionals is a unique opportunity to allow further growth in our specialty and is available in every medical environment. The literature allows the physician to see where we have been, where we are currently, and what the future holds. The physician can hold a piece of literature in the hand and review its message both in critical times, when patient management decisions must be made on a timely basis, and during leisure times, when a subject is studied and carefully measured against personal experience and knowledge acquired through professional contacts. It is hoped that this edition of *Plastic Surgery*, like its predecessors, can serve the purpose of literature in teaching. Its eight volumes contain more than 6800 pages of information carefully formulated by recognized experts in our specialty in plastic surgery. It is designed, as initially stated, to define the current knowledge of plastic surgery and to serve as a platform for future creativity to benefit the patient we see with congenital and acquired deformities.

Stephen J. Mathes, MD, 2005

✦ ACKNOWLEDGMENTS

So many talented and dedicated professionals are necessary to complete a text of this magnitude. It is impossible to really thank everyone adequately, since there are so many people behind the scenes who were silently working toward the completion of this project. However, I shall endeavor to acknowledge the people who provided scientific, technical, and emotional support to make this edition of *Plastic Surgery* possible.

My first contact with the publisher (Saunders, now Elsevier) started with my meeting with Allan Ross and Ann Ruzycka Anderson. Allan Ross, executive editor, was assigned to guide this text to publication. He is a dedicated publishing executive who was most supportive at the inception of this project. Ann Ruzycka Anderson, senior developmental editor, has been working in medical publishing for 20 years. This text was most fortunate to have Allan and Ann assigned as the guiding forces at the onset. Ann states that working on this text is "something exciting, worthwhile, and important" because she is helping to "produce the largest book in medical publishing history."

Because this book took 5 years to complete, there were changes in the personnel involved in the project. Joe Rusko, medical editor, assumed the responsibilities of guiding the development of the text, with Allan Ross taking on the role of consultant. Joe has great enthusiasm and provided great ideas for the format of this book and for associated advertising. During the past year, the project was turned over to the leadership of Sue Hodgson, currently the publishing director and general manager for Elsevier Ltd. With Sue living in London, the project took on a more international outlook, with Sue flying between London, Philadelphia, New York, and San Francisco to keep the project moving ahead to completion. Both Sue Hodgson and Allan Ross have a great deal of success in guiding complex publications to press. Sue has published highly successful books in dermatology, and now, it is hoped, she will be able to make the same claim for the field of plastic surgery. For sure, she can now lay claim to publishing the largest medical book in existence. Recently, Sue Hodgson summed up her role in the publishing industry as follows: "The opportunity to create new products to answer the market's educational needs and handling high-profile and demanding projects are what get me out of bed in the morning." All plastic surgeons who use this text are indebted to the perseverance and commitment of these publishing leaders: Allan Ross, Joe Rusko, and Sue Hodgson.

"The quality of a person's life is in direct proportion to their commitment to excellence, regardless of their chosen field of endeavor."

—Vince Lombardi

After the authors were selected for the 219 chapters, it was obvious that we needed someone special to serve as the editorial coordinator between the editors and the authors. Thanks to the advice of Allan Ross and Ann Ruzycka Anderson, Shireen Dunwoody was recommended for this position. Shireen is an accomplished computer programmer and musician and has served as a senior medical writer, media programmer/editor, and developmental editor since 1991. Among the high-profile medical texts on which she has worked are *Clinical Oncology* (Martin Abeloff et al., editors), *Surgery of the Liver and Biliary Tract* (Leslie Blumgart, editor), and *Fundamentals of Surgery* (John E. Niederhuber, editor). Shireen has worked closely with the editors and our assigned authors during every step of the process—obtaining the manuscripts (including a multitude of meetings and phone calls with authors), helping find artists when needed, confirming references, discovering historical information as related to the many subjects covered in *Plastic Surgery*, and coordinating all these data with the publishing staff in Philadelphia and New York. When asked to describe what this job was like, she described the process as follows: "At times, this project has been a struggle, but most of the time it has been a joy (kind of like raising eight children). On any given day, working on this project has given me a reason to (1) get up in the morning; (2) stay up all night; (3) despise the morning; (4) stay sober; (5) get drunk; (6) laugh; (7) cry; (8) live; (9) lie; (10) rejoice. Who could ask for anything more? It has certainly kept things interesting!" Shireen credits special members of the publishing staff for helping this immense project move ahead at a fairly steady pace. In Philadelphia, Linda Van Pelt, senior project manager, book production, and RoseMarie Klimowicz, freelance copyeditor, have been with this project since its inception. They have both dedicated vast amounts of blood, sweat, tears, and personal time. Ann Ruzycka Anderson has been dedicated to this project since the onset and has also worked closely with Shireen. Judy Fletcher, publishing director, provided the support needed for timely layouts and served as an advocate for this project even when layout or illustrations were changed to maintain the continuity and artistry of the chapters. Finally, Shireen acknowledges her two amazing assistants in Palm Springs, California, Donna Larson and Carla Parnell, who have helped her scan, copy, crop, sort, mail, and stay sane. Without the dedication and brilliance of Shireen Dunwoody in bringing out the best in the editors, publishers, authors, and artists, this text would not have the quality and completeness it now possesses.

My immediate family was always supportive of this project despite the time-consuming work associated with text preparation. I wish to acknowledge and thank my family for their exciting accomplishments, which are a source of pride and enjoyment: Mary, Norma, Paul, Leslie, Isabelle, Peter, David, Brian, Vasso, Zoe, Ned, Erin, Maggie, and Rick.

In any profession, the support and encouragement of one's colleagues are essential for productivity. I wish to thank the faculty in our division of plastic surgery for their specific contributions to the text and their active roles as outstanding teachers for our residents and students at the University of California in San Francisco. The faculty, both full time and clinical, include the following: Bernard Alpert, Jim Anthony, Ramin Behmand, Kyle Bickel, Greg Buncke, K. Ning Chang, Tancredi D'Amore, Keith Denkler, Issa Eschima, Robert Foster, Roger Friedenthal, Gilbert Gradinger, Ronald Gruber, William Hoffman, Clyde Ikeda, Gabriel Kind, Chen Lee, Pablo Leon, Mahesh Mankani, Robert Markeson, Mary McGrath, Sean Moloney, Douglas Ousterhout, John Owsley, Lorne Rosenfield, Vivian Ting, Bryant Toth, Philip Trabulsy, D. Miller Wise, and David Young.

During the time span in which this book was edited, a group of outstanding residents completed their plastic surgery residencies at UCSF. All these residents contributed to both the care of many of the patients included in the chapters written by our faculty and the development of concepts used in the chapters of this edition. Each resident listed has contributed to the advancement of our knowledge in plastic surgery: Delora Mount, Richard Grossman, Jeff Roth, Laura McMillan, Kenneth Bermudez, Marga Massey, Yngvar Hvistendahl, Duc Bui, Te Ning Chang, Hatem Abou-Sayed, Farzad Nahai, Hop Nguyen Le, Clara Lee, Scott Hansen, Jennifer Newman-Keagle, and Wesley Schooler. General surgery residents, research fellows, and students who participated in the project include Lee Alkureishi, Julie Lang, Edward Miranda, and Cristiane Ueno.

Without the dedication of our staff, the preparation of this text would not have been possible. Crystal Munoz served as our office manager during most of the preparation time. My patient coordinators, Marian Liebow and, later, Skye Ingham, are patient advocates and made the arrangements necessary to treat the patients discussed in our chapters. Our nurses, Janet Tanaka and, later, Ann Hutchinson, were essential to the overall care of patients presenting to our clinical practice. Our staff provides the support needed to allow the faculty to have the time necessary to participate in the creative activities expected in academic plastic surgery.

Plastic surgeons depend on visual assessment of problems; thus, illustrations are an essential part of our scientific literature. Numerous artists were involved in the chapters selected by the individual authors. However, two artists were available to all the contributors and provided outstanding art to accompany many of the chapters. Kathy Hirsh, located in Shanghai, China, and Scott Barrows, in Chicago, have worked diligently to provide accurate artistic interpretations of the surgical procedures recommended throughout this text.

"Mental toughness is many things. It is humility because it behooves all of us to remember that simplicity is the sign of greatness and meekness is the sign of true strength. Mental toughness is spartanism with qualities of sacrifice, self-denial, dedication. It is fearlessness, and it is love."

—Vince Lombardi

All the authors who contributed to these volumes exemplify mental toughness. To complete a chapter for a text is often considered an unappreciated task. However, thanks to the great reputation established by the prior editors of this comprehensive work, John M. Converse and Joseph G. McCarthy, and the previous editors of the hand volumes, William Littler and James May, the top plastic surgeons in their respective fields have given their time and efforts to maintain the excellence associated with past editions of this text. Thanks to these contributors, this book provides information at the forefront of innovation and current practice in the specialty of plastic surgery. The contributors and their families are thanked for their perseverance and sacrifice in the completion of these chapters and for their dedication to our specialty, plastic surgery.

SJM

✦ CONTENTS

✦ VOLUME II

The Head and Neck, Part 1

✦ VOLUME III

THE HEAD AND NECK, PART 2

✦ VOLUME IV
Pediatric Plastic Surgery

✦ VOLUME V
Tumors of the Head, Neck, and Skin

✦ VOLUME VII

The Hand and Upper Limb, Part 1

INTRODUCTION AND GENERAL PRINCIPLES 1

ACQUIRED DISORDERS— TRAUMATIC 151

Embryology of the Craniofacial Complex

Jill A. Helms, DDS, PhD ✦ Randall P. Nacamuli, MD
✦ Ali Salim, MD ✦ Yun-Ying Shi, BS

A man finds room in the few square inches of the face for the traits of all his ancestors; for the expression of all his history, and his wants.
                              —*Ralph Waldo Emerson*

In the last decade, we have made remarkable progress toward understanding the molecular and cellular foundations governing craniofacial morphogenesis. As a consequence, we have a better appreciation for the causes of many craniofacial anomalies. In some instances, intuition has been correct, and molecules with well-characterized roles in the regulation of cell proliferation, differentiation, and programmed cell death in other tissues serve similar functions in the development of the craniofacial structures. At times, the identification of a gene that is responsible for a particular craniofacial malformation comes as a complete surprise. This poses an interesting challenge because understanding a gene's unique function in the craniofacial tissues can shift existing paradigms of head development and lead to new insights into the pathogenesis of craniofacial birth defects. This chapter provides overviews of the basic embryology of head structures; our current understanding of the molecular events that specify and regulate the patterning, growth, and fusion of the craniofacial primordia; and the cellular events that regulate morphogenesis of the head skeleton. In addition, there is a discussion of current insights into the molecular basis for a number

of craniofacial defects. In summary, this chapter should provide the reader with an embryologic context in which to interpret the wide variety of normal and abnormal facial phenotypes observed in clinical practice today.

UNIQUE PROPERTIES OF CRANIOFACIAL DEVELOPMENT

One might legitimately wonder whether development of the craniofacial structures, despite their remarkable topologic complexity, is not actually a relatively straightforward process. After all, similar to other tissues and organs, craniofacial structures arise from the growth and fusion of a number of independent primordia whose initial organization is much simpler. One might then ask if there is reason to suspect that the factors controlling specification and morphogenesis in the head are different from those operating elsewhere in the body. In fact, a number of unique features of craniofacial development clearly distinguish morphogenesis of the head. One of these deals with the dual cellular origin of craniofacial tissues, and another lies in the unique spatial origins of cell populations that may ultimately come together. These unique characteristics of craniofacial development can confound analyses that seek to clarify how a single determinative event, such as a genetic mutation, relates to a particular craniofacial phenotype or how composite tissues heal after disease, dysmorphogenesis, or injury.

At the cellular level, craniofacial tissues are derived from two broad-based lineages, the neural crest and the cephalic mesoderm. Neural crest cells possess a repertoire of developmental programs rivaled only by the mesoderm. For example, neural crest cells give rise not only to neuronal and meningeal tissues but also to several skeletal components of the head. A question that continues to occupy center stage in this field of research is whether cranial neural crest cells carry out obligatory programs of patterning and differentiation or retain their cellular plasticity and therefore their ability to respond to changes in epithelium-derived signals.[1]

At the level of organization of the tissues, craniofacial morphogenesis is uniquely characterized by the massive relocation of cells, caused by both active cell migration and passive displacement. As a consequence, critically important developmental events that affect lineage-related cells can—and do—occur at spatially disparate points. Likewise, cells of different lineages can be brought into proximity by such relocations and form composite tissues and organs. This characteristic of head tissues will figure prominently in issues surrounding the healing and regenerative capacity of different regions of the cranial skeleton.

INITIATION OF CRANIOFACIAL DEVELOPMENT

Early Patterning of the Embryo

During the first week after fertilization of an ovum, the newly formed zygote divides repeatedly into a solid, mulberry-like cell mass known as a morula. As the morula traverses the fallopian tube and enters the uterus, cells continue to divide, and the morula develops into a blastocyst. A blastocyst contains a fluid-filled cavity that separates cells into inner and outer layers. Implantation of the blastocyst into the uterine endometrium occurs during the second week of development. The blastocyst's outer cell layer, known as the trophoblast, contributes to the formation of placental structures that support and nourish the developing embryo; the inner layer, known as the embryoblast, begins to differentiate into the embryo itself.

As the embryoblast grows, it divides into two and then three layers. This process of gastrulation ultimately results in the formation of three primary germ layers (ectoderm, mesoderm, and endoderm) by the third week. But even before this trilaminar disk of embryonic cells is established, it is apparent that the rostral or cranial region of the embryo is distinct from the caudal region. At the caudal end of the embryo, a group of cells known as the primitive streak grow cranially from a "primitive node." The gradually elongating column of cells (notochord process) grows cranially until it reaches the prechordal plate, which is the future site of the mouth. The notochordal process is the precursor to the notochord, around which the adult bony axial skeleton will form (Fig. 85-1).

Thus, by this time, the ectoderm has acquired properties that denote its rostral identity. The anterior primitive endoderm is partly responsible for these anterior properties in the overlying ectoderm. One signal emanating from the endoderm is the secreted protein Cerberus.[2] Recall that Cerberus is the three-headed dog that guards the gates of Hades in classical Greek mythology; this name was chosen for the secreted protein because of its unique role in governing head development. The Cerberus protein acts in part through its ability to regulate the expression of at least two homeodomain-containing transcription factors, Otx2 and Lim1, both of which are essential for forebrain and midbrain development. In the absence of Cerberus, rostral head development is severely compromised; likewise, the loss of its downstream targets Otx2 and Lim1 is associated with craniofacial malformations and the complete absence of head structures, respectively.[3] These types of studies indicate the critical nature of signals emanating from endoderm during early head development.

Shortly after neural plate induction, a host of other molecular signals begin to define dorsal and ventral identity in cells of the neural tube.[4] Disruptions in these molecular signals have devastating consequences on further development and frequently result in embryonic lethality in mice. It is highly probable that similar gene mutations in humans are responsible for many of the spontaneous abortions that occur within the first trimester of pregnancy. That there are such analogous consequences to gene disruptions in humans and mice underscores the usefulness of murine models for understanding human diseases. Some of these key molecules and the disorders and malformations resulting from their perturbations are discussed in the following section.

Holoprosencephaly and Sonic Hedgehog

Holoprosencephaly (HPE) is the most common structural malformation of the forebrain in humans; it occurs in an astonishing 1:250 human abortuses[5,6] and in 1 : 10,000 to 20,000 live births.[7] HPE is associated with a wide spectrum of craniofacial anomalies, the most severe of which includes cyclopia with a proboscis, cebocephaly, ethmocephaly, and median cleft lip.[8] Milder HPE phenotypes, known as microforms, include microcephaly, microphthalmia, ocular hypotelorism, midfacial hypoplasia, and cleft lip with or without cleft palate.[9,10] In some HPE microforms, affected individuals with relatively normal facial appearances exhibit only subtle dental abnormalities, such as the presence of a single, upper central incisor.[9] In some familial forms, obligate carriers exhibit a normal intellect and facial phenotype.[9,11] Human

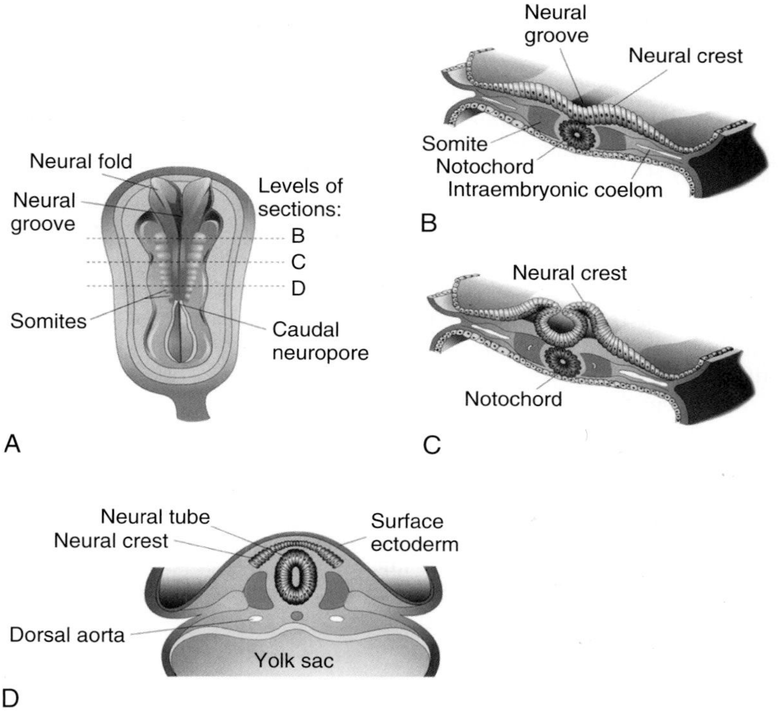

FIGURE 85-1. Diagrams illustrating the neural plate and folding of this structure into the neural tube. *A,* Dorsal view of an embryo of about 22 days. The neural folds have fused opposite the fourth to sixth somites but are widely spread apart at both ends. *B to D,* Transverse sections of this embryo at the levels indicated in *A* illustrating formation of the neural tube and its detachment from the surface ectoderm. Note that some neuroectodermal cells are not included in the neural tube but remain between it and the surface ectoderm as the neural crest. (Modified from Moore KL, Persaud TVN: The Developing Human: Clinically Oriented Embryology, 6th ed. Philadelphia, WB Saunders, 1998:452.)

HPE therefore manifests as an enormous variation in craniofacial form, ranging from a severe malformation to a normal appearance.

The etiology of HPE is equally heterogeneous. Mutations in Sonic hedgehog (*Shh*),[12-14] *Zic2,*[15] *Six3,*[8] and *Tgif*[16] are associated with human HPE. Fetal exposure to a variety of environmental agents can also elicit HPE-like defects (reviewed in reference 17). Preconceptional and gestational maternal diabetes,[18,19] maternal alcohol consumption,[20,21] and retinoic acid embryopathy[22] have been associated with HPE. These clinical data underscore the importance of genetic and environmental factors in the etiology of HPE but fail to provide clues about how genotypic changes result in the array of dysmorphisms associated with HPE.

Any embryonic process that requires complex morphogenetic movements is subject to disruption, the consequences of which are often manifested as craniofacial abnormalities. One of the most common of these defects is incomplete fusion of the neural tube. Such incomplete fusion events cause a host of fetal and postnatal defects ranging from spina bifida (incomplete fusion in the caudal end of the neural tube) to anencephaly (lack of fusion of the anterior neuropore) and a plethora of other anomalies.

Genesis of the Neural Crest

After specification and patterning of the neural plate, the tissue begins to invaginate and roll up to form the neural tube (see Fig. 85-1). This occurs through a complex morphogenetic process in which the notochordal process underlying the ectoderm is a source of signals that specify neural character in the ectoderm and thus delineate it from non-neural ectoderm. In considering how the craniofacial tissues achieve their ultimate arrangement, it is helpful to remember that those regions that were once positioned medially in the neural plate become positioned ventrally in the neural tube, and those regions that were lateral in the plate become dorsally located in the tube.

Just before fusion, a population of cells is generated from the area of the neural folds known as the neural crest. Their role in head development cannot be overestimated because these cells give rise to the majority of neural, odontogenic, and skeletogenic tissues of the head. Cranial neural crest cells give rise to a wide variety of neuronal and non-neuronal tissues, including ganglia of the dorsal root, the autonomic nervous system, and the cranial nerves; the meninges, pigment cells, and adrenal medulla are also derived from the neural crest.

Some of the molecular signals that instigate neural crest formation have been identified and include secreted proteins in the Wnt and bone morphogenetic protein (BMP) families. Wnts induce BMPs in the dorsal neural tube, and this starts the ball rolling in terms of neural crest induction. The ability of Wnts to stimulate neural crest cell formation from naive tissues raises the possibility that Wnt proteins may one day be used to induce the regeneration of cranial neural crest tissues.   .

The last century has brought a new understanding of how cranial neural crest cells get from "here," the dorsal part of the neural tube, to "there," the facial primordia. Experimentalists initially used coal dust sprinkled over the avian embryo to label migrating cells, which took up the particles along their way. Progressively more advanced techniques have been developed that allow us to ascertain just where cranial neural crest cells go after they leave home. By the now-classic approach of transplanting quail neural crest into a chick host embryo, investigators have been able to identify the migratory paths of subpopulations of the cranial neural crest in greater detail than had previously been possible.[23,24] Now, innovative visualization techniques provide us with a bird's-eye view of the migratory route of neural crest cells.[25] Why is there such interest in the movement of neural crest cells? The consequences of inaccurate or interrupted migration cannot be overemphasized; a plethora of craniofacial malformations have as their primary cause a perturbation in this cellular exodus. For example, genetic syndromes associated with aberrant neural crest cell migration include the DiGeorge and velocardiofacial syndromes as well as the pharyngeal arch syndromes. Teratogens such as retinoic acid and alcohol also affect neural crest cell migration, with well-documented craniofacial defects as a result.[26,27]

Much as an overseas trip can influence the course of a young person's life, signals encountered by neural crest cells during their migration to the facial primordia can alter their fate. During this trek, neural crest cells receive instructions from neighboring tissues and respond to these "roadside cues." Researchers have long suspected that signals from adjacent epithelia provide critical guidance information to migrating neural crest cells. Ephrins and the Eph receptors and semaphorin III/collapsin I appear to serve as migratory guidance cues.[28] One feature shared by these molecules is their well-documented role in axon path finding, suggesting that a common molecular mechanism coordinates the directed migration of multiple cell types.

MORPHOGENESIS OF THE FACIAL SKELETON

Development of the Branchial Structures

The fourth to eighth weeks are a significant period during development because precursors of all the major organs develop during this time. In addition to rapid growth, the embryo undergoes dramatic changes in shape. The brain expands significantly during this period, resulting in a prominent folding of the head,

and the cervical flexure becomes obvious and gives the embryo its characteristic C appearance.

Perhaps most critical to the development of craniofacial structures is the formation of five branchial (or pharyngeal) arches (Fig. 85-2). The arches are paired bulges on either side of the neck region that enlarge as neural crest cells migrate into the primordia and proliferate. Between each arch is a groove or cleft on the external surface of the embryo. This cleft forms a pouch of sorts that is lined by endoderm of the primitive pharynx. Thus, the ectoderm and endoderm are juxtaposed to one another at the opening of these pouches. Whereas the grooves are transient in nature (they disappear by week 7, giving the neck a smooth contour), the branchial arches contribute significantly to the development of head and neck structures. Stated another way, the contents of each branchial arch—a cartilaginous core and muscular portion, and an artery and nerve destined to supply the resulting tissues—contribute to derivative structures of that arch.

The first two branchial arches are most closely associated with development of the face and cranium. As outlined later, the first arch develops into the maxilla and mandible. The muscles of facial expression and mastication and other striated muscles in the head and neck are also derived from mesoderm in the first and second arches. The trigeminal and facial nerves originate from and supply structures derived from neural crest cells in the first and second arches.

Although the endoderm of the branchial pouches is not discussed in detail here, it is important to mention its contribution to key sensory and endocrine structures of the head and neck. Whereas the first pouch contributes to structures of the ear, including the eustachian tube and mastoid antrum, the second pouch differentiates into lymphoid tissues of the neck. The third pouch contributes to the inferior parathyroids and thymus; the fourth pouch develops into the superior parathyroid.

Organization of the Facial Primordia

The face proper is composed of four primordia: the midline frontonasal or median nasal process, which gives rise to the forehead, midline of the nose, philtrum, and primary palate; the maxillary processes, which contribute to the sides of the face, the upper lip, and the secondary palates; the lateral nasal processes, which give rise to the nares; and the mandibular process, which forms the lower jaw and lip (Fig. 85-3). The facial primordia must come into contact and fuse in a timely manner to establish the normal facial architecture. Fusion is therefore intimately linked to the proliferation and differentiation of cells in each primordium.

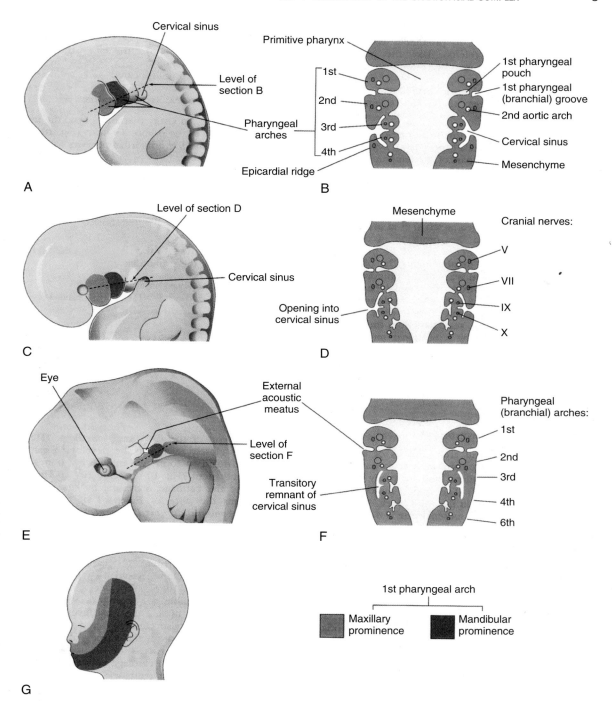

FIGURE 85-2. *A,* Lateral view of the head, neck, and thoracic regions of an embryo (about 32 days) showing the pharyngeal arches and cervical sinus. *B,* Diagrammatic section through the embryo at the level shown in *A* illustrating growth of the second arch over the third and fourth arches. *C,* An embryo of about 33 days. *D,* Section of the embryo at the level shown in *C* illustrating early closure of the cervical sinus. *E,* An embryo of about 41 days. *F,* Section of the embryo shown in *E* illustrating the transitory cystic remnant of the cervical sinus. Note that the anatomic fifth arch does not contribute to any adult structures, and thus the sixth arch is the fifth arch from a functional point of view. *G,* Drawing of a 20-week fetus illustrating the area of the face derived from the first pair of pharyngeal arches. (Modified from Moore KL, Persaud TVN: The Developing Human: Clinically Oriented Embryology, 6th ed. Philadelphia, WB Saunders, 1998:220.)

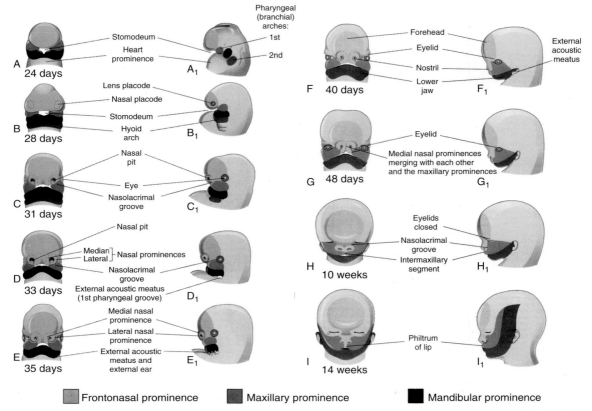

FIGURE 85-3. Diagrams illustrating progressive stages in the development of the human face. (Modified from Moore KL, Persaud TVN: The Developing Human: Clinically Oriented Embryology, 6th ed. Philadelphia, WB Saunders, 1998:237-238.)

FORMATION OF THE PRIMARY PALATE

The median nasal process gives rise to the primary palate. Despite the difference in the shape of the median nasal and frontonasal processes in avians, rodents, and humans, the expression of genes such as fibroblast growth factor 8 (*Fgf8*), *Shh*, *Bmp2*, and *Bmp4* is strikingly equivalent in these different species. After the initial establishment of these gene expression patterns, the outgrowth of the median nasal process begins to differ in the various species. In avians, the median nasal process begins to elongate, predicting the shape of the future beak; in rodents, the median nasal process develops as two lobes separated by a fissure, again predicting the shape of the future lip. In humans, the development of the median nasal process more closely resembles that of the mouse, although the fissure in the median nasal process is not as deep. In humans, this fissure is represented as the philtrum of the lip.

Interruptions in the rate, the timing, or the extent of proliferation in the frontonasal primordia lead to a failure in epithelial fusion and subsequently the formation of a cleft (Fig. 85-4). In patients with mild defects, the clefts may be limited to a notch in the vermilion border of the lip, which probably represents a failure of localized growth of the median nasal process. In patients with more severe defects, the cleft is through the tissues of the lip and can occur either unilaterally or bilaterally. In these patients, the cleft occurs because of a failure of fusion between the median nasal and maxillary processes. Clefts can also involve the side of the nose and therefore result from a failure in the fusion between the median nasal, lateral nasal, and maxillary processes. Although rare, clefts can also involve the sides of the face.

FORMATION OF THE SECONDARY PALATE

The secondary palate is a structure that separates the nasal passage from the pharynx and arises from condensations of neural crest mesenchyme within the maxillary primordia. These condensations undergo intramembranous ossification to form the palatal shelves, which initially extend vertically on either side of the tongue and subsequently rotate to a horizontal plane dorsal to the tongue. Initially, the shelves are

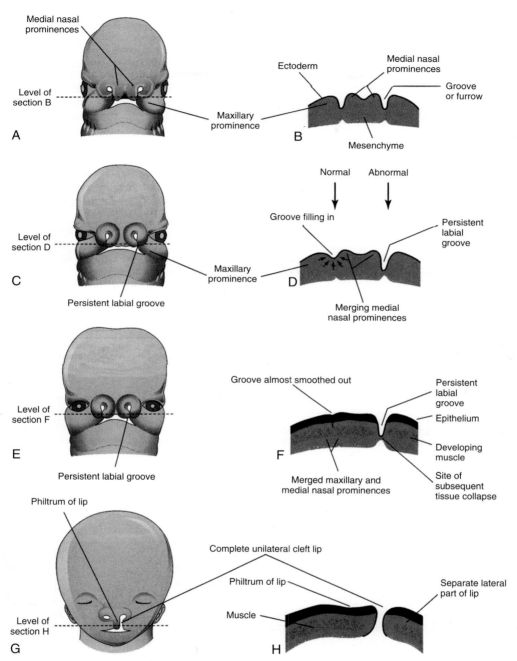

FIGURE 85-4. Illustrations depicting the embryologic basis of complete unilateral cleft lip. *A,* A 5-week embryo. *B,* Horizontal section through the head illustrating the grooves between the maxillary prominences and the merging medial nasal prominences. *C,* A 6-week embryo showing a persistent labial groove on the left side. *D,* Horizontal section through the head showing the groove gradually filling in on the right side after proliferation of mesenchyme *(arrows). E,* A 7-week embryo. *F,* Horizontal section through the head showing that the epithelium on the right has almost been pushed out of the groove between the maxillary and medial nasal prominences. *G,* A 10-week fetus with a complete unilateral cleft lip. *H,* Horizontal section through the head after stretching of the epithelium and breakdown of the tissues on the floor of the persistent labial groove on the left side, forming a complete unilateral cleft lip. (Modified from Moore KL, Persaud TVN: The Developing Human: Clinically Oriented Embryology, 6th ed. Philadelphia, WB Saunders, 1998:251.)

lined by an epithelium that is two cell layers thick. Before fusion of the palatal shelves, the outer peridermal layer is sloughed off, leaving the basal epithelial layer. The basal epithelial layer composes the medial edge epithelium of each shelf. The shelves grow toward the midline, and the medial edge epithelium of each shelf approximates and forms the midline epithelial seam. This seam is subsequently disrupted, which leads to mesenchymal confluence between the two shelves. Perturbations caused by genetic, mechanical, or teratogenic factors can occur at any of these steps and frequently result in a cleft secondary palate.

FUSION OF THE CRANIOFACIAL COMPLEX

Between the seventh and tenth weeks of human development, the palatal processes begin to fuse. Precisely how this fusion event occurs is still open to speculation. For example, medial edge epithelium cells may undergo a transdifferentiation event, changing from epithelial into mesenchymal cells that subsequently migrate from the fusion site and thereby produce a confluent mesenchyme. A second proposed mechanism by which fusion occurs is that epithelial cells simply migrate from the site of fusion without changing their phenotype. This is a less likely scenario simply because epithelial cells are not known for any migratory behavior. A third possibility is that medial edge epithelial cells undergo programmed cell death (apoptosis). It is evident that the removal of the epithelial seam is important because it allows the mesenchyme of the primordia to become confluent. Retained remnants of the epithelial seam are referred to as epithelial islands and generally do not interfere with function.

Fusions between any two primordia may appear identical at a cellular level but may be regulated by different molecules. For example, the secondary palatal shelves appear to fuse by the process of epithelial-mesenchymal transformation, although some earlier reports suggest that apoptosis plays a predominant role.[29] Whether this same process regulates fusion of the median nasal process seems unlikely because fusions between these two primordia are unaffected by mutations that inhibit secondary palatal fusion (see later). For illustrative purposes, the subsequent discussions focus on fusion events in the secondary palate because the majority of experiments have been carried out on this tissue. However, the molecular mechanisms underlying fusion of the palate may be generalized to other fusion events. Most notably, fusion of the dorsum of the penis is a normal occurrence in human embryos. Failure of this fusion to occur properly results in a condition known as hypospadias, which is frequently associated with facial clefting.[30]

Using a combination of experimental and genetic approaches, researchers are discovering the specific signaling events and cellular processes that often go awry in patients with craniofacial clefting. For example, some instances of human cleft palate have been associated with polymorphisms in the gene encoding transforming growth factor-α, an epidermal growth factor receptor (EGFR) ligand synthesized by facial epithelia. $Egfr^{-/-}$ mice have midline defects that produce an elongated primary palate, micrognathia, and a high incidence of cleft palate.[31] In vitro experiments suggest that a delay in epithelial degeneration occurs in the absence of EGFR signaling. The secretion of matrix metalloproteinases is also diminished in $Egfr^{-/-}$ explants, consistent with the ability of epidermal growth factor to increase matrix metalloproteinase secretion in other in vitro models.[32,33] These experimental and genetic results indicate that the role of EGFR signaling in craniofacial development is mediated, at least in part, through regulation of a matrix metalloproteinase.

Transforming growth factor-β3 is essential for fusion between palatal shelves because homozygous null $Tgfb3$ newborns exhibit a cleft secondary palate without other craniofacial abnormalities.[34,35] In $Tgfb3$ null mutants, the palatal shelves appear to approximate and adhere but the midline epithelial seam remains, and mesenchymal confluence does not occur. Precisely how the midline epithelial seam is normally removed remains controversial. There are at least three possible explanations for the disappearance of the seam. First, the medial edge epithelium cells may undergo programmed cell death and thus allow mesenchymal cells to move into the space previously occupied by the epithelial cells. However, ultrastructural studies[36] and fate mapping of the midline epithelial seam cells strongly suggest that programmed cell death does not account for the disappearance of the epithelial cells.[37,38] Second, epithelial cells may migrate from a midline position and become contiguous with the adjacent oral or nasal epithelium. Third, the midline epithelial cells may be transformed into mesenchymal cells. This type of genetic information is being used to develop more refined models of how craniofacial morphogenesis is normally regulated. These new data will undoubtedly form the basis for the treatment and ultimately the prevention of facial clefting.

THE CRANIOFACIAL SKELETON

The skeleton of the head is derived from cephalic and paraxial mesoderm as well as from the cranial neural crest. These cells form bone through both endochondral and intramembranous ossification. Accumulating evidence, however, suggests that the mechanisms initiating and controlling cranial skeletal development—and repair—are at least qualitatively different from those regulating appendicular or axial skeletogenesis.

Neurocranium

The neurocranium comprises that portion of the skull that encases the brain, functioning as a protective bony shell. The neurocranium can further be subdivided into two portions, the cartilaginous neurocranium and the membranous neurocranium, which form through two separate processes.

CARTILAGINOUS NEUROCRANIUM

The cartilaginous neurocranium, or chondrocranium, forms the base of the skull (Fig. 85-5). The bones that make up the basicranium include the sphenoid and ethmoid bones, the mastoid and petrous portions of the temporal bone, and the base of the occipital bone. These structures form through the process of endochondral ossification, whereby a cartilaginous condensation or anlage is replaced by bone. The chondrocranium is derived embryologically from occipital somites and somitomeres, which have their origin in the paraxial mesoderm.[39,40] The cartilages from which these bones derive include the parachordal cartilage and occipital sclerotomes (occipital base), the hypophyseal cartilages and the ala orbitalis and ala temporalis (sphenoid), the trabeculae cranii (ethmoid), and the periotic capsule (temporal).[41] Ossification and fusion of these cartilaginous structures lead to the formation of the skull base.

MEMBRANOUS NEUROCRANIUM

The membranous portion of the neurocranium forms the cranial vault. It is composed of seven bones: the paired frontal, squamosal, and parietal bones and a portion of the occipital bone (Fig. 85-5C). With the exception of the occipital bone, these bones form entirely through the process of intramembranous ossification, or direct bone formation without a cartilaginous precursor. The occipital bone is a composite, with the inferior portion forming by endochondral ossification and the superior portion by intramembranous ossification.

On histologic evaluation, these structures arise from a skeletogenic mesenchyme located between the surface ectoderm and the cerebral hemispheres.[39] Osteogenesis initiates in mesenchymal blastemas that are the precursors of the individual bones and expands radially as mesenchymal cells undergo differentiation and deposit the extracellular matrix that will subsequently undergo mineralization. Of the multitude of genes involved in the orchestration of bone formation, the most central is the transcription factor Runx2/Cbfa1.[42] Runx2 can be considered the "master switch" of osteoblast biology and directly turns on many genes required for the deposition and mineralization of osteoblast extracellular matrix, including collagen I, osteopontin, and osteocalcin. In $Runx2^{-/-}$ mice, there is absence of formation of the appendicular and axial skeleton due to failure of osteoblast differentiation.[43,44] Interestingly, mice that are $Runx2^{-/+}$ have a phenotype resembling the human disease cleidocranial dysplasia, characterized by deficiencies in intramembranous bone formation including wide, patent fontanels and hypoplasia of the clavicles.

Although histologically similar, the cells giving rise to the neurocranium are of mixed embryologic origin. On the basis of studies conducted in avians, the exact contributions of these cells to the craniofacial skeleton were unclear.[39,45] A genetic approach in mice has provided convincing data about the cellular origins of the cranial skeleton. Investigators took advantage of the fact that the gene Wnt1 is expressed in neural crest cells. By placing the Wnt1 promoter upstream of a Cre gene and crossing the mice with a reporter line, they succeeded in generating mice in which the neural crest cells were indelibly labeled with a reporter gene. This genetic "sleight of hand" permitted scientists to easily follow the fate of the labeled neural crest cells throughout the lifetime of the animal. These studies suggested that the frontal and squamosal bones are of cranial neural crest origin. The parietal bone is derived from paraxial mesoderm, and the occipital bone is derived from both.[46] In addition to establishing the contributions of neural crest cells to the face and jaw skeleton, the mouse has also firmly established the contribution of neural crest to another hard tissue in the head, the teeth.

Viscerocranium

The bones of the facial skeleton, including the mandible and the maxilla, compose the viscerocranium. These bones are derived primarily from the cranial neural crest cells of the first branchial arch. The dorsal portion of the first branchial arch, or maxillary process, develops into the maxilla, the zygomatic bone, and the squamosal portion of the temporal bone. The ventral portion, also known as the mandibular process, gives rise to the mandible as well as the ossicles of the ear. Whereas all the bones composing the face form by intramembranous ossification, the formation of the mandible occurs with one notable difference. Skeletogenic mesenchyme of the mandibular process condenses alongside a cartilaginous rod known as Meckel cartilage. This mesenchyme undergoes intramembranous ossification while at the same time Meckel cartilage disappears, presumably through resorption. The only remnant of this structure is the sphenomandibular ligament. Recent experiments in mice lacking cartilaginous structures of neural crest origin, including Meckel cartilage, demonstrate that morphogenesis and ossification of the mandible occur normally.[47] Thus, despite the physical proximity between Meckel cartilage and the skeletogenic mesenchyme of

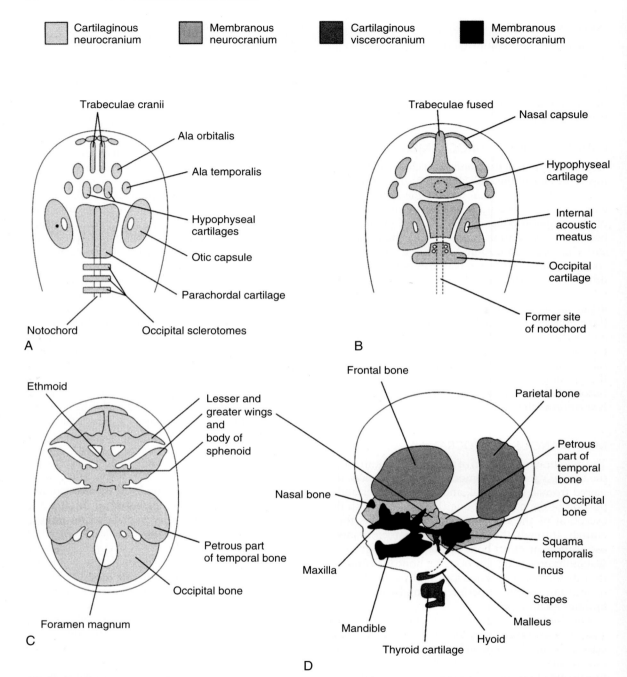

FIGURE 85-5. Diagrams illustrating stages in the development of the skull. *A* to *C* are views of the base of the developing skull (viewed superiorly). *D* is a lateral view. *A,* At 6 weeks, showing the various cartilages that will fuse to form the chondrocranium. *B,* At 7 weeks, after fusion of some of the paired cartilages. *C,* At 12 weeks, showing the cartilaginous base of the skull or chondrocranium formed by the fusion of various cartilages. *D,* At 20 weeks, indicating the derivation of the bones of the fetal skull. (Modified from Moore KL, Persaud TVN: The Developing Human: Clinically Oriented Embryology, 6th ed. Philadelphia, WB Saunders, 1998:415.)

the mandibular process, the mandible forms through intramembranous ossification.

A number of disorders arise from the disruption of normal development and morphogenesis of the first and second branchial arches.[48] Hemifacial microsomia is usually a unilateral congenital hypoplasia of the craniofacial structures derived from the first and second branchial arches and is thought to be due to trauma in utero to the developing arches between 30 and 45 days of gestation. Other possible explanations include damage to neural crest cells migrating into the arches and chromosomal aberrations. Treacher Collins syndrome, or mandibulofacial dysostosis, is an autosomal dominant disorder (genetic basis unknown) characterized by bilateral deficiencies in arch-derived structures.

Cranial Sutures

The cranial sutures are the fibrous joints found between the bones of the cranial vault. Sutures have several vital functions, including permitting the compression of the skull during birth and, most important, functioning as growth centers for the rapidly expanding neurocranium. The primary cranial sutures in humans are the interfrontal or metopic suture (between the frontal bones), the sagittal suture (between the parietal bones), the coronal suture (between the frontal and parietal bones), and the lambdoid suture (between the parietal and occipital bones). The transversely oriented coronal and lambdoid sutures are overlapping, whereas the osteogenic fronts of the interfrontal and sagittal sutures are not. Additional cranial sutures include the squamosal, sphenofrontal, sphenoparietal, sphenotemporal, and masto-occipital. Facial sutures include the palatal, frontomaxillary, frontozygomatic, zygomaticotemporal, zygomaticomaxillary, frontonasal, and nasomaxillary sutures. The intersection of two or more cranial sutures gives rise to the fontanels, the most well known being the anterior fontanel between the coronal, sagittal, and interfrontal sutures and the posterior fontanel between the sagittal and lambdoid sutures. Whereas most of these sutures remain patent until the third and fourth decade, the interfrontal suture is unique in that it undergoes physiologic fusion between the ages of 2 and 3 years.[49]

The definitive cranial sutures are formed when the osteogenic fronts of the developing neurocranial bones, initially widely spaced, begin to approach each other. The mesenchymal tissue separating the two bony fronts becomes more cellular and is recruited into the osteogenic fronts, presumably contributing to the osteoblasts and osteoblast precursors.[50] Thus, the main components of a cranial suture include the flanking osteogenic fronts, the intervening suture mesenchyme, and the underlying dura mater. How the suture is actually patterned remains unclear; no sole tissue, growth factor, or patterning gene has yet been identified that directly delineates suture formation. However, studies suggest that a gradient of growth or other regulatory factors is formed by the osteogenic fronts, suture mesenchyme, and dura mater.[51,52] This gradient, presumably, then regulates the balance between proliferation and differentiation of precursor cells in the suture mesenchyme. Osteogenic differentiation must be balanced by maintenance of the intervening suture mesenchyme; otherwise, bone bridging would occur, resulting in premature cranial suture fusion or craniosynostosis.

Studies in mice suggest that although the expression patterns of genes associated with the differentiation of osteoblasts are similar in the osteogenic fronts of patent and physiologically fusing sutures, genes implicated in the regulation of osteogenesis, such as *Fgf2* and BMP antagonists, are differentially regulated.[53-56] This would imply that the maintenance of suture patency is in part due to balancing of the differentiation and proliferation of precursor cells in the suture mesenchyme. Craniosynostoses result in numerous morphologic and physiologic abnormalities, including plagiocephaly, hydrocephalus, blindness, and airway compromise, because of the inability of the cranial vault to enlarge correctly during development.[48] Many of the mutations associated with the syndromic craniosynostoses occur in genes implicated in the control of proliferation and differentiation in osteoblasts. For example, patients with Boston-type craniosynostosis have a point mutation in *Msx2*, which codes for a transcription factor that may regulate differentiation of preosteoblasts.[57,58] Similarly, patients with Saethre-Chotzen craniosynostosis have mutations in *Twist,* a negative regulator of osteoblast proliferation.[59]

TERATOGENS AND CRANIOFACIAL BIRTH DEFECTS

What happens when craniofacial development goes awry? Genetic and teratogen-induced defects tell us a great deal about the regulation of normal facial development and offer insights into methods for diagnosis and prevention of craniofacial malformations. We are now entering into what was once the realm of science fiction, the repair of facial defects in utero. As techniques to diagnose craniofacial and other birth defects become increasingly reliable, we are confronted with the possibility of treating the milder forms of craniofacial birth defects in the fetus, thereby obviating the need for numerous surgical treatments because of postnatal scar tissue.

Craniofacial birth defects occur in almost 1 in 7 live births, an inordinately high frequency that begs the question of why these tissues are especially sensitive to teratogens. Part of the answer may be the unique character of head development; craniofacial morphogenesis is distinguished by the massive relocation of cells, and the timing, the rate, or the extent of cell migration has to be tightly regulated. By studying the molecular and cellular bases by which teratogens exert their effects, we can gain a better understanding of the regulation of normal development. Whereas the abnormalities that arise after exposure to a specific teratogen may be diverse and highly variable, they are usually reproducible because teratogens have distinct mechanisms of action and are selective with regard to their target cells, tissues, and organs.

Four factors may account for the range of phenotypic effects that can arise after exposure to a teratogenic agent.[60] These include differences in concentration or method of teratogen delivery, timing of exposure during embryonic development, variations in susceptibility of individuals due to diverse genetic backgrounds, and synergistic interactions among various compounds. All of these factors can lead to a continuum in the severity of birth defects in one species. Numerous substances have been identified that have teratogenic effects during craniofacial development.[60,61] As examples, two teratogens that disrupt the formation of the facial primordia and lead to clefting are described.

Retinoids and Retinoid-Induced Embryopathies

Clinical and experimental data generated during the past 60 years have clearly demonstrated that retinoic acid, a metabolite of vitamin A, can act as a powerful teratogen during embryogenesis. Both excesses and deficiencies of retinoic acid can lead to severe abnormalities in a variety of tissues.[62-65] The brain and the face appear to be especially sensitive to changes in the availability of retinoic acid during development.[64] Nervous system defects such as microphthalmia and holoprosencephaly as well as facial anomalies such as midfacial hypoplasia and cleft lip/palate are potential adverse outcomes of exposure to retinoic acid. The severity and extent of the craniofacial defects appear to relate to the developmental stage when the exposure occurred, the dosage of retinoic acid, and the particular tissue that is subjected to the exposure. For example, if embryos are exposed to high doses of retinoic acid at early stages of development, the frontonasal mass is disrupted and the derivatives (midline structures such as the nose and primary palate) are malformed. If older embryos are exposed to retinoic acid, the heart and limbs are primarily affected. Experimental evidence strongly suggests that this tissue sensitivity represents a dependency of the organ on endogenous retinoid sources, which are perturbed by excess retinoic acid.[65] This conclusion is supported by genetic experiments in which mutations in retinoic acid receptors give rise to a wide range of malformations in the neural tube and skull.[66]

Perturbations in Cholesterol Biosynthesis

The teratogenic effects of the plant *Veratrum californicum*, which is a potent inducer of holoprosencephaly, have been well documented during the last 40 years.[67] The active compounds in *V. californicum* have been traced to cyclopamine and jervine.[68] These molecules are steroidal alkaloids and may exert their teratogenic effect by perturbing cholesterol synthesis or transport.[69] Mutations of genes such as *megalin*, a member of the low-density lipoprotein receptor family, also produce defects that resemble holoprosencephaly.[70] Milder forms of holoprosencephaly are also observed in patients with Smith-Lemli-Opitz syndrome[71] that are caused by a defect in a cholesterol biosynthetic enzyme (reviewed in reference 60). Cholesterol is required for proper processing of the Shh protein,[69] and growing evidence indicates that disruptions in Shh signaling at multiple time points during development can account for the range of holoprosencephaly-like defects.[72]

CONCLUSION

Twenty years ago, investigators conjectured that the dividing line between mesoderm and cranial neural crest was significant in the development and repair of the cranial skeleton. More recent experimental results suggest that this is unlikely, since neural crest cells seem to be capable of responding to the same cues that promote skeletogenesis in mesoderm. In either instance, these data underscore the plasticity of cranial neural crest but raise the question of whether mesoderm and neural crest make osseous tissue by use of the same molecular pathways. Recent data from analyses of mice carrying mutations in the transcription factor encoded by *Twist* may provide insight into this question. Mice heterozygous for a mutation in *Twist* survive to adulthood but have a craniosynostotic phenotype similar to that of their human counterparts.[57] The *Twist*[+/−] skull bone defect is caused by the inappropriate intermixing of neural crest–derived cells in the frontal bone with mesoderm-derived cells in the parietal bones.[73] Given that humans with the same mutations exhibit nearly identical skeletal defects, it will prove interesting to determine if there is a way to circumvent such cranial skeletal defects.

REFERENCES

1. Helms JA, Schneider RA: Cranial skeletal biology. Nature 2003;423:326-331.

2. Piccolo S, Agius E, Leyns L, et al: The head inducer Cerberus is a multifunctional antagonist of Nodal, BMP and Wnt signals. Nature 1999;397:707-710.

3. Shawlot W, Min Deng J, Wakamiya M, Behringer RR: The cerberus-related gene, Cerr1, is not essential for mouse head formation. Genesis 2000;26:253-258.

4. Rubenstein JL, Beachy PA: Patterning of the embryonic forebrain. Curr Opin Neurobiol 1998;8:18-26.

5. Matsunaga E, Shiota K: Holoprosencephaly in human embryos: epidemiologic studies of 150 cases. Teratology 1977;16:261-272.

6. Croen LA, Shaw GM, Lammer EJ: Holoprosencephaly: epidemiologic and clinical characteristics of a California population. Am J Med Genet 1996;64:465-472.

7. Muenke M, Beachy PA: Genetics of ventral forebrain development and holoprosencephaly. Curr Opin Genet Dev 2000; 10:262-269.

8. Wallis DE, Muenke M: Molecular mechanisms of holoprosencephaly. Mol Genet Metab 1999;68:126-138.

9. McKusick VA: Online Mendelian Inheritance in Man, OMIM. McKusick-Nathans Institute for Genetic Medicine, Johns Hopkins University (Baltimore, Md) and National Center for Biotechnology Information, National Library of Medicine (Bethesda, Md). Available at: http://www.ncbi.nlm.nih.gov/omim/. Accessed August 20, 2002.

10. Muenke M: Holoprosencephaly as a genetic model for normal craniofacial development. Semin Dev Biol 1994;5:293-301.

11. Cohen MM Jr: Perspectives on holoprosencephaly. Part I. Epidemiology, genetics, and syndromology. Teratology 1989;40: 211-235.

12. Roessler E, Belloni E, Gaudenz K, et al: Mutations in the human Sonic Hedgehog gene cause holoprosencephaly. Nat Genet 1996;14:357-360.

13. Roessler E, Belloni E, Gaudenz K, et al: Mutations in the C-terminal domain of Sonic Hedgehog cause holoprosencephaly. Hum Mol Genet 1997;6:1847-1853.

14. Ming JE, Kaupas ME, Roessler E, et al: Mutations in PATCHED-1, the receptor for SONIC HEDGEHOG, are associated with holoprosencephaly. Hum Genet 2002;110:297-301.

15. Brown SA, Warburton D, Brown LY, et al: Holoprosencephaly due to mutations in ZIC2, a homologue of Drosophila odd-paired. Nat Genet 1998;20:180-183.

16. Gripp KW, Wotton D, Edwards MC, et al: Mutations in TGIF cause holoprosencephaly and link NODAL signalling to human neural axis determination. Nat Genet 2000;25:205-208.

17. Cohen MM Jr, Shiota K: Teratogenesis of holoprosencephaly. Am J Med Genet 2002;109:1-15.

18. Barr M Jr, Hanson JW, Currey K, et al: Holoprosencephaly in infants of diabetic mothers. J Pediatr 1983;102:565-568.

19. Martinez-Frias ML, Bermejo E, Garcia A, et al: Holoprosencephaly associated with caudal dysgenesis: a clinical-epidemiological analysis. Am J Med Genet 1994;53:46-51.

20. Ronen GM, Andrews WL: Holoprosencephaly as a possible embryonic alcohol effect. Am J Med Genet 1991;40:151-154.

21. Bonnemann C, Meinecke P: Holoprosencephaly as a possible embryonic alcohol effect: another observation. Am J Med Genet 1990;37:431-432.

22. Lammer EJ, Chen DT, Hoar RM, et al: Retinoic acid embryopathy. N Engl J Med 1985;313:837-841.

23. Noden DM: The control of avian cephalic neural crest cytodifferentiation. I. Skeletal and connective tissues. Dev Biol 1978;67:296-312.

24. Le Douarin NM, Dieterlen-Lievre F, Teillet M: Quail-chick transplantations. In Bronner-Fraser M, ed: Methods in Avian Embryology, vol 51. San Diego, Academic Press, 1996:23-59.

25. Birgbauer E, Sechrist J, Bronner-Fraser M, Fraser S: Rhombomeric origin and rostrocaudal reassortment of neural crest cells revealed by intravital microscopy. Development 1995;121:935-945.

26. Cartwright MM, Tessmer LL, Smith SM: Ethanol-induced neural crest apoptosis is coincident with their endogenous death, but is mechanistically distinct. Alcohol Clin Exp Res 1998;22:142-149.

27. Ahlgren SC, Thakur V, Bronner-Fraser M: Sonic hedgehog rescues cranial neural crest from cell death induced by ethanol exposure. Proc Natl Acad Sci U S A 2002;99:10476-10481.

28. McAllister AK: Conserved cues for axon and dendrite growth in the developing cortex. Neuron 2002;33:2-4.

29. Ferguson MW: Palate development. Development 1988; 103(suppl 10):41-60.

30. Yamada G, Satoh Y, Baskin LS, Cunha GR: Cellular and molecular mechanisms of development of the external genitalia. Differentiation 2003;71:445-460.

31. Miettinen PJ, Chin JR, Shum L, et al: Epidermal growth factor receptor function is necessary for normal craniofacial development and palate closure. Nat Genet 1999;22:69-73.

32. Suzuki M, Raab G, Moses MA, et al: Matrix metalloproteinase-3 releases active heparin-binding EGF-like growth factor by cleavage at a specific juxtamembrane site. J Biol Chem 1997;272:31730-31737.

33. Ellerbroek SM, Hudson LG, Stack MS: Proteinase requirements of epidermal growth factor–induced ovarian cancer cell invasion. Int J Cancer 1998;78:331-337.

34. Schmid P, Cox D, Bilbe G, et al: Differential expression of TGF beta 1, beta 2 and beta 3 genes during mouse embryogenesis. Development 1991;111:117-130.

35. Pelton RW, Saxena B, Jones M, et al: Immunohistochemical localization of TGF beta 1, TGF beta 2, and TGF beta 3 in the mouse embryo: expression patterns suggest multiple roles during embryonic development. J Cell Biol 1991;115:1091-1105.

36. Fitchett JE, Hay ED: Medial edge epithelium transforms to mesenchyme after embryonic palatal shelves fuse. Dev Biol 1989;131:455-474.

37. Griffith CM, Hay ED: Epithelial-mesenchymal transformation during palatal fusion: carboxyfluorescein traces cells at light and electron microscopic levels. Development 1992;116:1087-1099.

38. Shuler CF, Halpern DE, Guo Y, Sank AC: Medial edge epithelium fate traced by cell lineage analysis during epithelial-mesenchymal transformation in vivo. Dev Biol 1992;154:318-330.

39. Noden DM: The role of the neural crest in patterning of avian cranial skeletal, connective and muscle tissues. Dev Biol 1983;96:144-165.

40. Noden DM: Interactions and fates of avian craniofacial mesenchyme. Development 1988;103(suppl):121-140.

41. Langman J, Sadler TW: Langman's Medical Embryology, 7th ed. Baltimore, Williams & Wilkins, 1995.

42. Ducy P: Cbfa1: a molecular switch in osteoblast biology. Dev Dyn 2000;219:461-471.

43. Komori T, Yagi H, Nomura S, et al: Targeted disruption of Cbfa1 results in a complete lack of bone formation owing to maturational arrest of osteoblasts. Cell 1997;89:755-764.

44. Ducy P, Zhang R, Geoffroy V, et al: Osf2/Cbfa1: a transcriptional activator of osteoblast differentiation. Cell 1997;89: 747-754.

45. Couly GF, Coltey PM, Le Douarin NM: The triple origin of skull in higher vertebrates: a study in quail-chick chimeras. Development 1993;117:409-429.

46. Jiang X, Iseki S, Maxson RE, et al: Tissue origins and interactions in the mammalian skull vault. Dev Biol 2002;241:106-116.

47. Mori-Akiyama Y, Akiyama H, Rowitch DH, de Crombrugghe B: Sox9 is required for determination of the chondrogenic cell lineage in the cranial neural crest. Proc Natl Acad Sci U S A 2003;100:9360-9365.

48. Posnick JC: Craniofacial syndromes and anomalies. In Posnick JC, ed: Craniofacial and Maxillofacial Surgery in Children and Young Adults, vol 1. Philadelphia, WB Saunders, 2000:391-527.

49. Cohen MM Jr: Transforming growth factor betas and fibroblast growth factors and their receptors: role in sutural biology and craniosynostosis. J Bone Miner Res 1997;12:322-331.

50. Opperman LA: Cranial sutures as intramembranous bone growth sites. Dev Dyn 2000;219:472-485.

51. Opperman LA, Sweeney TM, Redmon J, et al: Tissue interactions with underlying dura mater inhibit osseous obliteration of developing cranial sutures. Dev Dyn 1993;198:312-322.

52. Roth DA, Bradley JP, Levine JP, et al: Studies in cranial suture biology. Part II. Role of the dura in cranial suture fusion. Plast Reconstr Surg 1996;97:693-699.

53. Nacamuli RP, Fong KD, Warren SM, et al: Markers of osteoblast differentiation in fusing and nonfusing cranial sutures. Plast Reconstr Surg 2003;112:1328-1335.

54. Greenwald JA, Mehrara BJ, Spector JA, et al: Regional differentiation of cranial suture–associated dura mater in vivo and in vitro: implications for suture fusion and patency. J Bone Miner Res 2000;15:2413-2430.

55. Mehrara BJ, Mackool RJ, McCarthy JG, et al: Immunolocalization of basic fibroblast growth factor and fibroblast growth factor receptor-1 and receptor-2 in rat cranial sutures. Plast Reconstr Surg 1998;102:1805-1817.

56. Warren SM, Brunet LJ, Harland RM, et al: The BMP antagonist noggin regulates cranial suture fusion. Nature 2003;422:625-629.

57. Satokata I, Ma L, Ohshima H, et al: Msx2 deficiency in mice causes pleiotropic defects in bone growth and ectodermal organ formation. Nat Genet 2000;24:391-395.

58. Liu YH, Tang Z, Kundu RK, et al: Msx2 gene dosage influences the number of proliferative osteogenic cells in growth centers of the developing murine skull: a possible mechanism for MSX2-mediated craniosynostosis in humans. Dev Biol 1999;205:260-274.

59. Lee MS, Lowe GN, Strong DD, et al: TWIST, a basic helix-loop-helix transcription factor, can regulate the human osteogenic lineage. J Cell Biochem 1999;75:566-577.

60. Gorlin RJ, Cohen MM, Levin LS: Syndromes of the Head and Neck, vol 1, 3rd ed. New York, Oxford University Press, 1990.

61. Shepard TH: Catalog of Teratogenic Agents, 8th ed. Baltimore, Johns Hopkins University Press, 1995.

62. Wedden SE: Effects of retinoids on chick face development. J Craniofac Genet Dev Biol 1991;11:326-337.

63. Richman JM, Tickle C: Epithelial-mesenchymal interactions in the outgrowth of limb buds and facial primordia in chick embryos. Dev Biol 1992;154:299-308.

64. Morriss-Kay G: Retinoic acid and craniofacial development: molecules and morphogenesis. Bioessays 1993;15:9-15.

65. Helms JA, Kim CH, Hu D, et al: Sonic hedgehog participates in craniofacial morphogenesis and is down-regulated by teratogenic doses of retinoic acid. Dev Biol 1997;187:25-35.

66. Lohnes D, Mark M, Mendelsohn C, et al: Function of the retinoic acid receptors (RARs) during development (I). Craniofacial and skeletal abnormalities in RAR double mutants. Development 1994;120:2723-2748.

67. Bryden MM, Perry C, Keeler RF: Effects of alkaloids of *Veratrum californicum* on chick embryos. Teratology 1973;8:19-25.

68. Keeler RF, Binns W: Teratogenic compounds of *Veratrum californicum* (Durand). V. Comparison of cyclopian effects of steroidal alkaloids from the plant and structurally related compounds from other sources. Teratology 1968;1:5-10.

69. Beachy PA, Cooper MK, Young KE, et al: Multiple roles of cholesterol in hedgehog protein biogenesis and signaling. Cold Spring Harb Symp Quant Biol 1997;62:191-204.

70. Willnow TE, Hilpert J, Armstrong SA, et al: Defective forebrain development in mice lacking gp330/megalin. Proc Natl Acad Sci U S A 1996;93:8460-8464.

71. Kelley RL, Roessler E, Hennekam RC, et al: Holoprosencephaly in RSH/Smith-Lemli-Opitz syndrome: does abnormal cholesterol metabolism affect the function of Sonic Hedgehog? Am J Med Genet 1996;66:478-484.

72. Cordero DR, Marcucio R, Gaffield W, et al: Temporal disruption in sonic hedgehog signalling mimics the phenotypic range of holoprosencephaly. Nat Med; in press.

73. Ishii M, Merrill AE, Chan YS, et al: Msx2 and Twist cooperatively control the development of the neural crest-derived skeletogenic mesenchyme of the murine skull vault. Development 2003;130:6131-6142.

Embryology, Classifications, and Descriptions of Craniofacial Clefts

JAMES P. BRADLEY, MD ✦ DENNIS J. HURWITZ, MD ✦ MICHAEL H. CARSTENS, MD

The plastic surgeon faces a difficult task of consoling the parents of a newborn with a craniofacial cleft when they foresee, for their child, a life of ridicule and discrimination. Although a majority of patients with craniofacial clefts have no mental deficiencies, without appropriate staged surgical correction, social interaction and advancement may prove impossible for those afflicted when others cannot get beyond their facial malformation.

Congenital craniofacial clefts are distortions of the face and cranium with deficiencies or excesses of tissue that cleave anatomic planes in a linear fashion. They are among the most disfiguring of all facial anomalies. Craniofacial clefts exist in varying degrees of severity and in a multitude of patterns. Although they appear strange and seem to defy description, most craniofacial clefts occur along predictable embryologic lines. They are expressed either unilaterally or bilaterally. In addition, one cleft type can be manifest on one side of the face while a different type is present on the other side.

EPIDEMIOLOGY

The precise incidence of craniofacial clefts has not been identified because of their rarity and because of the difficulty in characterizing physical findings in mild malformations. However, the incidence of craniofacial clefts has been estimated to be 1.4 to 4.9 per 100,000 live births.[1-3] The incidence of rare craniofacial clefts compared with common cleft lip and palate malformations may range from 9.5 to 34 per 1000.[3-5] In some of these reports, only one type of cleft was recorded per patient even when more facial clefts existed.

The intrauterine incidence of facial deformities of any type has been documented to be greater than the incidence at live births; this may also be true for craniofacial clefts. When spontaneously aborted or stillborn fetuses were examined for craniofacial malformations, a more frequent occurrence was found to exist than at live births. Fetuses of therapeutic abortions between 3 and 18 weeks of gestation were found to have craniofacial malformations at the rate of 42.5 per 1000. With the increasing use of prenatal ultrasonography, a more accurate incidence of intrauterine facial anomaly, including the incidence of rare craniofacial clefts, may be determined in the future.

ETIOLOGIC FACTORS

The majority of rare craniofacial clefts occur sporadically. However, heredity has a role in the causation of rare craniofacial clefts in Treacher Collins syndrome and in familial instances of Goldenhar syndrome. A dominant gene defect (*TCOF1*) causes Treacher Collins syndrome.[6,7] Although penetrance is somewhat variable, the malformation is consistent. In a *TCOF1* gene knockout animal model, regional massive cell death affected crest cell mesenchymal migration and resulted in zygomatic abnormalities.[8] Constriction limb deformities (amniotic band syndrome) have also been associated with rare facial clefting. Coady et al[9] found a statistically significant association between craniofacial clefts and limb ring constrictions. Animal and human clinical studies have shown that many environmental factors may contribute to the cause of facial clefts. On the basis of these investigations, four major categories group these factors: radiation,[10-14] infection,[15-17] maternal metabolic imbalances,[18,19] and drugs and chemicals.[20] A considerable number of drugs and chemicals have teratogenic potential.[21] The drugs and chemicals known to induce congenital malformations include anticonvulsants,[22,23] chemotherapeutic agents,[24,25] steroids,[26,27] and tranquilizers.[28,29] Although few have been shown to cause craniofacial malformations in humans, some medications, including those containing retinoic acid, are being looked at as a cause of facial malformations.[30]

Although the teratogenic potential of many drugs is well known, their effects on facial development may not be preventable. The critical phase of embryologic maturation occurs when the mother may be unknowingly pregnant. Teratologists are confronted with the problem of multiple factors acting on numerous pathways and have no simple answer that universally explains the formation of a particular cleft.

EMBRYOLOGIC CRANIOFACIAL DEVELOPMENT

The understanding of normal morphogenesis occurring in the embryo and fetus allows the clinician to better describe and classify craniofacial clefts of infants and adults.[31] Likewise, the study of rare craniofacial clefts lends clues to facial embryology and neuroembryology. A traditional summary of normal facial development and newer understanding of genetically determined development zones of the face based on neuroembryology is outlined here.

Early Development

The human genome is made of 3 billion base pairs of nucleotides encoding more than 40,000 protein alleles of genes that are transcribed and then translated into structural, regulatory, or enzymatic proteins necessary for differentiation of early pluripotential cells.[31] Critical to the process of cell proliferation, differentiation, migration, and programmed cell death (apoptosis) are growth factors and mitogens responsible for cell-cell and cell-extracellular matrix interactions. Pattern formation in the embryo whereby specific cell types are generated at appropriate locations and shape specifications is determined by homeobox (HOX) genes that regulate other genes involved with proliferation, migration, and differentiation.[32] For example, Sonic hedgehog (Shh) is associated with midline organization in the embryo, and interruption of Shh signals leads to cyclopia (a form of holoprosencephaly).[33]

The three primary germ layers—ectoderm, mesoderm, and endoderm—are the basis for tissue and organ formation.[34] The ectoderm forms a neural plate with bilateral folds that conjoin into a neural tube. During closure of the neural tube, neural crest cells (mesenchyme) migrate into underlying tissue, forming pluripotential stem cells.[35,36] The embryonic prominences of the face are formed by the migration of these neural crest cells. Segmental patterns of ventral migration of neural crest, termed rhombomeres, provide the precursors of cartilage, bone, muscle, and connective tissue of the face and head.[37,38] Any defect in the quantity and quality of this migrating ectomesenchyme is manifested as a craniofacial malformation from severe holoprosencephaly to minor clinical stigmata of craniofacial clefts like dimples or skin tags.[39] Another cause of dysplasias and dystopias (the abnormal formation and location of structures) is abnormal development or involution of embryologic arteries.[40]

Craniofacial Development

The important aspects of embryologic development of the face take place between 4 and 8 weeks of gestation.[34,41] During this time, the crown-rump length increases from approximately 3.5 mm to 28 mm. Five prominences (the frontonasal and paired maxillary and mandibular) formed by neural crest migration surround the stomodeum (Fig. 86-1).[42] The frontonasal prominence is formed by neural crest cells migrating ventrally from the mesencephalic region and contributes to the frontal and nasal bones. The maxillary and mandibular prominences are formed by more caudally located migrating neural crest cells that encounter pharyngeal endoderm in their ventral migration around the aortic arches.

Eye development begins when optic vesicles appear from lateral invaginations of the diencephalons. Lens placodes are induced in the ectoderm and neural crest migration to form the sclera. Defective optic vesicle formation results in microphthalmos or anophthalmos. The movement of this optic tissue from lateral to medial results from the narrowing frontonasal prominence and expansion of the lateral face. Inadequate transition of the eyes produces hypertelorism,

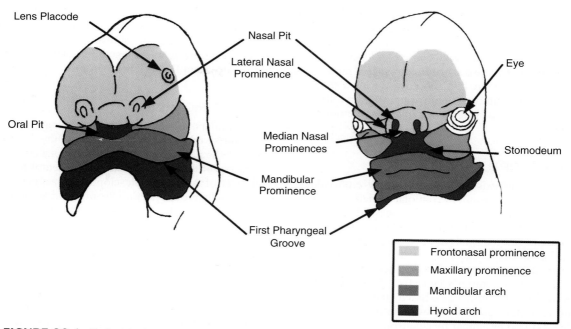

FIGURE 86-1. Embryologic facial formation: five facial prominences seen at 4 weeks *(left)* and 6 weeks *(right)*.

and overmigration produces hypotelorism or even median cyclopia.[43]

Nasal development begins when the nasal placodes arise from ectodermal tissue inferolateral to the frontonasal prominence and cephalad to the stomodeum. Nasal placodes invaginate into the face to form nasal pits, and elevations at the margins produce horseshoe-shaped median and lateral nasal prominences. The posterior aspect of each nasal pit is separated from the oral cavity by an oronasal membrane. Failure of this membrane to disintegrate normally leads to choanal atresia.[44] The paired median nasal processes merge with the frontonasal prominence to form the majority of the frontal process. These structures gradually enlarge and superiorly displace the frontonasal prominence. During the sixth week, the two median nasal processes coalesce in the midline, and their most caudal limbs, the premaxillary prominence, expand above the stomodeum. The nasal tip, philtrum, columella, cartilaginous septum, and primary palate are derived from these paired median elements. Cephalad to the medial nasal process, the frontonasal process persists to form the nasal dorsum and root. Elevation of the lateral nasal prominence promotes development of the nasal alae. Defects during this development may be midline and produce arrhinia or a bifid nose.[42]

The maxillary processes are paired mesodermal masses that lie cephalad to the mandibular arch and ventral to the optic neuroectoderm. These triangular masses enlarge, separate from the mandibular arch, and then migrate ventrally. The maxillary process

ultimately coalesces with the mesoderm of the globular processes (premaxillary prominence) to form the upper lip. The cheek, maxilla, zygoma, and secondary palate are also derived from the maxillary processes. Between the maxillary prominence and the lateral nasal prominence, a depression exists with a solid rod of epithelial cells.[42] The ends of this rod form a connection from the nasal pit to the conjunctival sac. This rod eventually becomes the nasolacrimal duct. With inadequate neural crest cell migration, a fissure within the line of this duct may persist as an oblique facial cleft.

The stomodeal aperture is reduced by migrating mesenchyme that fuses the maxillary and mandibular prominences to form the oral commissures. Inadequate neural crest cells results in macrostomia; excessive tissue produces microstomia or astomia. The mandibular prominence lies between the stomodeum and the first branchial groove, which delineates the caudal limits of the face. The paired, free ends of the mandibular arch enlarge and converge ventrally during the sixth week. The lower lip and mandible are developed from this arch. Paired, lateral pharyngeal elevations of the arch unite to form the anterior portion of the tongue.

The external ear and middle ear are also formed during the sixth week of gestation. The tragus and the crus of the helix are derived from three hillocks at the caudal border of the first branchial arch. The malleus and incus of the middle ear are also formed by the first branchial arch. The remainder of the external ear and the stapes of the middle ear are formed from three hillocks on the cephalic border of the second branchial arch.

In summary of early embryologic craniofacial development, there is a coordination of cell migration, cellular interaction, and apoptosis during a short 4-week period. Failure of this intricate program will result in clefts that usually fall along predictable embryonic lines.

FAILURE OF FUSION

Two theories exist that describe how embryologic failure or errors result in craniofacial cleft malformations. The fusion failure theory suggests that clefts are formed when fusion of facial processes fails.[45,46] The failure of mesodermal penetration theory implicates the lack of neuroectoderm and mesoderm migration and penetration into the bilaminar ectodermal sheets as the cause of craniofacial clefts.[47-49] Although most of the current knowledge is based on investigations of animal cleft lip and palate, rare craniofacial clefts may be produced by similar mechanisms.

The failure of fusion theory, proposed by Dursy[45] in 1869 and His[46] in 1892, purported that the free edges of the facial processes unite in the central region of the face. As various processes fuse, the face gradually forms. When epithelial contact is established between opposing facial processes, mesodermal penetration completes the fusion. Dursy suggested that the upper lip is formed when finger-like advancing ends of the maxillary process and the paired global process unite. He asserted that disruption of this sequence results in craniofacial cleft anomalies.

Proponents of the mesodermal penetration theory believed that the finger-like ends of the facial processes do not exist. Warbrick[50] and Stark and Ehrmann[51] suggested that the central facial processes are composed of bilamellar sheets of ectoderm. This bilamellar membrane is bordered by epithelial seams, which delineate the principal processes. During development, the mesenchymal tissue migrates and penetrates this double-layered ectoderm, called the epithelial wall.[52] Caudal to the stomodeum, the lower face is formed by the branchial arches. The arches consist of a thin sheet of mesoderm, which lies between the ectodermal and endodermal layers. The neural crest cells of neuroectodermal origin, which arise from the dorsolateral surface of the neural tube, migrate under the ectoderm and supplement the mesoderm of the frontonasal process and branchial arches.[53] Most of the craniofacial skeleton is believed to be formed by these neural crest cells. If neuroectoderm migration and penetration do not occur, the epithelium breaks down to form a facial cleft. The severity of the cleft is proportional to the failure of penetration by the neuroectoderm.

The precise nature of the proposed mechanisms in the formation of rare craniofacial clefts is not known. Nevertheless, the concepts of fusion and mesodermal penetration provide an understanding of the problems of the rare craniofacial cleft.

NEUROMERIC THEORY

Newer understanding of neuroembryology suggests that a direct relationship exists between the development of the nervous system and those structures to which its contents are dedicated. The neural tube is conceived of as a series of developmental zones within the central nervous system.[37] Six prosomeres provide a cartesian system to organize the tracts and nuclei of the prosencephalon (forebrain). The mesencephalon (midbrain) and rhombencephalon (hindbrain) are subdivided into 2 mesomeres and 12 rhombomeres, respectively. Each of these neuromeres is defined by a unique overlap of several genetic coding zones along the axis of the embryo. In the hindbrain and caudally to the coccyx, these neuromeric units are defined by the homeobox series of genes (HOX genes). In the forebrain, a more complex series of genes is used, such as Sonic hedgehog (Shh), Wingless (Wnt), and Engrailed (En).

The unique "barcode" for each neuromeric zone is shared with all cells exiting a particular level to form the mesoderm and endoderm of the embryo. For example, the HOX gene that codes for the rhombomeres 2 and 3 (which make up the first pharyngeal arch) is shared with the mesoderm that makes up those arches. This same HOX gene is also shared with the neural crest cells that subsequently move into the mesodermal "zones" of the first pharyngeal arch. The migrating neural crest cells then provide the instructions for differentiation into the appropriate facial tissues. Thus, all the bones and soft tissues of the face can be thought of as genetically determined "fields" with defined cellular content and a fixed position in space. With the folding of the embryo, these fields are placed into their correct topologic positions, and a three-dimensional form results.

This system permits the "mapping" of the face into developmental zones with distinct spatial origins in their precursor tissue units (Fig. 86-2). The midline mesoderm of the nasal and ocular fields has an origin, innervation, and blood supply different from all surrounding mesodermal elements. When all the developmental zones are accounted for, the occurrence of craniofacial clefts is nothing more than an orderly progression of deficiency states in the precursor fields resulting in varying degrees of absence of soft tissue functional matrix or underlying bone.[54] The anatomic and clinical observations of Tessier and his classification system are exactly compatible with this map. Variations include the following: clefts number

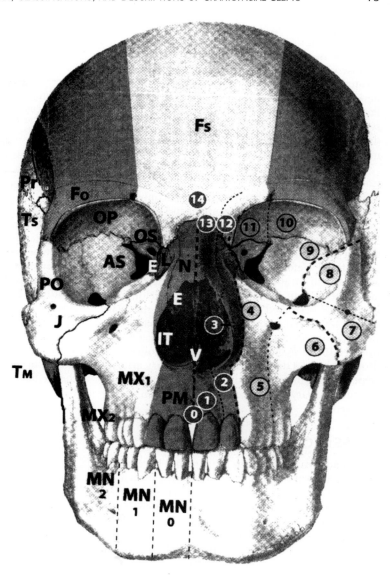

FIGURE 86-2. Neuromeric theory. Developmental fields depicted on the right side of the facial skeleton (left side of illustration) have a direct relationship with Tessier's numeric classification for craniofacial clefts on the contralateral side. Clefting is seen with failure of field boundaries (e.g., number 4 cleft) or deficiency of an axial field (e.g., number 5 cleft). AS, alisphenoid viscerocranial; E, ethmoid; Fs, frontal bone upper; Fo, frontal bone lower; IT, inferior turbinate; J, zygomatic field; MN, mandible field; MX₁, premolar zone; MX₂, molar zone; OS, orbito-sphenoid field; PM, premaxilla; PO, postorbital; Pr, parietal region; Tm, temporomandibular; Ts, temporo-squamous; V, vomer.

2 and number 3 fall within the same zone (cleft number 3 being more posterior); and clefts number 4 and number 5 represent varying degrees of involvement in the same zone of the maxilla. Tessier's classification system has been widely adopted by surgeons and other clinicians and has stood the test of time. However, geneticists and embryologists have been slow to embrace his numeric organization of craniofacial clefts because it could not previously be understood by existing theories of embryologic development. The consistency of these newer neuroembryologic theories with Tessier's classification of craniofacial clefts reinforces the importance of Tessier's descriptions. With progression of the neuromeric theory, the value of Tessier's organization of rare craniofacial clefts should become apparent to embryologists and geneticists.

PATHOGENESIS

Failure of ectodermal fusion and failure of mesodermal migration have been theorized to cause rare craniofacial clefts. Detrimental forces can interfere with cell formation, replication, or migration and produce craniofacial malformations including facial clefting. Also, drugs and other environmental factors disturb metabolic rate and cellular activity and may alter normal development. Intrauterine physical constrictions, such as in oligohydramnios, may interfere with fusion of facial processes by applying extrinsic mechanical restraint. Another proposed means of clefting is an alteration in the normal equilibrium between cell formation and spontaneous cell death (apoptosis). Warbrick[55] suggested that if the apoptosis fails to occur in the appropriate region during the appropriate time, mesenchymal tissue is not able to migrate normally. Arrest of neural crest cell migration is proposed as a cause of facial clefting. Johnston[56] experimentally produced a facial cleft by removing a portion of the neural crest cells before they began migration. Poswillo[57] demonstrated in animals that bilaterally symmetric facial clefts (such as in Treacher Collins syndrome) occur because the preotic neural crest cells migrating to the first branchial arch are disrupted.

Premature involution of embryonic arteries may lead to abnormal development of regional craniofacial tissues.[40] The stapedial artery is present only during day 33 to day 40 of fetal development and supplies the first and second branchial arches. Braithwaite and Watson[58] suggested that loss of the stapedial artery during this critical period causes ischemia and may cause facial clefting. Poswillo[59] induced clefting in animals with localized hemorrhage of the stapedial artery rather than an abnormal arterial development. Lockhard[60] described an anomaly of the maxillary artery that caused deformities of the zygoma, middle ear, and muscles of mastication. In addition, a dissection of a 10-week-old fetus with Treacher Collins syndrome showed a disruption of the maxillary artery.[61] Depending on the magnitude and timing of local tissue destruction, varying degrees of malformation may be observed.

CLASSIFICATIONS

Craniofacial malformations are rare and have multiple variations and a spectrum of severity. Individual reports in the literature have often been incomplete and add to the preexisting confusion. Different terminology to describe embryologic maldevelopment, genetic etiology, or anatomic landmarks has also been used to refer to the same or similar cleft anomalies. Organization of the seemingly heterogeneous clefting malformations is necessary for both morphogenetic understanding and knowledge of surgical anatomy for treatment. Therefore, orderly systems of classification have been described.

AMERICAN ASSOCIATION OF CLEFT PALATE REHABILITATION. The American Association of Cleft Palate Rehabilitation (AACPR) endorsed a classification system proposed by Harkins[62] in 1962. Craniofacial clefts are separated into four categories on the basis of pathologic location: mandibular process clefts, nasoocular clefts, oro-ocular clefts, and oro-aural clefts (Table 86-1). Mandibular process clefts group malformations of the mandible and lower lip. Naso-ocular clefts include malformations located between the nasal ala and the medial canthus. Oro-ocular clefts consist of clefting anomalies connecting the oral cavity to the orbit between the medial and lateral

TABLE 86-1 ✦ AMERICAN ASSOCIATION OF CLEFT PALATE REHABILITATION CLASSIFICATION OF CRANIOFACIAL CLEFTS

Mandibular process clefts
Naso-ocular clefts
Oro-ocular clefts
  *Type 1
  *Type 2   No 5 de Tessier
Oro-aural clefts

*Denotes subdivision of oro-ocular clefts described by Boo-Chai.

canthus. Oro-aural clefts describe anomalies involving the region from the oral commissure to the auricular tragus.

Boo-Chai[63] further defined the AACPR classification scheme, purely on the basis of surface anatomic landmarks, by including skeletal components. The oro-ocular clefts are subdivided on the basis of the infraorbital foramen into two types, oromedial canthus and orolateral canthus (see Table 86-1). Type 1 oro-ocular clefts begin lateral to Cupid's bow and extend up the cheek lateral to the nasal ala to involve the medial canthus. Type 1 skeletal involvement begins between the lateral incisor and canine and extends between the piriform aperture and infraorbital foramen. Type 2 oro-ocular clefts begin just medial to the oral commissure and extend to the lateral eyelid, often in the form of a coloboma. Type 2 skeletal involvement begins near the premolar dentition and passes lateral to the infraorbital foramen.

KARFIK CLASSIFICATION. The Karfik classification[64] has an embryologic and morphologic basis and is divided into five groups: group A, rhinencephalic malformations; group B, anomalies of the first and second branchial arch; group C, orbitopalpebral malformations; group D, craniocephalic malformations, such as Apert and Crouzon syndromes; and group E, atypical deformities from congenital tumors, atrophy, or hypertrophy and true oblique clefts that cannot be related to any embryologic fusion line (Table 86-2). Group A, the rhinencephalic malformations, is divided into two subtypes: group A1, axial malformations derived from the frontonasal prominence; and group A2, paraxial malformations adjacent to the nasal region. Group B, anomalies of the first and second branchial arch, is also divided into two subtypes: group B1 is composed of the lateral otocephalic malformations, including craniofacial microsomia, Treacher Collins syndrome, Pierre Robin sequence, and auricular malformations; group B2 includes the mandibular midline malformations.

VAN DER MEULEN CLASSIFICATION. The van der Meulen classification attempted to explain the

TABLE 86-2 ✦ KARFIK CLASSIFICATION OF CRANIOFACIAL CLEFTS

Group A: rhinocephalic disorders
  A1: Axial malformations (teratoma, glioma, median cleft lip, median cleft nasal defect)
  A2: Para-axial malformations (typical cleft lip, nasal atresia)

Group B: branchiogenic disorders
  B1: Lateral otocephalic malformations
  B2: Medial axial (lower lip cleft)–midline mandibular clefts

Group C: ophthalmo-orbital disorders (anophthalmos, ptosis, coloboma)

Group D: craniocephalic disorders (Apert syndrome, Crouzon syndrome, cutis aplasia)

Group E: atypical facial disorders (oblique facial clefts, hemifacial atrophy)

---

craniofacial clefts from an embryologic basis[65]; the term *dysplasia* is used because some of the malformations do not represent true clefts (Table 86-3). The defects are labeled by the name of the developmental area (facial processes and bones) that is involved. The mal-

TABLE 86-3 ✦ VAN DER MEULEN CLASSIFICATION OF CRANIOFACIAL CLEFTS (DYSPLASIAS)

Cerebrocranial dysplasias
  Anencephaly
  Microcephaly
Cerebrofacial dysplasias
  Rhinocephalic dysplasias
  Oculo-orbital dysplasias
Craniofacial dysplasias
  With clefting
    Lateral or medial nasomaxillary cleft
    Intermaxillary
    Maxillomandibular
  With dysostosis
  With synostosis
    Craniosynostosis
    Craniofaciosynostosis
    Faciosynostosis
  With dysostosis and synostosis
    Crouzon syndrome
    Apert syndrome
    Cloverleaf skull
  With dyschondrosis
    Achondroplasia
Craniofacial dysplasias with other origin
  Osseous (osteopetrosis, craniotubular dysplasia, fibrous dysplasia)
  Cutaneous (ectodermal dysplasia)
  Neurocutaneous (neurofibromatosis)
  Neuromuscular (Robin sequence)
  Muscular (glossoschisis)
  Vascular

---

formations are believed to occur before or during the fusion of the facial processes but before the start of ossification.

CLASSIFICATION OF MEDIAN FACIAL CLEFTS. Median facial clefts may be classified by tissue deficiency or tissue excess. Median tissue deficiency with a shortage of tissue and absence of parts has been called arrhinencephaly malformations.[66] The absence of olfactory bulbs and tracts was assumed to be the common malformation in this series of brain abnormalities. Subsequent investigators have established that the failure of the forebrain (prosencephalon) to undergo cleavage normally is the underlying developmental error.[67,68] DeMyer et al[69] proposed the term *holoprosencephalon* to denote an undivided prosencephalon. A relationship exists between the median facial structures and the forebrain; therefore, the severity of the facial abnormality is reflected in brain development. Elias et al[70] proposed a modification that describes a five-scaled classification for holoprosencephaly, with several subgroups, to categorize the wide range of these malformations. Groups I to III are associated with alobar brains; group IV is associated with lobar brains and group V with normal brains.

Median tissue excess is the second group of median facial clefts. This group of anomalies does not have a high correlation between the distorted face and the underlying brain. The spectrum of deformities ranges from a slight midline notch of the upper lip to the severest form of orbital hypertelorism. The midline facial clefts are characterized by seven features: orbital hypertelorism, V-shaped frontal hairline, cranium bifidum occultum, median cleft of the upper lip, median cleft of the primary palate, median cleft of the secondary palate, and telecanthus.[71] Mental development is typically normal except for a slight mental retardation when orbital hypertelorism is found in association with one or more of the other six features.

TESSIER CLASSIFICATION. In 1973, Tessier presented a classification of craniofacial clefts that was subsequently published in detail by Tessier[1] and Kawamoto.[2] Although other classification systems exist, Tessier's classification is the most complete and has withstood the test of time. The unique classification is based on the extensive personal experience of one investigator rather than a collection of examples from the literature. This enables the terminology to remain uniform and the characterizations to be detailed. In addition, the classification links the clinical observations with underlying skeletal deformity seen during surgery. Preoperative three-dimensional computed tomographic scans, more recently, have been useful in confirming skeletal findings. Correlation of the clinical appearance with the surgical anatomic findings improves the clinical utility of this system for the craniofacial surgeon.

During many years, Tessier developed a classification of rare craniofacial clefts based on a multitude of experiences and observations. The clefts are numbered 0 to 14 and follow well-defined "time zones" (Fig. 86-3). The eyelids and orbits define the primary axis of this functional system, dividing the face into upper and lower hemispheres. Tessier used these landmarks because the orbit belongs to both the cranium and the face. The orbit separates the cranial or "northbound" clefts from the facial or "southbound" clefts. All of the craniofacial clefts are formed by the combination of northbound and southbound clefts. In addition, the following combinations are clinically observed: 0 and 14, 1 and 13, 2 and 12, 3 and 11, 4 and 10, 5 and 9, and 6 and 8. Clefts 5 through 9 are considered lateral clefts because they pass lateral to the infraorbital foramen. Tessier cleft number 7 is the most lateral craniofacial cleft. Although the craniofacial clefts tend to coincide with these time zones, the vascular supply and embryonic processes do not necessarily follow the same pathways.

The clinical expression of the craniofacial cleft is highly variable. Tessier observed that hypoplasia did not evolve into facial clefts; however, clefts always possessed hypoplastic tissues. He perceived that the soft tissue and skeletal components were seldom affected to the same extent. Furthermore, the skeletal landmarks tend to be more constant and reliable than the soft tissue landmarks. Facial clefts medial to the infraorbital foramen had greater soft tissue involvement than did clefts found lateral to the foramen. By contrast, facial clefts lateral to the infraorbital foramen had greater bone disruption than did clefts found medial to the foramen. Finally, bilateral forms of the clefts are found in varying combinations.

DISTINCTIVE FEATURES

The craniofacial clefts are described by the Tessier classification. These groupings are treatment oriented and relate soft tissue clinical features to underlying bone involvement. The severity of involvement of

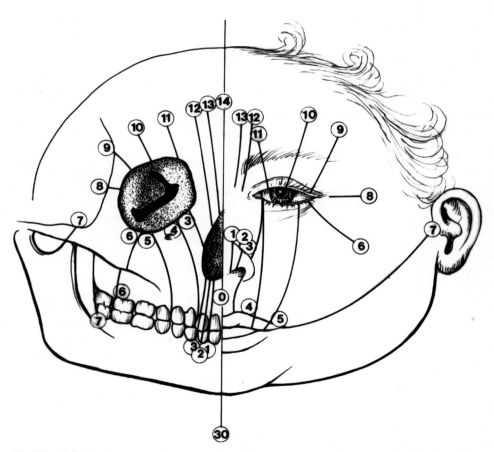

FIGURE 86-3. Tessier's classification of craniofacial clefts. The left half depicts the skeletal locations of numeric clefts, and the right half outlines the clinical locations of clefts on soft tissue landmarks. Facial clefts are numbered 0 to 7, and cranial clefts are numbered 8 to 14.

regional structures influences the therapeutic strategy. The order of description consists of facial clefts from medial to lateral followed by cranial clefts from lateral to medial.

Number 0 Cleft

The number 0 cleft has been referred to as median craniofacial dysrhaphia, centrofacial microsomia, frontonasal dysplasia, median cleft face syndrome, or holoprosencephaly.[65,68,71,72] Patients with this midline facial cleft may have a cranial extension or a number 14 cleft. The number 0 and number 14 Tessier craniofacial clefts are unique in that there may be either a deficiency or an excess of tissue.

DEFICIENCY OF MIDLINE STRUCTURES. A deficiency may manifest as hypoplasia or agenesis in which portions of midline facial structures are missing (Fig. 86-4). This developmental arrest may range from the mildest form with hypoplasia of the nasomaxillary region and hypotelorism to a severe form of cyclopia, ethmocephaly, or cebocephaly. This severe form is often fatal. DeMeyer[71] separated the spectrum of severity of midline clefts into five groups. These categories demonstrated that the severity of facial anomalies correlates well with the severity of brain abnormality and mental retardation. A computed tomographic scan of the brain can differentiate those patients with poor differentiation of the brain who may die in infancy from those with a better prognosis.

Soft tissue deficiencies with this midline facial cleft include the upper lip and nose (Fig. 86-4A). Agenesis or hypoplasia may result in a false median cleft lip and absence of philtral columns. When a wide central cleft exists, it typically extends the length of the upper lip and up into the nasal floor (Fig. 86-4B). With nasal anomalies, the columella may be narrowed or totally absent. The nasal tip may be depressed from lack of septal support. The septum is usually vestigial with no caudal attachment to the palate.

Skeletal deficiencies range from separation between the upper central canines to absence of the premaxilla and a cleft of the secondary palate. Nasal deficiencies include partial or total absence of nasal bones and the septal cartilages. The bone defect may extend cephalad into the area of the ethmoid sinuses and result in hypotelorism or cyclopia. The encephalocele may occur that fills the defect or void from the frontonasal junction back to the foramen cecum or sphenoid body.

EXCESS OF MIDLINE TISSUE. In the number 0 cleft, midline excess is noted as widening or duplications of structures.

Soft tissue midline excess tissue may be manifested as a true median cleft lip with broad philtral columns. A duplication of the labial frenulum may also exist. The nose may be bifid with a broad columella and

mid-dorsal furrow (Fig. 86-4C). The alae and upper lateral cartilages may be displaced laterally.

Skeletal excess in a widened number 0 facial cleft can be seen as a diastema between the upper central incisors (Fig. 86-4D). A duplicate nasal spine may exist. A characteristic keel-shaped maxillary alveolus is seen. Anterior teeth are angled toward the midline, creating an anterior open bite.[73] Central midface height is shortened. The cartilaginous and bony nasal septum is thickened or duplicated. The nasal bones and nasal process of the maxilla are broad, flattened, and displaced laterally from the midline. Ethmoid and sphenoid sinuses may be enlarged, contributing to symmetric widening of the anterior cranial fossa and hypertelorism.[74] The cribriform plate is low, and the breadth of the crista galli is exaggerated. The body of the sphenoid is broadened with displacement of the pterygoid plates away from the midline.

Number 1 Cleft

This paramedian facial cleft was first delineated by Tessier[1]; van der Meulen[65] classified this cleft as a type 3 nasoschisis nasal dysplasia. The number 1 facial cleft continues cranially as a number 13 cleft.

SOFT TISSUE INVOLVEMENT. The number 1 cleft, similar to the common cleft lip, passes through Cupid's bow and then the alar cartilage dome. Notching in the area of the soft triangle of the nose is a distinct feature (Fig. 86-5A). The columella may be short and broad. The nasal tip and nasal septum deviate away from the cleft. Soft tissue furrows or wrinkles may be present on the nasal dorsum if the cleft extends in a cephalic direction. The cleft is evident medial to a malpositioned medial canthus, and telecanthus may result. With a cranial extension as a number 13 cleft, vertical dystopia is present.

SKELETAL INVOLVEMENT. A keel-shaped maxilla with the anterior incisors facing toward the cleft forms an anterior open bite. An alveolar cleft is rare but passes between the central and lateral incisors. This paramedian cleft separates the nasal floor at the piriform aperture just lateral to the nasal spine (Fig. 86-5B). The cleft may extend posteriorly as a complete cleft of the hard and soft palate. Extension of the cleft in a cephalad direction is through the junction of the nasal bone and the frontal process of the maxilla. The nasal bones are displaced and flattened. Ethmoidal expansion leads to hypertelorism. There is also asymmetry of the greater and lesser sphenoid wings, pterygoid plates, and anterior cranial fossa.

Number 2 Cleft

SOFT TISSUE INVOLVEMENT. This other paramedian facial cleft may also begin in the region of the common

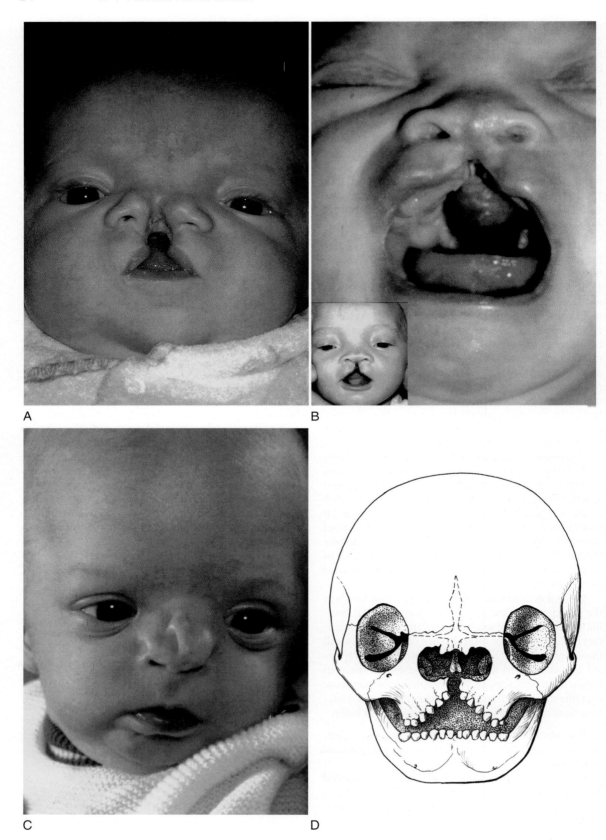

A

B

C

D

FIGURE 86-4. Number 0 cleft. *A,* Patient with a true median cleft lip, bifid nasal deformity, and extension to number 14 cleft with hypertelorism. *B,* Patient with agenesis of midline structures and absence of premaxilla and prolabium *(inset)*. Intraoral view demonstrates an encephalocele. Attempted cleft palate repair with a vomer flap should not be undertaken without imaging studies. *C,* Patient with excessive midline tissue manifested by bifid nose and an accessory band of skin on the nasal dorsum. *D,* Skeletal involvement causes separation between the central incisors, widening of the nasal region, and orbital hypertelorism.

---

cleft lip, yet the nasal deformity is in the middle third of the alar rim and distinguishes the number 2 cleft (Fig. 86-6). The ala is hypoplastic in the number 2 cleft, whereas the ala is merely notched at the dome in the number 1 cleft and the alar base is displaced in the number 3 cleft. The lateral aspect of the nose is flattened and the dorsum is broad. The eyelid is not involved; the cleft passes medially to the palpebral fissure. Although the medial canthus is displaced, the lacrimal duct is usually not involved. If the cleft continues in a cephalad direction as a cranial number 12 cleft, distortion of the medial brow is noted.

SKELETAL INVOLVEMENT. The number 2 cleft begins between the lateral incisor and the canine. It extends into the piriform aperture, lateral to the septum and medial to the maxillary sinus. A hard and soft palate cleft may occur. The nasal septum may be deviated away from the cleft. The cleft distorts the nasal bones as it passes between the nasal bones and the frontal process of the maxilla. Ethmoid sinus involvement may result in orbital hypertelorism. Asymmetry of the greater and lesser sphenoid wings and anterior cranial base is present.[73]

Number 3 Cleft

The number 3 cleft is the most common of the Tessier craniofacial clefts. Morian[75] was the first to report this

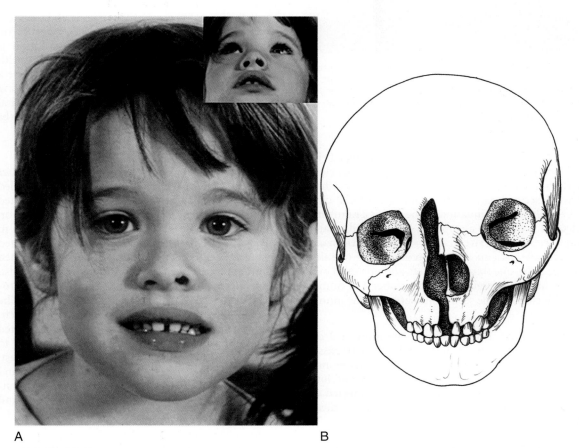

A   B

FIGURE 86-5. Number 1 cleft. *A,* Patient with notched alar dome and orbital hypertelorism. *B,* Skeletal involvement is through the piriform aperture just lateral to the nasal spine and septum. The orbit is displaced laterally.

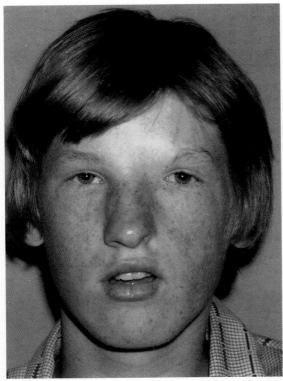

FIGURE 86-6. Number 2 cleft. Patient with hypoplasia of the middle third of the left nostril rim causing the appearance of alar base retraction. The lateral nose is flattened. The medial border of the eyebrow is also distorted as evidence of a number 12 cranial cleft.

disorder and later classified it as a Morian type I cleft. It is also referred to as a Tessier oro-naso-ocular cleft.[76] Others, including Davis,[77] Gunter,[78] and Boo-Chai,[63] have described patients with number 3 facial clefts. The cephalad continuation of the cleft is a number 11 cleft. In contrast to a common cleft lip and palate, a number 3 cleft has an equal distribution between male and female patients and an occurrence of one third on the right, one third on the left, and one third bilaterally. With bilateral clefting, a number 4 or number 5 facial cleft may be seen contralateral to the number 3 cleft.

SOFT TISSUE INVOLVEMENT. The number 3 cleft begins like a number 1 and number 2 cleft, passing through the philtral column and floor of the nose. Deficiency of tissue between the alar base and lower eyelid results in a shortened nose on the affected side (Fig. 86-7A). The cleft passes between the medial canthus and the inferior lacrimal punctum. The lacrimal system, particularly the lower canaliculus, is disrupted. Blockage of the nasolacrimal duct and recurrent infections of the lacrimal sac are common.[76] The inferior punctum is displaced downward, and drainage may occur directly onto the cheek instead of into the nasal cavity.

The medial canthus is inferiorly displaced and may be hypoplastic. Colobomas of the lower eyelid are medial to the inferior punctum. In mild forms, colobomas may be the only obvious evidence of this cleft. In patients with mild disease, it is important to check a computed tomographic scan for bone involvement and to maintain an index of suspicion for disruption of the lacrimal system. Involvement of the globe is rare, but microphthalmos may occur. The eye is typically malpositioned inferiorly and laterally. Injury to the normal eye, including corneal erosions, ocular perforation, and loss of vision in the affected eye, may result from desiccation unless the globe is protected (Fig. 86-7B).

SKELETAL INVOLVEMENT. Osseous characteristics of this facial cleft include involvement of the orbit and direct communication of the oral, nasal, and orbital cavities (Fig. 86-7C). The cleft begins between the lateral incisor and the canine. In contrast to the number 1 and number 2 facial clefts, the anterior maxillary arch is flat in the number 3 cleft. The number 3 cleft disrupts the frontal process of the maxilla and then terminates in the lacrimal groove. In the severest form, the cleft is bilateral and the skeletal disruption is significant (Fig. 86-7D). Alternatively, in patients with bilateral clefts, the contralateral facial cleft may be a number 4 or number 5 cleft. There may be narrowing of the ethmoid and sphenoid sinuses. Both the orbital floor and anterior cranial base are displaced inferiorly.

Number 4 Cleft

The number 4 cleft occurs lateral to the nose and other median facial structures. The cleft has been called meloschisis (separation of cheek). Dick[79] first reported the number 4 cleft in the English literature, and von Kulmus may have recorded the initial description in Latin in 1732. Tessier[1,76] and Kawamoto[79a] reported instances of number 4 clefts, and Boo-Chai[63] collected 23 other reports from the literature. The cleft has also been referred to as an oro-ocular cleft (AACPR), oro-facial cleft, and medial maxillary dysplasia.[1,62,65] The cranial continuation of the cleft is the number 10 cleft. For unilateral number 4 facial clefts, it is estimated that a distribution exists for right to left side of 2 to 1.3 and for male to female of 2.5 to 1. In contrast, bilateral clefts occur in equal numbers of male and female patients. Bilateral clefts are associated with contralateral craniofacial clefts number 3, number 5, and number 7.

SOFT TISSUE INVOLVEMENT. As opposed to facial clefts number 1, number 2, and number 3, the number 4 cleft begins lateral to Cupid's bow, between the tubercle (midline) and the oral commissure (Fig. 86-8A).

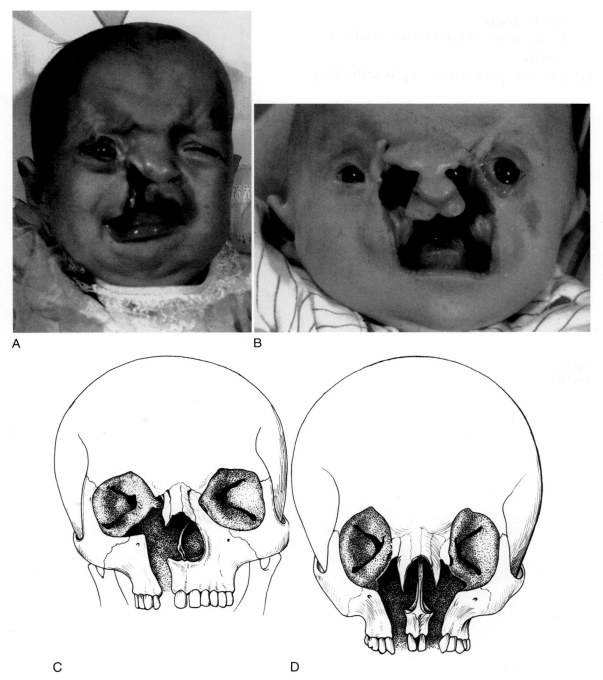

FIGURE 86-7. Number 3 cleft. *A,* Unilateral. Patient with complete form has a right-sided cleft lip and palate and severe shortening of tissues between the right alar base and medial canthus. The right nasal ala is displaced superiorly, the medial canthus is displaced inferiorly, and the nasolacrimal system is disrupted. *B,* Bilateral. Patient with significant midface distortion including bilateral cleft lip and palate and retraction of alar bases extending above the level of the medial canthi. *C,* Unilateral. Skeletal involvement is between the lateral incisor and the canine extending up through the lacrimal groove. The cleft enables communication among the orbital, maxillary sinus, nasal, and oral cavities. *D,* Bilateral. Skeletal defects are extensive; only the nasal septum divides the cavities of the midface.

Communication:
  - cavité orale
  - sinus maxillaire (paroi médiale intacte)
  - orbite
Médiale au foramen infra·orbitaire

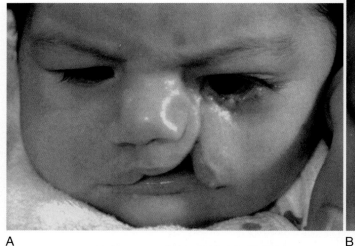

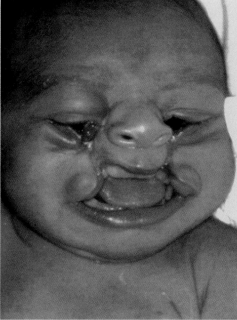

A

B

Orbicularis
oris = latéral

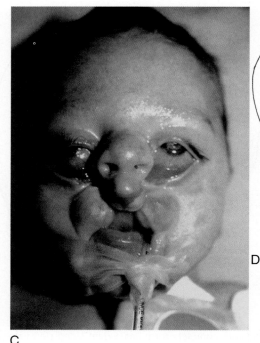

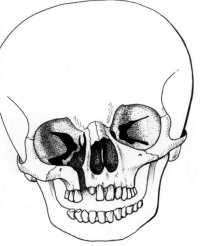

C

D

FIGURE 86-8. Number 4 cleft. *A,* Unilateral. Patient with left cheek cleft. The cleft lip begins lateral to Cupid's bow and terminates in the lower eyelid medial to the punctum. *B,* Bilateral. Patient with bilateral involvement has a cleft of the upper lip lateral to Cupid's bow and malar extension to the colobomas of the lower eyelids. Notching is also seen in the upper lids as evidence of a number 10 cranial cleft. *C,* Bilateral. Patient with complete bilateral involvement with premaxilla in protrusive position and nose displaced in a cephalad position. *D,* Unilateral. Skeletal involvement begins between the lateral incisor and canine and extends through the maxilla between the infraorbital foramen and the piriform aperture. The orbit, maxillary sinus, and oral cavities communicate.

The orbicularis oris muscle is located in the lateral lip element and gives a mass-like, bunching appearance. The cleft passes lateral to the nasal ala. Although the ala is not involved and the nose is intact, the alar base may be displaced superiorly. Bilateral involvement pulls the nose upward (Fig. 86-8B). The cleft extends through the cheek and into the lower eyelid lateral to the inferior punctum. The lower eyelid and lashes may extend directly into the lateral aspect of the cleft (Fig. 86-8C). The medial canthus and nasolacrimal system are normal. The globe is typically normal, but microphthalmos and anophthalmos may be seen.[80]

Skeletal Involvement. Skeletal involvement is usually less extensive than in the number 3 cleft. The alveolar cleft begins between the lateral incisor and the canine (Fig. 86-8D). The cleft extends lateral to the piriform aperture to involve the maxillary sinus. The medial wall of the maxillary sinus is intact. A confluence exists between the oral cavity, maxillary sinus, and orbital cavity but not the nasal cavity. The cleft then passes medial to the infraorbital foramen. This landmark defines the boundary between the medial number 4 facial cleft and the lateral number 5 facial cleft. The number 4 cleft terminates at the medial aspect of the inferior orbital rim. With an absent medial orbital floor and rim, the globe may prolapse inferiorly. In bilateral clefts, the medial midface and premaxilla are protrusive. The sphenoid body is asymmetric and the pterygoid plates are displaced, but the anterior cranial base is unaffected.[73]

Number 5 Cleft

This facial cleft is the rarest of the oblique facial clefts. It has been called the oculofacial cleft II, Morian III cleft, lateral maxillary dysplasia, or oro-ocular type 2 cleft (AACPR classification).[62,63,65] The cephalad progression of the number 5 cleft is the number 9 cleft. One fourth of these clefts are unilateral, one fourth are bilateral, and one half are combined with another facial cleft (Fig. 86-9A).

Soft Tissue Involvement. The number 5 facial cleft begins just medial to the oral commissure, courses along the cheek lateral to the nasal ala, and terminates

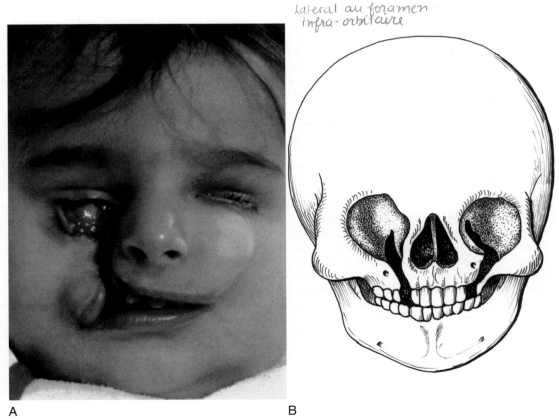

Lateral au foramen infra-orbitaire

A   B

FIGURE 86-9. Number 5 cleft (left side) and number 4 cleft (right side). *A,* The number 4 cleft begins lateral to Cupid's bow and extends up to the medial third of the lower eyelid; the number 5 cleft begins just medial to the oral commissure and extends up the lateral cheek to the middle of the eyelid. *B,* Skeletal involvement in the number 4 cleft begins between the lateral incisor and canine and passes medial to the infraorbital foramen. In the number 5 cleft, the cleft begins at the premolars and extends lateral to the infraorbital foramen.

in the lateral half of the lower eyelid. Although the globe is typically normal, microphthalmos may occur.

Skeletal Involvement. The alveolar cleft begins lateral to the canine in the region of the premolars. In contrast to the number 4 cleft, the number 5 cleft then courses lateral to the infraorbital foramen and terminates in the lateral aspect of the orbital rim and floor (Fig. 86-9B). Within the orbit, the cleft does not involve the inferior orbital fissure. The maxillary sinus may be hypoplastic. Prolapse of orbital contents through the lateral orbital floor defect into the maxillary sinus causes vertical orbital dystopia. The lateral orbital wall may be thickened and the greater sphenoid wing abnormal. The cranial base is normal.

Number 6 Cleft

This zygomatic-maxillary cleft represents an incomplete form of Treacher Collins syndrome. It was called maxillozygomatic dysplasia by van der Meulen.[65] Similar and often more severe cleft facial features are seen in Nager syndrome. Patients with Nager syndrome may also have radial club deformities of the upper extremities.

Soft Tissue Involvement. The cleft is often identified as a vertical furrow, due to hypoplastic soft tissue, from the oral commissure to the lateral lower eyelid (Fig. 86-10A). This line of hypoplasia runs through the zygomatic eminence along an imaginary line from the angle of the mandible to the lateral palpebral fissure. The lateral palpebral fissure is pulled downward. The lateral canthus is displaced inferiorly. This may cause a severe lower lid ectropion and an antimongoloid slant (Fig. 86-10B). Colobomas appear in the lateral lower eyelid and mark the cephalic end of the cleft.

Skeletal Involvement. The number 6 facial cleft is along the zygomatic-maxillary suture separating the maxilla and zygoma (Fig. 86-10C). There is no alveolar cleft, but a short posterior maxilla may result in an occlusal tilt. Choanal atresia is common. The cleft enters the orbit at the lateral third of the orbital rim and floor. It connects to the inferior orbital fissure. The zygoma is hypoplastic with an intact zygomatic arch. There is narrowing of the anterior cranial fossa. The sphenoid is normal.

Number 7 Cleft

This temporozygomatic facial cleft is the most common craniofacial cleft. Other descriptive terms of this cleft include craniofacial microsomia, hemifacial microsomia, otomandibular dysostosis, first and second branchial arch syndrome, auriculobranchiogenic dysplasia, hemignathia and microtia syndrome, oro-aural cleft (AACPR), group B1 lateral otocephalic branchiogenic deformity, and zygotemporal dysplasia.[58,64,65,81-84] Goldenhar syndrome (oculoauriculovertebral spectrum) is a more severe autosomal dominant form with epibulbar dermoids and vertebral anomalies.[85,86] The number 7 cleft is also seen in Treacher Collins syndrome. The incidence is approximately 1 in 5600 births. There is a slight (3:2) male predominance and bilateral involvement.[87]

Soft Tissue Involvement. The cleft begins at the oral commissure and runs to the preauricular hairline. The intensity of expression varies from a mild broadening of the oral commissure with a preauricular skin tag to a complete fissure extending toward the microtic ear (Fig. 86-11A). The cleft typically does not extend beyond the anterior border of the masseter. However, the ipsilateral tongue, soft palate, and muscles of mastication (cranial nerve V) may be underdeveloped. The parotid gland and parotid duct may be absent. Facial nerve weakness (cranial nerve VII) may be present. External ear deformities range from preauricular skin tags to complete absence. External ear and middle ear abnormalities have been documented by Longacre et al,[84] Grabb,[87] May,[88] and Converse et al.[89] Preauricular hair is usually absent in patients with craniofacial microsomia. Patients with Treacher Collins syndrome often have preauricular hair from the temporal region pointing to the oral commissure.[90] The ipsilateral soft palate and tongue are often hypoplastic.

Skeletal Involvement. Osseous anomalies in a number 7 cleft include a wide range. The skeletal cleft passes through the pterygomaxillary junction (Fig. 86-11B). Tessier believed that the cleft is centered in the region of the zygomaticotemporal suture. The posterior maxilla and mandibular ramus are hypoplastic in the vertical dimension, creating an occlusal plane that is canted cephalad on the affected side. The coronoid process and condyle are also often hypoplastic and asymmetric, which contributes to a posterior open bite on the affected side. The zygomatic body is severely malformed, hypoplastic, and displaced. In the most severe form, the zygomatic arch is disrupted and is represented by a small stump (Fig. 86-11C). The malpositioned lateral canthus is caused by a hypoplastic zygoma that results in the inferiorly displaced superolateral angle of the orbit. On occasion, severely deforming number 7 clefts can cause true orbital dystopia. The abnormal anterior zygomatic arch continues posteriorly as a normal zygomatic process of the temporal bone. The cranial base is asymmetric and tilts, causing an abnormally positioned glenoid fossa. The anatomy of the sphenoid is abnormal, and there can be a rudimentary medial and lateral pterygoid plate.

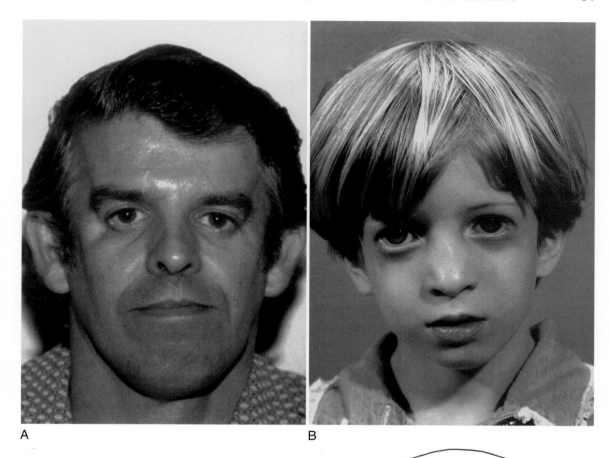

A

B

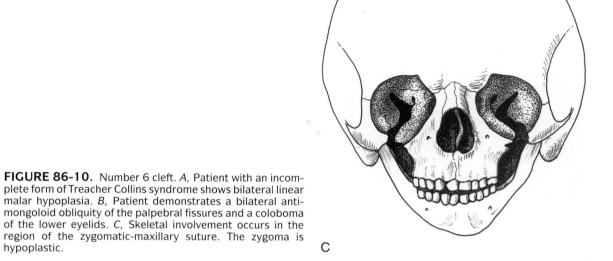

FIGURE 86-10. Number 6 cleft. *A*, Patient with an incomplete form of Treacher Collins syndrome shows bilateral linear malar hypoplasia. *B*, Patient demonstrates a bilateral antimongoloid obliquity of the palpebral fissures and a coloboma of the lower eyelids. *C*, Skeletal involvement occurs in the region of the zygomatic-maxillary suture. The zygoma is hypoplastic.

C

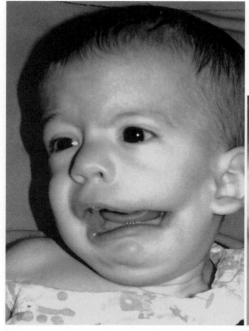

A

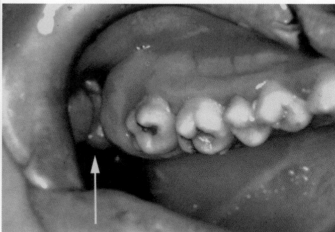

B

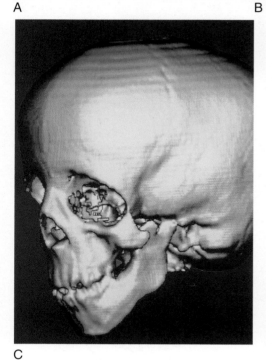

C

FIGURE 86-11. Number 7 cleft. *A,* Patient with a complete fissure of the oral commissure that extends toward the external ear, resulting in macrostomia. *B,* Cleft of posterior maxillary alveolus *(arrow)* between second and third molars. *C,* Skeletal involvement is seen in this three-dimensional computed tomographic scan that shows disruption of the zygomatic arch; the root shows only a small stump. The cleft is centered in the zygomatic-temporal suture line.

Number 8 Cleft

This frontozygomatic cleft at the lateral canthus is the equator of the Tessier craniofacial time zones (Fig. 86-12A). It is the temporal continuation of the orolateral canthus cleft (AACPR), the commissural clefts of the ophthalmo-orbital disorders, and zygofrontal dysplasia.[62,63,65] The number 8 cleft divides the facial clefts from the cranial clefts. The number 8 cleft rarely occurs alone but is usually associated with other craniofacial clefts. It appears to be the cranial extension of the number 6 cleft.

SOFT TISSUE INVOLVEMENT. The number 8 cleft extends from the lateral canthus to the temporal region. A dermatocele may occupy the coloboma of the lateral commissure. Hair markers can occasionally be seen along a line between the temporal area and the lateral canthus. The soft tissue malformation presents as a true lateral commissure coloboma (dermatocele) with absence of the lateral canthus (Fig. 86-12B). Abnormalities of the globe in the form of epibulbar dermoids are also often present, especially in Goldenhar syndrome.

SKELETAL INVOLVEMENT. The bone component of the cleft occurs at the frontozygomatic suture. Tessier noted a notch in this region in patients with Goldenhar syndrome (combination number 6, 7, and 8 clefts). In the complete form of Treacher Collins syndrome (combination number 6, 7, and 8 clefts), the zygoma may be hypoplastic or absent and the lateral orbital wall missing. Thus, the only support of the lateral palpebral fissure is the greater wing of the sphenoid, and downward slanting occurs. With this defect, there is soft tissue continuity of the orbit and temporal fossa.

Combination Number 6, 7, and 8 Clefts

The bilateral occurrence of the combination of number 6, number 7, and number 8 craniofacial clefts best describes the complete form of Treacher Collins syndrome (Fig. 86-13).[1,2] Clefting in the maxillozygomatic, temporozygomatic, and frontozygomatic regions results in the absence of the zygoma and lack of support for the lateral orbital tissues. Features of the patients with Treacher Collins syndrome may be explained with knowledge of facial clefts 6, 7, and 8. Features from number 6 cleft include coloboma of the lower eyelid and deficient eyelashes in the medial two thirds of the lid. Features caused by the number 7 cleft include absent malar bone, hypoplasia of the masseteric muscles, ear malformations (microtia), and anterior displacement of sideburns. Finally, the number 8 cleft causes an antimongoloid slant of the palpebral fissures or inferior displacement of the lateral canthus from lack of lateral orbital wall support. Unlike the

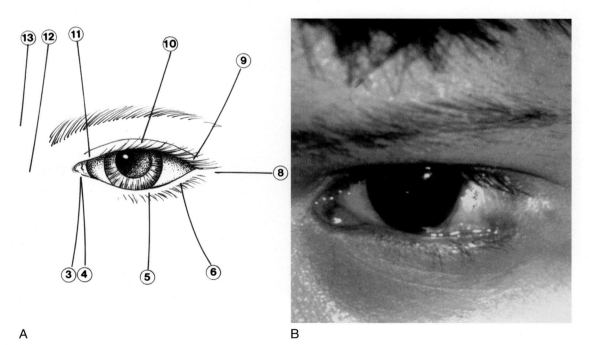

A   B

FIGURE 86-12. Number 8 cleft. A, This illustration depicts the number 8 cleft as the boundary or "equator" between the facial clefts (3, 4, 5, 6) and cranial clefts (9, 10, 11) that involve the eyelids and orbit. B, In this patient's left eye, the lateral commissure of the palpebral fissure is obliterated by a dermatocele.

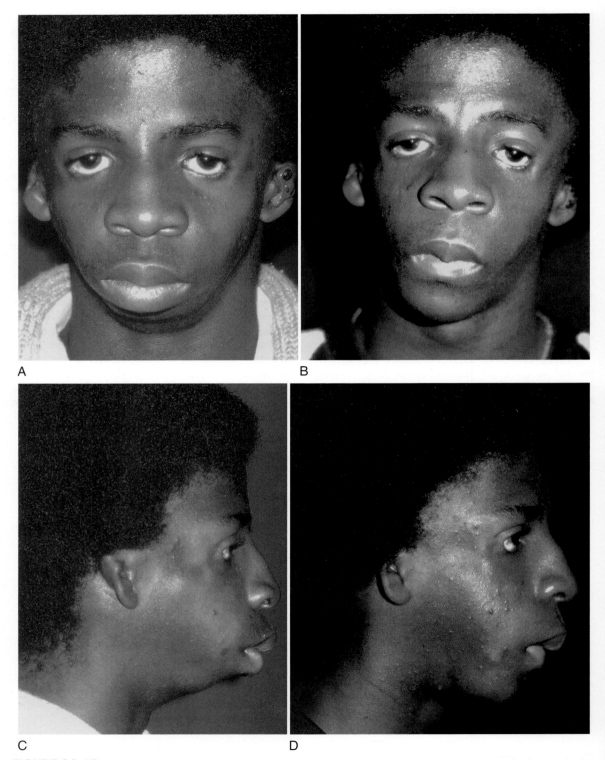

A

B

C

D

FIGURE 86-13. Combination number 6, 7, and 8 cleft. *A,* Frontal view of a patient with Treacher Collins syndrome preoperatively demonstrated malar hypoplasia and a severely retruded chin. *B,* Postoperative frontal view shows correction of chin. Upper to lower eyelid switch flap is planned. *C* and *D,* Lateral preoperative and postoperative views.

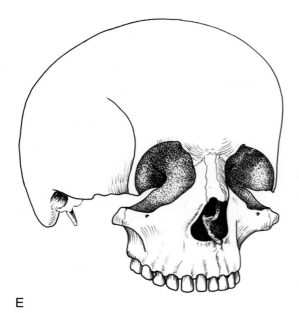

E

FIGURE 86-13, cont'd. *E*, Skeletal involvement in the complete form includes absence of the zygoma, lateral orbital wall (greater wing of sphenoid still remaining), and lateral orbital floor.

rim and orbital roof. Distortion of the upper part of the greater wing of the sphenoid, squamous portion of the temporal bone, and surrounding parietal bones may be present. This hypoplasia of the greater wing of the sphenoid results in a posterolateral rotation of the lateral orbital wall. Pterygoid plates may be hypoplastic. There may be a reduction in the anteroposterior dimension of the anterior cranial fossa.[73]

Number 10 Cleft

This upper central orbital cleft has also been classified as a frontal dysplasia group.[1,65] The number 10 cleft is the cranial extension of a number 4 cleft.

Soft Tissue Involvement. The number 10 cleft begins at the middle third of the upper eyelid and eyebrow (Fig. 86-15A). The lateral eyebrow may angulate temporally. The palpebral fissure may be elongated with an amblyopic eye displaced inferolaterally (Fig. 86-15B). The entire upper eyelid may be absent in severe forms (ablepharia). Colobomas and other ocular anomalies may be present. Frontal hair

bilateral symmetric pattern of Treacher Collins syndrome, unilateral involvement is typical in infants with Goldenhar syndrome. Whereas patients with Treacher Collins syndrome tend to have more severe bone abnormalities, patients with Goldenhar syndrome have more soft tissue malformations.

Number 9 Cleft

This upper lateral orbital cleft is the rarest of the craniofacial clefts. The number 9 cleft begins the march from lateral to medial of the cranial clefts. This defect was named frontosphenoid dysplasia by van der Meulen.[65] It is the cranial extension of the number 5 facial cleft.

Soft Tissue Involvement. The number 9 cleft is manifested by abnormalities of the lateral third of the upper eyelid and eyebrow. The lateral canthus is also distorted. In the severe form, microphthalmos is present (Fig. 86-14). The superolateral bone deficiency of the orbits allows lateral displacement of the globes. The cleft then extends cephalad into the temporoparietal hair-bearing scalp. The temporal hairline is anteriorly displaced, and a temporal hair projection is often seen in the number 9 cleft. Furthermore, a cranial nerve VII palsy in the forehead and upper eyelid is common.

Skeletal Involvement. The bone defect of the number 9 cranial cleft extends through the superolateral aspect of the orbit, involving the superior orbital

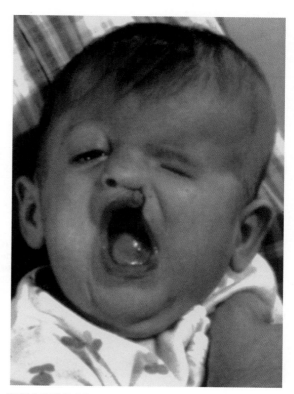

FIGURE 86-14. Number 9 cleft. Patient with right-side, rare number 9 cleft that goes through the superolateral orbital roof. The left cleft lip and microphthalmos are additional findings.

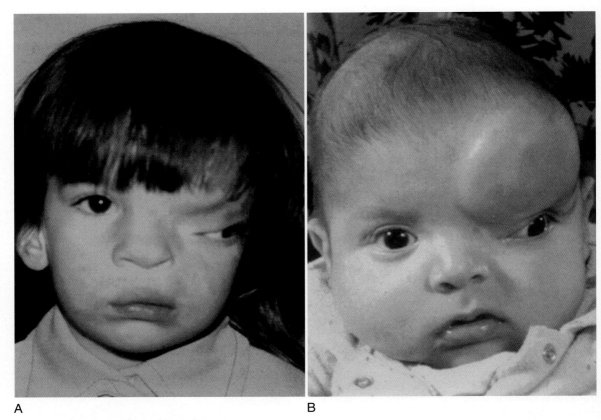

A   B

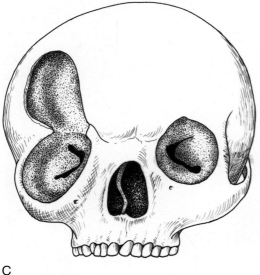

C

FIGURE 86-15. Number 10 cleft. *A,* Cleft through center of the left orbital roof produces asymmetric hypertelorism and a vertical dystopia. *B,* Patient with fronto-orbital encephalocele seen in the middle of the left forehead. This fills the void left by the cleft defect in the center of the left superior orbital rim. *C,* Skeletal defect and asymmetric hypertelorism are demonstrated on the right.

projection may connect the temporoparietal region to the lateral brow.

SKELETAL INVOLVEMENT. The bone component of the number 10 cranial cleft occurs in the middle of the supraorbital rim just lateral to the superior orbital foramen. An encephalocele often occupies the defect through the frontal bone, and a prominent bulge is observed in the forehead (Fig. 86-15*B*). The orbit may be deformed with a lateroinferior rotation. Orbital hypertelorism may result in severe disease. The anterior cranial base may also be distorted.

Number 11 Cleft

This upper medial orbital cleft is the cranial extension of the number 3 cleft. This malformation is included in the frontal dysplasia group of van der Meulen et al.[65]

SOFT TISSUE INVOLVEMENT. The medial third of the upper eyelid may show involvement with a coloboma (Fig. 86-16). The upper eyebrow may have a disruption that extends up to the frontal hairline. A tongue-like projection at the medial third of the frontal hairline may also be identified.

SKELETAL INVOLVEMENT. The number 11 cleft may be seen as a notch in the medial third of the supraorbital rim if it passes lateral to the ethmoid bone. If the cleft passes through the ethmoid air cells to produce extensive pneumatization, orbital hypertelorism is seen clinically. The cranial base and sphenoid architecture, including the pterygoid processes, are symmetric and normal.

Number 12 Cleft

The number 12 cleft is the cranial extension of the number 2 cleft.

SOFT TISSUE INVOLVEMENT. The soft tissue cleft lies medial to the medial canthus (Fig. 86-17A). There is a lateral displacement of the medial canthus, and telecanthus may result. With the number 12 cleft, there is no eyelid separation or clefting. Aplasia of the medial end of the eyebrow may exist. A short downward projection of the paramedian frontal hairline may exist, but the forehead skin is typically normal.

SKELETAL INVOLVEMENT. The number 12 cleft passes through the frontal process of the maxilla, giving a flattened appearance (Fig. 86-17B). In addition, an increase in the transverse dimension of the ethmoid air cells produces orbital hypertelorism (Fig. 86-17C). The frontal and sphenoid sinuses are usually also pneumatized and enlarged. The remainder of the sphenoid and frontal bones are not affected. The frontonasal angle is obtuse. The cleft is lateral to the olfactory groove; thus, the cribriform plate is normal in width. Encephaloceles have not been observed with this cleft. The anterior and middle cranial fossae are widened on the cleft side but otherwise normal.[73]

Number 13 Cleft

The number 13 cleft is the cranial extension of the paramedian, craniofacial number 1 cleft.

SOFT TISSUE INVOLVEMENT. There is typically a paramedian frontal encephalocele, which is between the nasal bone and the frontal process of the maxilla (Fig. 86-18). The soft tissue cleft is medial to intact eyelids and eyebrows. The medial end of the eyebrow, however, can be displaced inferiorly. A V-shaped frontal hair projection can also be seen.

SKELETAL INVOLVEMENT. Changes in the cribriform plate are the hallmark of a number 13 cleft. The paramedian bone cleft traverses the frontal bone and then courses along the olfactory groove (see Fig. 86-5B). There is widening of the olfactory groove, the cribriform plate, and the ethmoid sinus, which results in hypertelorism. A paramedian frontal encephalocele can cause the cribriform plate to be displaced inferiorly, leading to orbital dystopia. Unilateral and bilateral forms of the number 13 cleft exist, similar to most of the other craniofacial clefts. When the cleft is bilateral, some of the most severe instances of hypertelorism have been observed.[1]

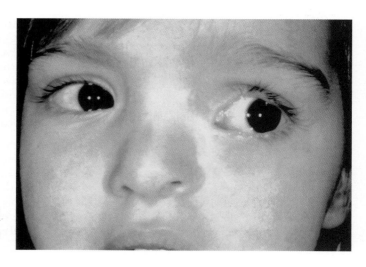

FIGURE 86-16. Number 11 cleft. Patient with small coloboma in medial third of left upper eyelid extending through the medial third of the eyebrow.

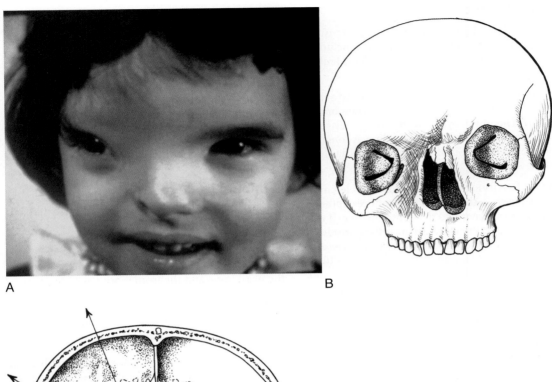

FIGURE 86-17. Number 12 cleft. *A*, Patient with right-sided cleft has orbital hypertelorism and a disturbance of the right medial eyebrow. *B*, Skeletal involvement is seen between the right nasal bone and the frontal process of the maxilla. Inferolateral displacement of the orbit is also demonstrated. *C*, Axial view of floor of the anterior cranial vault with lines demonstrating the axis of the orbit. As the ethmoid air cells widen medially, the orbit is displaced laterally, and hypertelorism results.

Number 14 Cleft

The number 14 cleft is the midline cranial cleft. The descriptions of the craniofacial clefts, outlined in the preceding, have come full circle around the entire orbit. The number 14 cleft has been termed median craniofacial dysraphia. It is the cranial extension of the number 0 cleft. This cranial cleft is similar to its facial counterpart in that it may consist of agenesis or an overabundance of tissue.

SOFT TISSUE AND SKELETAL TISSUE DEFICIENCY. Hypotelorism may be present with an agenesis in a number 14 cleft (Fig. 86-19*A*). A spectrum of holoprosencephalic disorders, which include cyclopia, ethmocephaly, and cebocephaly, may also be seen (Fig. 86-19*B*). With these malformations, the cranium is typically microcephalic. Cranial base structures may be completely absent so that the orbits coalesce. The severity of forebrain malformations is usually proportional to the degree of facial abnormality. An extensively involved number 14 cleft may have a poor prognosis with a life expectancy of hours to days. If the infant survives, severe disabilities may be observed.

SOFT TISSUE EXCESS. Hypertelorism may also be associated with the number 14 cleft (Fig. 86-19*C*). The terms frontonasal and frontonasoethmoid dysplasia were used by van der Meulen et al[65] to categorize this group. Lateral displacement of the orbits can be produced by midline masses, such as a frontonasal encephalocele or a midline frontal encephalocele (Fig. 86-19*D*). Cohen et al[91] thought that the

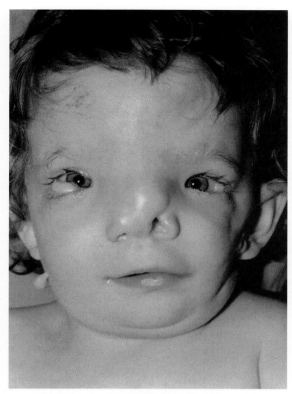

FIGURE 86-18. Number 13 cleft. Patient with a left-sided facial cleft that begins as a number 1 cleft through the alar dome, extends to the frontal bone to cause hypertelorism, and ends in a paramedian widow's peak. In addition, this patient has a nasal dorsal dermoid cyst, bilateral preauricular skin tags, conjunctival dermoid cysts, and lower eyelid colobomas.

basic fault in embryologic development lies in the malformation of the nasal capsule and that the developing forebrain remains in a low position. A morphokinetic arrest of the normal medial movement of the eyes occurs, and the orbits remain in their widespread fetal position. Flattening of the glabella and extreme lateral displacement of the inner canthi are also seen. The periorbita, including the eyelids and eyebrows, are otherwise normal. A long midline projection of the frontal hairline marks the superior extent of the soft tissue features of this midline cranial cleft.

Skeletal Tissue Excess. The frontal encephalocele herniates through a medial frontal defect (Fig. 86-19E). The caudal aspect of the frontal bone is flattened, giving the glabellar region a flattened and indistinct position. No pneumatization of the frontal sinus is evident; however, the sphenoid sinus is extensively pneumatized. The crista galli and the perpendicular plate of the ethmoid are bifid, and there is an increased distance between the olfactory grooves.

When the crista galli is severely enlarged, preservation of the olfactory nerve is often not possible during the surgical correction of hypertelorism. The crista galli and ethmoids are widened and caudally displaced. Consequently, the cribriform plate, which is normally 5 to 10 mm below the level of the orbital roof, can be causally displaced up to 20 mm.[92] The greater and lesser wings of the sphenoid are rotated and result in a relative shortening of the middle cranial fossa. The anterior cranial fossa is upslanting, causing a harlequin eye deformity on plain radiographs.

Number 30 Cleft

This median cleft of the lower jaw was first described by Couronné.[93] These clefts of the lower lip and mandible are caudal extensions of the number 14 cranial cleft and number 0 facial cleft. They may be included in the mandibular process clefts (AACPR classification), midline branchiogenic syndrome, and intermandibular dysplasia.[62,65,94]

Soft Tissue Involvement. Soft tissue involvement of this midline cleft may be as mild as a notch in the lower lip. However, the entire lower lip and chin may be involved. The anterior tongue may be bifid and attached to the split mandible by a dense fibrous band. Ankyloglossia and total absence of the tongue have also been reported with midline mandibular clefts.[95,96]

Skeletal Involvement. Skeletal involvement is typically a cleft between the central incisors extending into the mandibular symphysis. This anomaly is thought to be caused by failure of fusion of the first branchial arch. Neck anomalies are often associated but are thought to be caused by failure of fusion of other lower branchial arches. For instance, in many patients, the hyoid bone is absent and the thyroid cartilages may fail to form completely. Finally, the anterior neck strap muscles are often atrophic and replaced by dense fibrous bands that may restrict chin flexion.[97]

SUMMARY

The clinical expression of craniofacial clefts is highly variable and ranges from a mild, barely noticeable forme fruste (microform) to a disfiguring, complete defect of skeletal and soft tissue. Tessier's description of craniofacial clefts is based on bone and soft tissue landmarks. It provides a classification that can now also be validated by neuromeric theory of newer findings in neuroembryology. Far from being considered oddities, craniofacial clefts will allow plastic surgeons in the future to further understand the developmental architecture of the face and to refine their reconstructive techniques.

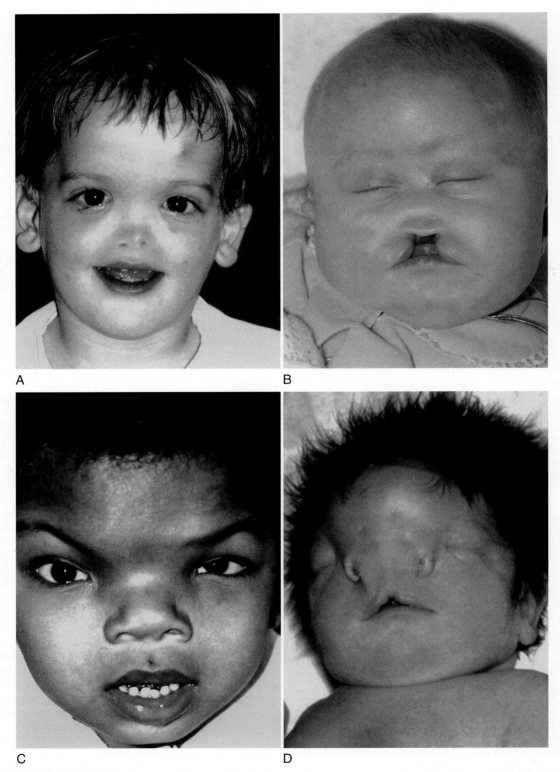

FIGURE 86-19. Number 14 cleft. *A*, Patient with midline cleft has nasal hypoplasia and hypotelorism. *B*, Patient with holoprosencephaly and failure of proper formation of the forebrain. *C*, Patient with a midline cleft has flattening in the glabella region and hypertelorism. *D*, Patient with a large frontonasal encephalocele has a true median cleft lip, a wide bifid nose, and orbital hypertelorism.

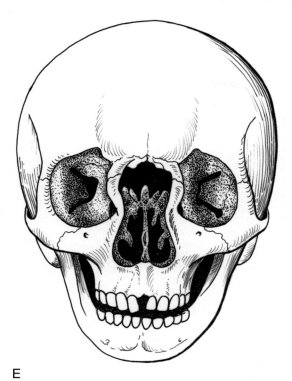

E

FIGURE 86-19, cont'd. *E,* Skeletal involvement shows displacement of the frontal process of the maxilla, nasal bones, and medial orbital walls laterally. This large defect is often occupied by an encephalocele.

REFERENCES

1. Tessier P: Anatomical classification of facial, cranio-facial and latero-facial clefts. J Maxillofac Surg 1976;4:69.
2. Kawamoto HK Jr: The kaleidoscopic world of rare craniofacial clefts: order out of chaos (Tessier classification). Clin Plast Surg 1976;3:529.
3. Kawamoto HK Jr: Rare craniofacial clefts. In McCarthy JG, ed: Plastic Surgery, vol 4. Philadelphia, WB Saunders 1990:2922-2973.
4. Burian F: Vzacne vrozene vady obliceje a lebky a jejich leceni [Seltene angeborene Defekte d. Gesichts u. d. Schadels u. ihre Behandlung]. Acta Universitatis Carolinae Praha, 1957.
5. Fogh-Andersen P: Rare clefts of the face. Acta Chir Scand 1965;129:275.
6. Dixon MJ: Treacher Collins syndrome. Hum Mol Genet 1996;5:1391.
7. Wise CA, Chiang LC, Paznekas WA, et al: TCOF-1 encodes a putative nucleolar phosphate that exhibits mutations in Treacher Collins syndrome throughout its coding region. Proc Natl Acad Sci USA 1997;94:310.
8. Dixon J, Hovanes K, Shiang R, Dixon MJ: Sequence analysis, identification of evolutionary conserved motifs and expression analysis of murine tcof1 provide further evidence for a potential function for the gene and its human homologue, TCOF1. Hum Mol Genet 1997;6:727.
9. Coady MSE, Moore MH, Wallis K: Amniotic band syndrome: the association between rare facial clefts and limb ring constrictions. Plast Reconstr Surg 1998;101:640.
10. Warkany J, Schraffenberger E: Congenital malformation induced in rats by roentgen rays. Am J Roentgenol 1947;57:455.
11. Callas G, Walker BE: Palate morphogenesis in mouse embryos after X-irradiation. Anat Rec 1963;145:61.
12. Poswillo D: The aetiology and surgery of cleft palate with micrognathia. Ann R Coll Surg 1968;43:61.
13. Neel JV: A study of major congenital defects in Japanese infants. Am J Hum Genet 1958;10:398.
14. Miller RW: Delayed radiation effects in atomic bomb survivors. Science 1969;166:569.
15. Ferm VH, Kilham L: Congenital anomalies induced in hamster embryos with H-1 virus. Science 1964;145:510.
16. Leck I, Hay S, Witte JI, Greene JC: Malformations recorded on birth certificates following A2 influenza epidemics. Public Health Rep 1969;84:971.
17. Gabka J: Beitrag zur Ätiologie der Lippen-Kiefer-Gaumenspalten unter besonder Beruchsichtigung der Toxoplasmose. Dtsch Stomatol 1953;3:294.
18. Tocci PM, Beber B: Abnormal phenylalanine loading test in mothers of children with cleft defects. Cleft Palate J 1970;7:663.
19. Langman J, Van Faassen F: Congenital defects in rat embryos after partial thyroidectomy of the mother animal: a preliminary report on eye defects. Am J Ophthalmol 1955;40:65.
20. Wilson JG: Abnormalities of intrauterine development in non-human primates. Acta Endocrinol Suppl (Copenh) 1972;166:261.
21. Wilson JG: Present status of drugs as teratogens in man. Teratology 1973;7:3.
22. Janz D, Fuchs U: Are antiepileptic drugs harmful when given during pregnancy? Dtsch Med Wochenschr 1964;89:241.
23. Spidel BD, Meadow SR: Maternal epilepsy and abnormalities of the fetus and newborn. Lancet 1972;2:839.
24. Braun JT, Franciosi RA, Mastri AR, et al: Isotretinoin dysmorphic syndrome. Lancet 1984;1:506.
25. Lammer EJ, Chen DT, Hoar RM, et al: Retinoic acid embryopathy. N Engl J Med 1985;313:837.
26. Frazer FC, Fainstat TD: Production of congenital defects in offspring of pregnant mice treated with cortisone. Pediatrics 1951;8:527.
27. Heiberg K, Kalter H, Fraser FC: Production of cleft palates in offspring of mice treated with ACTH during pregnancy. Biol Neonat 1959;1:33.
28. Smithells RW, Leck I: The incidence of limb and ear defects since the withdrawal of thalidomide. Lancet 1963;1:1095.
29. Safra MS, Oakley GP: Association between cleft lip with or without cleft palate and parental exposure to diazepam. Lancet 1975;2:478.
30. Webster WS, Johnston MC, Lammer EJ, Sulik KK: Isotretinoin embryopathy and cranial neural crest: an in vivo and in vitro study. J Craniofac Genet Dev Biol 1986;6:211.
31. Sperber GH: Craniofacial Embryology. London, Wright, 1989.
32. Sharpe PT: Homeobox genes and orofacial development. Connect Tissue Res 1995;32:17.
33. Chiang C, Litingtung Y, Lee E, et al: Cyclopia and defective axial patterning in mice lacking Sonic hedgehog gene function. Nature 1996;383:407.
34. Patten BM: Human Embryology, 3rd ed. New York, Blakiston, 1968.
35. Perris R, Perissinotto D: Role of the extracellular matrix during neural crest migration. Mech Dev 2000;95:3.
36. Chai Y, Jiang X, Ito Y, et al: Fate of the mammalian cranial neural crest during tooth and mandibular morphogenesis. Development 2000;127:11671.
37. Carstens M: Development of the facial midline. J Craniofac Surg 2002;13:129.

38. Muller F, O'Rahilly R: The timing and sequence of appearance of the neuromeres and their derivatives in staged human embryos. Acta Anat 1997;158:83.

39. Schutte BC, Murray JC: The many faces and factors of orofacial clefts. Hum Mol Genet 1999;8:1853.

40. Noden DM: Development of craniofacial blood vessels. In Feinberg RN, Sherer GK, Auerbach R, eds: The Development of the Vascular System. Basel, Karger, 1991:1-24. Issues in Biomedicine, vol 14.

41. Sperber G H: Pathogenesis and morphogenesis of craniofacial anomalies. Ann Acad Med Singapore 1999;28:703.

42. Sperber GH: Craniofacial Development. Hamilton, Ontario, BC Decker, 2001.

43. O'Rahilly R, Mueller F: Interpretation of some median anomalies as illustrated by cyclopia and symmelia. Teratology 1989;40:409.

44. English GM: Congenital anomalies of the nose, nasopharynx and paranasal sinuses. In English GM, ed: Otolaryngology. Philadelphia, JB Lippincott, 1990.

45. Dursy E: Zur Entwicklungsgeschichte des Kopfes des Menschen und der höheren Wirbelthiere. Tübingen, Lauppsche Buchhandlung, 1869:99.

46. His W: Die Entwicklung der menschlichen und thierischen Physiognomien. Arch Anat Physiol Anat Abt 1892;384.

47. Pohlmann EH: Die embryonale Metamorphose der Physiognomie und der Mundhöhle des Katzenkopfes. Morphol Jahrbuch Leipzig 1910;41:617.

48. Veau V, Politzer J: Embryologie du bec-de-lievre. Ann Anat Pathol 1936;12:275.

49. Stark RB: The pathogenesis of harelip and cleft palate. Plast Reconstr Surg 1954;13:20.

50. Warbrick JG: Early development of the nasal cavity and upper lip in the human embryo. J Anat 1938;94:459.

51. Stark RB, Ehrmann NA: The development of the center of the face with particular reference to surgical correction of bilateral cleft lip. Plast Reconstr Surg 1958;21:177.

52. Hochstetter F: Über die Entwicklung der Formverhältnisse des menschlichen Antlitzes. Denkschr Akad Wiss Wien 1953;109:1.

53. Johnston MC: A radioautographic study of the migration and fate of cranial neural crest cells in the chick embryo. Anat Res 1966;156:143.

54. Carstens MH: Functional matrix repair: a common strategy for unilateral and bilateral clefts. J Craniofac Surg 2000;11:437.

55. Warbrick JG: Aspects of facial and nasal development. Sci Basis Med Annu Rev 1963;84:99.

56. Johnston MC: Fetal malformations in chick embryos resulting from removal of neural crest. J Dent Res Suppl 1964;43:822.

57. Poswillo D: The pathogenesis of the Treacher Collins syndrome (mandibulofacial dysostosis). Br J Oral Surg 1975;13:1.

58. Braithwaite F, Watson J: Three unusual clefts of the lip. Br J Plast Surg 1949;2:38.

59. Poswillo D: The pathogenesis of the first and second branchial arch syndrome. Oral Surg 1973;35:302.

60. Lockhard RD: Variations coincident with congenital absence of the zygoma. J Anat 1929;63:233.

61. McKenzie J, Craig J: Mandibulo-facial dysostosis (Treacher Collins syndrome). Arch Dis Child 1955;30:391.

62. Harkins CS, Berlin A, Harding RL, et al: A classification of cleft lip and cleft palate. Plast Reconstr Surg 1962;29:31.

63. Boo-Chai K: The oblique facial cleft: a report of 2 cases and a review of 41 cases. Br J Plast Surg 1970;23:352.

64. Karfik V: Proposed classification of rare congenital cleft malformations in the face. Acta Chir Plast (Praha) 1966;8:163.

65. van der Meulen JC, Mazzola R, Vermey-Keers C, et al: A morphogenetic classification of craniofacial malformations. Plast Reconstr Surg 1983;71:560.

66. Kundrat H: Arhinencephalie als typische Art von Missbildung. Graz, Leuschner & Lubensky, 1882.

67. Yakovlev PI: Pathoarchitectonic studies of cerebral malformation. J Neuropathol Exp Neurol 1959;18:22.

68. DeMyer W: Cleft lip and jaw induced in fetal rats by vincristine. Arch Anat Histol Embryol 1964;48:179.

69. DeMyer W, Zeman W, Palmer CA: The face predicts the brain: diagnostic significance of median facial anomalies for holoprosencephaly (arrhinencephaly). Pediatrics 1964;34:256.

70. Elias DL, Kawamoto HK Jr, Wilson LF: Holoprosencephaly and midline facial anomalies: redefining classification and management. Plast Reconstr Surg 1992;90:951.

71. DeMyer W: The median cleft face syndrome. Differential diagnosis of cranial bifidum occultum, hypertelorism and median cleft nose, lip and palate. Neurology 1967;17:961.

72. Sedano HO, Cohen MM Jr, Jifasek J, Koplin R: Frontonasal dysplasia. J Pediatr 1970;76:906.

73. David DJ, Moore MH, Cooter RD: Tessier clefts revisited with a third dimension. Cleft Palate J 1989;26:163.

74. Converse JM, Ransohoff J, Mathews ES, et al: Ocular hypertelorism and pseudohypertelorism. Advances in surgical treatment. Plast Reconstr Surg 1970;45:1.

75. Morian R: Über die schrage Gesichtsspalte. Arch Klin Chir 1887;35:245.

76. Tessier P: Colobomas: vertical and oblique complete facial clefts. Panminerva Med 1969;11:95.

77. Davis WB: Congenital deformities of the face. Surg Gynecol Obstet 1935;61:201.

78. Gunter GS: Nasomaxillary cleft. Plast Reconstr Surg 1963;32:637.

79. Dick W: A case of hyperencephalous monstrosity. Lond Med Gaz 1837;19:897.

79a. Resnick JI, Kawamoto HK: Rare craniofacial clefts: Tessier No. 4 clefts. Plast Reconstr Surg 1990;85:843.

80. Rogalski T: A contribution to the study of anophthalmia with description of a case. Br J Ophthalmol 1944;28:429.

81. Franceschetti A, Zwahlen P: Un syndrome nouveau: la dysostose mandibulo-faciale. Bull Schweiz Akad Med Wiss 1944;1:60.

82. Caronni EP: Embryogenesis and classification of branchial auricular dysplasia. Transactions of the Fifth International Congress on Plastic and Reconstructive Surgery. Melbourne, Butterworth, 1971.

83. Stark RB, Saunders DE: The first branchial syndrome: the oral-mandibular-auricular syndrome. Plast Reconstr Surg 1962;29:299.

84. Longacre JJ, Stevens GA, Holmstrand KE: The surgical management of first and second branchial arch syndrome. Plast Reconstr Surg 1963;31:507.

85. Goldenhar M: Associations malformatives de l'oeil et de l'oreille: en particulier, le syndrome: dermoide épibulbaire-appendices auriculaires-fistula auris congenita et ses relations avec la dysostose mandibulo-faciale. J Genet Hum 1952;1:243.

86. Gorlin RJ, Jue KL, Jacobsen U, Goldschmidt E: Oculoauriculovertebral syndrome. J Pediatr 1963;63:991.

87. Grabb WC: The first and second branchial arch syndrome. Plast Reconstr Surg 1965;36:485.

88. May H: Transverse facial clefts and their repair. Plast Reconstr Surg 1962;29:240.

89. Converse JM, Coccaro PJ, Becker M, Wood-Smith D: On hemifacial microsomia. Plast Reconstr Surg 1973;51:268.

90. Moore MH, David DJ, Cooter RD: Hairline indicators of craniofacial clefts. Plast Reconstr Surg 1988;82:589.

91. Cohen MM Jr, Jirasek JE, Guzman RT, et al: Holoprosencephaly and facial dysmorphia: nosology, etiology and pathogenesis. Birth Defects 1971;7:125.

92. Tessier P: Orbital hypertelorism. 1. Successive surgical attempts, material and methods, causes and mechanisms. Scand J Plast Reconstr Surg 1972;6:135.

93. Couronné A: Clin Soc Med Prot Montpellier 1819;107.
94. Cosman B, Crikelair GF: Midline branchiogenic syndromes. Plast Reconstr Surg 1969;44:41.
95. Millard DR Jr, Lehman JA Jr, Deane M, Garst WP: Median cleft of the lower lip and mandible: a case report. Br J Plast Surg 1971;24:391.
96. Rosenthal R: Aglossia congenital: report of a case of the condition combined with other congenital malformations. J Dis Child 1932;44:383.
97. Monroe CW: Midline cleft of the lower lip, mandible, tongue with flexion contracture of the neck: case report and review of the literature. Plast Reconstr Surg 1966;38:312.

Classification, Varieties, and Pathologic Anatomy of Primary Labial Clefts

PETER D. WITT, MD ✦ JAY RAPLEY, MD

The broad spectrum of differences in the morphologic expression of labial clefting reminds us of the hackneyed phrase "a cleft is not a cleft is not a cleft." Clefts of the lip may be unilateral or bilateral. They may be complete or incomplete. They may be right or left sided, and they may occur with or without cleft palate. They may be associated with syndromes or occur sporadically. The morphologic heterogeneity observed in cleft lip reflects aberrations in both the molecular and embryologic bases of development.

Virtually every conceivable combination and permutation of facial clefting is possible. For example, some unilateral complete clefts of the lip and palate exhibit wide separation of the palatal shelves. Others exhibit less separation, and the segments actually overlap in some cases. A clear understanding of the various hard and soft tissue components associated with facial clefts is necessary to achieve high-quality, consistent treatment outcomes for affected patients. Many of the anatomic and physiologic complexities of the cleft lip and its variations have been recognized for centuries. Many of these observations have been applied to current surgical therapy algorithms.

Recognition of the wide varieties of labial clefts is important for prognostic determination. Accurate diagnosis helps in deciding the number of stages necessary for repair of the cleft lip. It helps in providing parents and ancillary care providers judgments about the timing of those operations. It helps in understanding how the severity of a given cleft affects subsequent dental and orthodontic care as well as the nasal configuration. This chapter examines the classification, morphologic variations, and pathologic anatomy of labial clefts. It also describes how labial clefting affects the underlying palatal arch configuration and how the severity of labial clefting correlates with the severity of the associated classic nasal deformity.

Specific operative techniques, long-term clinical outcomes, and detailed comments about clefts of the secondary palate are not the subject of this chapter. Likewise, detailed information about subjects with more complicated facial cleft variations, including those patients having syndromic conditions or malformation sequences, is beyond the scope of this chapter.

DEFINITIONS

By convention, the primary palate consists of premaxilla, anterior septum, and soft tissues of the lip. The secondary palate is separated from the primary palate by the incisive foramen. The secondary palate consists of the structures posterior (dorsal) to the incisive foramen, including the remaining hard palate, the soft palate, and the uvula (Fig. 87-1).

EMBRYOLOGY

Virtually every cleft classification system is based on anatomy, which in turn depends on embryology. Clefts

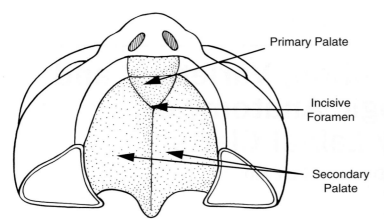

Primary Palate

Incisive Foramen

Secondary Palate

FIGURE 87-1. The incisive foramen lies in the anterior midline, just dorsal to the central incisal teeth. The primary palate refers to the anatomic region ventral to the incisive foramen. The secondary palate (posterior palate) refers to the anatomic region dorsal to the incisive foramen. The uvula represents the most posterior portion of the secondary palate.

of the lip (with or without clefts of the palate) must be distinguished from "cleft palate only" because the embryogenesis of these entities is believed to be entirely different.[1,2] Interestingly, both of these distinct patterns of clefting may be caused by similar phenomena, including chromosome aberrations, environmental teratogens, and multifactorial inheritance.

Cleft lip may result from failure of an epithelial contact to be maintained because of failure of mesodermal penetration from the maxillary and nasal processes. Without mesodermal penetration, there is subsequent breakdown of the epithelium, resulting in a cleft of the lip. The abnormal sequence of lip development may have a deleterious effect on tongue position and, as a consequence, palatal development. For example, high tongue position may mechanically interfere with palatal fusion and thereby produce a cleft palate (Fig. 87-2).

CLASSIFICATION OF CLEFT TYPES

Standardized documentation of the cleft lip and cleft palate morphologic expressions began in the late 1950s when Kernahan and Stark suggested a classification scheme.[3] Their system was comprehensible to a broad-based audience, but it lacked detail. Other classification

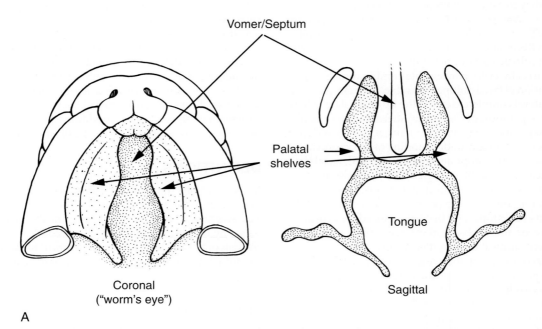

Vomer/Septum

Palatal shelves

Tongue

Coronal ("worm's eye")

Sagittal

A

FIGURE 87-2. *A* to *C,* Normal embryologic sequence. The lateral palatal shelves reorient from a vertical position to a horizontal position.

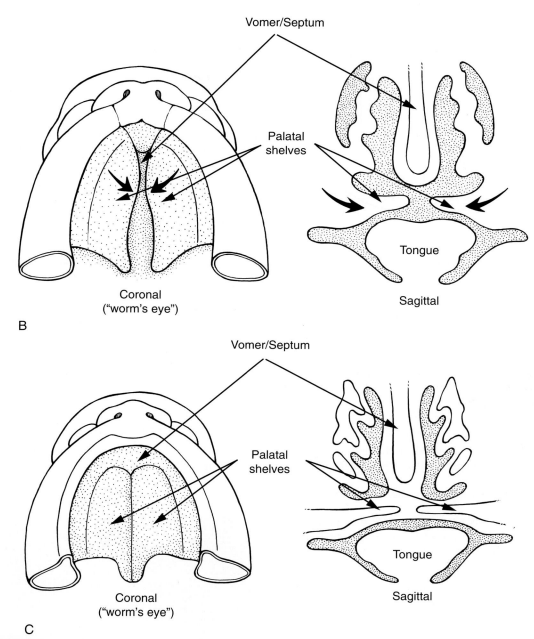

FIGURE 87-2, cont'd.

systems have been proposed[4-6] that assume or exclude varying degrees of sophistication, complexity, and ease with which data can be entered into a computer database. Kernahan's striped Y, which draws attention to the incisive foramen as the key anatomic landmark, has withstood the test of time and is probably the most popular schematic used in contemporary cleft-related registries and databases (Fig. 87-3).[7,8]

Processus palatins deviennent horizontaux
G après D ⟹ +de fentes labiales G que D

MORPHOLOGIC VARIETIES OF LABIAL CLEFTS

Cleft lip and cleft palate occur in combinations too numerous to describe conveniently. However, Berkowitz[9] has suggested that the bewildering variations observed in cleft lip and palate anatomy may segregate into four general categories:

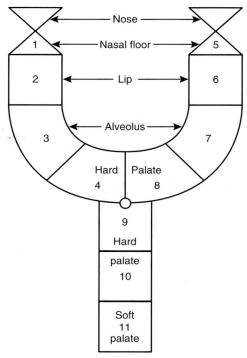

FIGURE 87-3. Kernahan's striped Y classification scheme. (Redrawn from Millard R, ed: Cleft Craft, vol 1. Boston, Little Brown, 1977.)

1. Clefts involving the lip and alveolus
2. Clefts involving the primary palate (lip) and secondary palate
3. Clefts in which only the secondary palate is affected
4. Clefts involving congenital insufficiency of the palate (non-cleft-related velopharyngeal dysfunction, submucous cleft palate)

This chapter focuses on category 1, clefts involving the lip and alveolus. The remaining categories are not covered extensively in this chapter, except as they occur in conjunction with labial clefts (such as category 2).

Clefts Involving the Lip and Alveolus

MINIMAL CLEFT LIP

A cleft of the lip may be complete (extending from the vermilion free border of the lip to the ventral floor of the nose) or incomplete. There is a wide spectrum of "incompleteness." For example, the most rudimentary labial cleft, the minimal cleft lip (so-called forme fruste cleft lip), may involve the vermilion border of the lip only (Fig. 87-4). At first glance, it would appear that there is virtually no disruption of the underlying orbicularis oris muscle.

Burt and Byrd[10] have noted that the microform cleft lip variation has three components, although not all components need be present for the diagnosis to be established: (1) a small vermilion notch; (2) a visible band of fibrous tissue extending from the edges of the red lip to the nostril floor; ostensibly, these bands mimic the normal philtral columns, but on close inspection, they stream cephalad in a lateral direction compared with the normal lip—they converge on the midnostril floor instead of on the basilar flair of the columella; and (3) an irregularity of the ala on the side of the notch or band.

Most of the time, these minimal clefts of the lip require surgical treatment. The objectives of surgical repair are to eliminate the vermilion notch, to correct the minimally flattened ala, and to restore orbicularis oris muscle continuity. Of course, these same goals apply to the repair of essentially all labial clefts, even the widest ones. What makes minimal cleft lip a surgical challenge is accomplishing these goals with minimal scarring. Some microform cleft lips show subtle deviations from normal anatomy. In such cases, sound surgical judgment should be exercised in regard to the decision to operate or not. It is wise to remember the most fundamental of medical treatment dictums, *primum non nocere* (of first importance, do no harm).

UNILATERAL INCOMPLETE CLEFT LIP AND CLEFT ALVEOLUS

Incomplete labial clefts may run all the way from the vermilion free border to the nose, sparing only a thin

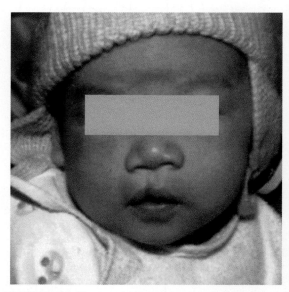

FIGURE 87-4. Microform cleft lip. Notice that there is no apparent orbicularis oris disruption.

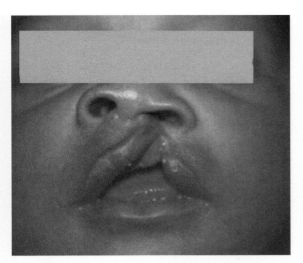

FIGURE 87-5. Incomplete cleft involving the lip.

cases. The soft tissue connection bridging the cleft and noncleft sides, however small, may serve as an important restraining force in limiting anterior projection of the premaxilla.

UNILATERAL COMPLETE CLEFT LIP AND CLEFT ALVEOLUS

With complete cleft lip and cleft alveolus (secondary palate intact) (Fig. 87-6), the premaxillary portion of the noncleft segment is rotated anterolaterally. The underlying alveolus is completely cleft, not merely notched. In cases in which lateral displacement of the lateral alveolar segments is observed, the premaxilla in the larger segment advances forward in the facial skeleton.[11]

BILATERAL INCOMPLETE CLEFT LIP

If the labial cleft is bilateral, it may or may not involve both sides of the labial soft and hard tissues equally (Fig. 87-7). Such asymmetric bilateral cleft lips may pose vexing management problems. In bilateral clefts, the prolabial-premaxillary segments may be tiny or large, outwardly rotated or relatively normally positioned (i.e., the greater and lesser maxillary alveolar arches may be relatively well aligned). The median prolabial portion of lip is isolated in the midline and remains attached to the premaxilla and the columella. With increasing severity of the bilateral labial cleft, the premaxilla often protrudes considerably forward when it is viewed in profile, producing the so-called flyaway

band of soft tissue (Simonart band) (Fig. 87-5). The bridge of tissue connecting the medial and lateral lip elements contains only mucous membrane, skin, and fibrous connective tissue. In these cases, there is usually a complete diastasis of the orbicularis oris muscle. The alveolar ridge may show partial expression of the clefting process with a notch. Alveolar notching may cause minor dental crossbite, but bone grafting at a later time is often unnecessary in these

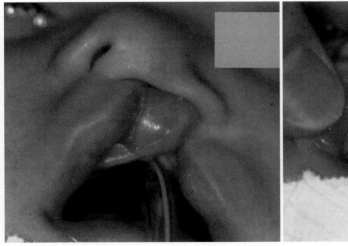
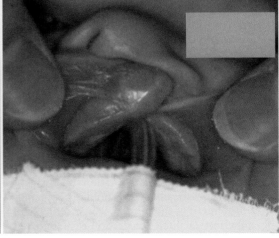

A   B

FIGURE 87-6. Complete unilateral cleft involving the lip and alveolus. Anterior view *(A)* and retracted view *(B)* are shown. With complete unilateral clefts of the lip and palate, the premaxillary portion of the noncleft segment is rotated anterolaterally. The underlying alveolus is completely cleft, not merely notched. In cases in which lateral displacement of the lateral alveolar segments is observed, the premaxilla in the larger segment advances forward in the facial skeleton.

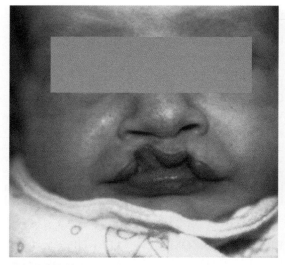

FIGURE 87-7. Bilateral incomplete cleft lip.

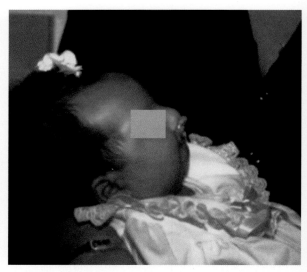

FIGURE 87-8. So-called flyaway prolabium of the complete bilateral cleft lip.

premaxillary configuration (Fig. 87-8). The underlying alveolus is completely cleft, not merely notched. In cases in which lateral displacement of the lateral alveolar segments is observed, the premaxilla in the larger segment advances forward in the facial skeleton.[11]

Clefts Involving the Lip and Palate

UNILATERAL COMPLETE CLEFT LIP AND CLEFT PALATE

With complete labial clefts (Fig. 87-9), the combination of osseous defects in both the alveolus and the palate contributes to instability of the dental arch and sometimes collapse of the lateral segments. When this process occurs in utero, the infant is born with medial collapse of the lesser alveolar segment and lateral rotation of the greater cleft segment. The direction and magnitude of this pathologic change are variable. In such instances, patients may benefit from staged surgical closure with a preliminary lip adhesion,[12] along with fabrication of a passive alveolar molding appliance.[13] Lip adhesion provides a continuous force of soft tissue, which offsets the tendency for outward rotation (buccal inclination) of the premaxilla. The molding appliance controls movement of the maxilla, which, along with the lip adhesion, facilitates migration of the greater and lesser cleft segments into anatomic abutment. Using this protocol for complete clefts of the lip and palate, the authors have observed salutary reorientation of the maxillary frenum toward the dental midline and correction of the displaced sagittal relationships.

BILATERAL COMPLETE CLEFT INVOLVING THE LIP, ALVEOLUS, AND PALATE

The premaxilla may be small or large, symmetric or asymmetric. The number of incisor teeth contained in the premaxillary segment is directly related to the size and shape of the premaxilla. When cleft lip is complete on both sides (i.e., bilateral), the premaxilla projects considerably forward from the facial aspect of the maxilla and the alar-facial junctions on both sides (Fig. 87-10). With complete bilateral clefts of the lip, the premaxilla often protrudes considerably forward

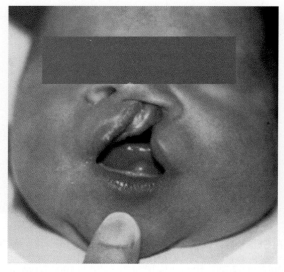

FIGURE 87-9. Unilateral complete cleft involving the lip, alveolus, and palate.

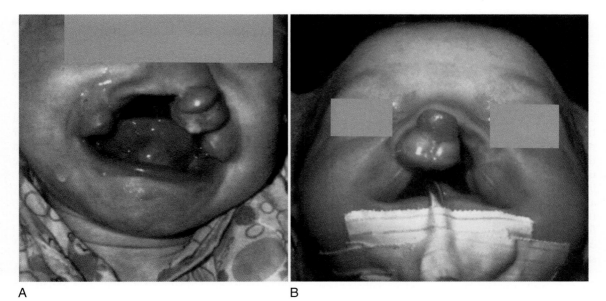

A   B

FIGURE 87-10. *A and B,* Examples of premaxilla rotated and ventrally projected.

when it is viewed in profile, producing the so-called flyaway premaxillary configuration (see Fig. 87-8). This anterior protrusion is less evident if the lip is incompletely cleft on one or both sides.

The premaxilla is attached to a stalk-like vomer and to the nasal septum. The columella appears to be deficient if not completely absent, and the alar cartilages are flattened on both sides. Mulliken[14] has pointed out that "the columella is in the nose" and that substantial improvement in facial aesthetics can result from surgical repositioning of the alar cartilages medially in infancy, at the time of primary cheiloplasty.

With complete bilateral cleft lip and palate, both nasal chambers are in direct communication with the oral cavity. The palatal processes are divided into two virtually identical parts, and on intraoral inspection, the turbinates are clearly visible within both nasal cavities. The nasal septum forms a midline structure that is firmly attached to the base of the skull but is fairly mobile ventrally, where it supports the premaxilla and the columella. Cephalometric radiographs demonstrate the existence of the premaxillary vomerine suture.[9] This suture serves an important function in facial growth. It is also a point of flexion for the premaxilla on the vomer.

How Cleft Lip Configuration Relates to the Alveolus

There is an intimate relationship between the extent of labial clefting and the extent of deformation of the underlying alveolar process. Defects in the alveolus affect the eruption pattern of the deciduous and

permanent dentition. The dental defect may be assessed in terms of the number of teeth, their shape, and their structure as well as by the position of the teeth in the dental arch.[9] Irregularities in the alveolar process range from small dimples, as observed in association with minor clefts of the lip, to actual grooves in the alveolar process and, in extreme cases, total loss in the alveolar ridge and displacement of the premaxillary segment toward the noncleft side. Small dimples or grooves in the alveolar ridge tend to fill in as the jaw grows. The deciduous and lateral incisors that are in this area, however, may be T shaped, or otherwise misshapen, and malpositioned in the line of occlusion.

PATHOLOGIC ANATOMY
Osseous Considerations

Pathologic unilateral cleft lip osseous morphology may be summarized as follows:

1. The premaxilla is outwardly rotated and projecting (see Fig. 87-10).
2. The lateral maxillary element is retropositioned and collapsed medially.

Soft Tissue Considerations

Unilateral cleft lip soft tissue dysmorphology may be summarized as follows[10]:

1. The orbicularis oris muscle in the lateral lip element cants upward at the margin of the cleft and inserts into the alar wing. In cases of incomplete clefting, the muscle does not cross the cleft

unless the bridge is at least half the height of the lip.
2. The philtrum is short.
3. Two thirds of Cupid's bow, one philtral column, and a dimple hollow are preserved.

The muscle anatomy of unilateral and bilateral cleft lip has been described; however, conflicting observations have been reported. Dado and Kernahan[15] found no distinct muscle bundles parallel to the cleft margin that were inserted into the opposite base of the columella. They observed that the muscle bulk composing complete and incomplete cleft lips consisted of a haphazard arrangement of muscle fibers running transversely, obliquely, and anteroposteriorly. These findings contrast with those of Fara,[16] in which the orbicularis oris muscle orientation was seen to be smooth and generally parallel.

The orbicularis oris muscle consists partially of fibers derived from facial muscles and partially of fibers that originate on bone. Anatomically and functionally, there are two distinctive layers, superficial and deep. Nicolau[17] distinguishes the superficial and the deep as two well-defined anatomically separate parts of orbicularis oris muscle. The deep layer of orbicularis oris muscle consists of fibers that arise from other facial muscles. Many fibers arise from the buccinator muscle. The upper muscle fibers decussate into the lower lip, and the lower muscle fibers decussate into the upper lip. Other muscle fibers arise from the levator and depressor anguli muscles. The deep component has a sphincteric function that acts in concert with the oral-pharyngeal muscle apparatus.

The superficial portion associates with the maxilla and septum above and the mandible below. In the upper lip, these connections consist of the lateral muscle bands, which originate from the alveolar border of the maxilla, and the medial bands, which connect the upper lip to the septum. Between the two medial bands is the philtrum. In the lower lip, the superficial layer is composed of slips arising from either side on the midline lip and inserting into the mandible. It is believed that the superficial component functions during facial expression and provides the precise movements of the lips necessary for speech production. Some authors believe that a detailed understanding of this complex muscle arrangement is important because it influences operative technique. For example, Randall et al[18] have advocated interdigitation of the muscle slips at primary cheiloplasty.

Mulliken et al[19] detailed the gross and microscopic anatomy of the skin-mucosal junction (white roll of Gillies) at the Cupid's bow in infants with both normal and cleft lips. In cleft lip specimens, the white roll is absent. In addition, there is both hypoplasia and disorientation of the underlying pars marginalis component of the orbicularis oris muscle, decreased

vermilion width on the medial side of the cleft, and normal to slightly increased width of the vermilion laterally. These observations support the logic of Noordhoff's recommendation[20,21] for use of a tiny lateral vermilion flap during cleft lip repair to augment the deficient medial vermilion.

Slaughter et al[22] detailed the blood supply of the unilateral and bilateral cleft lip. To various degrees, labial clefting interrupts the normal anastomoses that occur among the superior labial artery, anterior ethmoid artery, posterior septal artery, and greater palatine artery.

How Lip Configuration Affects the Cleft Nasal Deformity

The cardinal features of the unilateral cleft nasal deformity have been outlined.[23] In cases of increasing severity of the cleft lip, the nasal alar cartilage on the cleft side is increasingly displaced and flattened, and the tip of the nose is increasingly deviated toward the noncleft side. The spectrum of pathologic changes observed in the lip parallels those pathologic changes observed in the nose. These variations include any of the following:

The inferior edge of the septum is dislocated out of the vomerine groove and is present with the nasal spine in the floor of the normal nostril.

There is unilateral shortness in the vertical height of the columella, varying from three fourths to even half that of the normal size.

The lower lateral (alar) cartilage is attenuated, its medial crus is lower in the columella, and its dome is separated from the opposite alar cartilage to rest inferiorly. The lateral segment is flattened and spread across the cleft at an obtuse angle. There is variable kinking in the alar margin.

The alar base is rotated outwardly in a flare.

The alar rim is invariably distorted by a skin curtain (without cartilage) that droops over the alar rim like a web and further reduces the apparent height of the columella.

The vestibular lining is deficient on the cleft side. This deficiency is readily observed in primary cheiloplasty on repositioning of the alar-facial junction. A triangular defect opens in the lateral vestibular wall as the alar-facial junction is repositioned mesially over the premaxilla.

GENERAL AXIOMS

- There are many varieties of labial clefts.
- A classification system for cleft lip is important so that clinicians can organize and communicate their knowledge effectively.
- The Kernahan striped Y is a simple diagrammatic classification scheme useful to describe discrete

cleft anatomy, including the severity and sidedness of the labial cleft.

- The more severe the cleft lip, the greater the influence of the cleft on the deformity of the underlying alveolus.
- The more severe the cleft lip, the more severe the cleft nasal deformity.
- The less severe the labial cleft deformity, the higher the parental expectations for treatment outcome.

REFERENCES

1. Carter C: Principles of polygenic inheritance. Birth Defects 1976;13:69.
2. Ferguson M: Palate development. Development 1988; 103(suppl):41.
3. Kernahan DA, Stark RB: A new classification for cleft lip and palate. Plast Reconstr Surg 1958;22:435.
4. Schwartz S, Kapala JT, Rajchgot H, Roberts GL: Accurate and systematic numerical recording system for the identification of various types of lip and maxillary clefts (RPL system). Cleft Palate Craniofac J 1993;30:330.
5. Harkins CS: A classification of cleft lip and cleft palate. Plast Reconstr Surg 1963;29:31.
6. Friedman H, Sayetta RB, Coston GN, Hussey JR: Symbolic representation of cleft lip and palate. Cleft Palate Craniofac J 1991;28:252.
7. Kernahan DA: The striped Y: A symbolic classification for cleft lips and palates. Plast Reconstr Surg 1971;47:469.
8. Kernahan DA: On cleft lip and palate classifications. Plast Reconstr Surg 1973;51:578.
9. Berkowitz S: Cleft Lip and Palate: With an Introduction to Other Craniofacial Anomalies. San Diego, Singular, 1996.
10. Burt J, Byrd H: Cleft lip: unilateral primary deformities. Plast Reconstr Surg 2000;105:1043.
11. Huebener D, Liu J: Maxillary orthopedics. Clin Plast Surg 1993;20:723.
12. Randall P: A lip adhesion operation in cleft lip surgery. Plast Reconstr Surg 1965;35:371.
13. Witt P, Hardesty R: Rotation-advancement repair of the unilateral cleft lip: one center's perspective. Clin Plast Surg 1993;20:633.
14. Mulliken J: Bilateral complete cleft lip and nasal deformity: an anthropometric analysis of staged to synchronous repair. Plast Reconstr Surg 1995;96:9.
15. Dado D, Kernahan D: Anatomy of the orbicularis oris muscle in incomplete unilateral cleft lip based on histological examination. Ann Past Surg 1985;15:90.
16. Fara M: Anatomy and arteriography of cleft lips in stillborn children. Plast Reconstr Surg 1968;42:29.
17. Nicolau P: The orbicularis oris muscle: a functional approach to its repair in the cleft lip. Br J Plast Surg 1983;36:141.
18. Randall, P, Whitaker L, LaRossa D: The importance of muscle reconstruction in primary and secondary cleft lip repair. Plast Reconstr Surg 1974;54:316.
19. Mulliken J, Pensler J, Kozakewich H: The anatomy of Cupid's bow in normal and cleft lip. Plast Reconstr Surg 1993;92:395.
20. Noordhoff M: Reconstruction of vermilion in unilateral and bilateral cleft lips. Plast Reconstr Surg 1984;73:52.
21. Noordhoff MS, Chen YR, Chen KT, et al: The surgical technique for the complete unilateral cleft lip-nasal deformity. Operative Techniques Plast Reconstr Surg 1995;2:167.
22. Slaughter W, Henry J, Berger J: Changes in Blood vessel patterns in bilateral cleft lip. Plast Reconstr Surg 1960;26:166.
23. Huffman W, Lierle D: Studies on the pathologic anatomy of the unilateral harelip nose. Plast Reconstr Surg 1949;4:225.

Classification and Anatomy of Cleft Palate

ANIL P. PUNJABI, DDS, MD ✦ ROBERT A. HARDESTY, MD

CLASSIFICATION

The diverse complexity of cleft lip and palate anomaly has resulted in various classification systems, but only a few have been adapted to clinical practice. An ideal system should be comprehensive, based on sound embryologic and anatomic principles, and yet be user friendly, visually easy to document and overcoming language barriers.[1]

In the first generally accepted classification by Davis and Ritchie,[2] congenital clefts were grouped into three according to the position of the cleft in relation to the alveolar process (Table 88-1). This did not adequately describe the lip deformity and could not describe a cleft of the primary palate with intact secondary palate.[1]

Veau[3] described a classification divided into four groups (Fig. 88-1):

Group 1 Cleft of the soft palate
Group 2 Cleft of the hard and soft palates up to the incisive foramen, involving the secondary palate
Group 3 Complete unilateral cleft, extending from the uvula to the incisive foramen in the midline, then deflecting to one side and extending through the alveolus at the position of the future lateral incisor tooth
Group 4 Complete bilateral cleft, resembling group 3 with two clefts projecting forward from the incisive foramen through the alveolus; the small anterior segment of the palate, the premaxilla, remains suspended from the nasal septum

Kernahan and Stark[4] based their classification on embryology. They divided the palate into primary and secondary. The primary palate is that segment of the palate anterior to the incisive foramen or its vestige, the incisive papilla; the secondary palate is the part distal or posterior to the incisive foramen. A cleft of the secondary palate is further described as complete or incomplete with regard to the involvement of the soft or hard palate. Kernahan subsequently proposed a visual classification, the striped Y classification, which is the most widely adapted classification in use (Fig. 88-2). Elsahy[4a] modified the Y by adding triangular peaks to the ends of the prongs to denote the nasal floor. Millard[5] added another inverted triangle to denote the nasal deformity (Fig. 88-3).

Friedman et al[6] proposed a modification of the Kernahan Y classification by incorporating elements that are affected by the cleft and assigning a scale according to the severity. The features that were coded for the severity of involvement of various components of the cleft are shown in Table 88-2. Smith et al[1] proposed yet another modification of the Y (Fig. 88-4). Their system allows a compact alphanumeric description of any cleft. The first set of numerals describes the most anterior aspect of the cleft, and the second set of numerals describes the most posterior extent of the cleft.

Ortiz-Posadas[7] developed a mathematical expression to characterize clefts of the primary palate, including the magnitude of palatal segment separation and the added complexity of bilateral clefts, yielding a numerical score that reflects the overall complexity of the cleft. Clefts of the secondary palate are also considered in a separate score. The numerical score thus obtained provides a means for expressing the severity of the cleft but does not give a visual depiction of the cleft. The RPL system of Schwartz et al[8] is a three-digit numbering system that takes into account only the

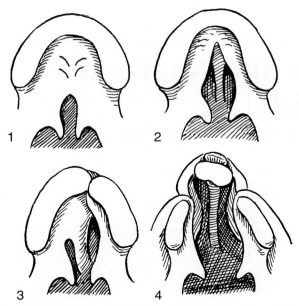

FIGURE 88-1. The Veau classification of the clefts of the lip and palate: group 1, cleft of soft palate only; group 2, cleft of the soft and hard palate as far forward as the incisive foramen; group 3, complete unilateral alveolar cleft, usually involving the lip; and group 4, complete bilateral alveolar cleft, usually associated with bilateral clefts of the lip. (From McCarthy JG, Cutting CB, Hogan VM: Introduction to facial clefts. In McCarthy JG, ed: Plastic Surgery, vol 4. Philadelphia, WB Saunders, 1990:2443.)

number of anatomic components affected by the cleft in each of the three regions originally described by Kernahan.[4] There is no mechanism for characterizing the severity of the cleft.[6]

Kriens[9] proposed the LAHSHAL classification system. The cleft of the lip (L), alveolus (A), and hard

TABLE 88-1 ✦ DAVIS AND RITCHIE CLASSIFICATION

Prealveolar cleft (cleft lip only)	Group 1
Unilateral	Subset 1.1
Median	Subset 1.2
Bilateral	Subset 1.3
Postalveolar clefts (cleft palate only)	Group 2
Soft palate	1/3
	2/3
	3/3
Hard palate	1/3
	2/3
	3/3
Alveolar clefts (cleft lip, alveolus, and palate)	Group 3
Unilateral	Subset 3.1
Median	Subset 3.2
Bilateral	Subset 3.3

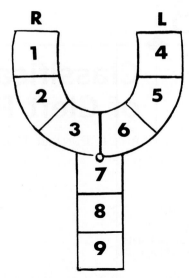

FIGURE 88-2. The striped Y classification. This provides visual demonstration of the site and extent of cleft involvement. (From Kernahan DA: The striped Y—a symbolic classification for cleft lip and palate. Plast Reconstr Surg 1971;47:469.)

palate (H) are paramedian, joined by the median soft palate (S) (Fig. 88-5). The velar area serves to bring the two sagittal paramedian areas LAH and HAL into the same line as S. Thus, LAHSHAL is the anatomic paraphrase of a complete bilateral cleft lip and palate. The letter S represents the middle, and LAHSHAL is read like a radiograph: the right side of the patient is

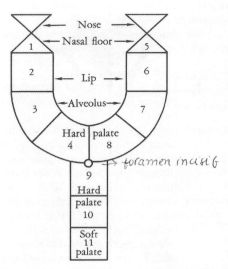

FIGURE 88-3. The inverted triangles at the apex denote the nasal floor. (From Millard DR Jr: Cleft Craft: The Evolution of Its Surgery, vol 1. The Unilateral Deformity. Boston, Little, Brown, 1977:52.)

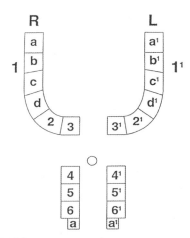

FIGURE 88-4. Smith modification of the Kernahan striped Y classification. (From Smith AW, Khoo AK, Jackson IT: A modification of the Kernahan "Y" classification in cleft lip and palate deformities. Plast Reconstr Surg 1998;102:1842.)

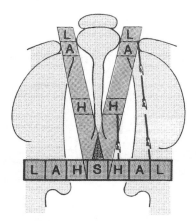

FIGURE 88-5. The locations of cleft lip, alveolus, hard palate, and soft palate are marked by the first letter of each region. The two paramedian prongs LAH and HAL are rotated laterally on one line with S, that is, the median velar cleft region. Thus, the definition of the cleft side has become mandatory. (From Kriens O: LAHSHAL: a concise documentation system for cleft lip, alveolus and palate diagnosis. In Kriens O, ed: What Is a Cleft Lip and Palate? New York, Thieme, 1989:32.)

on the left side of the formula and vice versa. For example, L- is a complete cleft lip of the right side, and -L stands for one on the left side. Complete clefts are defined by capital letters, partial clefts by lowercase letters, and microforms by asterisks.

ANATOMY
Bones of the Palate

The premaxilla is situated anterior to the incisive foramen and includes the anterior nasal spine and four incisor teeth. The paired maxillae form the anterior portion of the palate, and the paired palatal bones form the posterior palate including the posterior nasal spine. The palatine bones also contain the major and minor palatine foramina. The palatine bone articulates with the medial plate of the pterygoid, from which projects the pterygoid hamulus, which acts as a pulley for the tensor veli palatini (Figs. 88-6 and 88-7).[10]

Muscles of the Palate

The extrinsic muscles of the palate are those that have a portion of their origin or insertion in the palate. They include the levator veli palatini, tensor veli palatini, palatopharyngeus, palatoglossus, salpingopharyngeus, and superior constrictor. The only intrinsic muscle is the musculus uvulae (Figs. 88-8 to 88-10

TABLE 88-2 ✦ FRIEDMAN MODIFICATION

Deformity	Rating
Deformity of the nostril	0-4
Prolabial and premaxillary	0-3
Protrusion	not rated
Upper lip deformity	0-4
Alveolar deformity	0-3
Preincisive foraminal trigone	0-2
Hard palate deformity	0-3
Soft palate or velum deformity	0-5

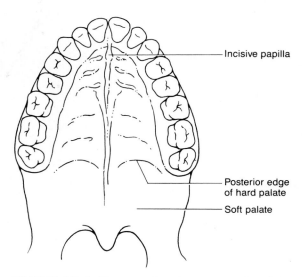

FIGURE 88-6. The normal surface topography of the palate. Although the mucosa of the hard palate is thick, it is easy to identify the major palatal vessels and the posterior nasal spine. (From Randall P, LaRossa D: Cleft palate. In McCarthy JG, ed: Plastic Surgery, vol 4. Philadelphia, WB Saunders, 1990:2723-2752.)

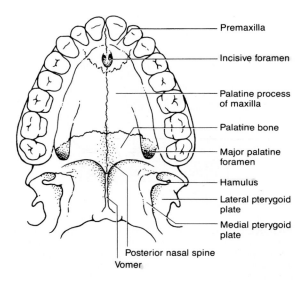

Premaxilla

Incisive foramen

Palatine process
of maxilla

Palatine bone

Major palatine
foramen

Hamulus

Lateral pterygoid
plate

Medial pterygoid
plate

Posterior nasal spine

Vomer

FIGURE 88-7. The normal bony topography of the palate. The major palatine foramen, the incisive foramen, and the hamulus are important surgical landmarks. (After Millard DR Jr: Cleft Craft, vol 3. Boston, Little, Brown, 1980:19. From Randall P, LaRossa D: Cleft palate. In McCarthy JG, ed: Plastic Surgery, vol 4. Philadelphia, WB Saunders, 1990:2723-2752.)

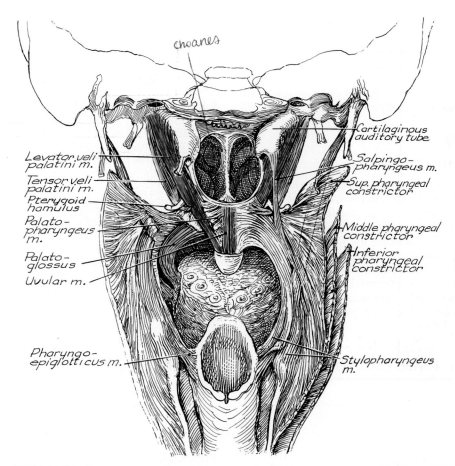

choanes

Levator veli
palatini m.

Tensor veli
palatini m.

Pterygoid
hamulus

Palato-
pharyngeus
m.

Palato-
glossus

Uvular m.

Pharyngo-
epiglotticus m.

Cartilaginous
auditory tube

Salpingo-
pharyngeus m.

Sup. pharyngeal
constrictor

Middle pharyngeal
constrictor

Inferior
pharyngeal
constrictor

Stylopharyngeus
m.

FIGURE 88-8. Muscles of the palatopharyngeal region, nasal view. (From Fara M: The musculature of cleft lip and palate. In McCarthy JG, ed: Plastic Surgery, vol 4. Philadelphia, WB Saunders, 1990:2598-2626.)

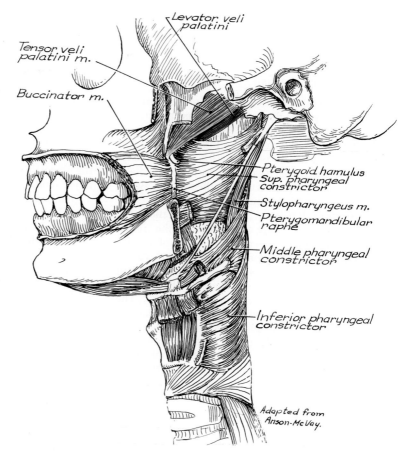

Levator:

Origine - Cartilage de la trompe
         d'Eustache
       - Portion pétreuse de
         l'os temporal

Insertion : aponévrose palatine

Tensor :

Origine - Fosse scaphoïde de la
         plaque ptérygoïdienne
         médiale
       - Épine du sphénoïde
       - Cartilage de la trompe
         d'Eustache

Insertion : aponévrose palatine

FIGURE 88-9. Muscles of the palatopharyngeal region, lateral view. (From Fara M: The musculature of cleft lip and palate. In McCarthy JG, ed: Plastic Surgery, vol 4. Philadelphia, WB Saunders, 1990:2598-2626.)

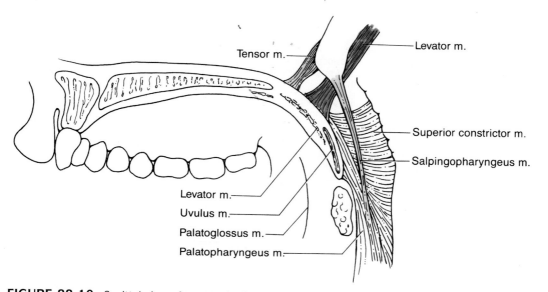

FIGURE 88-10. Sagittal view of a normal adult palate indicating the relationships of the levator, the uvulus, and the palatoglossus muscle within and beyond the palate. The adjacent superior pharyngeal constrictor muscle is also shown. (After Millard DR Jr: Cleft Craft, vol 3. Boston, Little, Brown, 1980:opposite 36. From Randall P, LaRossa D: Cleft palate. In McCarthy JG, ed: Plastic Surgery, vol 4. Philadelphia, WB Saunders, 1990:2723-2752.)

and Table 88-3). The salpingopharyngeus and the palatoglossus make minimal or no contribution to velar function.

LEVATOR VELI PALATINI

The levator veli palatini is a cylindrical muscle forming a sling that suspends the soft palate from the cranial base (Fig. 88-11). Its superior attachment is the posteromedial part of the eustachian tube at the junction of its cartilaginous and bony portions.[11] The muscle bundle descends on each side anteriorly and medially toward the soft palate, occupying the space between the superior constrictor and the cranial base.

The levator veli palatini lies inferior and medial to the eustachian tube except at each end. At the cranial end, the muscle turns superior and posterior around the tube to attach to its posteromedial aspect. At the pharyngeal end, it curves slightly anterior so that it lies inferior to the membranous portion and anterolateral to the cartilaginous part of the tube.[11] The levator enters the velum by fanning out between the two heads of the palatopharyngeus. In the velum, the fibers spread over the posterior three fourths of the velum. Huang et al[12] found that the intravelar portion of the levator occupied the middle 50% of the velar length measured from the posterior nasal spine

to the tip of the uvula. These fibers cross the midline to meet the fibers from the opposite side. Anteriorly, it is attached to the posterior margin of the aponeurosis of the tensor veli palatini.[12] Within the soft palate, the levator veli palatini is the most superior muscle with the exception of the musculus uvulae.[13]

The levator veli palatini is hypoplastic and thin in the cleft palate. The posterior bundles run posterolaterally toward the palatopharyngeus. The medial bundles radiate into the margin of the cleft. The anterior bundles attach to the triangular tendinous area to the posterior edge of the palate or are directly linked to the tendon of the tensor veli palatini.[14]

The function of the levator is velar elevation and retrodisplacement during speech and swallowing. This function is due to the sling-like structure formed by its cylindrical bundles, which suspend the soft palate from the cranial base. The downward, forward, and medial path of its axis is consistent with the upward, backward, and lateral pull that the velum is subjected to during velopharyngeal closure.[12] The levator also brings about a medial, posterior, and superior displacement of the torus tubarius, which is usually incidental and does not contribute to velopharyngeal closure.[12]

The role of the levator veli palatini in eustachian tube function is controversial. Anatomic and

TABLE 88-3 ✦ MUSCLES OF THE PALATE

Muscle	Origin	Insertion	Blood Supply	Nerve Supply	Function
Levator veli palatini	Posteromedial eustachian tube tube	Palatal midline	APA, RPA	IX, X	Elevates velum; eustachian tube dilation
Tensor veli palatini	Scaphoid fossa of sphenoid	Aponeurosis on the posterior hard palate	Maxillary	V	Eustachian tube dilation
Palatopharyngeus	Posterior border of aponeurosis and levator	Lateral pharynx and larynx	APA, RPA, maxillary	IX, X	Antagonistic to levator; helps in velopharyngeal closure
Musculus uvulae	Anteriorly to the aponeurosis in the midline	Posterior connective tissue of the midline velum	APA	IX, X	Forms the knee in velopharyngeal closure
Superior constrictor	Medial pterygoid plate	Pharyngeal ligament	AphA, APA, RPA	IX, X	Medial displacement of lateral pharynx
Salpingopharyngeus	Posteroinferior tip of eustachian tube	Palatopharyngeus	Unknown	IX, X	Vestigial
Palatoglossus	Transverse bundles of tongue	Muscle of palate	APA, maxillary	IX, X	Lifts tongue and propels food

APA, ascending palatine artery; AphA, ascending pharyngeal artery; RPA, recurrent pharyngeal artery.

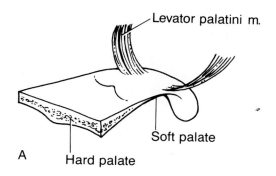

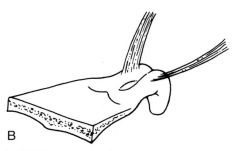

FIGURE 88-11. The levator muscle is the critical muscle involved in velopharyngeal closure. Note that the pull is approximately 45 degrees superiorly and posteriorly. *A,* At rest. *B,* After contraction. (From Randall P, LaRossa D: Cleft palate. In McCarthy JG, ed: Plastic Surgery, vol 4. Philadelphia, WB Saunders, 1990:2723-2752.)

physiologic studies point to a dilatory effect on the eustachian tube.[15-20] Others have postulated that the levator veli palatini has no effect on the eustachian tube.[21-23]

Huang et al[11] concluded that the levator veli palatini causes an upward medial and posterior displacement of the medial tubal cartilage by muscle isotonic contraction with a superior and posterior displacement of the levator sling, resulting in the opening of the lumen of the tube. The effect on the membranous part of the eustachian tube is also a dilatory one (Fig. 88-12).

Serous otitis media in patients with cleft palate is due to the dysfunction of the paratubal muscles, particularly the levator veli palatini.[14,24-26] The ability of the levator veli palatini to dilate the eustachian tube is lost in the unrepaired cleft owing to its substantial anterior bony insertion on the posterior margin of the hard palate. Repositioning of the levator veli palatini during an intervelar veloplasty and the Furlow double opposing Z-plasty restores the velar suspensory apparatus, allowing dilation of the eustachian tube.[10]

TENSOR VELI PALATINI

The tensor veli palatini has an oblique origin from the scaphoid fossa of the greater wing of the sphenoid between the superior end of the medial pterygoid plate and the spine of the sphenoid as well as the adjacent superolateral aspect of the cartilaginous and membranous parts of the entire length of the eustachian tube.[10] The muscle is triangular with a fleshy belly and tendinous at each end. The angle between the axis of the tensor veli palatini and the eustachian tube is about 30 to 40 degrees. The tendon of the tensor veli palatini hooks around the anterior aspect of the hamulus, forming a 90-degree turn as it enters the soft palate. In the soft palate, the tendon spreads out to become the horizontal sheet-like aponeurosis occupying the anterior quarter of the velar length and extending from the posterior nasal spine to the tip of the uvula.

The tensor veli palatini is thinner in the newborn cleft. A few fibers are attached to the hamulus. The front parts of its bundles extend along the rudimentary palatine aponeurosis toward the posterior nasal spine or run laterally to the posterior edge of the palatine bone. The main tendon arches backward to the cleft margin and ends in two different manners: (1) the tendon, occasionally, is partially dispersed, and a triangular portion passes into the anterior bundles of the levator; or (2) the tendon does not disperse and passes anteriorly into the levator veli palatini to form a thick musculotendinous bundle.[13]

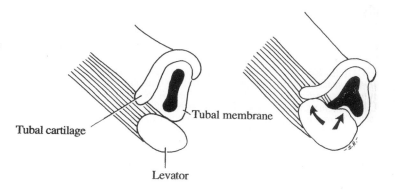

FIGURE 88-12. Postulated role of levator veli palatini in tubal biomechanics. *Left,* At rest. Note shape of tubal lumen. *Right,* During contraction. Posterior, superior, and medial displacement of medial tubal cartilage and superior displacement of tubal membrane result in tubal dilation. (From Martin HS, Lee ST, Rajendran K: A fresh cadaveric study of the paratubal muscles: implication for eustachian tube function in cleft palate. Plast Reconstr Surg 1997;100:838.)

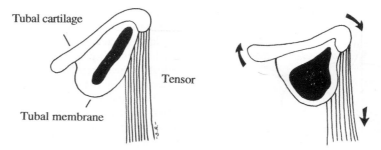

FIGURE 88-13. Postulated action of tensor veli palatini on eustachian tube. *Left,* At rest. Note shape of tubal lumen. *Right,* Contraction of tensor results in anterolateral traction on tubal membrane and superior rotation of medial tubal cartilage by means of the pull on lateral tubal cartilage. Both actions open tubal lumen. (From Martin HS, Lee ST, Rajendran K: A fresh cadaveric study of the paratubal muscles: implication for eustachian tube function in cleft palate. Plast Reconstr Surg 1997;100:840.)

The function of the tensor veli palatini is to dilate the eustachian tube. Its effect on the tube is to pull it inferiorly, laterally, and anteriorly. In concert with the levator veli palatini acting on the medial aspect of the eustachian tube, the tensor augments the opening and may have pumping action that milks the tube of its contents (Fig. 88-13).[12,27,28] Complete hamular fracture or division of the tensor tendon may reduce the effectiveness of the tubal dilatation by the tensor veli palatini (Fig. 88-14).[10]

SALPINGOPHARYNGEUS

This vestigial muscle occupies the salpingopharyngeal fold. Its superior attachment is the posteroinferior

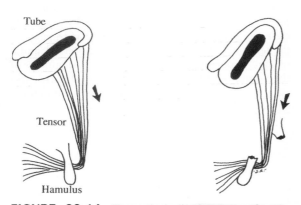

FIGURE 88-14. Theoretical disadvantage of completely fracturing the hamulus. *Left,* Before hamular fracture. Note normal vector of action of tensor veli palatini on eustachian tube. *Right,* After total hamular fracture. Distal hamular fragment is displaced medially, leading to impairment of ability of tensor to open tube from loss of mechanical advantage. (From Martin HS, Lee ST, Rajendran K: A fresh cadaveric study of the paratubal muscles: implication for eustachian tube function in cleft palate. Plast Reconstr Surg 1997;100:841.)

tip of the medial end of the eustachian tube, to both the cartilaginous and membranous components. The muscle descends posteriorly and inserts into the palatopharyngeus at the junction of the velum and lateral pharyngeal wall.

The functions attributed to the salpingopharyngeus include closing the eustachian tube, opening it, lateral pharyngeal wall elevation, and elevation of the velum.[14,29,30] However, the vestigial form of the muscle and its diminutive size and its actions have minimal functional significance.[10,31]

MUSCULUS UVULAE

The musculus uvulae is a paired muscle running longitudinally in the nasal midline of the velum, attached anteriorly to the aponeurosis and posteriorly to the base of the uvula, which itself is devoid of muscle fibers. Its function consists of a passive space-occupying role that prevents attenuation of the midline bulk caused by the lateral traction from the levator during velopharyngeal closure; augmentation of this passive role by active contraction that increases its diameter and midline velar bulk, particularly at the apex of the contracted soft palate, thus contributes to the levator eminence and velar extension, which also enhances midline contact in velopharyngeal closure (Fig. 88-15). This muscle should be preserved during intervelar veloplasty, and it is invariably divided and reoriented in a nonanatomic position in the Furlow double opposing Z-plasty.[32]

PALATOPHARYNGEUS

The palatopharyngeus is an extensive sheet extending between the velum superiorly, the larynx inferiorly, and the pharyngeal wall posteriorly.[11] It occupies the central 50% of the velar length and consists of two heads separated by the levator veli palatini, with one

FIGURE 88-15. Functions of musculus uvulae. *Left,* At rest. Note sagittal contour of muscle. *Right,* During velar elevation. On contraction, maximal sagittal thickness occurs in region of posterior two thirds of muscle. Shortening of the muscle also results in velar extension. Both effects enhance midline velopharyngeal contact. Both the levator and musculus uvulae are responsible for the levator eminence. (From Huang MH, Lee ST, Rajendran K: Structure of the musculus uvulae: functional and surgical implications of an anatomic study. Cleft Palate Craniofac J 1997;34:466.)

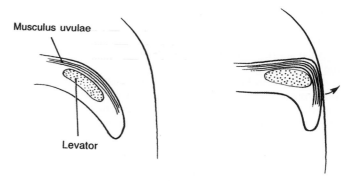

head lying on the oral aspect and the other on the nasal side of the levator. Hence, the two heads of the palatopharyngeus embrace the levator in the velum, with the palatal head being more developed than the nasal. In the paramedian zone, the fibers of the palatopharyngeus thin out and merge with those of the levator. Lateral to the levator, the two heads of the palatopharyngeus blend to form a broad sheet of muscle. Most of these fibers run posteriorly, forming the posterior faucial pillar, and inferiorly fuse with the fibers of the superior constrictor. The remainder insert inferiorly into the larynx.

The palatopharyngeus forms the cleft muscle of Veau along with the fibers of the levator. The fibers of the palatopharyngeus in the cleft palate insert along the posterior edge of the hard palate.

The palatopharyngeus in conjunction with the antagonistic action of the levator modulates velar position, size, and shape <u>to optimize velopharyngeal closure</u> (Fig. 88-16). <u>Along with the superior constrictor, it causes medial displacement of the lateral pharyngeal walls and also contributes to the Passavant ridge</u> (Fig. 88-17).[11]

PALATOGLOSSUS

This slender muscle arises from the transverse muscle fibers of the tongue, passing superiorly in the ante-

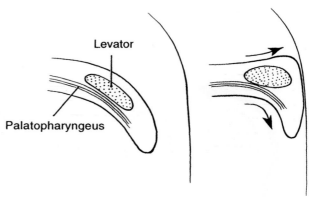

FIGURE 88-16. Effect of the palatopharyngeus on velar position. The inferior vector of action of the palatopharyngeus antagonizes the superior pull of the levator. The net result is velar retrodisplacement with enhanced velopharyngeal contact. (From Huang MH, Lee ST, Rajendran K: Anatomic basis of cleft palate and velopharyngeal surgery: implications from a fresh cadaveric study. Plast Reconstr Surg 1998;101:613.)

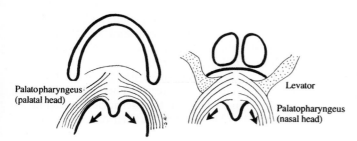

FIGURE 88-17. Effect of the palatopharyngeus on velar size and shape. *Left,* Oral view. *Right,* Nasal view. Contraction of both heads stretches the velum inferiorly and laterally to increase the available velar surface area and to optimize velar shape for contact with the posterior pharyngeal wall. (From Huang MH, Lee ST, Rajendran K: Anatomic basis of cleft palate and velopharyngeal surgery: implications from a fresh cadaveric study. Plast Reconstr Surg 1998;101:613.)

rior faucial pillar and inserting fan shaped into the muscles of the soft palate.[13] It functions to narrow the pharyngo-oral isthmus and forms the anterior pretonsillar sphincter. It lifts the tongue and helps propel the food.

In clefted newborns, it passes into the cleft margin at the posterior edge of the hard palate. It is the most superficial of the soft palate muscles and extends anteriorly into the oral periosteum of the hard palate.[13]

SUPERIOR CONSTRICTOR

This quadrangular muscle arises anteriorly from the posterior border of the medial pterygoid plate from the level of the hard palate to the tip of the hamulus. This origin continues on a downward and forward slope along the pterygomandibular ligament. The muscle then sweeps around the pharynx, forming its lateral and posterior walls, and inserts posteriorly into the pharyngeal ligament. It is the deepest of the pharyngeal constrictors. In both normal and cleft conditions, there is a close intermingling of its fibers with those of the palatopharyngeus.

The superior constrictor functions to bring about the medial excursion of the lateral pharyngeal walls by a sphincteric mechanism, which also involves the palatopharyngeus (Fig. 88-18). It causes the anterior displacement of the posterior pharyngeal wall by fibers that meet across the posterior midline. It is also the main component of the Passavant ridge.

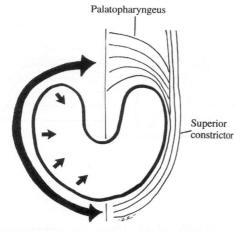

Palatopharyngeus

Superior constrictor

FIGURE 88-18. Nasal view of palatopharyngeus-superior constrictor sphincter. The two muscles in continuity form a hemisphincteric mechanism on each side, which provides a mechanical basis for medial excursion of the lateral pharyngeal walls. (From Huang MH, Lee ST, Rajendran K: Anatomic basis of cleft palate and velopharyngeal surgery: implications from a fresh cadaveric study. Plast Reconstr Surg 1998;101:613.)

Blood Supply of the Palate

The blood vessels of the hard and soft palates are found in the plane of the glandular tissue.[33] This plane of connective tissue is situated between the mucosa and periosteum in the hard palate and between the mucosa and the velar muscles in the soft palate. The network of anastomosing vessels is extensive on the oral surface of the palate compared with the nasal surface.[32]

Broomhead[34] reported that the greater palatine artery supplies the oral surface of the hard palate and gives off branches that pierce the maxilla and supply the nasal mucosa. The lesser palatine artery supplies the anterior half of the oral surface of the soft palate. The ascending palatine artery, a branch of the facial artery, is the largest vessel entering the soft palate. This artery ascends on the lateral aspect of the superior constrictor and supplies branches to the levator and tensor veli palatini. Its two terminal branches supply the uvula posteriorly and anteriorly run along the anterior border of the levator. Branches of the tonsillar and the ascending pharyngeal artery also reach the soft palate.

Huang et al[32] confirmed the blood supply and clarified that hard palate, soft palate, and superior part of the pharynx are supplied by the four branches of the external carotid artery in the ascending order of the ascending palatine branch of the facial artery, the ascending pharyngeal artery, a previously undescribed vessel named the recurrent pharyngeal artery, and the maxillary artery.

The ascending palatine artery is a branch of the facial artery arising at the angle of the mandible. It runs superiorly between the palatoglossus and the palatopharyngeus, and it supplies the velar portion of the levator veli palatini. Along its way, it gives a branch to the palatoglossus, a tonsillar branch, and a branch to the palatopharyngeus. It also supplies branches to the musculus uvulae, which is entirely dependent on it for its blood supply.[32]

The ascending pharyngeal artery is a branch of the medial aspect of the external carotid artery arising close to the bifurcation. As it ascends vertically, it gives branches to the lateral pharyngeal wall, the superior constrictor, the palatopharyngeus, and the salpingopharyngeus.[32] Mercer and MacCarthy[35] reported that only the ascending palatine artery supplied the soft palate and that the ascending pharyngeal artery supplied only the superior constrictor and the pharyngeal part of the palatopharyngeus. This is in agreement with the findings of Huang et al.[32]

The recurrent pharyngeal artery, a distinct branch of the external carotid artery, originates from the level of the upper third of the sternocleidomastoid as described by Huang et al[33] in their dissections of five adult cadavers of Asian origin. It ascends vertically to the base of the skull, sending a small meningeal branch, and then turns down in a recurrent fashion along the posterolateral path of the levator veli palatini. It supplies branches to the eustachian tube, the extravelar portion of the levator veli palatini, the palatopharyngeus, and the tensor veli palatini. The blood supply to the extravelar part of the levator veli palatini was attributed to the ascending pharyngeal artery by Freedlander[36] and to the ascending palatine artery by Mercer and MacCarthy,[35] which is in variance with the findings of Huang et al.

The maxillary artery branches from the external carotid artery at the level of the mastoid, giving off a muscle branch to the tensor veli palatini.[33] Before entering the pterygomaxillary fissure, the maxillary artery gives its lesser palatine branch, emerging from the lesser palatine foramen to supply the oral surface of the aponeurosis of the tensor veli palatini. The lesser palatine artery anastomoses substantially with the branches of the greater palatine artery, which arises from the third part of the maxillary artery in the pterygopalatine fossa and exits through the greater palatine foramen. It provides the branches to the bony palate and alveolus.

Nerve Supply of the Palate

The sensory branches to the palate are supplied by the maxillary division of the trigeminal nerve. The facial nerve provides secretory and sympathetic fibers to the maxillary division through the sphenopalatine ganglion. The greater palatine nerve descends through the greater palatine canal, emerges through the greater palatine foramen, and runs anteriorly to supply the bony palate and mucous membrane and glands of the hard palate. It sends the branches throughout the palatine process to the inferior concha and the middle and inferior meatuses.[37] Branches of the sphenopalatine nerve emerge from the incisive foramen to the anterior hard palate. The lesser palatine nerves descend through the greater palatine foramen and supply the uvula, soft palate, and tonsil.

The motor supply to the tensor veli palatini is different from that of the other velopharyngeal muscles. The tensor is innervated by the internal pterygoid nerve, a branch of the mandibular nerve, the third division of the trigeminal nerve (X).

Broomhead[34] described important anatomic findings for cleft surgery. He presented that the glossopharyngeal nerve (IX) and the pharyngeal branch of the vagus nerve (X) supply the pharyngeal constrictors, the levator veli palatini, the palatoglossus, and the nerve to the medial pterygoid muscle. He also showed the course of the nerves to the palatoglossus

and palatopharyngeus on the medial side of the superior constrictor.

Broomhead[34] cautioned against damage inflicted on the nerve to the tensor veli palatini during operative repair, resulting in paralysis. The lesser palatine nerves are sectioned, resulting in anesthesia of the soft tissue and paralysis of the musculus uvulae. The nerves to the palatoglossus, palatopharyngeus, and levator veli palatini muscle are usually not affected.

Nishio et al[38] concluded that the levator veli palatini, uvula, and superior constrictor muscles are dually innervated by the facial nerve and branches of the pharyngeal plexus derived from the glossopharyngeal and vagus nerves and that the facial nerve plays an important role as one of the motor nerves in the movements responsible for velopharyngeal closure. They also proposed that the nasal grimacing during phonation in patients with velopharyngeal insufficiency not only compensates for velopharyngeal incompetence but also augments the firing of the facial nerve to complement velopharyngeal movements.

Palatal Anatomy with Magnetic Resonance Imaging

The muscles of the palate, especially the levator veli palatini, can be evaluated by magnetic resonance imaging (MRI).[39-41] A Siemens 1.5-tesla scanner was used with fast spin echo proton density-weighted imaging for all sessions. Compared with either T1-weighted or T2-weighted images, the proton density-weighted images provided better contrast of the levator veli palatini muscle in relation to the surrounding soft tissue structures. Oblique coronal and sagittal images were obtained (Fig. 88-19).[41]

The levator veli palatini can be seen originating along the medial aspect of the eustachian tube, with the tensor veli palatini along the lateral eustachian tube (Fig. 88-20). The encapsulated musculus uvulae can be visualized, cradled by the levator sling; the musculus uvulae is based dorsally on the nasal aspect (Fig. 88-21). Kuehn et al[39] have recommended the use of MRI as a diagnostic tool to evaluate the velopharynx before surgery in patients with occult submucous clefts. The velopharyngeal anatomy of patients with velocardiofacial syndrome was evaluated by MRI, and the findings show that the levator is attenuated and the origin from the cranial base is obtuse.[41] The levator is based more anteriorly and thus is situated in a position that is mechanically disadvantageous during function. As the quality of the MRI technology improves, it will play an important role in clinical diagnosis and surgical treatment planning.

1) All muscles with "glossus" → NC XII (except palatoglosse → NC X)
2) All muscles with "palat" → NC X (except tensor veli palatini → V₃)

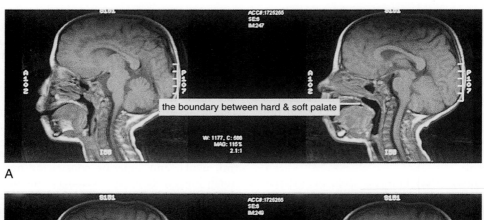

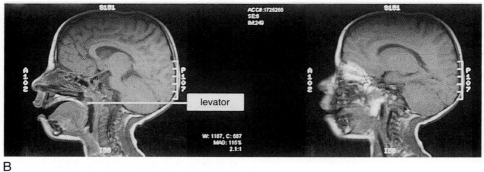

FIGURE 88-19. *A,* A sagittal MRI showing the boundary between the hard and soft palates. *B,* A sagittal MRI showing the levator as it descends from the cranial base and folds into the velum.

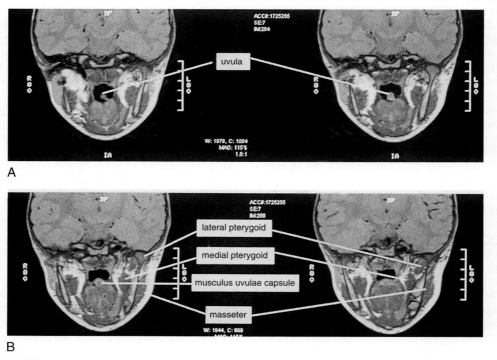

FIGURE 88-20. *A,* A coronal MRI of the uvula. *B,* Coronal MRI showing the muscles of mastication and intrinsic musculus uvulae of the velum.

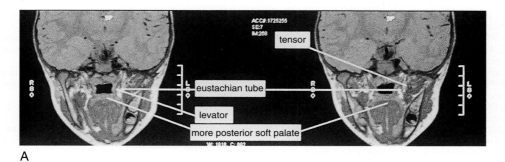

A

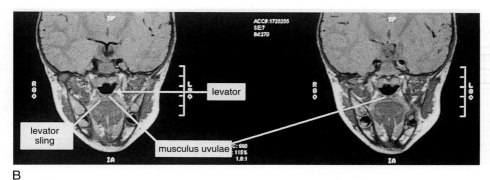

B

FIGURE 88-21. *A,* Coronal MRI showing the relationship of the levator veli palatini, eustachian tube, and tensor veli palatini. *B,* Coronal MRI showing the levator sling cradling the dorsally located musculus uvulae.

REFERENCES

1. Smith AW, Khoo AK, Jackson IT: A modification of the Kernahan "Y" classification in cleft lip and palate deformities. Plast Reconstr Surg 1998;102:1842.
2. Davis JS, Ritchie HP: Classification of congenital cleft of the lip and palate. JAMA 1922;79:1323.
3. Veau V: Division palatine. Paris, Masson, 1931.
4. Kernahan DA, Stark RB: A new classification for cleft lip and cleft palate. Plast Reconstr Surg 1958;22:435.
4a. Elsahy NL: The modified striped Y—a systematic classification for cleft lip and palate. Cleft Palate J 1973;10:247–250.
5. Millard DR Jr: Cleft Craft: The Evolution of Its Surgery, vol 1. The Unilateral Deformity. Boston, Little, Brown, 1977.
6. Friedman HL, Sayeta RB, Coston GN, Husey JR: Symbolic representation of cleft lip and palate. Cleft Palate Craniofac J 1991;28:252.
7. Ortiz-Posadas MR, Vega-Alvarado L, Maya-Behar J: A new approach to classify cleft lip and palate. Cleft Palate Craniofac J 2001;38:545.
8. Schwartz S, Kapela JT, Rajchgot H, Roberts GI: Accurate and systematic numerical recording system for the identification of various types of lip and maxillary clefts. Cleft Palate Craniofac J 1993;30:330.
9. Kriens O: LAHSHAL: a concise documentation system for cleft lip, alveolus and palate diagnosis. In Kriens O, ed: What Is a Cleft Lip and Palate? New York, Thieme, 1989:32-33.
10. Randall P, LaRossa D: Cleft palate. In McCarthy JG, ed: Plastic Surgery, vol 4. Philadelphia, WB Saunders, 1990:2723-2752.
11. Huang MH, Lee ST, Rajendran K: A fresh cadaveric study of the paratubal muscles: implications for eustachian tube functions in cleft palate. Plast Reconstr Surg 1997;100:833.
12. Huang MH, Lee ST, Rajendran K: Anatomic basis of cleft palate and velopharyngeal surgery: implications from a fresh cadaveric study. Plast Reconstr Surg 1998;101:613.
13. Millard DR Jr: Cleft Craft: The Evolution of Its Surgery, vol 3. Alveolar and Palatal Deformities. Boston, Little, Brown, 1980:19-50.
14. Fara M: The musculature of cleft lip and palate. In McCarthy JG, ed: Plastic Surgery, vol 4. Philadelphia, WB Saunders, 1990:2598-2626.
15. Simkins CS: Functional anatomy of the eustachian tube. Arch Otolaryngol 1943;3:473.
16. Seif S, Dellon AL: Anatomic relationships between the human levator and tensor veli palatini and the eustachian tube. Cleft Palate J 1978;15:329.
17. Rood SR, Doyle WJ: The nasopharyngeal orifice of the auditory tube: implications for tubal dynamics anatomy. Cleft Palate J 1982;19:199.
18. Shprintzen RJ, Croft CB: Abnormalities of the eustachian tube orifice in individuals with cleft palate. Int J Pediatr Otolaryngol 1981;3:15.
19. Swartz JD, Rood SR: The morphometry and three-dimensional structure of the adult eustachian tube: implication for function. Cleft Palate J 1990;27:374.
20. Spauwen PH, Hillen B, Lommen E, Otten E: Three-dimensional computer reconstruction of the eustachian tube and paratubal muscles. Cleft Palate J 1991;28:217.
21. Doyle WJ, Rood SR: Comparison of the anatomy of the eustachian tube in the rhesus monkey *(Macaca mulatta)* and man: implications for physiologic modeling. Ann Otol Rhinol Laryngol 1980;89:49.
22. Honjo L, Okazaki N, Nozoe T: The role of the tensor veli palatini in movement of the soft palate. Acta Otolaryngol 1979;88:137.
23. Finklestein Y, Talmi YP, Nachmani A, et al: Levator veli palatini muscle and eustachian tube function. Plast Reconstr Surg 1990;85:684.
24. Latham RA, Long RE, Latham EA: Cleft palate velopharyngeal musculature in a five-month-old infant: a three-dimensional histological reconstruction. Cleft Palate J 1980;17:1.

25. Doyle WJ, Kitajari M, Sando I: The anatomy of the auditory tube and paratubal musculature in a one-month-old cleft palate patient. Cleft Palate J 1983;20:218.

26. Doyle WJ, Reilly JS, Jardini L, Rovnak S: Effect of palatoplasty on the function of the eustachian tube in children with cleft palate. Cleft Palate J 1986;23:63.

27. Ross MA: Functional anatomy of the tensor palatini: its relevance in cleft palate surgery. Arch Otolaryngol 1971;93:1.

28. Rood SR, Doyle WJ: Morphology of tensor veli palatini, tensor tympani and dilator tubae muscles. Ann Otol Rhinol Laryngol 1978;87:202.

29. Fara M, Dvorak J: Abnormal anatomy of the muscles of palatopharyngeal closure in cleft palates. Plast Reconstr Surg 1970;46:488.

30. Bosma JF: A correlated study of the anatomy and motor activity of the upper pharynx by cadaver dissection and by cinematic study of patients after maxillofacial surgery. Ann Otol 1953;62:51.

31. Dickson DR: Anatomy of the normal velopharyngeal mechanism. Clin Plast Surg 1975;2:235.

32. Huang MH, Lee ST, Rajendran K: Structure of the musculus uvulae: functional and surgical implications of an anatomic study. Cleft Palate Craniofac J 1997;34:466.

33. Huang MH, Lee ST, Rajendran K: Clinical implications of the velopharyngeal blood supply. Plast Reconstr Surg 1998;102:655.

34. Broomhead IW: The nerve supply of the muscles of the soft palate. Br J Plast Surg 1951;4:1.

35. Mercer NS, MacCarthy P: The arterial supply of the palate: implications for closure of cleft palates. Plast Reconstr Surg 1995;96:1038.

36. Freedlander E: The blood supply of the levator and tensor veli palatini muscles: implications for closure of cleft palates. Clin Anat 1988;1:300.

37. Williams PL, Warwick R, eds: Gray's Anatomy. London, Churchill Livingstone, 1980:1065.

38. Nishio J, Matsuya T, Machida J, Miyazaki T: The motor nerve supply of the velopharyngeal muscles. Cleft Palate J 1976;13:20.

39. Kuehn DP, Ettema ST, Goldwasser MS, et al: Magnetic resonance imaging in the evaluation of occult submucous cleft palate. Cleft Palate J 2001;38:421.

40. Ettema SL, Kuehn DP, Perlman A, Alperin N: Magnetic resonance imaging of the levator veli palatini muscle during speech. Cleft Palate J 2002;39:130.

41. Punjabi AP, Hoshouser BA, D'Antonio LL, Kuehn DP: Magnetic resonance imaging of the velopharynx in patients with velocardiofacial syndrome. Presented at the American Cleft Palate-Craniofacial Association Annual Meeting, Seattle, Washington, May 1, 2002.

Anatomy and Classification of Alveolar and Palatal Clefts

David M. Kahn, MD ✦ Stephen A. Schendel, MD, DDS

ANATOMY OF ALVEOLAR AND PALATAL CLEFTS

In approaching any surgical problem, one must have an understanding of both normal and aberrant anatomy. This holds true for clefts of the alveolus and palate, in which reconstruction of the abnormal anatomy is critical to restoration of proper functioning of the velopharyngeal mechanism. In this chapter, the normal and abnormal anatomy of the palate and velopharynx is reviewed. In the second portion, various classification systems used to categorize different types of clefts of the lip, alveolus, and palate are examined.

Surface Anatomy

On examination of the oral cavity, the mucosa of the anterior portion of the hard palate has an irregular surface covered by rugae. The posterior portion of the hard palate and the soft palate are covered by a smooth mucosal surface. The incisive papilla is just posterior to the alveolar ridge. The median raphe originates at the incisive papilla and extends posteriorly to the uvula, dividing the palate in half. The soft palate ends with the uvula, which hangs in the oropharyngeal opening.

There are two folds on the surface of each side of the posterolateral walls of the oral cavity. These are known as the tonsillar pillars (also referred to as arches). The palatoglossal muscle forms the anterior pillar. The palatopharyngeal muscle forms the posterior pillar. The palatine tonsil resides between these two pillars.

A horizontal ridge may occasionally be noted on the posterior wall of the pharynx during active muscle movement. This ridge, named for Passavant, who described it in 1869,[1] may be noted in normal individuals.[2,3] More commonly, it is found in those patients with a cleft of the palate[1] or with some other reason for incompetence of the velopharyngeal mechanism. Debate exists among authors as to whether the superior pharyngeal constrictor[4,5] or the horizontal fibers of the palatopharyngeus form Passavant ridge.[6]

The hard palate is covered by a keratinized stratified squamous epithelium.[7] This mucosa is tightly adherent to the underlying periosteum. The epithelial surface in this region is well adapted to handle the abrasive nature of forming the food bolus. Markus[8] divided the hard palate mucosa into three zones. The palatal fibromucosa composes the central portion of the palate. It is thin centrally and thickens laterally to where the palate begins to curve downward. At this downward curve is the transition into the maxillary fibromucosa. This portion of the mucosa is thicker and contains the neurovascular bundle. The mucosa then thins into the gingival fibromucosa, which is the vertical portion of the mucosa between the teeth and the lateral border of the maxillary fibromucosa. In the newborn, the gingival fibromucosa covers only the alveolar ridge.

The soft palate mucosa is composed of a nonkeratinized stratified squamous epithelium[9] on its oral surface. The nasal mucosa of the palate is covered by a ciliated columnar epithelium suited for respiratory functions.[7] The anterior portion of the nasal surface of the velum is covered by a pseudostratified ciliated columnar epithelium.[9] This respiratory epithelium abruptly makes a transition into stratified squamous epithelium at 40% to 60% of the soft palate's length. This stratified squamous epithelium then covers the remaining 30% of the nasal surface of the velum. Thus, the epithelium in the anterior portion of the velum is suited for respiration, whereas the posterior portion is suited more for the abrasive action of abutting the posterior pharyngeal wall as occurs during the act of closure of the velopharynx.[9] Laterally, a band of transitional epithelium composed of a mixture of stratified and ciliated epithelium exists between the two different mucosal types.

Skeletal Anatomy

The bones of relevance to the hard palate and velopharyngeal apparatus are the maxilla, palatine, vomer, sphenoid, and temporal (Figs. 89-1 and 89-2). The palatine process of the maxilla forms the anterior portion of the hard palate. The posterior portion of the hard palate is formed by the horizontal laminae of the palatine bone. The maxilla and palatine bones meet at the transverse palatine suture (palatomaxillary suture). Both the palatine process of the maxilla and the horizontal plates of the palatine bones join the vomer in the midline. In cleft of the hard palate, the vomer can be seen in the midline in the nasal cavity. In a unilateral cleft palate, the vomer remains attached to the noncleft side of the palate.

The premaxilla, the anterior portion of the maxilla, develops from the frontonasal process. The palatal shelves of the maxilla, the posterior portion (also referred to as the lateral segment), are derived from the maxillary processes. The incisive suture marks the junction of the premaxilla and the palatal shelves of the maxilla. The median palatine suture divides the palate in half and runs from between the central incisors anteriorly to the posterior nasal spine. The Y formed by the incisive sutures and the posterior portion of the median palatine suture marks the course of epithelial fusion between the palatal shelves and the premaxilla.[10] Clefts of the alveolus and hard palate occur along these suture lines. The median palatine suture plays an important role in the transverse growth of the maxilla and is the site of the osteotomy for palatal expansion.

The incisive foramen is located in the premaxilla-derived portion of the palate. The nasopalatine nerve

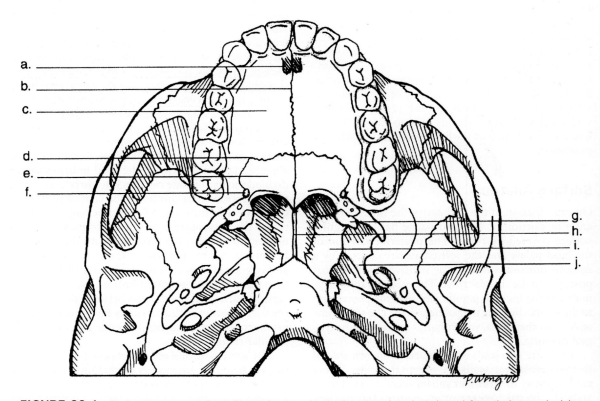

FIGURE 89-1. Skeletal anatomy of maxilla, palate, and velopharyngeal region viewed from below. a, incisive foramen; b, median palatine suture; c, horizontal plate of the maxilla; d, transverse palatine suture; e, horizontal plate of the palatine bone; f, greater palatine foramen; g, pterygoid hamulus; h, vomer; i, medial pterygoid plate; j, lateral pterygoid plate.

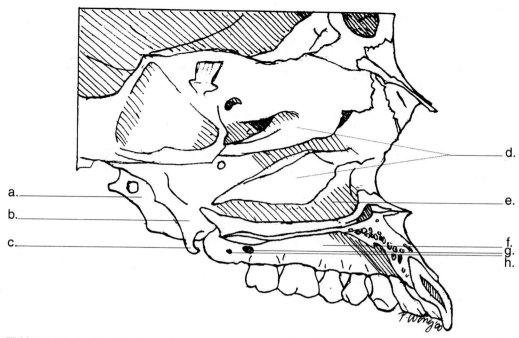

a.
b.
c.

d.
e.
f.
g.
h.

FIGURE 89-2. Sagittal view of bone anatomy of maxilla, palate, and velopharyngeal region. a, lateral pterygoid plate; b, medial pterygoid plate; c, pterygoid hamulus; d, nasal conchae; e, maxilla; f, alveolar process of the maxilla; g, greater palatine foramen; h, lesser palatine foramen.

and the posterior septal branch of the sphenopalatine artery reach the palate through the incisive foramen to supply the premaxilla.

The alveolar process is the ridge of bone on the maxilla that provides support for the teeth. This bone develops with tooth eruption and resorbs when teeth are lost. The central and lateral incisors are located in the premaxillary segment. The canines, bicuspids, and molar teeth are located in the lateral segments of the maxilla. Clefts of the palate form along the epithelial fusion plane between the premaxilla and the lateral segments of the maxilla. Thus, when a cleft is present in the alveolar ridge of the maxilla, there is a risk for involvement of the lateral incisor in the cleft process.

The horizontal plate of the palatine bone makes up the posterior portion of the hard palate. The greater palatine and lesser palatine foramina are located in the posterolateral portion of the bone. The greater and lesser palatine neurovascular bundles, respectively, pass through these foramina. The palatal aponeurosis attaches to the posterior border of the palatine bones.[11]

The sphenoid and temporal bones of the cranial base are also relevant to the structure of the palate and velopharynx. These two bones serve as the origin for several of the muscles involved in the functioning of the velopharyngeal apparatus. The sphenoid is posterior to the palatine bones. It has two vertical processes, the medial and lateral pterygoid plates. The pterygoid hamulus extends from the inferior portion of the medial pterygoid plate and serves as a pulley for the tensor veli palatini muscle. The temporal bone is posterior and lateral to the sphenoid bone. It contains the orifice to the bony portion of the eustachian tube. The cartilaginous portion of the eustachian tube takes its origin from the bony portion and travels inferior, medial, and anterior to reach the pharynx. The opening of the eustachian tube is just above the level of the hard palate on the lateral pharyngeal wall. The torus tubarius, the enlarged pharyngeal end of the eustachian tube, is an inbulging of the pharyngeal wall posterior to the tubal opening.

Anomalies of the cranial base have been found in association with clefts of the palate. This has suggested to some that cleft palate may be part of a craniofacial syndrome.[12] Maue-Dickson[13] reported that cleft palate is associated with an abnormally wide cranial base. In her studies, the eustachian tube lumens were found to be narrower and smaller than in noncleft individuals. In addition, the tubal cartilage was enlarged and more widely separated than in the normal individuals. The pterygoid plates were found to be widely separated; the pharyngeal width was increased, with the pharyngeal height being reduced. She believed that this could have a negative impact on the functioning of the eustachian tube.

Soft Tissue and Muscle Anatomy

The muscles in the velopharyngeal region play a role in swallowing, speech production, and auditory tube function. Four of the muscles that insert into the soft palate have their origins extrinsic to the velum; these are the tensor veli palatini, the levator veli palatini, the palatoglossus, and the palatopharyngeus. These muscles form opposing slings that meet in the soft palate raphe (Figs. 89-3 and 89-4). The tensor veli palatini and the levator veli palatini each form a superior sling, and the palatoglossus and the palatopharyngeus each form inferior ones. The origins of these muscles are unaffected in the cleft process. The musculus uvulae is the only muscle whose origin is intrinsic to the velum. Also of note are the superior pharyngeal constrictor, the salpingopharyngeus, and the stylopharyngeus muscles. These three muscles are located in the walls of the pharynx.

Between the two epithelial layers of the soft palate, the histologic composition of the velum varies (Fig. 89-5).[9] The oral aspect of the anterior half of the soft palate is composed of seromucous glands and adipose tissue that decrease in amount as one moves posteriorly. On the nasal side of the soft palate, the opposite is true. Seromucous glands and adipose tissue are less prevalent in the anterior portion of the velum and increase in number as one moves toward the uvula.

The tensor veli palatini tendon, which makes the transition into the palatal aponeurosis, is closer to the nasal portion of the velum, occupying the anterior 20% of soft palatal length. Kuehn and Kahane[9] hypothesized that the tensor tendon may act to relieve the stress due to movement at the junction between the hard and soft palates. They liken the aponeurosis to the protective collar at the junction of an electrical plug and the wire cord extending from the plug. The collar protects the wire from breakage due to stressful movement at the interface between the stiff and mobile structures.

The levator veli palatini muscle begins in the most anterior portion of the soft palate. It is sandwiched between the tensor veli palatini tendon and the seromucous glands on the oral side of the palate. It is most prominent at 20% to 30% of the palate's length until about 60% of palatal length. Fibers from the palatoglossus and palatopharyngeus (palatothyroideus) muscles can be found to intermingle with those of the levator in the medial third of soft palatal length.

The musculus uvulae, the only intrinsic muscle of the palate, is superior to the levator veli palatini muscle and is cradled by it. It begins at approximately 25% and disappears at about 70% of velar length. A surrounding ring of collagenous fibers adds intrinsic support to the musculus uvulae.

The pendulous uvula occupies the last 20% of the soft palate's length. A highly vascular structure, it contains few if any muscle fibers. It is predominantly composed of adipose, collagen, and glandular tissues.

Elastic fibers exist in the subepithelial layer of the anterior half of the velum. These fibers are believed to help restore velar shape after its deformation by a food bolus. These elastic fibers may also assist in keeping the nasopharyngeal mechanism patent during sleep.[14]

The tensor veli palatini originates from the spine and scaphoid fossa of the sphenoid bone as well as from the lateral side of the cartilaginous portion of the eustachian tube. The muscle travels in an inferior and anterior direction to take a right-angle turn around the pterygoid hamulus, assuming a horizontal orientation as it passes into the substance of the velum. Within the velum, the tendon of the tensor veli palatini fans into the palatal aponeurosis, joining with the fibers from the aponeurosis of the opposite side. It is underneath the nasal mucosa and occupies the anterior 25% of the soft palate. It attaches anteriorly to the posterior border of the hard palate. Some have reported that the aponeurosis serves as an anterior insertion point for the levator veli palatini, palatopharyngeus, and musculus uvulae[15]; others disagree on this point.[16] The tensor veli palatini is the only velar muscle innervated by the trigeminal nerve through its mandibular branch. The other muscles of the palate are innervated by the pharyngeal plexus composed of branches from the glossopharyngeal nerve (IX), the vagus nerve (X), and the accessory nerve (XI).

Variability exists among authors in the description of this muscle. Some authors have described superior extensions of the muscle to join the tensor tympani muscle.[17] Attachments have also been described from the muscle to the hamulus[18] and to the maxillary tuberosity.[17,19]

Three factors are necessary for eustachian tube function: the opening of the tube, a pressure differential between the middle ear and the pharynx, and the production of surfactant to overcome the surface tension within the tube. The primary function of the tensor veli palatini muscle is to open the eustachian tube. As will be elaborated on later, the levator veli palatini may also play a role in eustachian tube function. If the tensor does indeed insert into the hamulus as some believe, complete fracture of the hamulus to achieve mobility of the soft tissues during palate repair may have a detrimental effect on the tensor's ability to open the eustachian tube.[20]

Some have also postulated that the muscle plays a role in tensing the velum. Although no physiologic evidence exists to support this possible function, it cannot be ruled out on the basis of the anatomic course and position of the muscle.[16] More likely, though, the aponeurosis acts to reinforce the transition between the immobile hard palate and the mobile soft palate.

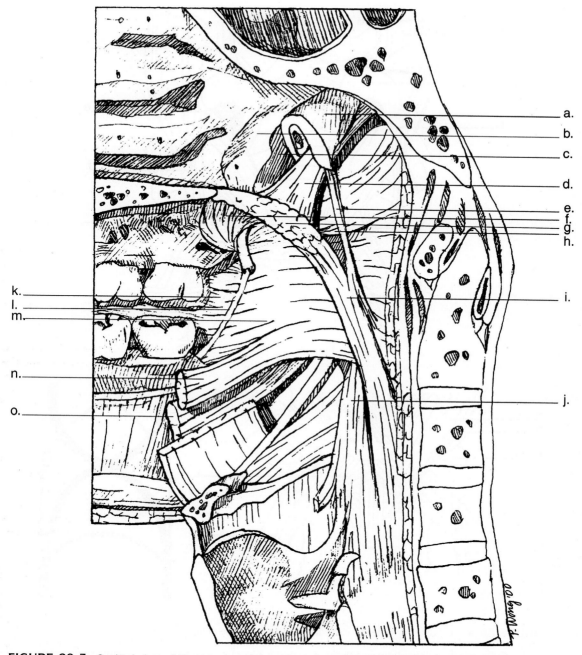

FIGURE 89-3. Sagittal view of the muscles of the velopharyngeal mechanism. a, eustachian tube; b, medial pterygoid plate; c, tensor veli palatini; d, levator veli palatini; e, salpingopharyngeus; f, palatine aponeurosis; g, confluence of the muscles of the soft palate; h, location of Passavant ridge; i, palatopharyngeus; j, stylopharyngeus; k, buccinator; l, pterygomandibular raphe; m, superior pharyngeal constrictor; n, glossopharyngeus; o, styloglossus.

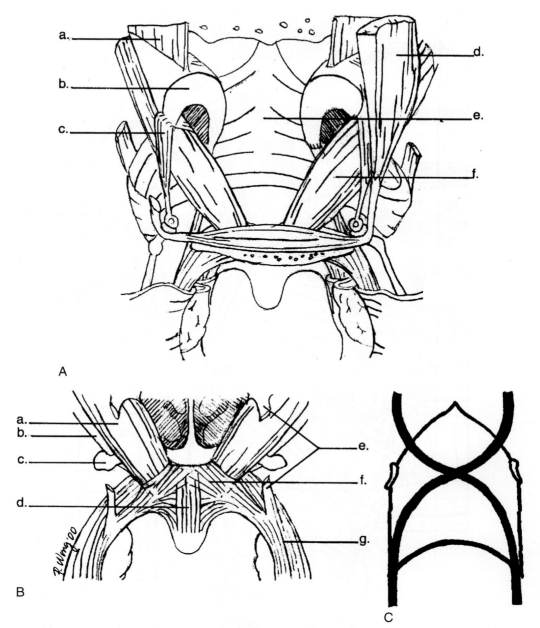

A

B

C

FIGURE 89-4. *A,* Posterior-anterior view of the muscles of the velopharyngeal mechanism. a, superior tubal ligament; b, eustachian tube; c, tensor veli palatini (pulls hook of eustachian cartilage downward); d, tensor veli palatini (tenses palate); e, superior pharyngeal constrictor; f, levator veli palatini. (After Proctor B: Anatomy of the eustachian tube. Arch Otolaryngol 1973;97:2.) *B,* Opposing slings formed by the tensor veli palatini and levator veli palatini muscles above and the palatoglossus and palatopharyngeus muscles below. a, levator veli palatini; b, tensor veli palatini; c, hamulus; d, musculus uvulae; e, salpingopharyngeus (cut); f, palatothyroideus; g, palatopharyngeus. *C,* Simplified diagram illustrating opposing slings. (After Millard DR: Anatomy of the palate. In Millard DR: Cleft Craft: The Evolution of Its Surgery, vol III. Alveolar and Palatal Deformities. Boston, Little, Brown, 1980:19.)

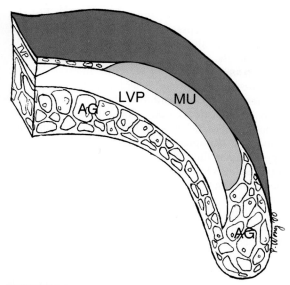

FIGURE 89-5. Histology of the soft palate. AG, adipose and glandular tissue; LVP, levator veli palatini; MU, musculus uvulae; TVP, tensor veli palatini. (After Kuehn DP, Kahane JC: Histologic study of the normal human adult soft palate. Cleft Palate J 1990;27:26.)

The levator veli palatini originates from the petrous portion of the temporal bone just below the eustachian tube[16] and from the posteromedial aspect of the junction of the bony and cartilaginous portions of the eustachian tube.[20] From its origin, it passes alongside the eustachian tube and then lateral to the torus tubarius to enter the soft palate. Within the substance of the soft palate, the muscle fibers pass inferior to the musculus uvulae and join the levator fibers from the opposite side to form a muscular sling in the intermediate 40% of velar length.[21] Muscle fibers from the palatoglossus and palatopharyngeus (palatothyroideus) muscles penetrate into the levator and intermingle with its fibers. Dimples visualized on the oral surface of the soft palate while an "ah" sound is made represent the point at which the levator and palatopharyngeal muscle fibers intermingle.[22]

The function of the levator muscle is to elevate and lengthen the velum toward the posterior pharyngeal wall for closure of the velopharyngeal mechanism. Authors have also postulated that the muscle effects lateral pharyngeal wall movement in the region of the torus tubarius.[16] Whereas some have postulated a role for the levator in eustachian tube function,[20] others have refuted this function of the muscle.[12] If the levator does play a role in eustachian tube function, it appears to be as a tubal dilator.[20] Malpositioning of the muscle in the individual with cleft palate compromises this function and may even obstruct the opening of the tube.[19] This levator pathologic process has been con-

sidered to play a role in the development of serous otitis media in the patient with cleft palate.

The palatoglossus muscle arises from the dorsum and sides of the tongue. It travels up through the anterior tonsillar pillar to enter into the soft palate. Its fibers intermingle with those of the levator veli palatini muscle in the substance of the velum. The direction of this muscle is opposite to that of the levator. Thus, it has been postulated that its action is to pull the soft palate forward and down.[16] Electromyographic evidence[23] suggests rather that the role of the palatoglossus is in tongue functioning. Thus, the muscle probably plays a role in the swallowing mechanism and tongue resting position.

In the palate, the palatopharyngeus muscle inserts into the posterior border of the hard palate and palatine aponeurosis as well as having fibers that intermingle with the levator muscle fibers. The muscle also forms a sling by joining fibers from the opposite side. The palatopharyngeus travels through the posterior tonsillar pillar. In the pharyngeal walls, the muscle fibers commingle with the fibers of the superior pharyngeal constrictor. The muscle also has an insertion into the thyroid cartilage. For this reason, some authors have advocated calling the horizontally oriented muscle fibers the palatopharyngeus muscle and the vertically oriented fibers a separate muscle, the palatothyroideus.[7]

The anatomic position of the muscle suggests that it functions to depress the soft palate or to elevate and constrict the oropharynx. Thus, the muscle would play a role in the pharyngeal stage of swallowing. Some have suggested that the muscle acts to assist the levator by providing a proper vector for the velum during closure of the velopharyngeal mechanism. Research has not confirmed this role for the muscle.[16] It has also been suggested that the muscle may contribute to lateral pharyngeal wall movement.[6,11] It may be that the palatothyroideus is a depressor of the soft palate and the palatopharyngeus moves the pharyngeal walls.[7]

The musculus uvulae is the only intrinsic muscle of the palate. It is a paired muscle that is the most superiorly located of the muscles of the velum. It is longitudinally oriented and resides on the nasal side of the levator veli palatini. The musculus uvulae originates from the palatine aponeurosis and reaches an indistinct termination at the base of the uvula, with some studies suggesting muscle fibers that penetrate into the substance of the uvula. In general, the bulk of the muscle occupies the middle 40% of velar length.

The musculus uvulae assists the levator in obtaining closure of the velopharyngeal apparatus. Electromyographic studies have confirmed that the muscle is active during all speech tasks and often parallels the activity of the levator.[24] Solitary contraction of the levator results in a midline concavity in the velum. With closure of the velopharyngeal mechanism, however, a bulge is seen on the nasal surface of the soft palate. This "levator eminence" (also referred to as uvulus eminence or velar knee) is probably formed by both the musculus uvulae and the levator veli palatini muscles.[25] Loss of this eminence in individuals with velopharyngeal incompetence, whether from submucous or overt clefts of the palate, is likely to be due to abnormalities of both the levator and the musculus uvulae.

Whether the musculus uvulae plays a passive role as a bulk of tissue to fill a space or an active role as a velar extensor or a stiffness modifier to prevent velopharyngeal insufficiency is unclear and debatable.[24,25] Blockade of the lesser palatine nerve, the nerve to the musculus uvulae, did not cause velopharyngeal incompetence or have an effect on the nasoendoscopic appearance of the velopharyngeal mechanism during phonation.[21] This lends support for a passive role of the musculus uvulae in velopharyngeal function. A short-term block, however, does not mimic the condition of an atrophied, hypoplastic muscle. Nevertheless, abnormalities of the musculus uvulae may contribute to velopharyngeal insufficiency.[12]

Three other muscles warrant consideration in a discussion of the velopharyngeal apparatus. They are the superior pharyngeal constrictor, the salpingopharyngeus, and the stylopharyngeus. The superior pharyngeal constrictor muscle originates from the posterior pharyngeal raphe and courses downward and forward to insert into the pterygoid hamulus, the lateral pterygoid plate, the pterygomaxillary ligament, the mandible, and the floor of the mouth. This muscle exists below the level of the hard palate, and thus it probably does not play a role in velopharyngeal function during speech production. The salpingopharyngeus resides within the salpingopharyngeal fold. Many authors have not found any true muscle fibers to exist within the fold, and if any are present, their functional significance is unknown.[16] This muscle originates from the posterior surface of the end of the cartilaginous eustachian tube and ends inferiorly by mingling with the pharyngeal portion of the palatopharyngeus muscle. The stylopharyngeal muscle arises from the styloid process of the temporal bone. It inserts between the fibers of the superior and middle pharyngeal muscles into the pharyngeal wall. It does not have a role in velopharyngeal closure for speech.

When a cleft of the soft palate is present, the anatomic abnormalities of the musculature (Fig. 89-6) are confined to the portion that is within the substance of the palate.[6,23] In the process, the muscles are displaced anterolaterally and the palatal aponeurosis is displaced laterally.[26] The extrinsic velar portions of the muscles are normal. The pathologic process is a failure of the fusion of the components of the soft palate in the midline, which occurs in an anterior to posterior direction. Varying degrees of the cleft defect may exist. These range from a submucous cleft palate,

in which the mucosa of the palate is intact but the muscles fail to decussate in the midline, to a complete cleft of the lip, alveolus, hard palate, and soft palate. Instead of the muscle fibers being transverse in orientation and decussating with the fibers from the opposite side, they are oriented anteriorly.[19] The muscles of the palate and the palatal aponeurosis are often hypoplastic as well.[6] The thinner the muscle bellies are, the thicker is the layer of loose connective tissue that occupies the muscle bed.[6] Koch et al[27] reported that the palatal aponeurosis exists in cleft patients but is folded on itself. Their paper advocated the unfolding of the aponeurosis during the repair of the velum.

The muscle fibers of each hemipalate converge along the medial border of the cleft. This is the cleft muscle described by Veau[5] in 1931. It is composed of the fibers of the musculus uvulae, the levator veli palatini, and the palatopharyngeus. The fibers from the musculus uvulae and the medial fibers of the palatopharyngeus insert into fibrous tissue along the medial border of the velar cleft. Lateral fibers from the palatopharyngeus travel forward to insert into the palatal aponeurosis and the medial border of the cleft of the hard palate.[19] These fibers end just short of the transverse palatomaxillary suture. The tensor veli palatini (the palatal aponeurosis) and palatoglossus muscles insert along the posterior border of the hard palate.

In repair of the cleft of the velum, the goal is to develop normal soft palate anatomy and the opposing muscle slings. To accomplish this, the surgeon must release the muscles from their abnormal attachments to the posterior and medial edges of the hard palate. The muscles must then be reoriented transversely. The exception is the musculus uvulae, which needs to remain longitudinally oriented but repositioned to the nasal side of the velum. Of note, the Furlow double opposing Z-plasty incorrectly reorients the musculus uvulae in an oblique direction.[25]

Vascular Anatomy

The maxilla, alveolus, teeth, and hard palate are included in the segment mobilized when a Le Fort I osteotomy is performed. Many authors have studied the vascular supply of this region (Fig. 89-7).[28-33] An anastomotic network exists between the maxillary artery, the facial artery, and the ascending pharyngeal artery to bring blood supply to this segment. The branches of the maxillary artery, in particular its third or pterygopalatine portion, are the predominant vascular supply to the segment (i.e., the alveolus, maxilla, teeth, and hard palate). These branches include the descending palatine artery, the sphenopalatine artery, the posterior superior alveolar artery, and the infraorbital artery. The facial artery contributions to the network include the superior labial artery and the

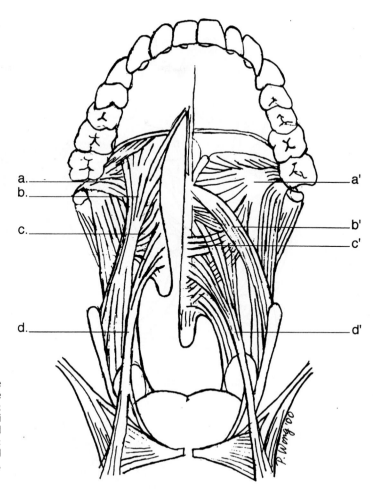

FIGURE 89-6. Normal palate muscle anatomy (x′) versus cleft palate muscle anatomy (x). a, palatine aponeurosis; b, palatopharyngeus muscle; c, levator veli palatini; d, palatoglossus. (After Millard DR: Anatomy of the palate. In Millard DR: Cleft Craft: The Evolution of Its Surgery, vol III. Alveolar and Palatal Deformities. Boston, Little, Brown, 1980:19.)

buccal branches of the facial artery, which together contribute supply to the Le Fort I segment. The ascending palatine branch of the facial artery and the ascending pharyngeal artery, which enter through the soft palate, also contribute to this vast interconnected network of vessels.

The descending palatine artery, a branch of the maxillary artery, travels through the pterygopalatine canal within the posterior wall of the maxillary sinus to reach the palate. In its course through the canal, the descending palatine artery divides into the greater and lesser palatine arteries and has branches that supply the bony hard palate.[23] The greater palatine artery is the predominant blood supply to the hard palate (Fig. 89-8). It enters the oral side of the palate through the greater palatine foramen. It then proceeds anteriorly in the mucoperiosteal layer of the hard palate toward the incisive foramen. Posteriorly, anastomoses exist between the greater palatine artery and the ascending palatine artery, which is the vascular supply of the soft palate.[29] Interconnections also exist between the right and left greater palatine arteries across the median raphe. The

lesser palatine artery turns posteriorly to supply the oral side of the anterior half of the velum.[30] This vessel, however, has not been found to be a major contributor to the blood supply of the soft palate.

The sphenopalatine artery, like the descending palatine artery, is a branch of the maxillary artery. The nasopalatine branch of the sphenopalatine artery travels along the vomer to reach the incisive canal, which it enters to supply blood to the premaxilla. The posterior septal branches of the nasopalatine artery supply the nasal side of the palate. Most authors report anastomoses between the greater palatine artery and the nasopalatine artery once it exits the incisive foramen.[31] In addition, numerous osseous perforating vessels were found connecting the nasal mucosal vasculature to the oral palatal mucoperiosteal vasculature, again linking the nasopalatine arterial supply to the greater palatine arterial supply. Thus, the blood supply to the bony hard palate arrives from two sources, the descending palatine artery and its greater palatine branch and the sphenopalatine artery and its nasopalatine branch. This dual blood supply is what allows

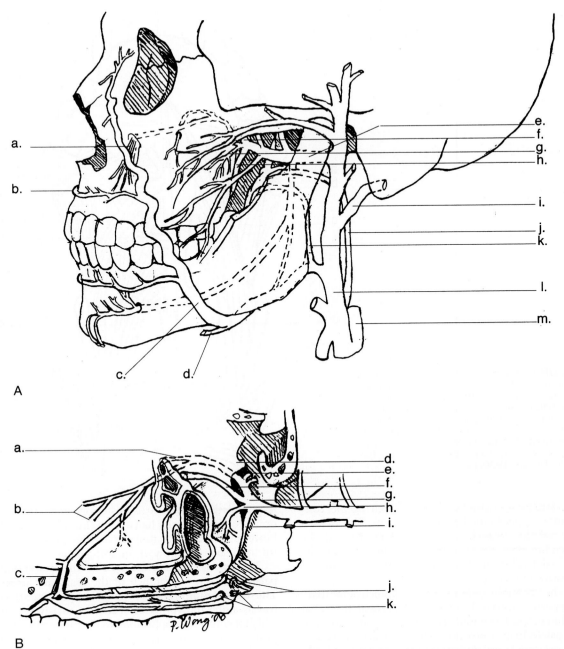

FIGURE 89-7. *A,* Arterial anatomy of the Le Fort I segment. a, infraorbital artery; b, superior labial artery; c, facial artery; d, inferior alveolar artery; e, maxillary artery; f, sphenopalatine artery; g, posterior superior alveolar artery; h, descending palatine artery; i, occipital artery; j, ascending pharyngeal artery; k, ascending palatine artery; l, external carotid artery; m, internal carotid artery. *B,* Close-up view of the bone relationships to the branches of the maxillary artery. a, posterior lateral nasal artery; b, posterior septal branches of the sphenopalatine artery; c, nasopalatine artery and incisive canal; d, sphenopalatine artery; e, sphenopalatine foramen; f, infraorbital artery; g, maxillary artery; h, posterior superior alveolar artery; i, descending palatine artery in the pterygopalatine fossa; j, lesser palatine arteries; k, greater palatine artery. (After Millard DR: Anatomy of the palate. In Millard DR: Cleft Craft: The Evolution of Its Surgery, vol III. Alveolar and Palatal Deformities. Boston, Little, Brown, 1980:19.)

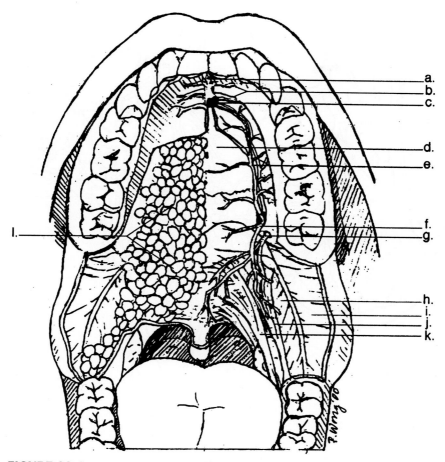

FIGURE 89-8. Arterial anatomy of the hard palate. a, incisive papilla; b, transverse palatine folds; c, incisive fossa; d, palatine process of the maxilla; e, greater palatine artery and nerve; f, lesser palatine artery; g, lesser palatine nerve; h, buccinator; i, superior pharyngeal constrictor; j, palatoglossus; k, palatopharyngeus; l, palatine glands. (After Millard DR: Anatomy of the palate. In Millard DR: Cleft Craft: The Evolution of Its Surgery, vol III. Alveolar and Palatal Deformities. Boston, Little, Brown, 1980:19.)

the oral mucoperiosteal flap to be elevated for palatal closure with the continued viability of the bony hard palate. Studies by Welsh cited in Millard's text *Cleft Craft*[23] failed to confirm the anastomosis between the nasopalatine and greater palatine vessels.

The posterior superior alveolar artery arises either directly from the maxillary artery or from the maxillary artery by a short common trunk it shares with the infraorbital artery. This vessel arises from the maxillary artery within the pterygopalatine fossa. It travels anteriorly along the maxilla to the alveolar ridge, where it supplies the maxillary dentition as far forward as the central incisors.

The infraorbital artery arises from the maxillary artery, travels through the infraorbital canal, and exits the infraorbital foramen. Branches of the infraorbital artery also contribute to the anastomotic network

between the maxillary and facial arteries that supply the Le Fort I segment. Some authors describe an anterior superior alveolar branch of the infraorbital artery, which brings blood to the anterior alveolar ridge and teeth. Other authors, however, have failed to confirm the existence of this vessel.[31]

The vast anastomotic system formed by the arteries around the Le Fort I segment terminates as a vascular plexus within the gingiva and mucosa.[28] These vessels penetrate the cortical bone to anastomose with the periodontal plexus (Fig. 89-9). Branches of this periodontal plexus as well as the interosseous dental alveolar branches of the superior alveolar vessels supply the dental pulps of the maxillary dentition.

This network is important to maintenance of blood supply to the developing and permanent maxillary dentition during surgery in this region. Bell[28]

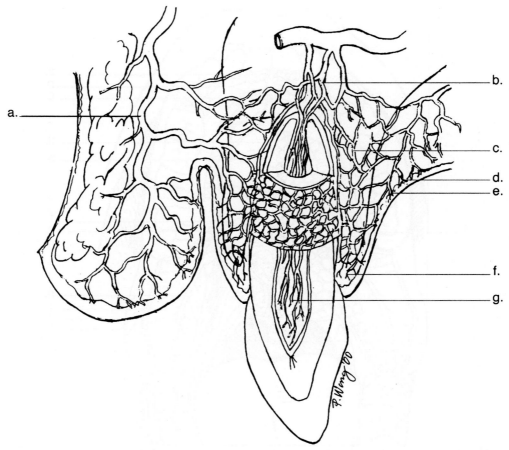

FIGURE 89-9. Alveolar and dental arterial anatomy. a, labial artery; b, apical vessels; c, intra-alveolar vessels; d, palatal plexus; e, periodontal plexus; f, gingival plexus; g, pulp vessels. (After Bell WH: Biologic basis for maxillary osteotomies. Am J Phys Anthropol 1973;38:279. Reproduced with permission of Wiley-Liss, Inc., a subsidiary of John Wiley & Sons, Inc.)

demonstrated that the viability of the maxillary dental alveolar segments is maintained even if the vessels entering through the incisive canal or the greater palatine artery are sacrificed. For example, this occurs when the lateral incisions are made for the medial mobilization of the hard palate mucoperiosteal flaps during cleft palate repair. During this maneuver, the contributions of the greater palatine artery are divided; however, viability of the developing dentition is maintained. In addition, Bell demonstrated that the viability of the teeth is not compromised by subapical or interdental osteotomies as long as the bone cuts are placed away from the apices of the teeth and either the lingual or buccal mucoperiosteal attachments are maintained to the mobilized segment. In both instances, the viability of the teeth is maintained by the numerous other contributions to the anastomotic vascular network.

The soft palate and its musculature are supplied primarily by the ascending palatine artery.[29,30] This vessel is a branch of the facial artery in the majority of people.[29] It may also originate from the ascending pharyngeal artery, from the maxillary artery, or directly from the external carotid artery. After its origin, the vessel courses by the styloid musculature, ascending on the lateral side of the superior constrictor muscle to enter the lateral pharyngeal space. In this space, branches of the ascending palatine artery supply the origins of both the tensor and levator veli palatini muscles. The vessel continues dividing into an anterior and posterior branch, both of which enter the soft palate. The anterior branch of the ascending palatine artery travels along the anterior border of the levator, passing within 1 mm of the hamulus. It terminates in the anterior third of the soft palate. This vessel is at risk for injury when a lateral relaxing incision is performed and during manipulation of the hamulus to achieve medial mobilization of the palate to allow a tension-free repair. There is also a risk for injury to this vessel when the musculature of the soft palate is dissected off the posterior border of the hard palate to allow the reorientation of these muscles in the transverse direction.[29] This area, the junction of the hard and soft palates, is also farthest from the blood supply and at an increased risk for ischemia with more extensive dissection.

The predominant blood supply of the soft palate comes from the posterior branch of the ascending palatine artery. This vessel has a variable course in relation to the levator veli palatini in the soft palate. The vessel may course above, below, or through the muscle itself. Extensive dissection of the levator muscle during intravelar veloplasty can place the vessel and hence the blood supply to the velum at risk. Once it is past the levator, the artery adopts a superficial position below the nasal mucosa on its way to supply blood to the musculus uvulae. The location where the artery penetrates the musculus uvulae can be variable. The more anterior it is in its entrance to the musculus uvulae, the greater the risk of damage to the vessel (i.e., from mobilization of the levator veli palatini). This may result in atrophy of the muscle and failure of it to function normally after repair.[29]

Some authors have reported a secondary extrapalatal arterial supply to the soft palate from the ascending pharyngeal artery and from the accessory meningeal artery. Girgis[34] noted branches of the ascending pharyngeal artery or direct branches from the external carotid artery that ascended in the posterior tonsillar pillar to supply blood to the uvular region of the soft palate. Freedlander[35] reported that a dual blood supply exists for the tensor and levator veli palatini. The tensor veli palatini received its blood supply from the ascending palatine artery and the accessory meningeal artery. In the levator veli palatini, dual supply was from the ascending palatine artery and the ascending pharyngeal artery. In five patients, the ascending pharyngeal artery was the exclusive blood supply to the levator. Mercer and MacCarthy[29] did not find significant vascular contributions to exist from the accessory meningeal artery to the tensor or from the ascending pharyngeal artery to the levator. Obviously, some variability does exist in velar blood supply.

Also of importance to the cleft palate surgeon is the relationship of the internal carotid artery to the structures of the velopharyngeal apparatus. This vessel travels lateral to the lateral pharyngeal wall and has been demonstrated to lie within 1 to 1.5 cm of the typical incisions used for pharyngeal flaps in the adult.[36] It has also been demonstrated that the vessel may deviate from its normal course in children with velocardiofacial syndrome. Preoperative imaging studies have been advocated to evaluate the location of the vessel before pharyngoplasty surgery is performed.

Maher[31] also studied the cleft palate vascular supply. The only effect on the vascular network is that the connections between vessels across the cleft are not present. Instead, he demonstrated that the palate and mucoperiosteal blood supply wrapped around the bony border of the cleft to anastomose with vessels from the nasal mucosal side instead of the vessels from the contralateral palate.

Nerve Supply

The muscles related to the soft palate perform two functions, regulation of pressure of the middle ear by way of the eustachian tube and movement of the velopharynx. Neural innervation of the muscles involved in these two separate actions differs. The tensor tympani and tensor veli palatini both work to aid in pressure equalization in the middle ear. The mandibular branch of the trigeminal nerve (cranial nerve V) innervates the tensor veli palatini. The tensor tympani is also innervated by the trigeminal nerve. This similar innervation seems to allow the coordinated actions of these two muscles and lends further evidence to the role of the tensor veli palatini in eustachian tube function.

The remaining muscles of the soft palate participate in the functioning of the velopharyngeal apparatus. These muscles share a common innervation that may play a role in coordinating their action on velar movement. In the cat, the cell bodies in the region of the brain known as the nucleus ambiguus control soft palate movement.[37] These cell bodies contribute to the glossopharyngeal nerve (IX), the pharyngeal branch of the vagus nerve (X), and the accessory nerve (XI). These nerves have been shown through human cadaver dissection to collectively form the pharyngeal plexus. Nerve fibers from this plexus innervate the muscles involved in the movement of the velum.[30,38,39] The musculus uvulae receives innervation from the glossopharyngeal nerve by way of the lesser palatine nerve.[38] Nishio[39] noted activity in the facial nerve with the action of the levator, musculus uvulae, and superior pharyngeal constrictor in monkeys. Whether contributions of the facial nerve play a role in humans is unclear; other authors have not confirmed this finding.

The motor nerves to the soft palate, with the exception of the nerve to the tensor veli palatini, reach their respective muscles by coursing behind the lateral pharyngeal walls. Thus, extensive dissection in this region would place these nerves at risk for injury. Similarly, extensive intravelar dissection at the junction of the hard and soft palates would place the lesser palatine nerve at risk. Injury to this nerve would have an effect on functioning of the musculus uvulae and could lead to atrophy of this muscle. This could lead to velopharyngeal incompetence.

Sensory innervation to the alveolus and the hard and soft palates is derived primarily from the infraorbital branch of the maxillary portion of the trigeminal nerve. Branches from the infraorbital nerve contribute to the formation of the pterygopalatine ganglion. The greater and lesser palatine nerves arise from the pterygopalatine ganglion and travel with their respective arteries to reach the hard and soft palates. The greater palatine nerve emerges from the greater palatine foramen and receives sensation from the posterior portion of the hard palate. The lesser palatine nerves emerge from the lesser palatine foramen and receive sensory information from the oral surface of the soft palate. The nasopalatine branch of the infraorbital nerve passes through the incisive foramen to reach the anterior hard palate (the premaxilla).

The alveolus and teeth receive sensory innervation from fibers of the anterior, middle, and posterior superior alveolar nerves. The posterior and middle superior alveolar nerves arise from the infraorbital nerve after it leaves the pterygopalatine fossa. The anterior superior alveolar nerve is a branch of the infraorbital nerve after it exits the infraorbital foramen. Branches of these nerves are divided when a maxillary vestibular incision is made, such as in orthognathic surgery of the maxilla. This contributes to the temporary numbness of the dentition and gingiva noted by many of these patients in the postoperative period.

Summary

Clefts of the palate are caused by a failure of mesodermal penetration in the primary palate and a failure of fusion of the palatal shelves in the secondary palate. If one does not have a thorough knowledge and understanding of the normal and pathologic anatomy of this region, the risks for injury to the structures involved and the chances of failure of any procedure to correct the underlying pathologic process are increased.

CLASSIFICATION OF ALVEOLAR AND PALATAL CLEFTS

The purpose of a classification system is to arrange clefts into groups on the basis of defined criteria for documentation and record keeping. This system can then be used as a guide in treatment planning or for prognostic information with regard to outcomes and results. A classification system is essential to allow communication between the various members of the cleft palate team as well as between cleft teams. Ideally, for a classification system to be effective, it must be universally adopted. It should be concise and easy to use. The terms used must be adequately defined, and it should be reproducible and uniform such that any evaluator would classify a cleft into the same group. Several classification systems have been proposed over time. These have been arranged along morphologic, anatomic, and embryologic guidelines.

Davis and Ritchie[40] reported one of the earliest systems of classification in the *Journal of the American Medical Association* in 1922. They proposed a system based on morphologic characteristics. Clefts were categorized on the basis of the alveolar process, which they believed formed the foundation for a surgical grouping. Clefts were divided into three groups: group I, prealveolar clefts; group II, postalveolar clefts; and group III, all clefts involving the alveolar process. Group I and group III were subdivided into unilateral, bilateral, and median clefts. Group II was subdivided into clefts of the hard and soft palates. In 4% of the patients analyzed by Davis and Ritchie, patients had a prealveolar and postalveolar cleft but with a normal alveolus. This type of cleft could be categorized into group I, group II, or both. Last, the cleft could then be described in terms of degree as complete or incomplete.

Veau,[5] in his 1931 book *Division Palatine*, proposed a four-group classification system based on morphologic features (Fig. 89-10). Group 1 included clefts of the soft palate only. Group 2 contained clefts of the soft and hard palates. Complete unilateral clefts of the lip, alveolus, and palate were placed into group 3, and bilateral clefts of the lip, alveolus, and palate were placed into group 4.

Pruzansky[41] proposed a classification that divided clefts into four general categories: lip only; lip and palate; palate alone; and congenital insufficiency of the palate. Within each category, terminology (e.g., complete, incomplete, soft) could be used to further describe each cleft. His analysis was based on the

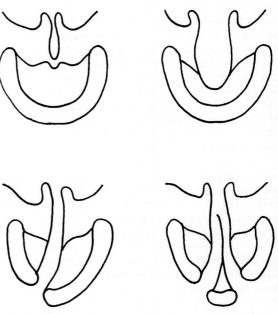

FIGURE 89-10. Veau's classification of cleft lip and palate. (After Veau V: Division palatine: anatomie, chirurgie, phonetique. Paris, Masson et Cie, 1931.)

evaluation of cephalometric radiographs and casts of the face and jaws of more than 350 patients. No special consideration was given to the alveolar process in this organization, and its involvement did not constitute a unique category. Pruzansky based this on his observation that a constant relationship existed between the degree of cleft formation in the lip and the extent of involvement of the alveolar process. Thus, the more complete the cleft in the lip, the greater the degree of involvement in the alveolar process. He believed this was due to the embryologic development of the lip and palate. The fourth category in the Pruzansky classification, congenital insufficiency of the palate, comprised velopharyngeal incompetence of any etiology (e.g., submucous clefts of the palate, congenitally short palate). This was one of the first systems to categorize clefts with consideration of embryology and physiology as well as anatomy.

Kernahan and Stark[42] developed a classification system based on embryologic development. They noted that the incisive foramen was the site of junction between the primary palate formed by mesodermal penetration and the secondary palate formed by fusion of the palatal shelves in the midline, which begins at the incisive foramen and proceeds posteriorly. Thus, the dividing point between groups in their system became the incisive foramen and not the alveolar process. Clefts were categorized as follows: anterior to the incisive foramen (as a result of failure of mesodermal penetration in the primary palate); posterior to the incisive foramen (as a result of failure of fusion of the secondary palate); or combination of the two embryologic events. Again, more descriptive terms could be added to detail the cleft (Table 89-1).

In an effort to come to a consensus on a universally accepted classification of cleft lip and palate, the American Association for Cleft Palate Rehabilitation formed the Nomenclature Committee. The report released by Harkins et al[43] (Fig. 89-11) provided a "basic plan" to divide all clefts into two major categories with subheadings:

Prepalate
    Lip
    Alveolar process (to incisive foramen)
Palate
    Soft palate
    Hard palate (to incisive foramen)

As with the other classification systems, provisions were made under each subheading for more descriptive terminology. Velopharyngeal incompetence was included as well. Unlike in the earlier classification schemes, however, included here were facial clefts other than those of the prepalate and palate. In addition, whereas many described hard palatal clefts as left, right, or bilateral with regard to the

TABLE 89-1 ✦ CLASSIFICATION SYSTEM OF KERNAHAN AND STARK

Clefts of primary palate (lip and premaxilla) only
  Unilateral (right or left)
    Total
    Subtotal
  Median
    Total (premaxilla absent)
    Subtotal (premaxilla rudimentary)
  Bilateral
    Total
    Subtotal

Clefts of the secondary palate only
  Total
  Subtotal
  Submucous

Clefts of the primary and secondary palates
  Unilateral (right or left)
    Total
    Subtotal
  Median
    Total
    Subtotal
  Bilateral
    Total
    Subtotal

From Kernahan DA, Stark RB: A new classification for cleft lip and cleft palate. Plast Reconstr Surg 1958;22:435.

relationship to the vomer, the Committee viewed all hard palatal clefts as midline. This system combined an embryology-based division with recording of the area of the anatomic defect.

Spina[44] proposed a modification of the classification system of Kernahan and Stark and that of Harkins et al. Again, with the incisive foramen as the reference point, four groups were proposed: group I, perincisive foramen clefts, which could be subdivided into unilateral, bilateral, or median as well as total or partial; group II, transincisive foramen clefts, which could be described as unilateral or bilateral; group III, postincisive foramen clefts, which could be described as total or partial; and group IV, rare facial clefts.

In addition to the descriptive classifications, many authors have presented documentation systems based on codes or symbolic representation. Villar-Sancho,[45] using the Latinized letters of Greek words for the defect to be described, proposed a coding system for cleft lip and palate (Table 89-2 and Fig. 89-12). This system of documentation proved to be too complex for general acceptance.

Kernahan[46] proposed a symbolic classification (Fig. 89-13) based on his earlier work with Stark. The lip and palate are represented by a Y, with each limb being composed of three squares. A circle at the junction of the limbs represents the incisive foramen. Squares 1

CLEFTS OF PREPALATE

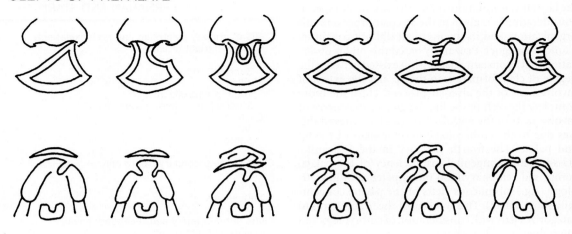

CLEFTS OF PALATE

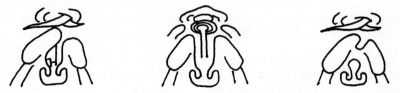

CLEFTS OF PREPALATE AND PALATE

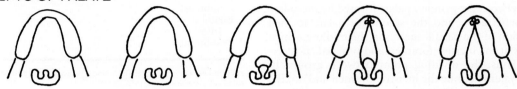

FACIAL CLEFTS OTHER THAN PREPALATAL AND PALATAL

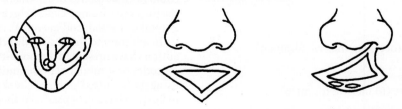

FIGURE 89-11. Classification of the American Association for Cleft Palate Rehabilitation. (After Harkins CS, Berlin A, Harding RL, et al: A classification of cleft lip and palate. Plast Reconstr Surg 1962;29:31.)

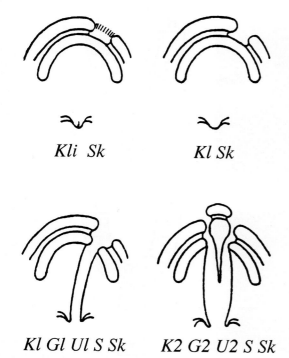

Kli Sk   *Kl Sk*

Kl Gl Ul S Sk   *K2 G2 U2 S Sk*

FIGURE 89-12. Classification of Villar-Sancho. (After Villar-Sancho B: A proposed new international classification of congenital cleft lip and palate. Plast Reconstr Surg 1962;30:263.)

of the Y to represent the nasal floor. The purpose of this was to differentiate complete from incomplete clefts. A complete cleft of the lip is represented by stippling of the nasal triangle and lip square. An incomplete cleft of the lip is represented by stippling of the lip square only. Blackening of the alveolar square represents collapse of the lateral maxillary segment. If there is no collapse of the segment, the square is stippled. In the modified striped Y classification, the squares representing the hard palate, 9 and 10, are represented by double lines at the border as opposed to the soft palate, which is represented by a single line. Arrows are used to represent the direction of displacement of the palatal segments, if indicated. Velopharyngeal competence is represented by a line drawn to connect the stem of the Y to the circle numbered 12, which symbolizes the posterior pharyngeal wall. For incompetence of the velopharyngeal mechanism, no line is drawn. Last, the circle 13 symbolizes the premaxilla. An arrow drawn from the crotch of the Y to the circle represents the degree of protrusion of the premaxillary segment.

Kriens[26] proposed the LAHSHAL code to represent clefts of the lip, alveolus, and palate based on the anatomic structures involved. The LAHSHAL formula is a concise, descriptive code that is amenable to computer data processing. In the formula (Fig. 89-15), L represents the lip, A the alveolus, H the hard palate, and S the soft palate. Kriens noted that clefts are sagittal malformations from the lip to the uvula. Because clefts of the lip, alveolus, and hard palate can occur bilaterally, they form the two prongs in the formula; clefts of the soft palate are midline malformations. Thus, the soft palate acts as a hinge in the formula for the two prongs. Capital letters represent complete clefts, and lowercase letters incomplete ones. An asterisk in the location of the letter involved notes microform clefts (Table 89-3).

and 4 represent the lip, 2 and 5 the alveolus, and 3 and 6 the primary palate from the alveolus to the incisive foramen. Squares 7, 8, and 9 are posterior to the incisive foramen and represent the hard and soft portions of the secondary palate. The degree of stippling of each square corresponds to the degree of cleft formation. Crosshatching of a box represents a submucous section or, in the lip, a Simonart band.

Elsahy[47] proposed further refinement of the striped Y classification in an effort to illustrate clefts in greater detail (Fig. 89-14). He added a triangle to the top limbs

Over time, many documentation and classification systems have been proposed for use in the categorization of clefts of the lip and palate. Each has its merits and deficiencies. As with any system of its type, however, the main problem has been universal acceptance and use of one coding and classification system as the standard. The ideal system would be concise and easy to use, sufficiently descriptive to encompass most clefts, and amenable to computer data entry and handling by a database. In addition, independent evaluators of a cleft would consistently assign patients with cleft palate to the same groups. Once it is in place, a worldwide standard would ideally allow not just use within a cleft team but transmission of data between teams. In the end, it is hoped that this will aid in research toward the etiology and embryology of clefts of the lip and palate as well as provide better insight into the best methods of treatment to ensure the optimal outcome.

TABLE 89-2 ✦ VILLAR-SANCHO PROPOSED CODING SYSTEM FOR CLEFT LIP AND PALATE

K	*keilos*	lip
G	*gnato*	maxillary process/alveolus
U	*urano*	hard palate
S	*stafilos*	soft palate

The letter followed by Sk (the first letters of the Greek word for cleft, *skisis*) describes a complete cleft; 2, bilateral; d, right; l, left; and o, operated. By use of a combination of these letters, various clefts could be described.

From Villar-Sancho B: A proposed new international classification of congenital cleft lip and palate. Plast Reconstr Surg 1962;30:263.

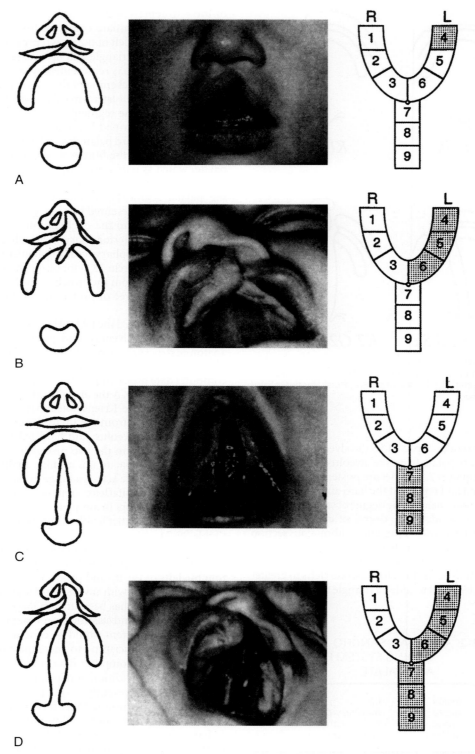

FIGURE 89-13. The striped Y classification of Kernahan. (After Kernahan DA: The striped Y—a symbolic classification for cleft lip and palate. Plast Reconstr Surg 1971;47:469.)

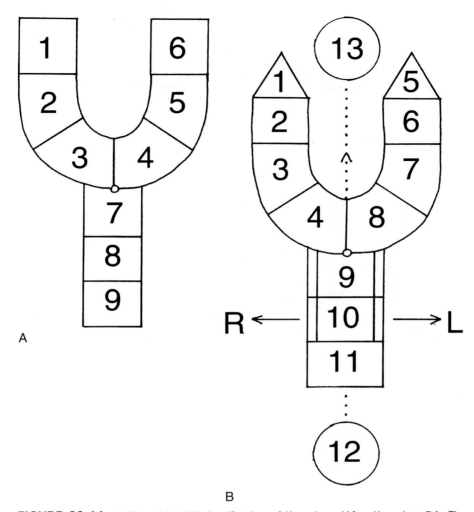

FIGURE 89-14. *A,* The striped Y classification of Kernahan. (After Kernahan DA: The striped Y—a symbolic classification for cleft lip and palate. Plast Reconstr Surg 1971;47:469.) *B,* The modified striped Y classification. (After Elsahy NI: The modified striped Y—a systematic classification for cleft lip and palate. Cleft Palate J 1973;10:247.)

TABLE 89-3 ✦ EXAMPLES OF THE LAHSHAL CLASSIFICATION

Computer Code	Written Diagnosis of Cleft	Handwritten Code
L......	Complete cleft of right lip only	L–
......L	Complete cleft of left lip only	–L
L.....L	Complete bilateral cleft lip	L-L
LAHS	Complete right unilateral cleft of the lip, alveolus, and hard and soft palates	LAHS
I......	Partial right cleft lip only	I–
..sss..	Submucous velar cleft	sss
LA....I	Complete right cleft lip and alveolus and incomplete left cleft lip	LAl
LAHSHAL	Complete bilateral cleft of the lip, alveolus, and palate	LAHSHAL
*...SHAL	Microform of cleft lip on the right and complete cleft of the lip, alveolus, and hard and soft palates on the left	*SHAL

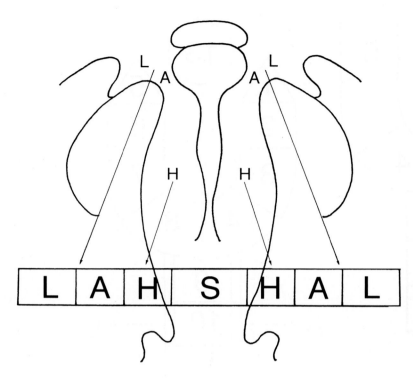

FIGURE 89-15. The LAHSHAL classification of Kriens. (After Kriens O: Documentation of cleft lip, alveolus, and palate. In Bardach J, Morris HL, eds: Multidisciplinary Management of Cleft Lip and Palate. Philadelphia, WB Saunders, 1990:127.)

REFERENCES

1. Passavant G: Über die Verschliessung des Schlundes beim Sprechen. Arch Pathol Anat Physiol Klin Med 1869;64:1.
2. Calnan J: Modern views on Passavant's ridge. Br J Plast Surg 1957;10:89.
3. Fletcher S: A cinefluoroscopic study of the posterior wall of the pharynx during speech and deglutition [master's thesis]. University of Utah, Salt Lake City, 1957.
4. Kriens O: Anatomy of cleft palate. In Bardach J, Morris HL, eds: Multidisciplinary Management of Cleft Lip and Palate. Philadelphia, WB Saunders, 1990:287.
5. Veau V: Division palatine: anatomie, chirurgie, phonetique. Paris, Masson et Cie, 1931.
6. Fara M, Dvorak J: Abnormal anatomy of the muscles of palatopharyngeal closure in cleft palates. Plast Reconstr Surg 1970;46:488.
7. Cassell MD, Moon JB, Elkadi H: Anatomy and physiology of the velopharynx. In Bardach J, Morris HL, eds: Multidisciplinary Management of Cleft Lip and Palate. Philadelphia, WB Saunders, 1990:366.
8. Markus AF, Smith WP, Delaire J: Primary closure of cleft palate: a functional approach. Br J Oral Maxillofac Surg 1993;31:71.
9. Kuehn DP, Kahane JC: Histologic study of the normal human adult soft palate. Cleft Palate J 1990;27:26.
10. Lisson JA, Kjaer I: Location of alveolar clefts relative to the incisive fissure. Cleft Palate Craniofac J 1997;34:292.
11. Boorman JG, Freedlander E: Surgical anatomy of the velum and pharynx. In Jackson IT, Sommerlad BC, eds: Recent Advances in Plastic Surgery, No. 4. Edinburgh, Churchill Livingstone, 1992:17.
12. Maue-Dickson W, Dickson DR: Anatomy and physiology related to cleft palate: current research and clinical implications. Plast Reconstr Surg 1980;65:83.
13. Maue-Dickson W, Dickson DR, Rood SR: Anatomy of the eustachian tube and related structures in age-matched human fetuses with and without cleft palate. Trans Am Acad Ophthalmol Otolaryngol 1976;82:159.
14. Kuehn DP, Azzam NA: Anatomical characteristics of palatoglossus and the anterior faucial pillar. Cleft Palate J 1978;15:349.
15. Ruding R: Cleft palate: anatomical and surgical considerations. Plast Reconstr Surg 1964;33:132.
16. Dickson DR: Anatomy of the normal velopharyngeal mechanism. Clin Plast Surg 1975;2:235.
17. Lupin A: The relationship of the tensor tympani and tensor palati muscles. Ann Otol 1969;78:792.
18. Ross ME: Functional anatomy of the tensor palati—its relevance to cleft palate surgery. Arch Otolaryngol 1971;93:1.
19. Latham RA, Long RE Jr, Latham EA: Cleft palate velopharyngeal musculature in a five-month-old infant: a three dimensional histologic reconstruction. Cleft Palate J 1980;17:1.
20. Huang MH, Lee ST, Rajendran K: A fresh cadaveric study of the paratubal muscles: implications for eustachian tube function in cleft palate. Plast Reconstr Surg 1997;100:833.
21. Boorman JG, Sommerlad BC: Musculus uvulae and levator palati: their anatomical and functional relationship in velopharyngeal closure. Br J Plast Surg 1985;38:333.
22. Boorman JG, Sommerlad BC: Levator palati and palatal dimples: their anatomy, relationship and clinical significance. Br J Plast Surg 1985;38:326.
23. Millard DR: Anatomy of the palate. In Millard DR, ed: Cleft Craft: The Evolution of Its Surgery, vol III. Alveolar and Palatal Deformities. Boston, Little, Brown, 1980:19.
24. Kuehn DP, Folkins JW, Linville RN: An electromyographic study of the musculus uvulae. Cleft Palate J 1988;25:348.
25. Huang MH, Lee ST, Rajendran K: Structure of the musculus uvulae: functional and surgical implications of an anatomic study. Cleft Palate Craniofac J 1997;34:466.

26. Kriens O: Documentation of cleft lip, alveolus, and palate. In Bardach J, Morris HL, eds: Multidisciplinary Management of Cleft Lip and Palate. Philadelphia, WB Saunders, 1990: 127.

27. Koch KH, Grzonka MA, Koch J: Pathology of the palatal aponeurosis in cleft palate. Cleft Palate Craniofac J 1998;35: 530.

28. Bell WH: Biologic basis for maxillary osteotomies. Am J Phys Anthropol 1973;38:279.

29. Mercer NS, MacCarthy P: The arterial supply of the palate: implications for closure of cleft palates. Plast Reconstr Surg 1995;96:1038.

30. Broomhead IW: The nerve supply of the muscles of the soft palate. Br J Plast Surg 1951;4:1.

31. Maher WP: Distribution of palatal and other arteries in cleft and non-cleft human palates. Cleft Palate J 1977; 14:1.

32. Siebert JW, Angrigiani C, McCarthy JG, et al: Blood supply of the Le Fort I maxillary segment: an anatomic study. Plast Reconstr Surg 1997;100:843.

33. You ZH, Zhang ZK, Xia JL: A study of maxillary and mandibular vasculature in relation to orthognathic surgery. Chin J Stomatol 1991;26:263.

34. Girgis IH: Blood supply of the uvula and its surgical importance. J Laryngol Otol 1966;80:397.

35. Freedlander E: The blood supply of the levator and tensor palatini muscles: implications for cleft palate surgery. Clin Anat 1988;1:300.

36. Dingman RO, Grabb WC, Bloomer HH: Posterior pharyngeal flap. Some anatomical considerations and an evaluation of patients. Transactions of the Third International Congress of Plastic Surgery. Amsterdam, Excerpta Medica, 1963:220. International Congress Series No. 66.

37. Keller JT, Saunders MC, van Loveren H, et al: Neuroanatomical considerations of palatal muscles, tensor and levator veli palatini. Cleft Palate J 1984;21:70.

38. Broomhead IW: The nerve supply of the soft palate. Br J Plast Surg 1957;4:81.

39. Nishio J, Matsuya T, Machida J, Miyazaki T: The motor nerve supply of the velopharyngeal muscles. Cleft Palate J 1976;13:20.

40. Davis JS, Ritchie HP: Classification of congenital clefts of the lip and palate. JAMA 1922;79:1323.

41. Pruzansky S: Description, classification, and analysis of unoperated clefts of the lip and palate. Am J Orthod 1953;39:590.

42. Kernahan DA, Stark RB: A new classification for cleft lip and cleft palate. Plast Reconstr Surg 1958;22:435.

43. Harkins CS, Berlin A, Harding RL, et al: A classification of cleft lip and palate. Plast Reconstr Surg 1962;29:31.

44. Spina V: A proposed modification for the classification of cleft lip and palate. Cleft Palate J 1973;10:251.

45. Villar-Sancho B: A proposed new international classification of congenital cleft lip and palate. Plast Reconstr Surg 1962;30:263.

46. Kernahan DA: The striped Y—a symbolic classification for cleft lip and palate. Plast Reconstr Surg 1971;47:469.

47. Elsahy NI: The modified striped Y—a systematic classification for cleft lip and palate. Cleft Palate J 1973;10:247.

Craniofacial Syndromes

Craig A. Vander Kolk, MD ✦ John Menezes, MD

The purpose of this chapter is the review of craniofacial syndromes and the important concepts related to their treatment. This includes an overview of the general concepts of genetic etiology, pathogenesis, and specific syndromes that are frequently encountered in the field of craniofacial surgery. These syndromes have been separated into two categories, those that are cranial with a facial component and those that are mostly facial. In addition to basic concepts of normal cranial and facial development, growth and surgery are also reviewed. This provides the reader with a basic framework for discussion of abnormalities in genetics, development, growth, and reconstruction of craniofacial syndromes.

HISTORY

A historic review of European, American, Asian, and African cultures shows a ubiquitously negative attitude toward individuals with congenital malformations throughout time. According to extensive ethnologic studies mostly done in the second half of the last century, people from a variety of ethnic backgrounds have often reacted similarly to an abnormal newborn—with disposal of the malformed infant immediately after birth, usually by drowning, strangulation, suffocation, or live burial.[1] Although the

results were similar, the reasoning behind the actions and the acts themselves were often quite different.

In pre-Colombian and contemporary American Indian cultures, ritual infanticide was frequently practiced, most often by the Aztecs. Congenital malformations were believed to be due to transgression of the mothers during pregnancy. The mother often killed the deformed child immediately after the birth, stating that she was, by their customs, obliged to do this.[1]

In Far East Indian cultures, the handling of malformed children was dictated by religious tradition as opposed to legal practice. Because the existence of a child was not officially recognized until the third day of life, the family had 3 days after the birth of a disfigured child to decide whether to raise the infant. The choice was often to leave the child for 3 days without food and shelter on a bundle of rags. If the child survived, which seldom happened, the parents then felt obligated to raise the child. The predominant tendencies regarding children with birth defects in ancient non-European cultures were in favor of abandonment with delegation of responsibility to supernatural authorities.[2]

In some African cultures, one finds a dichotomy of belief; most minor abnormalities were seen as a sign of majesty or power, whereas grossly abnormal facial features were believed to signify criminality. Instances of child abandonment and infanticide relating to congenital deformity have not been heavily documented in ancient African cultures.

In ancient Roman and Greek cultures, the decision to nurture or to dispose of a newborn was left to the father in the belief that no father should have to raise a child he did not want. In ancient Greece, a malformed adult, if one survived, was often selected by the community to be the ritual projection center (ritual impersonation) of all misdeeds having happened in the city during the year. The poor individual was then escorted by citizens, in a procession, to the city gates and banished from the city, and with him, all of the evil.[1] One cannot help but wonder at the degree of ignorance to the cause of these conditions that led to such ongoing practices.

ETIOLOGY AND CLASSIFICATION

The term *craniofacial anomalies* has been used to describe a diverse group of congenital disorders. These disorders include but are not limited to complex syndromes marked by multiple sutural fusions (e.g., Crouzon, Saethre-Chotzen, and Apert syndromes), clefts of the lip and palate, simple craniosynostoses involving single fusions (e.g., sagittal synostoses), and hemifacial microsomia. This vast array of dysmorphic syndromes involve abnormalities of craniofacial development that vary from minor anomalies of the facial features to major abnormalities of the skull and facial skeleton and its appendages.

Although certain cranial deformities arise from mechanical or functional causes (e.g., plagiocephaly and hydrocephaly), the molecular basis of the majority of the dysmorphic syndromes, including craniofacial abnormalities, is becoming increasingly evident through advancements in molecular biology. Early explanations of cranial suture fusion included anecdotal associations with intrauterine constraint, uterine malformation, decreased amniotic fluid, or breech presentation. Ozaki et al[3] performed an ultrastructural analysis of sagittal sutures in the process of fusion, and although they were unable conclusively to show a mechanical cause, their analysis revealed several new facts:

1. Premature fusion of sutures was found to begin centrally in the suture.
2. It began endocranially as opposed to both endocranially and ectocranially in normal sutures.
3. It exhibited a disorganized ultrastructure of lower density than in normal sutures.

Bradley et al[4] examined the question of a mechanical cause by placing a plate across one coronal suture in developing sheep. This study showed more definitively that mechanical compression across a cranial suture results in plagiocephaly and deformation similar to unicoronal synostosis, but the suture remained histologically open.

Following the explanation of the genetic basis of Crouzon syndrome by Rearden et al,[5] many researchers have concentrated their efforts on investigating the genetic basis of the craniosynostosis syndromes and the functional consequences of mutations involving the fibroblast growth factor receptor (FGFR) gene. In addition, mutations in certain homeobox (HOX) genes have been linked to particular craniofacial disorders. HOX genes are a key family of genes that are involved in designation of the body plan and pattern formation. They subdivide the early embryo into fields of cells with the potential for becoming distinct tissues and organs; therefore, mutations in these genes can lead to phenotypic abnormalities in the craniofacial region.[6]

Molecular biology has now taken us beyond the speculative explanations of mechanical causes to the roots of abnormal suture development. This progression is particularly evident among the autosomal dominant syndromic craniosynostoses. The first gene mutation identified was for Boston-type craniosynostosis, a familial form of cranial deformity noted in New Englanders of Irish decent.[7] A single mutation (Pro148→His) in the homeobox gene *MSX2* will cause this transcription factor to have increased DNA-binding affinity. This results in craniosynostosis in addition to cleft soft palate and triphalangeal thumb.[8]

The other principal syndromes with autosomal dominant transmission have also had their genetic origins identified—the fibroblast growth factor family of glycoprotein transmembrane receptors (FGFR1, FGFR2, and FGFR3) with immunoglobulin-like binding regions. On activation, these regions form dimers, activating the intracellular tyrosine kinase (Fig. 90-1).[9] Subsequent downstream effects on the nucleus influence cellular proliferation, differentiation, and migration. Each of the factors appears to be important both spatially and temporally in the developing cranium.[10] A mutation in Crouzon syndrome, for instance, leads to cross-linking and dimerization in the immunoglobulin-like region and constitutive activation.[11] In Apert syndrome, the mutation may cause enhanced binding of ligand, whereas in Pfeiffer syndrome, there may be an enhanced response to binding.[12,13] Crouzon, Pfeiffer, and Apert syndromic *FGFR2* and *FGFR3* mutations have also shown a bias for male gametes. This association is likely to be secondary to advancing paternal age and the number of sperm versus egg divisions that take place over time.[14] Saethre-Chotzen syndrome is caused by a mutation in the *TWIST* gene, which results in a loss of function of a gene product that may be required for FGFR signaling (Table 90-1).[15]

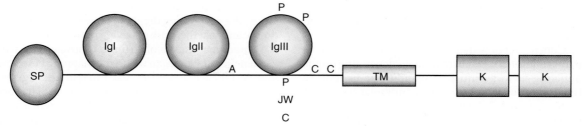

FIGURE 90-1. Fibroblast growth factor receptor with locations of point mutations for Apert (A), Pfeiffer (P), Jackson-Weiss (JW), and Crouzon (C) syndromes. SP, signal peptide; Ig, immunoglobulin-like domains; TM, transmembrane region; K, split tyrosine kinase domains. Point mutations result in constitutive activation of the fibroblast growth factor receptor. (Modified from Jabs EW, Li X, Scott AF, et al: Jackson-Weiss and Crouzon syndromes are allelic with mutations in fibroblast growth factor receptor 2. Nat Genet 1994;8:275-279; and DeLeon VB, Jabs EW, Richtsmeier J: Craniofacial growth: genetic basis and morphogenetic process in craniosynostosis. In Achauer BM, Eriksson E, Guyuron B, et al, eds: Plastic Surgery: Indications, Operations, and Outcomes. St. Louis, Mosby, 2000:627.)

Whereas characterization of specific mutations in genes that cause craniofacial malformations is a giant step toward understanding the mechanism of normal and abnormal development of the craniofacial region, multifarious approaches of research in this area are still needed to help unravel the complex interaction of gene products that participate in signaling pathways, to understand the function of their target genes, and to understand gene-environment interactions.[16] The eventual goal is to have a genetic diagnosis for each clinically characterized craniofacial anomaly as well as a molecular pathway for its genesis.

INTRODUCTION TO CRANIOFACIAL ANOMALIES

In general, it is agreed that most congenital anomalies can be divided into three types—disruptions, deformations, and malformations.[17] Malformations are the most common anomalies and include polydactyly, congenital heart anomalies, and cleft lip. A malformation is generally considered a morphologic defect in an organ area of the body from an intrinsically abnormal developmental process. A deformation is typically thought to occur secondary to mechanical forces of a lesser degree than those mechanical forces that result in disruption. This would be the pathogenesis of a common deformity such as a clubfoot. Cleft palate, secondary to Robin sequence, may be related to a deformational force. Robin sequence can occur in the setting of oligohydramnios, which results in limited extension of the face and jaw. This then keeps the tongue from dropping down, and in its original position between the palatal shelves, the tongue keeps the shelves in their vertical position. This results in a U-shaped as opposed to a V-shaped cleft palate. Posterior plagiocephaly may also have its origin in deformational mechanical forces due to the position of the fetal head low in the pelvis before birth. This may predispose to problems with further growth when the child is placed in a supine or lateral position. Finally, a disruption is the rare anomaly related to breakdown of the

TABLE 90-1 ✦ GENETIC ABNORMALITIES ASSOCIATED WITH SYNDROMIC CRANIOSYNOSTOSIS

Craniofacial Syndrome	Clinical Features	Genetic Abnormality
Crouzon	Proptosis, beaked nose, conductive hearing loss	*FGFR2, FGFR3*
Apert	Syndactyly, low IQ, cleft palate	*FGFR2*
Pfeiffer	Syndactyly, broad thumbs and toes	*FGFR1, FGFR2, FGFR3*
Jackson-Weiss	Midface hypoplasia, abnormal feet, similar to Pfeiffer	*FGFR2*
Saethre-Chotzen	Ptosis, low frontal hairline, midface hypoplasia	*TWIST*
Craniosynostosis, Boston type	Multiple suture, Irish background, cleft soft palate, triphalangeal thumb	*MSX2*
Nonsyndromic coronal suture		*FGFR3*
Nonsyndromic other sutures		Unknown

Modified from Raymond GV: Craniofacial genetics and dysmorphology. In Achauer BM, Eriksson E, Guyuron B, et al, eds: Plastic Surgery: Indications, Operations, and Outcomes. St. Louis, Mosby, 2000:616; and Wilkie AO, Morriss-Kay GM: Genetics of craniofacial development and malformation. Nat Rev Genet 2001;2:458-468.

original, normal fetal developmental process. An example of this is craniofacial clefting resulting from amniotic bands.

Cohen[18] reports that the Robin sequence may be malformational or deformational, "depending on the initiating factors—intrinsic mandibular hypoplasia (malformational) or extrinsic mandibular constraint (deformational)." This makes the interrelationship between anomalies complex. Surgeons typically report anomalies as deformities when they are not true deformations. In fact, deformations can occur secondary to malformations, such as in cleft lip and cleft palate. The initial anomaly of cleft lip and cleft palate is further extended after birth by various mechanical factors. A baby's sticking his tongue between the alveolar segments of a cleft can further exacerbate the problem. Conversely, surgical repair of a cleft lip and cleft palate can cause deformational, mechanical, and subsequent deformational changes that result in mandibular or maxillary hypoplasia.

A syndrome is traditionally characterized by multiple malformations that occur during fetal development. In medical genetics, a "syndrome" is recognized as representing multiple malformations occurring in embryonically noncontiguous areas. Many syndromes have multiple phenotypic expressions. They can vary by the presence or absence of a particular malformation or even the degree of the malformation. The craniofacial field is unique in that the more common craniofacial syndromes are readily identifiable by their appearance. This is true for cleft lip and palate, Treacher Collins syndrome, hemifacial microsomia, Apert syndrome, and Crouzon syndrome. There are, however, several important syndromes for which diagnosis is more difficult. These are Stickler syndrome, 22q syndromes including DiGeorge syndrome and velocardiofacial syndrome, Saethre-Chotzen syndrome, and Jackson-Weiss syndrome.

The prevalence of malformation syndromes is difficult to ascertain. This is based on several factors. First, there are frequently many physicians treating these anomalies in multiple institutions that see patients from a wide geographic area. The second reason is that many malformations can result in fetal death and early pregnancy loss. This makes the overall incidence and prevalence difficult to ascertain. Perhaps the best source for these craniofacial numbers is the report of Cohen.[19]

The field of genetics has realized an explosion of knowledge. This is based on the in-depth understanding of DNA and the ability to map the human genome. Whereas much of this information is helpful in the delineation of a cause-effect relationship and the overall pathogenesis of important craniofacial syndromes, clinical geneticists also help establish the diagnosis and may assist in understanding and predicting surgical outcomes.[20] Even more important, the geneticist helps families understand that most commonly there is nothing they have done to cause the syndrome and that their risk of having more children with such an anomaly can be, often times, relatively predicted.

Genetic studies began with gene mapping based on linkage. Linkage recognizes that different loci of genes occupy the same region of a chromosome. The loci can result in phenotypic expression of genetic characteristics. When these characteristics are expressed within families and the frequency of the characteristic is determined, calculations can be performed to determine the distance between two loci on a particular chromosome. This ultimately leads to a further understanding of the location of genes on chromosomes. This technique is still used in attempts to identify the genetic basis of less common anomalies that have less completely understood genetic influence (e.g., cleft lip and palate).

With the ability to further analyze DNA by recombinant techniques, geneticists have been able to identify specific mutations.[7] This has not been particularly successful in the oral-facial cleft anomalies; however, it has been the key to finding the clues to complex craniosynostosis syndromes. Although a mutation is at the heart of the overall cause of a syndrome, the cause-effect relationship and overall pathogenesis are less well understood. Part of this arises out of genetic heterogeneity. Different genes, on different chromosome locations, may result in the same disorder. This is true for Pfeiffer syndrome and Crouzon syndrome.[21] However, in Apert syndrome, there appear to be, at least at present, only two mutations that result in this deformity.[22]

Because we now know that many of the craniofacial anomalies result from fibroblast growth factor mutations, it is hoped that analyses of these gene mutations and the effect they have on fetal development will provide a better understanding of the pathogenesis. This will be important in understanding growth and development and help determine the best options for treatment.[20]

Whenever significant technological advances occur, new ethical dilemmas frequently arise, particularly in clinical medicine. Identifying gene mutations early can provide an opportunity for pregnancy termination. Whereas this is generally more acceptable for life-threatening and lethal genetic disorders, craniofacial abnormalities present a more ethical dilemma. Physicians in Israel reported that the technological advance of transvaginal ultrasonography provided an opportunity to make a diagnosis of cleft lip and cleft palate in 26 fetuses of more than 10,000 ultrasound examinations. Subsequently, parents made the decision to terminate the pregnancies for cleft lip and cleft palate in 15 of the 16 fetuses identified.[23]

This poses a unique question to the treating physicians: What is the perception of treatment outcomes for families, such as with cleft lip and cleft palate and craniosynostosis? Obviously, some families would consider the outcome of cleft lip and cleft palate unacceptable. This may presuppose their consideration of the ethical opinion of termination or abortion. However, it behooves the practicing physician to inform parents, patients, pediatricians, and obstetricians that the long-term outcome in such anomalies is excellent. The author has had direct experience of such an ethical dilemma for a family with cleft lip and cleft palate. A child was treated with cleft lip and palate whose mother also had an associated cleft lip and palate. The overall outcome was excellent. In fact, the mother subsequently went on to have further revision of her cleft lip and cleft palate. When the child became 6 years old, the overall outcome of speech, development, and appearance was essentially normal. However, at that time, the twin sister of the mother, who did not have a cleft lip and palate, underwent an ultrasound examination during the second trimester of her pregnancy in which a cleft lip and palate was diagnosed. This mother had the difficult decision presented to her of whether to proceed with an abortion. Obviously, she knew directly what living with a cleft lip and palate was like, having grown up with her identical twin sister. In addition, she knew firsthand what medical treatment was required for a child with cleft lip and palate. Ultimately, the decision came down to the sister affected with a cleft telling the other sister that if she had undergone an abortion, she would not have her 6-year-old child, who is a unique, loving, and normal child. With this information, the mother went on to deliver her child, who is in the process of undergoing surgical treatment. As a result of this example and ethical dilemma, the cleft palate team at Johns Hopkins has established the mission statement that the goal of treatment is to help the child "be all that you can be," which in general terms means helping each child become a normal, productive infant, child, adolescent, and adult.

Technological advances have also resulted in the consideration of fetal surgery. Whereas there has been much research into understanding fetal surgery and its unique scarless healing,[24] it is natural that it would proceed to consideration in the treatment of cleft lip and cleft palate. However, the major aspect of cleft lip and cleft palate is not the scarring but the shape and symmetry of the reconstruction. Therefore, repair of a cleft lip in utero, just to limit scarring, would not be expected to offer significant advantages to outweigh the considerable overall risk to mother and child. However, if it could improve the overall disruptive secondary effects due to the secondary mechanical force affecting growth, perhaps it could be considered in the future. To date, there has been one report of an attempt at intrauterine cleft lip repair, which was unsuccessful because it led to the death of the infant and major morbidity to the mother (F. Ortiz-Monasterio, personal communication).

CRANIOFACIAL GROWTH

Craniofacial syndromes have significant alterations in craniofacial growth. These growth alterations occur in utero, during infancy, and throughout childhood. They are important considerations in understanding the treatment of craniofacial anomalies because surgical intervention is thought to unlock growth and to improve the deformational changes that occur in the craniofacial complex. The growth in the facial region occurs during a longer period and is less understood than in the cranium.

Most of the treatment of craniofacial anomalies stems from the treatment of the underlying skeletal structures. Manipulation of the skeletal framework results in movement of the overlying soft tissues. In addition, it can have an effect on associated craniofacial structures and underlying function. Soft tissues, although they heal with scar formation, generally do not limit facial growth unless there is a significant amount of absence of the soft tissues. This is most common in bilateral cleft lip and palate and with a very wide unilateral cleft lip and palate. Treatment and repair of the soft tissues result in some growth restrictions secondary to the limited amount of tissues that are available for reconstruction. Obviously, there are various degrees to which this has an effect. A very wide cleft palate that requires extensive undermining and leaves raw surfaces can result in the formation of significant scar tissue, which will limit the underlying skeletal growth.

However, other associated facial structures have a significant influence on craniofacial growth. In general, the eye grows in a normal fashion, resulting in the associated growth of the surrounding structures. When the eye is missing, the orbit and the associated soft tissue, such as the eyelids, will not grow in a normal fashion. It does appear that placement of an expander to establish some normal volume growth can improve the overall development of the surrounding tissues. The development of teeth will also result in some associated growth and development of the mandible and maxilla. A major influence on maxillary growth is the development of the maxillary sinus; the maxilla and mandible are greatly influenced by surrounding muscle growth and development of the secondary or permanent teeth.

Perhaps the most complex area of understanding and interaction comprises the brain, dura, periosteum, suture, cranial vault, and cranial base. Essentially all craniofacial syndromes have as their main anomaly an abnormality of the individual sutures and synchondroses of the cranium and cranial base. It has become obvious that the genetic mutation results in abnormalities of both the bone and suture and perhaps of the underlying dura. Finally, the development of the brain is what drives the development of the cranial base and cranial vault and has some direct influence on cranial growth. Underlying brain abnormalities are not completely understood in regard to their influence on underlying craniofacial growth and development. This is true for such abnormalities as hydrocephalus, Chiari formations, and developmental abnormalities like the ones that affect IQ in Apert syndrome.

The general theories of craniosynostosis have historically involved all of these observations and findings. Virchow[25] thought that the underlying abnormality was the suture itself. Moss[26] however, thought that it was secondary to the growth of the other functional surrounding structures, such as brain, airway, and muscle attachments extending out from an abnormality of the cranial base. Finally, Park and Powers[27] suggested that it was abnormalities in the mesenchymal blastema that resulted in craniosynostosis abnormalities. Most likely, it is a combination of all of these different factors that results in the wide variety of manifestations of craniosynostosis, both isolated and syndromic. Virchow was the first to note abnormal cranial growth patterns associated with early sutural fusion. However, the complex deformations that extend to the cranial base, orbit, and other regions of the cranium are not fully explained by the idea that growth is restricted to the plane perpendicular to the synostosis. Delashaw[28] has taken these facts and developed them into four rules:

1. Cranial bones act as a single bone plate across the fused suture with restricted growth potential for the entire plate.
2. Abnormal and asymmetric growth occurs at perimeter sutures, with increased bone deposition directed away from the synostotic bone plate. This is in evidence with the characteristic expansion of the contralateral frontal and parietal bones and the ipsilateral squamosal region for unicoronal synostosis.
3. Along both edges of the suture contiguous with the fused suture, enhanced symmetric bone deposition occurs. In unicoronal synostosis, this results in frontal bossing from the normal contiguous, contralateral coronal suture.
4. Adjacent sutures show greater compensatory growth than do perimeter sutures (Fig. 90-2).

Enlow[29] contributed to the understanding of craniofacial growth and development. His research demonstrated that growth of the skeletal structures responded to both intrinsic and extrinsic forces. The craniofacial skeleton grows through two basic mechanisms. Most initial growth occurs at growth centers by expansion at sutures and synchondroses; this is particularly true of the neurocranium. Bone remodeling is accomplished through deposition on the outer surface of the bone and resorption on the inner surface; this occurs in the neurocranium but is most obvious in the facial region. Both mechanisms of growth allow enlargement and displacement of the underlying structures.

DIAGNOSIS AND CLASSIFICATION

Diagnosis of a syndrome is often based on the clinical observation of abnormal body parts and proportions or simply an unusual appearance. Placement of various deformities into known complexes allows the clinician to further diagnose the patient's condition. The correct diagnosis of a syndrome enables the physician to provide the patient and family with treatment options, possible preventive measures, prognosis, and genetic counseling in regard to pathogenesis and recurrence risk.[30]

In the presence of obvious structural defects, such as visible clefts or unilateral disruptions, this initial diagnosis provides little challenge to the trained clinician, although the inceptive clinical impression could often be misleading and must be validated by quantitative criteria and analytical methodology. A thorough phenotypic assessment not only involves an impression of the overall view of the face at rest and during crying, smiling, and frowning, it also includes detailed measurement of many craniofacial dimensions.[30]

However, for many congenital syndromes with subtle but unique patterns of facial variation, physical observation may provide little or no help in identification and classification of a particular syndrome or its severity. Through the introduction of techniques such as computed tomography (CT), magnetic resonance imaging (MRI), ultrasound studies, and stereoscopic imaging, the ability to describe and categorize facial morphology has significantly improved. Although more elementary techniques such as cephalometry, anthropometry, and photogrammetry continue to provide unique advantages in the identification of craniofacial deformities, the use of modern modalities, especially the expertise of a geneticist, enables further identification and counseling for the family.

MULTIDISCIPLINARY TEAM MANAGEMENT

The word *team* can be defined as a group of individuals on the same side who have agreed to work together for a common goal.[31] In the early 1970s, after the success of French plastic surgeon Paul Tessier in surgical correction of congenital deformities previously deemed untreatable, plastic surgeons from

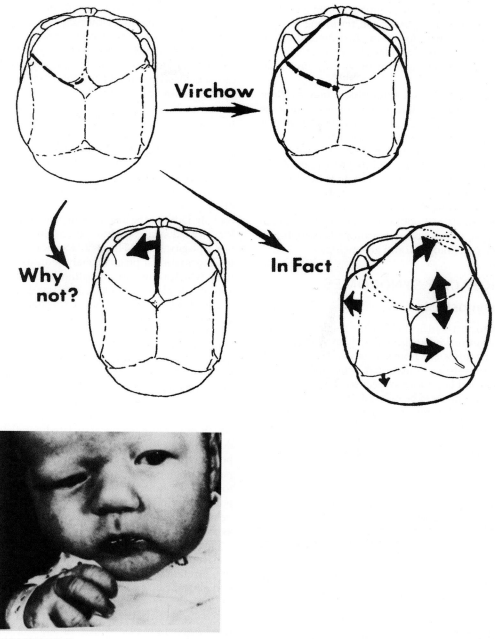

FIGURE 90-2. Virchow predicted restricted growth perpendicular to the fused suture. Why does the metopic suture not compensate? Instead, the local cranial bones act as a single bone plate across the fused suture with restricted growth potential for the entire plate. Along both edges of the suture contiguous with the fused suture, enhanced symmetric bone deposition occurs. In unicoronal synostosis, this results in frontal bossing from the normal contiguous, contralateral coronal suture. The photograph is of a patient with left unicoronal synostosis. (From Delashaw JB, Persing JA, Jane JA: Cranial deformation in craniosynostosis. A new explanation. Neurosurg Clin North Am 1991;2:611-620.)

the United States and other countries rushed to Paris to study this new discipline.[32] On returning to their native countries, many of them attempted to establish multidisciplinary craniofacial centers to care for those children suffering from previously untreated anomalies.

It is now known and understood that children who have complex craniofacial anomalies require the skills of a variety of medical professionals for assessment of their development and formulation of a comprehensive treatment plan. The wide variety of potential problems found in children with craniofacial syndromes makes it desirable for them to be observed by a multidisciplinary team composed of many providers, including plastic surgeons, neurosurgeons, otolaryngologists, orthodontists, oral surgeons, speech pathologists, social workers, orthopedists, ophthalmologists, psychologists, and geneticists.[33]

CRANIOFACIAL SYNDROMES

Craniosynostosis

Craniosynostosis can be divided into single-suture and multiple-suture synostosis. Generally speaking, single-suture synostoses are nonsyndromic. These include metopic synostosis, unicoronal synostosis, sagittal synostosis, and lambdoid synostosis. These deformities generally appear to be isolated and have a low incidence of familial occurrence, generally considered to be less than 5%. The highest incidence of familial occurrence is with sagittal synostosis, which has been reported to be as high as 8% (Table 90-2).

TABLE 90-2 ✦ EPIDEMIOLOGY OF CRANIOSYNOSTOSIS

Craniosynostosis	Rate/Relative Prevalence
Overall	1 in 2500
Syndromic	1 in 25,000 to 1 in 100,000
Sagittal	40% (2% familial)
Unicoronal	15%
Bicoronal	20% (10% familial)
Coronal and sagittal	10%
Total (microcephaly)	10%
Metopic	7%
Lambdoid	1%-2%
Plagiocephaly without synostosis	5%-25% of normal births
Crouzon	4.8%, 16.5/1,000,000
Apert	4.0%, 13.7/1,000,000

Data from JC Posnick: Craniofacial and Maxillofacial Surgery. Philadelphia, WB Saunders, 2000:127; Cohen MM Jr, Kreiborg S: Birth prevalence studies of the Crouzon syndrome: comparison of direct and indirect methods. Clin Genet 1992;41:12-15; Cohen MM Jr, Kreiborg S, Lammer EJ, et al: Birth prevalence study of the Apert syndrome. Am J Med Genet 1992;42:655-659; and Cohen MM Jr, Kreiborg S: Perspectives on craniofacial syndromes. Acta Odontol Scand 1998;56:315-320.

Each of the single-suture synostoses has a typical phenotypic expression. However, whereas unicoronal synostosis has a fairly standard presentation (whether right or left), metopic and sagittal synostoses have a wider variation in their phenotypic expression. Sagittal synostosis can present as a total sagittal deformity or an anterior or posterior deformity. Metopic synostosis has the widest variation, extending from a minimal metopic ridge to a more pronounced frontal deformity with anterior narrowing. In the most severe presentation, the deformity includes an extension into the temporal region with lateral orbital retrusion and associated hypotelorism.

Unicoronal synostosis should not be confused with other presentations of anterior or posterior plagiocephaly. Differential diagnosis in plagiocephaly (Greek for "twisted skull") includes torticollis and deformational plagiocephaly. The major location of abnormality in deformational plagiocephaly is a posterior deformity, which results in a twisting of the cranial base, anterior displacement of the ipsilateral ear with posterior displacement of the contralateral ear, and varying degrees of frontal deformation. It is unknown whether this is related to an underlying abnormality of the sutures or caused by a deformation in late pregnancy with the positioning of the fetus in the pelvis and then further complicated by supine positioning of the infant.

Posterior positional plagiocephaly should not be confused with unicoronal or unilambdoid synostosis, which does not have the associated parallelogram as described by Bruneteau and Mulliken.[34] In general, positional plagiocephaly improves with time and the patient's being able to roll from front to back and back to front. In patients with more severe deformities, a positioning pillow can be helpful. Finally, molding helmets can be used and result in improvement as long as they are instituted at an early age (e.g., 3 months).

Torticollis occurs from shortening or injury and scarring of the sternocleidomastoid muscle, resulting in a limitation in movement of the head to one side and a head tilt. Twisting of the skull and asymmetry of growth are secondary to these fetal or infant mechanical restrictive and deformational forces. Torticollis generally occurs in 1 in 300 live births. The majority of patients respond to conservative treatment with physical therapy to improve range of motion, both rotation of the skull and tilt from side to side. If there is progressive deformity and incomplete motion with aggressive physical therapy, then toward the latter half of the first year of life, surgical release of the sternocleidomastoid may need to be considered. Cervical spine subluxations can be related to torticollis. They occur at the C1-2 level and are otherwise known as axial rotary subluxations. The differential diagnosis of a head tilt includes a nerve palsy or abnormality of the superior oblique muscle. Both of these diagnoses should be considered in evaluation of patients with plagiocephaly.

Apert Syndrome

Apert syndrome is one of the more distinctive and severe craniofacial syndromes. It has multiple moderate to severe anomalies that affect the cranial, facial, and extremity regions. In addition, it has a significant potential for delayed development and a low IQ. Treatment and reconstructive procedures are difficult and usually require multiple operations.

Apert syndrome has been studied extensively and has been clearly defined on a genetic level. It is generally sporadic; however, it can be inherited in an autosomal dominant fashion.[17] Although it is readily identified clinically by its typical phenotypic expression, the diagnosis can now be confirmed by the recent molecular genetic advances. This research has identified abnormalities of the fibroblast growth factor receptor gene for many craniofacial syndromes. There have been only a limited number of mutations in Apert syndrome. This is in contrast to Crouzon syndrome, which has many reported mutations.

The typical phenotypic expression is easy to recognize but difficult to describe. The cranium is brachycephalic, consistent with bicoronal synostosis. However, this brachycephaly is not only anterior; it is also seen posteriorly with variable bilateral lambdoid synostosis. There is usually a large triangular, anteriorly displaced anterior fontanel. The brachycephaly extends to the orbital region with superior orbital retrusion. Interorbital distance is usually increased and occasionally results in moderate hypertelorism. Compensatory changes in the cranium secondary to the brachycephaly result in a degree of parietal expansion and increased vertical height (turricephaly).

Orbital retrusion extends to the entire orbit and results in exophthalmos that can require ophthalmologic intervention (tarsorrhaphy) or orbital advancement to protect the eye and cornea. The orbits tend to have a lateral rotation. The orbital deformity extends to the soft tissues and the lateral canthus, which has an antimongoloid orientation. Extension of the orbital retrusion to the midface levels leads to maxillary hypoplasia. This midface hypoplasia can result in significant airway obstruction. In many instances, this requires a tracheostomy. All patients demonstrate a high arched palate and a central groove; 30% of patients have an associated cleft palate.[17] The nasal airway can be further compromised by the small size of the nose and the parrot beak type of deformity. Thickening of the nasal skin is often noted, and acne vulgaris can be seen in the facial region.

Other malformations are typically characterized in Apert syndrome. Complex syndactyly of the fingers and toes is severe in nature, especially when it includes the thumb. In addition, central nervous system malformations include macrocephaly, hydrocephalus, and significant developmental delay in many children with a tendency toward a lower than average IQ. Developmental delays and the potential for increased intracranial pressure always need to be monitored, although the large anterior fontanel and open metopic suture protect the brain until the time of closure at a later date. Because hydrocephalus affects 5% to 10% of children with Apert syndrome, ventricular-peritoneal shunting may need to be performed. In older patients with airway abnormalities, Chiari malformations need to be ruled out because foramen decompression may be necessary.

Options for reconstruction need to prioritize functional restoration, followed by the aesthetic concerns of the patient and family. Delay of surgery for as long as possible has been thought by many authors to be advantageous to obtain the best possible result. This limits the need for multiple or more frequent surgeries, and the bone is generally more mature for better stabilization and positioning. Several surgeons, however, suggest that early surgery can unlock the potential for cranial and brain growth. They recommend surgery at an early age (e.g., before 6 months). Currently, the authors recommend surgery in the latter part of the first year of life, which can involve orbital advancement and frontal-orbital-temporal reshaping. This is followed by careful monitoring of cranial vault growth because these patients may require a posterior cranial reconstruction at a later date. Midface advancement before the ideal age of 4 to 5 years may need to be considered for earlier problems, such as airway obstruction or removal of a tracheostomy.

Crouzon Syndrome

Crouzon syndrome is the most common form of craniofacial dysostosis. It is characterized by a wide variation in presentation despite its autosomal dominant inheritance pattern. Crouzon syndrome is caused by multiple mutations in the fibroblast growth factor gene (*FGFR2*). Parents who carry the gene frequently demonstrate mild deformities that are subsequently noted when a child is born with more severe deformities and Crouzon syndrome is diagnosed. Bicoronal synostosis is the most frequent finding; there may be other associated cranial vault suture involvement. Midface hypoplasia has a variable presentation, as does the orbital proptosis, secondary to face and orbital retrusion.

In general, the functional concerns that are present with craniofacial dysostosis syndromes are typically not seen in infants and children with Crouzon syndrome. However, as opposed to Apert syndrome, which has a large area for decompression of pressure with a large anterior fontanel, Crouzon syndrome has a potential for increased intracranial pressure. This is often manifested by optic nerve compression and papilledema, and it can result in optic atrophy and partial blindness. This appears to be possible throughout childhood and requires careful, frequent ophthalmologic monitoring.

Hydrocephalus appears to affect 5% to 10% of patients with Crouzon syndrome,[17] although it is generally thought to be less severe than with Apert syndrome. Crouzon syndrome generally can have conductive hearing loss, which may be related to cranial base abnormalities and may be manifested by frequent middle ear infections. This needs to be closely monitored. Treatment is usually less involved than in Apert syndrome and is more variable, depending on the findings and presentation.

Pfeiffer Syndrome

Pfeiffer syndrome generally appears to be closer to Crouzon syndrome than are many of the other dysostosis syndromes. However, it is thought to have an autosomal dominant inheritance pattern with incomplete penetrance. Although there are similarities to Crouzon and Jackson-Weiss syndromes, the deformities are distinct. Cohen[19] reports three clinical subtypes.

Pfeiffer syndrome type I is the classic form of the syndrome with nearly normal intelligence, bilateral coronal synostosis, and variable midface involvement. The degree of proptosis is generally minimal, and the overall growth expectation is good.

Pfeiffer syndrome type II has more severe midface deficiency and ocular proptosis with an associated cloverleaf skull. Typical findings also include hydrocephalus, central nervous system findings, elbow ankylosis, broad thumbs, and broad great toes. This is the most severe form of the subtypes.

Pfeiffer syndrome type III is a variation of type II, without a cloverleaf skull. Patients have severe proptosis secondary to decreased anterior cranial base length, shallow orbits, and midface deficiency. In general, these children have neurologic compromise and a limited life span.

The broad toes and broad thumbs characterize the diagnosis. Differential diagnosis may be confused with Saethre-Chotzen syndrome, which also has broad toes; however, the great toe of Pfeiffer type III is more triangular and bulbous in shape and in the valgus position. Jackson-Weiss syndrome does not have broad thumbs but may have broad great toes similar to those of Pfeiffer syndrome.[17]

Saethre-Chotzen Syndrome

Saethre-Chotzen syndrome has an autosomal dominant inheritance pattern with high penetrance and extensive variable expressivity of the craniofacial deformity. This is because craniosynostosis is facultative rather than obligatory. When synostosis is seen, it is most commonly bicoronal synostosis with brachycephaly. Other malformations include low-set frontal hairline, upper lid ptosis, facial asymmetry, brachydactyly, and partial cutaneous syndactyly.

Jackson-Weiss Syndrome

In 1976, Jackson and Weiss reported a syndrome in 138 affected individuals that consisted of an autosomal dominant inheritance, craniosynostosis, midface hypoplasia, and abnormalities of the feet. The variability in presentation of this extended family was so extensive that there were examples similar to all of the craniofacial dysostosis acrocephalosyndactylies. This makes Jackson-Weiss syndrome difficult to diagnose clinically. The key appears to be the molecular differentiation of these syndromes.

Carpenter Syndrome

Carpenter syndrome is autosomal recessive and characterized by variable suture synostosis and complex cranial deformities. As with other craniofacial syndromes, mental deficiency and extremity anomalies are frequently seen. As opposed to other craniofacial syndromes, Gorlin reports that Carpenter syndrome is more commonly characterized by middle to posterior deformities with sagittal and lambdoid synostosis to a greater degree. In addition, unilateral synostosis can result in cranial asymmetry. Finally, the most common syndrome is pansynostosis or cloverleaf deformity (Kleeblattschädel). Hand and feet abnormalities are common. The fingers are short and wide, as are the hands. Syndactyly is common, as is clinodactyly. The feet have varus deformities, preaxial polysyndactyly, duplication of the great toe or second toe, and two phalanges in each toe. Cardiovascular anomalies are seen in one third of patients.[17]

FACIAL SYNDROMES
Treacher Collins Syndrome

Treacher Collins syndrome, also known as mandibulofacial dysostosis and Francheschetti-Zwahlen-Klein syndrome, has a distinctive facial appearance that is well known. This bilateral facial deformity has etiology in anomalies of the structures derived from the first branchial arch, groove, and pouch. The deformity is centered around the middle portion of the face as opposed to hemifacial microsomia, which is secondary to abnormalities of the first and second branchial arches and therefore usually centered around the lower face and mandible.

Treacher Collins syndrome is generally considered to be autosomal dominant in its inheritance with variable expressivity. The characteristic appearance revolves around the deformity in the lower lateral orbit and medial zygoma. There is frequently an absence of the bone in this region, which many think is consistent with a craniofacial cleft. However, the deformity extends outward from this area to the maxilla and mandible in such a way that it is much more severe than the malformation seen even in complex facial clefts. This suggests a more extensive underlying pathophysiologic process. Basic science animal investigation has produced similar malformations in animals with teratogenic doses of vitamin A and isotretinoin. The histologic findings demonstrated neurocrest development abnormalities.[35]

The maxilla, from the nasomaxillary region, is caudally rotated. This results in clockwise rotation of the mandible, which is also retrognathic and micrognathic. These abnormalities in the facial skeletal framework displace the associated soft tissues, resulting in many other deformities. The palpebral fissures are short and slanted downward. The lateral canthus is inferiorly displaced, and there is usually an associated coloboma of the lower eyelid. The nose has a parrot beak deformity made more noticeable by its small size. The underlying nasal, oral, and pharyngeal airway is narrowed and compromised, resulting in airway obstruction and the need for a tracheostomy in patients with more severe disease. Other malformations include cleft palate in 35% of patients and macrostomia in 15%.[17] Finally, there frequently are auricular abnormalities that are both internal and external in nature. Because the ear anomaly is bilateral, most patients require a bone conduction hearing aid. Cochlear hearing devices that are anchored to bone have been introduced. The patient usually undergoes costochondral external ear reconstructions for complete microtia.

Nager syndrome is similar to Treacher Collins syndrome but with hypoplastic or absent thumbs, radius and ulna fusion, or radial and metacarpal hypoplasia or aplasia. Other aspects in the differential diagnosis of Nager syndrome are a lower incidence of coloboma, a higher incidence of cleft palate, and more severe hypoplasia of the mandible.

Hemifacial Microsomia

Hemifacial microsomia is the most common name for a syndrome that is most likely the second most common facial deformity after cleft lip and palate. Poswillo[36] and Grabb[37] estimated the incidence at 1 of 3500 and 1 of 5600, respectively, with a slight predilection for males over females (3:2) and the right side. Other terms used for this heterogeneous group of disorders include oculoauriculovertebral syndrome, craniofacial microsomia (because the deformity occasionally includes the orbital and lower cranial region), and first and second branchial arch syndrome. Goldenhar syndrome is a separate diagnosis that characteristically includes epibulbar dermoid and vertebral anomalies.

Most instances of this deformity are thought to be sporadic with some familial association. Numerous associated chromosome abnormalities have been reported, including deletions (5p), (6q), and (39a) along with trisomy 7, 9, and 18 to name just a few.[17] Poswillo[38] demonstrated in animals that early vascular disruption and hematoma in utero resulted in similar deformities. The development of the skeletal and soft tissue anomalies of the first and second branchial arches would point to a process that has an effect at 30 to 45 days of gestation.

There is marked variability in presentation, which has resulted in several classification systems of the ear deformity, mandibular hypoplasia, cranial nerve VII (marginal mandibular branch) involvement, and soft tissue hypoplasia.[39,40] The severity of one tissue group deformity is not always related to the severity in another associated tissue group. Fifty percent of patients have other anomalies. These can include eye findings such as blepharoptosis, palpebral shortening, and even anophthalmia or microphthalmia. Epibulbar dermoids are thought to occur in 35% of patients and usually occur in the infratemporal region of the eye. Oral findings include macrostomia, which is more common in Goldenhar syndrome. This often has the appearance of a lateral cleft of the lip. Conventional unilateral and bilateral cleft lip is seen in 7% to 15%; cleft palate alone is twice as common as cleft lip with or without cleft palate. Velopharyngeal insufficiency has been reported and is probably secondary to ipsilateral velum paresis. Other reported cranial nerve involvement includes I, II, III, IV, VI, VIII, IX, and X.[17]

Treatment is centered around the three major components of the syndrome: the ear, mandible, and soft tissues hypoplasia. Ear tags or sinuses are frequently seen, and the ear is generally a complete microtia. Hearing loss is common secondary to the abnormal development of the middle ear associated with first branchial arch development. Sensorineural hearing loss can be as high as 15%. The major difficulty in reconstruction of the external ear is the position of the hairline and the lobule. This is related to the soft tissue deficiency and the underlying skeletal asymmetry. Modified ear reconstruction techniques are frequently required for the hairline and the soft tissue reconstruction, and support needs to be performed before costochondral ear reconstruction. Perhaps the first thing to address in major reconstruction planning is the mandible. The traditional classification is type 1, 2, and 3 with subcategorizations for the degree of condylar and glenoid fossa hypoplasia. Distraction osteogenesis has been a major advance in providing an opportunity for early skeletal reconstruction so that soft tissue and ear reconstruction can proceed at a relatively early age.

Robin Sequence/Syndrome

Terminology of and references to Pierre Robin syndrome have been changed to Robin sequence. This is based on the understanding that the diagnosis encompasses the findings of cleft palate, micrognathia, and glossoptosis; this is due to a cascade of events in utero that results in these findings. It is not a syndrome because each of the deformities is tied to the same pathophysiologic events. Early in gestation, the palatal shelves are vertically oriented and separated by the developing tongue. If the fetal head does not extend sufficiently to allow the tongue to drop down, the continued presence of the tongue between the palatal shelves keeps them from changing position and a U-shaped cleft palate occurs. In addition, the mandible growth is retarded. Because the tongue is supported by the incompletely advancing and growing mandible, the tongue is retrodisplaced and can in turn result in airway obstruction and the observation that the tongue is small and ptotic. Whereas this sequence of events seems to account for the majority of children with these findings, there are occasionally other findings and malformations that make it clear there is a syndromic component to this diagnosis. Hanson and Smith[41] reported that a specific syndrome was noted in 25% of Robin children; 35% had multiple anomalies but without an identifiable syndrome, leaving 40% of patients with isolated Robin sequence. These patients usually have truncal abnormalities along with delayed growth and development, which is greater than what would be expected with the classic triad of deformities.

The degree of deformity determines the extent of treatment that is required. When the anatomic findings of the tongue and the mandible are moderate to severe, airway obstruction occurs. Most patients will respond to conservative therapy of positioning and alternative feeding regimens. However, when the findings are severe and unresponsive to conservative therapy, surgical intervention must take place. This can include tracheostomy, mandibular advancement with distraction osteogenesis, and tongue-lip adhesion, depending on the experience and preference of the surgeon. Cleft palate treatment is usually delayed if the airway is compromised. Most surgeons think that the results of palatoplasty for the U-shaped palatal cleft are less successful. Finally, as the child grows, the mandibular growth is carefully monitored. In patients with mild deformities, there may be additional growth that allows the mandible to "catch up"; this may result in a deformity consisting mostly of microgenia. In patients with more severe "syndromic like" deformities, growth is limited and mandibular advancement required.

Stickler Syndrome

Cleft palate with the possibility of eye abnormalities prompts cleft palate teams and surgeons to rule out Stickler syndrome. Because the eye abnormalities can include retinal detachment and cataracts, ophthalmologic evaluation should at least be considered in all patients with cleft palate. This is especially true when there is myopia, which is usually severe in Stickler syndrome. Other findings include a flat midface, hearing loss, and mild spondyloepiphyseal dysplasia. Gorlin reports that 30% of children with Robin sequence will be diagnosed with Stickler syndrome.[17] The syndrome is autosomal dominant and appears to have an abnormality of a gene that is close to the type II collagen gene on chromosome 12.[42]

Velocardiofacial Syndrome and DiGeorge Syndrome

Shprintzen[43] in 1978 reported a syndrome with a cleft palate, cardiovascular anomalies, and characteristic facies that is now termed velocardiofacial syndrome. Further analysis has demonstrated that this is an autosomal dominant syndrome associated with a 22q chromosome abnormality. The diagnosis can be confirmed by fluorescent in situ hybridization. There is a close association between velocardiofacial syndrome and DiGeorge syndrome, which generally includes immunologic findings such as absent or small thymus, tonsils, and adenoids and hypocalcemia.[17]

The palate abnormality can be mild and manifested by palatal weakness, or it can be a submucous or complete cleft of the palate. The characteristic facies are manifestations of vertical maxillary excess, malar flattening, relative mandibular retrusion, narrow palpebral fissures, and small ears. The cardiovascular abnormalities are usually cardiac and multiple. They include ventricular septal defect, tetralogy of Fallot, and right-sided aortic arch. The most important finding for surgeons is medial displacement of the carotid artery into the pharynx,[44] which must be considered in planning of pharyngeal flap surgery. Finally, a learning disability is almost universally seen in these children, and the children can have behavioral and psychological problems. These findings support the need for a low index of suspicion for the diagnosis and close monitoring of development.

Van der Woude Syndrome and Cleft Lip and Palate

Whereas cleft lip with or without cleft palate is the most frequently encountered facial deformity, it is infrequently associated with a syndrome. This is in contrast to cleft palate, which is part of a syndrome or at least has other malformations in up to 50% of patients. The most common syndrome that is seen with cleft lip and palate is Van der Woude syndrome. The incidence is between 1 in 35,000 and 1 in 100,000 white individuals, and it occurs in 1% to 2% of patients with facial clefts.[45] The syndrome is autosomal dominant with variable expressivity. The diagnostic finding in Van der Woude syndrome is bilateral paramedian lower lip pits. These pits are oval or transverse sinuses that are present at the dry and wet vermilion junction. They typically traverse the underlying orbicularis muscle and end in a blind pouch that communicates with the underlying minor salivary glands. Gorlin reports that there is controversy about the associated clefts seen in Van der Woude syndrome. It is suggested that 33% of patients with pits have cleft lip and palate, 33% have cleft palate, and 33% do not have a cleft.[17] Although it is difficult to confirm the percentage of isolated pits from the clinical experience in a cleft clinic, it is the authors' opinion that the majority of patients with lip pits have cleft lip and palate and not cleft palate alone.

SURGICAL TREATMENT

The field of craniofacial surgery has existed only a short time in the overall history of medicine. Of course, the patients have always been there, with a birth prevalence of craniosynostoses of approximately 343 in 1 million[46]; but it is only since Paul Tessier began his pioneering work in the late 1960s that the field has developed. Since his protégés helped develop the field in the United States during the 1970s, the specialty of craniofacial surgery has grown to include multidisciplinary teams treating a wide variety of patients. Also, whereas Tessier treated mainly adults in a single stage of therapy, today's interventions occur in the very young, in multiple stages, and during many years of growth and development.

For the physician evaluating a patient with a craniofacial syndrome, the process of presurgical work-up and procedural planning has been developed. The risks and benefits are known and can be explained. Many of the surgical outcomes are known. The need for certain secondary procedures can also be predicted and explained to the family before they begin the reconstructive path.

The surgical procedures themselves have changed. Tongue-in-groove techniques of bone advancement stabilized with sutures or stainless steel wire have given way to titanium or Vitallium plating systems. The toxicity of these systems has been brought into question.[47] In addition, hardware migration, infection, palpability, and other issues have occasionally required their removal.[48] This has led to the development of resorbable systems. Plating systems composed of a combination of polylactic acid and polyglycolic acid allow stabilization of the initial construct, followed by slow resorption.

Indications

Craniosynostosis can be divided into two broad categories, simple or nonsyndromic and syndromic. In nonsyndromic patients, individual cranial sutures may be fused, resulting in an abnormality of shape requiring fronto-orbital advancement, but the midface is generally unaffected. In syndromic craniofacial dysostoses, in addition to cranial suture abnormalities, the cranial base is abnormal, resulting in an abnormal midface. The reasons for surgical intervention in the nonsyndromic group are primarily aesthetic; in the syndromic group, they are multifactorial. Aesthetic considerations are more difficult to quantify than is the objective value of protecting vision, reducing intracranial pressure, or improving occlusion, for instance. Nevertheless, the benefits of improving appearance on psychosocial adjustment have been evaluated across many different populations. The timing of this improvement is also important. Pertschuk[49] studied the psychosocial impact of surgery on two groups of craniofacial patients. If corrective surgery was performed after the age of 4 years, the children were more introverted and had poorer self-concept compared with normal control subjects. If surgical intervention was undertaken before the age of 4 years, no differences were found.

Aesthetic and psychosocial considerations aside, one must consider the functional benefits of corrective surgery. Exorbitism is a significant component for the syndromic patients with craniosynostosis. Hypoplastic orbits and a retruded midface cause globe and corneal exposure, which can result in corneal injury and exposure keratitis. The majority of orbital problems occur relatively early, in the first 5 years of life—the main period of orbital growth.[50] Early protection of the eye, before 6 months of age, is achieved with lubricants and maneuvers such as lid taping at night. This is a temporary measure performed until the child is of sufficient age to undergo orbital advancement.

Elevated intracranial pressure is also associated with craniosynostosis. Renier[51] provided the first major study to measure preoperative and postoperative differences in intracranial pressure. Nonsyndromic patients overall had a 14% incidence of elevated intracranial pressure before surgery, which fell to within normal limits in all but 7% after surgery. Severity of disease also affects the probability that intracranial pressure will be elevated. Preoperatively, if the patient had only one cranial suture involved, 8.9% had elevated intracranial pressure; multiple sutures, 45%; Crouzon syndrome, 66%; and Apert syndrome, 44%. The effect of craniosynostosis, elevated intracranial pressure, and syndromic disease on resulting intelligence is less clear. In general, for most nonsyndromic patients, intelligence is normal with single-suture involvement (>90%) but decreases with multiple suture involvement (78%).[52] For syndromic patients, the degree of developmental delay is highly variable, depending on the syndrome and severity of disease. For patients with Crouzon syndrome, intelligence is generally normal; in patients with Apert syndrome, mean IQ has been reported as 74.[53]

Although no conclusive evidence is available to show the benefit of decreasing intracranial pressure on intelligence, it is generally accepted that operative decompression may arrest further deterioration in intelligence.

Timing of Surgery

The advancements in pediatric anesthesia and intensive care have made available to younger children the extensive cranial reconstructions that during the early period of craniofacial surgery were available only to adolescents and adults. Concerns for the effect of early intervention on skeletal growth were reduced by studies demonstrating that in syndromic patients, midface growth was deficient whether patients had early surgery or not.[54,55] McCarthy and Cutting[56] propose that the first procedure, cranial vault remodeling and fronto-orbital advancement, be performed between 6 and 9 months of age. At an earlier age, the bone is more fragile; at a later age (>18 months), residual calvarial defects will fail to reossify. Early surgery is also important because of rapid growth of the brain, which more than doubles in volume during the first year of life.[57] Later procedures also delay the potential benefits of early decompression. For the patient with coronal synostosis, this means bilateral fronto-orbital advancement with frontotemporal cranial remodeling. It involves a two-team approach; neurosurgeons perform the frontal craniotomy, and plastic surgeons perform the orbital osteotomy, cranial remodeling, and advancement. To enhance stabilization of the advanced segment, a separate temporoparietal bone graft may be used behind the advanced segment.[50] Metopic synostosis is treated with remodeling of the frontal bone flap. Sagittal synostosis is treated with strip craniectomy if the deformity is limited or extensive cranial vault remodeling for significant anterior-posterior lengthening with narrow bitemporal width.

Midface hypoplasia will often become a significant factor by the age of 3 to 4 years. It is during this period that plans are made for Le Fort III or monobloc advancement of the midface. The Le Fort III is an extracranial procedure that advances the entire midface, nose, lower orbits, and zygoma. Correction of occlusal abnormalities is not the main goal during this stage of reconstruction because continued growth deficiency of the midface will result in Angle class III malocclusion and require further orthognathic surgery on completion of skeletal growth. Should the

TABLE 90-3 ✦ TIMING OF SURGERY

Procedure	Age at Intervention
Fronto-orbital advancement	6-12 months
Monobloc/Le Fort III	3-8 years
Le Fort I/bilateral sagittal split osteotomy	14-18 years
Revision advancement (for elevated intracranial pressure or resynostosis)	2-8 years

forehead require concomitant advancement, a monobloc advancement is the procedure of choice.

Orbital hypertelorism, or wide intercanthal distance, is a characteristic physical finding of both Crouzon and Apert patients. There is also an associated nasal deformity with widening of the upper third of the nose. The displaced nasal bones and cartilages result in a short, wide nose. The timing of surgical correction is more individualized than for primary treatment of cranial suture fusion, but it is generally not performed before 2 years of age.[58] The widened intercanthal distance can also be addressed with three- or four-wall osteotomy.

The third stage of reconstruction follows the end of facial and tooth development. It is now known that Le Fort I advancement can correct the discrepancy between mandibular and midface enlargement, as can rhinoplasty or genioplasty (Table 90-3).

Surgical Outcomes and Secondary Surgery

Abnormalities of facial growth that are present preoperatively in syndromic patients persist postoperatively as well. Depending on the degree of growth deficiency or the amount of relapse after initial correction, minor revision or even secondary readvancement may be required. Kreiborg and Aduss[59] observed a series of patients during 10 years and evaluated preoperative and postoperative facial growth in Apert and Crouzon patients requiring Le Fort III maxillary advancement. They found the lack of maxillary sutural growth and patterns of abnormal remodeling similar to those of preoperative patients. Advancements were 9 to 19 mm, and there was no evidence of relapse. However, the basic abnormalities of midfacial growth in these syndromic patients result in maxillary deficiency in three planes, which may progress despite surgery. The degree of developmental deformity is highly variable among patients, but the overall conclusion is that further orthognathic intervention will be required for the majority of patients on completion of growth. In a review comparing 167 syndromic and nonsyndromic patients during 3 years of

TABLE 90-4 ✦ THE WHITAKER CLASSIFICATION

Whitaker Category	Secondary Procedures
Category I	No refinements or surgical revision considered necessary
Category II	Soft tissue or lesser bone-contouring revisions able to be performed on an outpatient basis or minimal 2-day hospital stay
Category III	Major secondary osteotomies or bone graft repositioning, onlay bone grafts, Le Fort advancement; the listed procedures are not as extensive as the original operation
Category IV	A major craniofacial reconstruction, duplicating or exceeding the original procedure

From Whitaker LA, Bartlett SP, Schut L, Bruce D: Craniosynostosis: an analysis of the timing, treatment, and complications in 164 consecutive patients. Plast Reconstr Surg 1987;80:195-212.

follow-up, Williams et al[60] had 12 patients requiring reoperation of a magnitude equal to or greater than the original operation (7%). Overall reoperation rates were 27.3% for syndromic patients and 5.9% for nonsyndromic patients. McCarthy[61,62] and Whitaker,[63] using similar surgical approaches, have reported greater reoperation and complication rates in syndromic patients (Table 90-4). The Johns Hopkins experience during the 1990s has confirmed the higher rate of major secondary procedures among syndromic patients without the significantly greater early and late complication rate (unpublished data).

The majority of series evaluating outcomes in the surgical correction of craniosynostosis do not address psychosocial outcomes. Purely surgical outcomes are available for both syndromic and nonsyndromic populations. These have been the basis for early surgical intervention. Many also use Whitaker's method of evaluating the degree of and need for secondary procedures and are retrospective. Wagner et al[64] described 22 nonsyndromic patients with a morbidity of 23%, similar to other series. He also noted that overall, 14% required revisional cranial recontouring or cranioplasty to achieve a satisfactory aesthetic outcome. Of note, a trend was found that reoperation was higher if operations were performed at an age of 5 months or earlier. McCarthy[62] provided one of the most comprehensive experiences available by examining 20 years' worth of results in 76 syndromic and 104 nonsyndromic patients. Among nonsyndromic patients undergoing primary fronto-orbital advancement at a mean age of 8 months, 87% required no or minimal revisional procedures. This is significantly different from the group of patients with syndromes or panfacial synostoses. Major secondary procedures were required in 36.8%

versus 13.5%. Perioperative complications were also higher (11.3% versus 5.0%). Some of these differences are attributable to ongoing abnormalities of development, and turribrachycephaly developed in some of the syndromic patients despite primary correction. Whereas rates of significant need for major secondary procedures are lower in nonsyndromic patients, early age at primary surgery may play a role as well. An evaluation of nonsyndromic patients with sagittal synostosis revealed that 3 of 85 patients had poor results. All of these patients had their procedures performed before 3 months of age.[65] Resynostosis is likely to be related to the cause of the original sutural fusion, and therefore one would anticipate higher rates of major reoperation for syndromic patients.

Resorbable Versus Nonresorbable Rigid Internal Fixation

Achieving stability of osseous segments in craniofacial surgery, as in the treatment of facial or other fractures, is essential for proper bone healing. During the early development of craniofacial techniques, this stability was obtained from techniques similar to carpentry; the advanced segments were stabilized against one another with mortise and tenon, or other joints, and then secured with wires. Methods of rigid fixation have evolved over the years, with the advancement of materials, toward rigid internal fixation with biocompatible metallic plates and screws. Facial fractures are now routinely stabilized with 1.0- to 2.0-mm-thick titanium or Vitallium (cobalt-chromium alloy) miniplates. The use of these systems in the treatment of craniofacial fractures maintains the three-dimensional restoration of the bone segment and facilitates healing.[66,67] Any system of fixation must overcome soft tissue forces and maintain the repositioned bone in position long enough for it to heal. Bone to bone contact is also important because contact healing is superior to gap healing.[68] This same technology has been adapted for use in the craniofacial patient. With widespread use of metallic hardware, problems have been identified that have led to the development of alternative systems. Tissue toxicity varies according to the material. Although silicone, titanium, Vitallium, and stainless steel wire are generally compatible with biologic systems, the relative inflammatory response of the brain was examined. Titanium has the earliest inflammatory response (2 weeks). The late tissue inflammation (26 weeks) was greatest with stainless steel wire. Titanium and Vitallium incited a similar inflammatory response that was greater than the response found with silicone elastomer but less than that with stainless steel wire. This study, performed in rabbits, resulted in no neurologic damage.[47] Titanium alone has not been shown to cause malignant transformation, but compounds with chromium, nickel, and cobalt are carcinogenic in animals. Only 11 clinical instances of malignant neoplasia associated with metal alloys have been reported in humans and are generally soft tissue sarcomas.[67] Artifact on MRI and CT, infection, palpability, pain, and temperature sensitivity have been associated with permanent plating systems. Because these procedures are performed in children, bone growth and remodeling will be affected and may result in growth retardation and transcranial migration of the plates. Translocation of the plates has been reported to occur in up to 50% of pediatric patients.[69] Migration of the plates also makes secondary procedures more difficult, necessitating their removal for bone repositioning. Permanent plating systems have also been implicated in disturbances of growth, and although the subject remains controversial, several studies support this view.[70-72] Many of these problems require secondary procedures. Orringer et al[48] described 55 patients, both congenital craniofacial and adult trauma patients, in whom internal fixation devices required removal. Common reasons for removal were palpable or prominent hardware (35%), loosening of plates and screws (25%), infection (23%), pain (25%), and hardware exposure (20%). The majority of these problems occurred during the first year after surgery. Infection, palpability, and pain remain the most significant reasons for hardware removal in other studies as well.[73]

Polylactic acid, polyglycolic acid, and polydioxanone polymers have been in use as resorbable suture material for more than 20 years. As sutures, they have been used to secure bone segments in craniofacial surgery, but they have the same disadvantages of wire fixation in terms of rigidity and stability.[74] The first reported use of these materials for plate fixation of facial fractures was in 1987 by Bos,[75] who showed effective healing of unstable zygomatic fractures. Since then, material advances have led to copolymer plating systems that offer the strength characteristics of one compound with the rapid resorption properties of another. Polylactic acid and polyglycolic acid are naturally occurring substances in the human body. Polyglycolic acid is characterized by flexural strength but rapid resorption (6 weeks); polylactic acid has much greater strength and a longer period for degradation (5 to 6 years). Current variations offer periods of resorption between 6 months and several years.[76] Ideally, these materials should have sufficient strength and stability for bone healing and then be degraded by the body such that the space previously occupied by the plate is replaced with bone. The use of these plating materials is a relatively recent development, encompassing approximately the last 5 years. A few studies are now available reporting early outcomes. In a review of 51 patients undergoing craniofacial surgery with an average follow-up of 2 years, Kurpad et al[77] reported no complications and no relapse of the advanced orbital reconstruction. A second report described 85 patients with

1 to 2 years of follow-up after fixation with resorbable plates and either metallic screws or resorbable material, depending on calvarial thickness. Similarly good results were found, with no plate complications, excellent bone healing, and no evidence of inhibition of growth as evidenced radiologically by separation of the fixed segments. In a third study, 54 children with disease involving the upper and middle craniofacial skeleton were examined. Anatomic union was the focus of this study and was achieved in 96% of the patients studied. The two patients who experienced malunion had undergone revisional procedures in which bone grafting was not used.[78] Many described a learning curve in the molding of the materials and appropriate drilling and tapping of the holes compared with metal systems. Although palpability was an early problem, this resolved with resorption of the plates and screws. Resorbable systems, in general, appear to offer the advantages of metallic plating systems without many of the major disadvantages, including a lack of toxicity and radiopacity on MRI or CT.

NONSYNDROMIC MALFORMATIONS

Frontonasal Malformation

Beyond syndromic malformations of the craniofacial skeleton, several nonsyndromic malformations are important, including frontonasal malformation (also known as median cleft facial syndrome or median face syndrome). Frontonasal dysplasia was the term first used by Sedano and Gorlin in 1970 and subsequently modified to frontonasal malformation by the same authors in 1988 as a more general way of referring to this condition of uncertain pathogenesis.[79,80] A universal feature of this malformation is hypertelorism. The spectrum of clinical expression includes anterior cranium bifidum occultum; broad nasal root; median cleft of the nose or the nasal tip, upper lip, and premaxilla; occasional median cleft palate; and widow's peak in the hairline.[81] Central nervous system abnormalities may also be present with an anterior encephalocele, sphenoethmoidal encephalocele, or absent corpus callosum. For the majority of patients with a sphenoethmoidal encephalocele, optic disc abnormalities such as hypoplasia are also present. It was suggested in one study that the presence of a midline cleft and optic disc abnormalities in a child should alert the clinician to the possibility of a basal encephalocele.[82] Cardiac malformations do occur, albeit not commonly, in particular tetralogy of Fallot (Fig. 90-3).[83]

The etiology of the frontonasal malformation is not known. The anterior neurocranium and most of the facial bones are formed by a migration of neural crest cells—a mesenchymal tissue that subsequently undergoes intramembranous ossification.[84] It appears that this condition is morphologically a failure of the

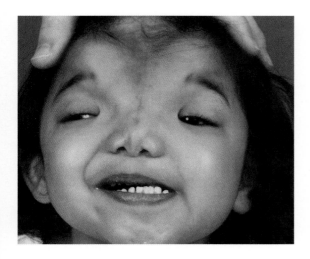

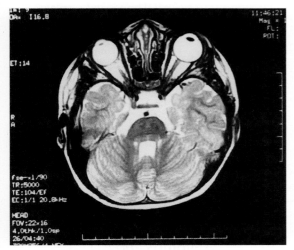

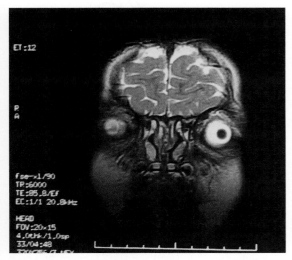

FIGURE 90-3. Hypertelorism in a young girl with frontonasal dysplasia. On MRI, note the duplication of midline structures between the orbits, which must be reduced during correction of the deformity and centralization of the orbits.

frontonasal process and medial nasal processes to develop and fuse. One explanation of this failure of fusion is a late embryonic failure of cellular degeneration that interferes with fusion.[85] Alternatively, an early ischemic episode or failure of neural crest cell migration has been suggested as the cause.[86,87]

Craniofrontonasal dysplasia is recognized as a form of frontonasal malformation. It was first described by Cohen[88] in 1979 as a familial disorder with an unusual X-linked pattern. Originally believed to be autosomal dominant, it has been shown to be X-linked dominant (mapping to Xp22), whereby all daughters of males are affected and none of their sons is affected.[89] The majority of affected individuals are female; males have a milder form of the disorder. It is defined as the combination of frontonasal dysplasia and coronal craniosynostosis with varying extracranial manifestations. Accompanying the expected hypertelorism, broadened nose, and bifid nasal tip are frontal bossing and brachycephaly secondary to the synostosis. Many of the affected individuals also have characteristically curly hair and nails with longitudinal grooves. Other physical findings may include soft tissue syndactyly in the hands and feet, shoulder and hip derangements, and occasionally cleft lip and palate.[88,90]

MIDLINE FRONTONASAL MASSES

A spectrum of malformations in the frontonasal region is a reflection of varying degrees of altered embryologic development. Frontal dermoid cyst, sinus track, glioma, and encephalocele all progress along a similar anatomic tract extending from the foramen cecum into the prenasal space. As the frontonasal process develops between the third and eighth weeks of life, an evagination of dura exists below the ectoderm. If this dural extension does not retract and the foramen cecum fails to close, a sinus or cyst may result (Fig. 90-4).

Dermoid

A dermoid cyst is a sequestration of ectodermal tissue and is therefore lined with epithelial tissue with adnexal elements. It represents a failure of the underlying dural process to completely separate from its dermal attachments. Varying degrees of captured adnexal tissues result in varying degrees of heterogeneity of the cyst contents, including hair and pilonidal glandular structures. Dermoids may occur throughout the body; nasal cysts account for 1% of all types, and 3% to 12% are head and neck cysts.[91] They may be located anywhere between the glabella and the nasal tip and can present as a dimple or pore in the skin. It is possible for them to become infected, but they rarely act as a source for intracranial abscess; intracranial extension occurs in 36% of all midline dermoids according to Posnick.[92]

Whereas the more laterally located brow dermoids can be simply excised, frontonasal dermoids require

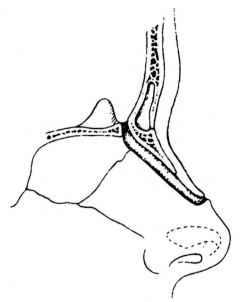

FIGURE 90-4. The common pathway for dermoid, glioma, and encephalocele is an evagination of dura through the foramen cecum, which normally regresses. This occurs in the prenasal space between the skin and the nasal cartilages. (From Bauer BS: Benign tumors and conditions of the head and neck. In Coleman JJ, Wilkins EG, VanderKam VM: Head and Neck Surgery. St. Louis, Mosby, 2000:1135. Achauer BM, Eriksson E, Guyuron B, et al, eds: Plastic Surgery: Indications, Operations, and Outcomes; vol 3.)

CT or MRI evaluation and neurosurgical consultation. Their excision may require combined intracranial and extracranial excision.

Glioma

Nasal gliomas are heterotopic neural tissue (glial fibers) thought to be encephaloceles that have lost their intracranial attachment. A connecting stalk to the intracranial space may persist in 20%. Nasal gliomas may be external, intranasal, or a combination. On histologic examination, they resemble encephaloceles but are often very vascular, making them easily mistaken clinically for hemangiomas.[93] The most common areas of presentation are in the area of the cribriform plate at the nasal root (nasal glioma) and the bridge of the nose (extranasal). They are generally firm and may be distinguished from vascular lesions or encephalocele by the patient's performance of a Valsalva maneuver. They may present as a nasal obstruction, and the work-up and treatment are similar to those for frontonasal dermoids (Fig. 90-5).

ENCEPHALOCELE

An encephalocele is a herniation of dura, cerebrospinal fluid, and often brain tissue through a defect in the cranium. Encephaloceles are generally categorized into anterior, parietal, or occipital; occipital is the most common. Encephaloceles of the frontonasal region are relatively uncommon in Western civilizations with a birth prevalence of 1 in 35,000, whereas the condition approaches 1 in 5000 births in Asian countries. If not directly visible, they are termed basal; the visible types are called sincipital. Charoonsmith[94] divides them into the following groups:

Nasofrontal encephalocele	The midline cranial defect is between the orbits at the nasal root. The medial orbital walls are laterally displaced.
Nasoethmoidal encephalocele	The cranial defect is between the frontal and ethmoid bones. The frontal lobe herniates between the nasal bones and cartilages. Again, the medial orbital walls are displaced.
Naso-orbital encephalocele	The brain herniates through a medial orbital wall defect. The frontal and nasal bones are normal.

It is also possible for there to be combinations of these subtypes. In general, the goal of surgical treatment is the early management of elevated intracranial

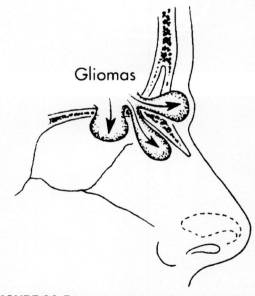

FIGURE 90-5. Pathways for extranasal and intranasal gliomas can traverse the frontonasal suture, foramen cecum, or cribriform plate. (From Bauer BS: Benign tumors and conditions of the head and neck. In Coleman JJ, Wilkins EG, VanderKam VM: Head and Neck Surgery. St. Louis, Mosby, 2000:1136. Achauer BM, Eriksson E, Guyuron B, et al, eds: Plastic Surgery: Indications, Operations, and Outcomes; vol 3.)

pressure if it is present. Beyond this, Holmes et al[95] also recommend measures to prevent sac rupture, urgent closure of skin defects, removal of nonfunctional extracerebral tissue, and watertight dural closure. Bone correction usually means frontal remodeling, nasal bone grafting with attention to prevention of the "long-nose" deformity, and correction of the telecanthus with transnasal wire. Correction of dystopia or hyper-telorism can be performed in the same stage.

HYPERTELORISM

Displacement of the craniofacial skeleton secondary to frontonasal malformation or midline masses results in varying degrees of deformity. Malposition of the orbital structures spans the spectrum from a mild appearance of telecanthus to true hypertelorism. The nasal root is widened. The nose itself can become elongated, and structures may occasionally be duplicated, resulting in a bifid septum. With frontonasal dysplasia, there is often true hypertelorism with lateral displacement of the entire orbit; with midline mass lesions, only the medial orbital wall is displaced laterally, resulting in telecanthus.

Mulliken[96] defines hypertelorism as greater than two standard deviations from age- and gender-matched means for interorbital distance and outer orbital distance. Interorbital distance is defined as the bone measurement between the junction of the frontal lacrimal bones. Outer orbital distance is defined as the distance between the lateral orbital rims at the same level. Orbital hypertelorism is defined as an abnormal increase in both measures, whereas interorbital hypertelorism is merely an increase in interorbital distance. Among these various categories, orbital hypertelorism is usually present in frontonasal malformation; interorbital hypertelorism is a result of midline mass effect as seen with encephalocele.

Tessier[97] ranked the severity of deformity in adults by measuring the interorbital distance and placed it in three categories:

First-degree:	30 to 34 mm
Second-degree:	34 to 40 mm
Third-degree:	>40 mm

For children, of course, these standards need to be adjusted. Farkas[98] has established normative data for myriad facial anthropometric dimensions. Mean inter-canthal width in the first year of life ranges from 25 to 27 mm; outer orbital distance ranges from 74 to 76 mm. By 5 years of age, these distances have increased to 27 to 30 mm and 76 to 80 mm. For those older than 20 years, mean intercanthal width is 31 to 33 mm; mean outer orbital distance is 87 to 91 mm.

Another method of grading severity of disease based on CT scan is provided by Munro.[99] He noted four categories of medial orbital wall and ethmoidal

deformity based on coronal views of the orbits. Types I and II are the more common forms and are differentiated from types III and IV in that the latter forms have their widest dimension posterior to the globe and therefore a more technically difficult correction of the hypertelorism (Fig. 90-6).

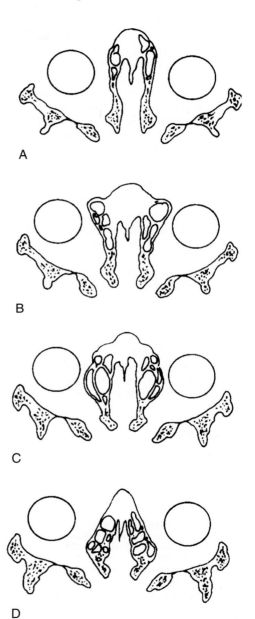

A

B

C

D

FIGURE 90-6. Types of medial orbital wall deformity seen in hypertelorism. *A,* Type I, parallel medial orbital walls. *B,* Type II, wedge shaped posteriorly. *C,* Type III, oval. *D,* Type IV, wedge shaped anteriorly. Types III and IV are the rarest and most difficult to repair because the maximum width is located posteriorly. (From Munro IR, Das SK: Improving results in orbital hypertelorism correction. Ann Plast Surg 1979;2:499-507.)

Hydrocephalus should be corrected as early as possible with placement of a ventriculoperitoneal shunt. Correction of gross deformity and bone grafting can occur concomitantly with neurosurgical elimination of the hernia sac. If no emergent neonatal surgery is required for imminent central nervous system exposure, the first reconstruction can be deferred to a period when the child is larger and can more easily tolerate blood loss and general anesthesia—at 4 to 5 months. Nasal bone grafts in this period may not grow to the same extent as the rest of the face.

The second stage of reconstruction with further correction of the anterior cranial vault, hypertelorism, or nose is recommended as needed before school age at 4 to 6 years. With the completion of facial growth in the teenage years, rhinoplasty and any necessary orthognathic surgery can be considered.

CONCLUSION

The history of human craniofacial malformation and its treatment spans many cultures across the centuries. Although this medium cannot encompass every known syndromic malformation in depth, it does provide a broad overview that brings into focus the most recent view, including the genetic origins of these complex processes. With ongoing research, we will continue to better educate patients, parents, and the public and to address not only the medical and surgical outcomes but the psychosocial ones as well.

Special Acknowledgment

We would like to acknowledge Jaleh Pourhamidi, DMD, MDS, Assistant Professor and Orthodontist, University of Nevada, Las Vegas, School of Dental Medicine, for her contributions to the historical sections of the chapter.

REFERENCES

1. Sailer HF, Kolb E: Influence of craniofacial surgery on the social attitudes toward the malformed and their handling in different cultures and at different times: a contribution to social world history. J Craniofac Surg 1995;6:314-326.
2. Kinney BA: Infant abandonment in early China. Early China 1993;18:107-138.
3. Ozaki W, Buchman SR, Muraszko KM, Coleman D: Investigation of the influences of biomechanical force on the ultrastructure of human sagittal craniosynostosis. Plast Reconstr Surg 1998;102:1385-1394.
4. Bradley JP, Shahinian H, Levine JP, et al: Growth restriction of cranial sutures in the fetal lamb causes deformational changes, not craniosynostosis. Plast Reconstr Surg 2000;105:2416-2423.
5. Reardon W, Winter RM, Rutland P, et al: Mutations in the fibroblast growth factor receptor 2 gene cause Crouzon syndrome. Nat Genet 1994;8:98-103.
6. Cohen MM Jr: Craniofacial disorders caused by mutations in homeobox genes MSX1 and MSX2. J Craniofac Genet Dev Biol 2000;20:19-25.
7. Jabs EW, Muller U, Li X, et al: A mutation in the homeodomain of the human MSX2 gene in a family affected with autosomal dominant craniosynostosis. Cell 1993;75:443-450.
8. Ma L, Golden S, Wu L, Maxson R: The molecular basis of Boston-type craniosynostosis: the Pro148→His mutation in the N-terminal arm of the MSX2 homeodomain stabilizes DNA binding without altering nucleotide sequence preferences. Hum Mol Genet 1996;5:1915-1920.
9. Jabs EW, Li X, Scott AF, et al: Jackson-Weiss and Crouzon syndromes are allelic with mutations in fibroblast growth factor receptor 2. Nat Genet 1994;8:275-279.
10. Kim HJ, Rice DP, Kettunen PJ, Thesleff I: FGF-, BMP- and Shh-mediated signalling pathways in the regulation of cranial suture morphogenesis and calvarial bone development. Development 1998;125:1241-1251.
11. Neilson KM, Friesel RE: Constitutive activation of fibroblast growth factor receptor-2 by a point mutation associated with Crouzon syndrome. J Biol Chem 1995;270:26037-26040.
12. Robertson SC, Meyer AN, Hart KC, et al: Activating mutations in the extracellular domain of the fibroblast growth factor receptor 2 function by disruption of the disulfide bond in the third immunoglobulin-like domain. Proc Natl Acad Sci USA 1998;95:4567-4572.
13. Anderson J, Burns HD, Enriquez-Harris P, et al: Apert syndrome mutations in fibroblast growth factor receptor 2 exhibit increased affinity for FGF ligand. Hum Mol Genet 1998;7:1475-1483.
14. Crow JF: The origins, patterns and implications of human spontaneous mutation. Nat Rev Genet 2000;1:40-47.
15. El Ghouzzi V, Legeai-Mallet L, Aresta S, et al: Saethre-Chotzen mutations cause TWIST protein degradation or impaired nuclear location. Hum Mol Genet 2000;9:813-819.
16. Nuckolls GH, Shum L, Slavkin HC: Progress toward understanding craniofacial malformations. Cleft Palate Craniofac J 1999;36:12-26.
17. Lee S, Seto M, Sie K, Cunningham M: A child with Saethre-Chotzen syndrome, sensorineural hearing loss, and a TWIST mutation. Cleft Palate Craniofac J 2002;39:110-114.
18. Cohen MM Jr: The Robin anomalad—its nonspecificity and associated syndromes. J Oral Surg 1976;34:587-593.
19. Cohen MM Jr: Craniosynostosis: Diagnosis, Evaluation and Management. New York, Raven Press, 1986.
20. Dufresne C, Richtsmeier JT: Interaction of craniofacial dysmorphology, growth, and prediction of surgical outcome. J Craniofac Surg 1995;6:270-281.
21. Kress W, Collmann H, Busse M, et al: Clustering of FGFR2 gene mutations in patients with Pfeiffer and Crouzon syndromes (FGFR2-associated craniosynostoses). Cytogenet Cell Genet 2000;91:134-137.
22. Park WJ, Theda C, Maestri NE, et al: Analysis of phenotypic features and FGFR2 mutations in Apert syndrome. Am J Hum Genet 1995;57:321-328.
23. Bronshtein M, Blumenfeld I, Blumenfeld Z: Early prenatal diagnosis of cleft lip and its potential impact on the number of babies with cleft lip. Br J Oral Maxillofac Surg 1996;34:486-487.
24. Chang J, Siebert JW, Schendel SA, et al: Scarless wound healing: implications for the aesthetic surgeon. Aesthetic Plast Surg 1995;19:237-241.
25. Virchow R: Über den Cretinismus, namentlich in Franken, und über pathologische Schädelformen. Verh Phys Med Gesellsch Wurzburg 1851;2:230.
26. Moss ML: The functional matrix hypothesis revisited. 3. The genomic thesis. Am J Orthod Dentofacial Orthop 1997;112:338-342.
27. Park EA, Powers GF: Acrocephaly and scaphocephaly with symmetrically distributed malformations of the extremities: a study of the so-called "acrosyndactylism." Am J Dis Child 1920;20:235.
28. Delashaw JB, Persing JA, Jane JA: Cranial deformation in craniosynostosis. A new explanation. Neurosurg Clin North Am 1991;2:611-620.

29. Enlow DH, Han M: Essentials of Facial Growth. Philadelphia, WB Saunders, 1996.

30. Allanson JE: Objective techniques for craniofacial assessment: what are the choices? Am J Med Genet 1997;70:1-5.

31. Webster's Dictionary. Springfield, Mass, Meriam-Webster, 1999.

32. Tessier P, Guiot G, Rougerie J, et al: Cranio-naso-orbito-facial osteotomies. Hypertelorism. Ann Chir Plast 1967;12:103-118.

33. Kline RM Jr: Management of craniofacial anomalies. J S C Med Assoc 1997;93:336-341.

34. Bruneteau RJ, Mulliken JB: Frontal plagiocephaly: synostotic, compensational, or deformational. Plast Reconstr Surg 1992;89:21-31.

35. Sulik KK, Smiley SJ, Turvey TA, et al: Pathogenesis of cleft palate in Treacher Collins, Nager, and Miller syndromes. Cleft Palate J 1989;26:209-216.

36. Poswillo D: The pathogenesis of the first and second branchial arch syndrome. Oral Surg 1973;35:302-329.

37. Grabb WC: The first and second branchial arch syndrome. Plast Reconstr Surg 1965;36:485-508.

38. Poswillo D: Hemorrhage in development of the face. Birth Defects 1975;11:61-81.

39. Kaban LB, Moses MH, Mulliken JB: Surgical correction of hemifacial microsomia in the growing child. Plast Reconstr Surg 1988;82:9-19.

40. David DJ, Mahatumarat C, Cooter RD: Hemifacial microsomia: a multisystem classification. Plast Reconstr Surg 1987; 80:525-535.

41. Hanson JW, Smith DW: U-shaped palatal defect in the Robin anomalad: developmental and clinical relevance. J Pediatr 1975;87:30-33.

42. Francomano CA, Liberfarb RM, Hirose T, et al: The Stickler syndrome: evidence for close linkage to the structural gene for type II collagen. Genomics 1987;1:293-296.

43. Shprintzen RA: New syndrome involving cleft palate, cardiac anomalies, typical facies, and learning disabilities: velocardiofacial syndrome. Cleft Palate Craniofac J 1978;15:56-62.

44. D'Antonio LL, Marsh JL: Abnormal carotid arteries in the velocardiofacial syndrome. Plast Reconstr Surg 1987;80:471-472.

45. Burdick AB: Genetic epidemiology and control of genetic expression in van der Woude syndrome. J Craniofac Genet Dev Biol Suppl 1986;2:99-105.

46. Posnick JC: Craniofacial dysostosis. Staging of reconstruction and management of the midface deformity. Neurosurg Clin North Am 1991;2:683-702.

47. Mofid MM, Thompson RC, Pardo CA, et al: Biocompatibility of fixation materials in the brain. Plast Reconstr Surg 1997;100:14-20.

48. Orringer JS, Barcelona V, Buchman SR: Reasons for removal of rigid internal fixation devices in craniofacial surgery. J Craniofac Surg 1998;9:40-44.

49. Pertschuk MJ, Whitaker LA: Psychosocial considerations in craniofacial deformity. Clin Plast Surg 1987;14:163-168.

50. Vander Kolk CA, Toth BA: Syndromic craniosynostosis: craniofacial dysostosis. In Achauer BM, Eriksson E, Guyuron B, et al, eds: Plastic Surgery: Indications, Operations, and Outcomes. St. Louis, Mosby, 2000.

51. Renier D: Intracranial pressure in craniosynostosis: pre- and postoperative recordings—correlation with functional results. In Persing J, Edgerton MT, Jane JA: Scientific Foundations and Surgical Treatment of Craniosynostosis. Baltimore, Williams & Wilkins, 1989.

52. Renier D: Longitudinal assessment of mental development in infants with nonsyndromic craniosynostosis with and without cranial release and reconstruction: discussion. Plast Reconstr Surg 1993;92:840.

53. Lefebvre A, Travis F, Arndt EM, Munro IR: A psychiatric profile before and after reconstructive surgery in children with Apert's syndrome. Br J Plast Surg 1986;39:510-513.

54. Coccaro PJ, McCarthy JG, Epstein FJ, et al: Early and late surgery in craniofacial dysostosis: a longitudinal cephalometric study. Am J Orthod 1980;77:421-436.

55. Kreiborg S, Aduss H: Pre- and postsurgical facial growth in patients with Crouzon's and Apert's syndromes. Cleft Palate J 1986;23(suppl 1):78-90.

56. McCarthy JG, Cutting CB: The timing of surgical intervention in craniofacial anomalies. Clin Plast Surg 1990;17:161-182.

57. DiRocco C, Velardi F: Surgical management of craniosynostosis. In Galli G: Craniosynostosis. Boca Raton, Fla, CRC Press, 1984.

58. Salyer KE, Hubli EH: Orbital hypertelorism. In Achauer BM, Eriksson E, Guyuron B, et al, eds: Plastic Surgery: Indications, Operations, and Outcomes. St. Louis, Mosby, 2000.

59. Kreiborg S, Aduss H: Pre- and postsurgical facial growth in patients with Crouzon's and Apert's syndromes. Cleft Palate J 1986;23(suppl 1):78-90.

60. Williams JK, Cohen SR, Burstein FD, et al: A longitudinal, statistical study of reoperation rates in craniosynostosis. Plast Reconstr Surg 1997;100:305-310.

61. McCarthy JG, Glasberg SB, Cutting CB, et al: Twenty-year experience with early surgery for craniosynostosis: II. The craniofacial synostosis syndromes and pansynostosis-results and unsolved problems. Plast Reconstr Surg 1995;96:284-295.

62. McCarthy JG, Glasberg SB, Cutting CB, et al: Twenty-year experience with early surgery for craniosynostosis: I. Isolated craniofacial synostosis—results and unsolved problems. Plast Reconstr Surg 1995;96:272-283.

63. Whitaker LA, Bartlett SP, Schut L, Bruce D: Craniosynostosis: an analysis of the timing, treatment, and complications in 164 consecutive patients. Plast Reconstr Surg 1987;80:195-212.

64. Wagner JD, Cohen SR, Maher H, et al: Critical analysis of results of craniofacial surgery for nonsyndromic bicoronal synostosis. J Craniofac Surg 1995;6:32-37.

65. Boop FA, Chadduck WM, Shewmake K, Teo C: Outcome analysis of 85 patients undergoing the pi procedure for correction of sagittal synostosis. J Neurosurg 1996;85:50-55.

66. Francel TJ, Birely BC, Sadove AM: The fate of plates and screws after facial fracture reconstruction. Plast Reconstr Surg 1992;90:568-573.

67. Altobelli DE, Yaremchuk MJ, Gruss JS, Manson PN: Implant materials in rigid fixation: physical, mechanical, corrosion, and biocompatibility considerations. In Yaremchuk MJ, Gruss JS, Manson PN, eds: Rigid Fixation of the Craniomaxillofacial Skeleton. Boston, Butterworth-Heinemann, 1992:28-56.

68. Yaremchuk MJ, Gruss JS, Manson PN: Rigid Fixation of the Craniomaxillofacial Skeleton. Boston, Butterworth-Heinemann, 1992.

69. Goldberg DS, Bartlett S, Yu JC, et al: Critical review of microfixation in pediatric craniofacial surgery. J Craniofac Surg 1995;6:301-307.

70. Eppley BL, Platis JM, Sadove AM: Experimental effects of bone plating in infancy on craniomaxillofacial skeletal growth. Cleft Palate Craniofac J 1993;30:164-169.

71. Fearon JA, Munro IR, Bruce DA: Observations on the use of rigid fixation for craniofacial deformities in infants and young children. Plast Reconstr Surg 1995;95:634-637.

72. Yaremchuk MJ: Experimental studies addressing rigid fixation in craniofacial surgery. Clin Plast Surg 1994;21:517-524.

73. Francel TJ, Birely BC, Ringelman PR, Manson PN: The fate of plates and screws after facial fracture reconstruction. Plast Reconstr Surg 1992;90:568-573.

74. Bos RR, Rozema FR, Boering G, et al.: The potential of resorbable biomaterials for skeletal fixation. In Yaremchuk MJ, Gruss JS, Manson PN, eds: Rigid Fixation of the Craniomaxillofacial Skeleton. Boston, Butterworth-Heinemann, 1992:57-62.

75. Bos RR, Boering G, Rozema FR, Leenslag JW: Resorbable poly (L-lactide) plates and screws for the fixation of zygomatic fractures. J Oral Maxillofac Surg 1987;45:751-753.

76. Imola MJ, Hamlar DD, Shao W, et al: Resorbable plate fixation in pediatric craniofacial surgery: long-term outcome. Arch Facial Plast Surg 2001;3:79-90.

77. Kurpad SN, Goldstein JA, Cohen AR: Bioresorbable fixation for congenital pediatric craniofacial surgery: a 2-year follow-up. Pediatr Neurosurg 2000;33:306-310.

78. Eppley BL, Sadove AM, Havlik RJ: Resorbable plate fixation in pediatric craniofacial surgery. Plast Reconstr Surg 1997; 100:1-7.

79. Sedano HO, Cohen MM Jr, Jirasek J, Gorlin RJ: Frontonasal dysplasia. J Pediatr 1970;76:906-913.

80. Sedano HO, Gorlin RJ: Frontonasal malformation as a field defect and in syndromic associations. Oral Surg Oral Med Oral Pathol 1988;65:704-710.

81. Nevin NC, Leonard AG, Jones B: Frontonasal dysostosis in two successive generations. Am J Med Genet 1999;87:251-253.

82. Hodgkins P, Lees M, Lawson J, et al: Optic disc anomalies and frontonasal dysplasia. Br J Ophthalmol 1998;82:290-293.

83. De Moor MM, Baruch R, Human DG: Frontonasal dysplasia associated with tetralogy of Fallot. J Med Genet 1987;24:107-109.

84. Wilkie AO, Morriss-Kay GM: Genetics of craniofacial development and malformation. Nat Rev Genet 2001;2:458-468.

85. Poelman RE, Vermeij-Keers C: Cell degeneration in the mouse embryo: a prerequisite for normal development. In Muller-Berat V: Progress in Differentiation Research. New York, American Elsevier, 1976.

86. Cohen MM Jr, Sedano HO, Gorlin RJ, Jirasek JE: Frontonasal dysplasia (median cleft face syndrome): comments on etiology and pathogenesis. Birth Defects Orig Artic Ser 1971;7:117-119.

87. Mazzola RF: Congenital malformations in the frontonasal area: their pathogenesis and classification. Clin Plast Surg 1976;3:573-609.

88. Cohen MM Jr: Craniofrontonasal dysplasia. Birth Defects Orig Artic Ser 1979;15:85-89.

89. Feldman GJ, Ward DE, Lajeunie-Renier E, et al: A novel phenotypic pattern in X-linked inheritance: craniofrontonasal syndrome maps to Xp22. Hum Mol Genet 1997;6:1937-1941.

90. Grutzner E, Gorlin RJ: Craniofrontonasal dysplasia: phenotypic expression in females and males and genetic considerations. Oral Surg Oral Med Oral Pathol 1988;65:436-444.

91. Bratton C, Suskind DL, Thomas T, Kluka EA: Autosomal dominant familial frontonasal dermoid cysts: a mother and her identical twin daughters. Int J Pediatr Otorhinolaryngol 2001;57:249-253.

92. Posnick JC, Bortoluzzi P, Armstrong DC, Drake JM: Intracranial nasal dermoid sinus cysts: computed tomographic scan findings and surgical results. Plast Reconstr Surg 1994;93:745-754.

93. Jaffe BF: Classification and management of anomalies of the nose. Otolaryngol Clin North Am 1981;14:989-1004.

94. Charoonsmith T, Suwanwela C: Frontoethmoidal encephalomeningocele with special reference to plastic reconstruction. Clin Plast Surg 1974;1:27-47.

95. Holmes AD, Meara JG, Kolker AR, et al: Frontoethmoidal encephaloceles: reconstruction and refinements. J Craniofac Surg 2001;12:6-18.

96. Tan ST, Mulliken JB: Hypertelorism: nosologic analysis of 90 patients. Plast Reconstr Surg 1997;99:317-327.

97. Tessier P: Orbital hypertelorism. I. Successive surgical attempts. Material and methods. Causes and mechanisms. Scand J Plast Reconstr Surg 1972;6:135-155.

98. Farkas LG: Anthropometry of the Head and Face, 2nd ed. New York, Raven Press, 1994.

99. Munro IR, Das SK: Improving results in orbital hypertelorism correction. Ann Plast Surg 1979;2:499-507.

Craniofacial Microsomia

Joseph G. McCarthy, MD ✦ Richard A. Hopper, MD
✦ Barry H. Grayson, DDS

Canton, in 1861, described the clinical association of ipsilateral congenital mandible and ear anomalies. Since that time, various names have been used to designate this condition, including the first and second branchial arch syndrome,[1,2] otomandibular dysostosis,[3] oculoauriculovertebral sequence,[4] Goldenhar syndrome,[5] lateral facial dysplasia,[3] hemifacial microsomia,[4] and craniofacial microsomia.[6] Because the dysmorphology can be bilateral in 5% to 30% of cases, the terms *unilateral* and *bilateral craniofacial microsomia* (CFM) are preferred. Goldenhar syndrome, or oculoauriculovertebral sequence, is considered a variant of CFM, constituting approximately 10% of patients. It is differentiated by the presence of ocular abnormalities (lipoma, lipodermoid, epibulbar dermoid, or coloboma) and cervical spine anomalies.[5,7,8]

The reported incidence of CFM ranges from 1 in 3500 to 1 in 26,550 live births,[9] with a commonly quoted incidence of 1 in 5600 live births.[2,10] It is the second most common craniofacial anomaly after cleft lip and palate.[11] Grabb[2] reported a male predominance, with a male-to-female ratio of 63:39, and Rollnick[8] reported a similar ratio of 191:103. The clinical series of Horgan et al[12] reported an equal sex ratio of 59 males to 62 females.

ETIOPATHOGENESIS

The underlying cause or etiopathogenesis of CFM remains a subject of debate. Until recently, the prevailing theory was that CFM is a sporadic event, possibly precipitated by exposure to teratogens.[13-17] Other studies have instead suggested a fundamental role for genetic transmission in some patients.[18,19] The etiology of CFM is probably heterogeneous among individuals, with variable contributions from extrinsic and intrinsic factors.

Teratogen Theory

Support for a teratogenic etiology of CFM is based largely on animal studies. Poswillo exposed mouse embryos to triazine by maternal administration of the drug, causing CFM-like phenotypes (Fig. 91-1). Focal hematomas arising from disruption of the stapedial artery were also observed. Although a "stapedial artery hemorrhage etiology" is attractive because the vessel is a second branchial arch derivative, a causative association between the bleeding and the deformities has not been made. The hemorrhages occurred 14 days after administration of the teratogen, and there was no clear temporal relationship between the hemorrhage appearance and the associated deformity. Louryan et al exposed mice to triazine later in development (10 days of gestation).[20] All animals developed deformities; however, only a third showed evidence of a hematoma. The authors concluded that triazine has a direct teratogenic effect and that the stapedial artery findings were simply a side effect. In contrast to those described by Poswillo, these animals demonstrated more evidence of bilateral deformities and inner ear anomalies. The mouse may not be an appropriate

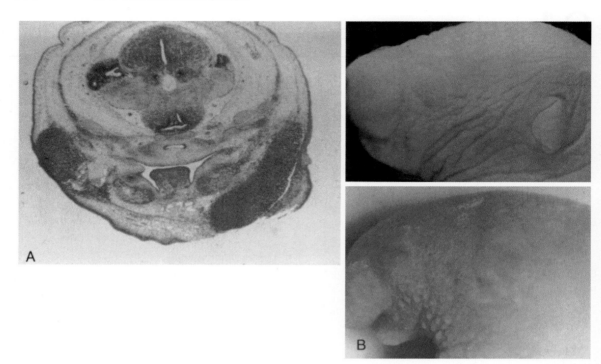

FIGURE 91-1. Mouse phenocopy of craniofacial microsomia induced by the administration of triazine. *A,* Histologic section of the head showing bilateral hematomas. The smaller one is in the ear region *(right),* and the large one encompasses the ramus and angle of the mandible *(left). B, Upper panel,* Normal ear-jaw relationship at full term in the normal animal. *Lower panel,* The diminutive helix and abnormal mandible in the unilateral craniofacial microsomia phenocopy. (From Poswillo D: The pathogenesis of the Treacher Collins syndrome [mandibulofacial dysostosis]. Br J Oral Surg 1975;13:1.)

model of CFM.[20] Intermittent occlusion of the internal carotid system of fetal sheep late in gestation has been shown to result in deformities similar in appearance to CFM.[21] The vascular disruption hypothesis, therefore, cannot be excluded.

Jacobsson[16] exposed rats to etretinate, a retinoic acid derivative, to cause deformities comparable to the first and second branchial arch syndromes. This finding is consistent with the finding that neural crest cells express large amounts of retinoic acid-binding proteins. Furthermore, when retinoic acid is administered early in development, it interferes with cell migration. When administered later in gestation, however, retinoic acid kills ganglionic placodal cells, resulting in a deformity similar to mandibulofacial dysostosis (Treacher Collins).[20] Human case studies also support a teratogen-based etiology for CFM. Thalidomide,[22] ethanol,[23] and gestational diabetes[14] have been implicated.

Genetic Theory

Support of a genetic etiology of CFM has come from both animal and human studies. A transgenic mouse model for CFM with an insertional deletion on mouse chromosome 10 has been described with an autosomal dominant mode of transmission and 25% penetration.[24,25] The affected animals display low-set ears, unilateral microtia, and jaw asymmetry, without middle ear abnormality. Second branchial arch hematomas were also observed in the embryos. Human genetics studies have documented a positive family history in 9.4% of 32 probands,[26] 21% of 57 probands,[27] 26% of 88 probands,[28] and 44% of 82 probands.[29] Kaye et al[18] performed segregation analysis on 74 families of probands with CFM and rejected the hypothesis that genetic transmission is not a causative factor. The evidence favored autosomal dominant inheritance; however, recessive and polygenic models were not distinguishable. Despite the suggestion of autosomal dominant transmission, they found only a 2% to 3% overall recurrence rate in first-degree relatives. This figure compares to the 10% recurrence risk in first- and second-degree relatives reported by the same group in an earlier study of 294 individuals with CFM.[8] Graham et al described a family with a strong autosomal dominant transmission of Goldenhar-like phenotype with linkage to a mutation at locus 8q13.

The high variability and low penetrance of CFM may be explained in terms of genetic transmission by a number of theories.[30] Compensation of defective genes by adjacent normal genes has been described in a cleft palate mouse model, and it may explain the variability of CFM.[31] Another mechanism may be "maternal rescue," by which transplacental transfer of a normal maternal gene product may compensate for an abnormal fetal gene.[32] The low penetrance of CFM may be explained by differential expression of maternal and paternal DNA sequences (genomic imprinting)[33,34] or by only a limited number of cells possessing the abnormal gene (mosaicism).[35] A number of cellular random events are also known to modify the expression of a defective gene.[36]

Twin Studies

Studies on the incidence and expression of craniofacial anomalies in twins have provided insight into the etiology of CFM. Mulliken's group in Boston described 10 twin pairs with CFM.[37] Only one of the pairs, who were monozygotic, was concordant for the anomaly. Other twin studies have noted a high level of discordance of CFM among monozygotic twins.[38-40] Even among concordant monozygotic twins, the anomaly can be mirror image.[41] One theory to explain the discordant findings is that vascular insufficiency of the first and second branchial arch occurs in monozygotic twins with a shared placenta (monochorionic) and unequal circulation.[37] Arguing against this is the observation that discordance is not limited to monochorionic twins but is also observed in dichorionic pairs.[39] Monozygotic discordance would appear to refute the teratogen theory of CFM; however, monozygotic twins have been reported to respond to in utero teratogens in a discordant manner.[42]

In summary, the exact etiology of CFM is not known. It is likely to involve a number of factors ranging from abnormal genes with various intrinsic modifiers to extrinsic insults such as teratogens or vascular events. It is also probable that like patients with cleft palate, the population of patients with CFM is a heterogeneous group. Some individuals with the phenotype may be part of a family with a dominant abnormal gene expression, in which case the recurrence risk would approach 50%. In other individuals with a purely environmental etiology, recurrence would be negligible. The empirically stated recurrence rate of 2% to 3% for CFM[18] should be recognized as a group summary and placed in context when an individual or family with this phenotype is counseled.

EMBRYOLOGY

The ear serves as a frame of reference in this syndrome because of its developmental relationship with the jaw.[43] A brief review of the phylogeny and ontogeny of the auricle and hearing apparatus is helpful in understanding the embryogenesis of the malformation in the patient with CFM.

The two principal divisions of the organ of hearing are derived from different embryonic anlagen. The sensory organ in the inner ear is derived from the ectodermal otocyst; the sound-conducting apparatus in the external and middle ear comes from the gill structures.

The membranous labyrinth has its beginning in the $3\frac{1}{2}$-week-old human embryo as a thickening of the ectoderm in the side of the head—the otic placode. This area is enfolded to become the otic pit and is subsequently pinched off to become the otocyst. By means of a series of folds, the otocyst differentiates in the 3-month-old fetus into the endolymphatic duct and sac, the semicircular endolymphatic ducts, the utricle, the saccule, and the organ of Corti. By the fifth month of fetal life, the sensory end organ of the ear attains adult form and size as the cartilaginous otic capsule ossifies.

It is speculated that the aquatic ancestors of humans swam in seas not yet as salty as today's oceans and that endolymph, entrapped by the enfolding otocyst, closely resembles in chemical composition the dilute salt water of the primeval sea. Our ancient aquatic forebears did not require any special mechanism to transmit sound to the inner ear. As in today's fish, sound was readily transmitted from the sea through the skin to the fluid of the inner ear.

When these ancestors struggled out of the seas onto dry land, a new problem appeared. A mechanical device was needed to convert air vibrations of large amplitude and small force into fluid vibrations of small amplitude and large force. The gill structures, no longer needed for breathing, became converted into such a mechanism. The first branchial groove became the external auditory meatus and canal; the first pharyngeal pouch became the eustachian tube and middle ear. Instead of the branchial groove and pharyngeal pouch connecting to become a gill cleft, a thin intervening layer of tissue remained to form the tympanic membrane.

The mandible, incus, and malleus develop from the cartilage of the first branchial arch (Meckel cartilage) (Fig. 91-2); the stapes (with the exception of the footplate, which originates from the otic capsule), styloid process, and hyoid bone develop from the cartilage of the second branchial arch (Reichert cartilage). The large area of the tympanic membrane, connected by the lever system of the ossicular chain to the small area of the oval window, provides the ear with an effective mechanism to overcome the sound barrier between air and water.

By the third fetal month, the external auricle has been formed from the first and second branchial arches on either side of the first branchial groove, which is the primary shallow, funnel-shaped external auditory meatus (Fig. 91-3). From the inner end of the primary meatus, a solid cord of ectodermal cells extends farther

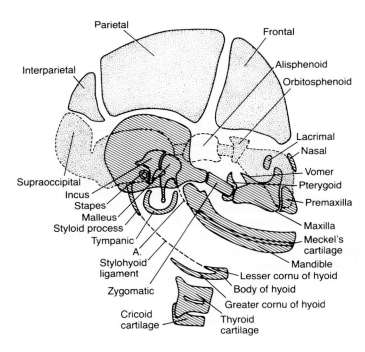

FIGURE 91-2. In this schematic drawing, the visceral arch cartilages are designated by oblique hatching; the cranial base cartilages are heavily stippled and outlined by broken (dashed) lines. The remaining skeletal elements are the intramembranous bones of the face and cranial vault. (From Hamilton WJ, Mossman H: Human Embryology, 4th ed. Cambridge, England, W. Heffer & Sons, 1972.)

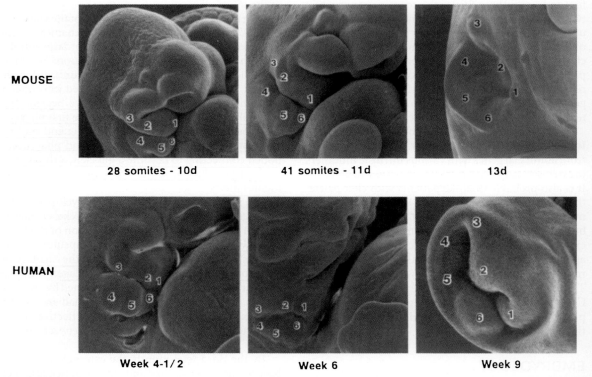

FIGURE 91-3. Comparison of external ear development in the mouse *(upper panel),* on which most experimental studies have been conducted, and the human *(lower panel).* The various growth centers (auricular hillocks, which are six in number) are virtually the same in the two species. (From Jarvis BL, Sulik KK, Johnston MC: Congenital malformations of the external, middle, and inner ear produced by isotretinoin exposure in fetal mouse embryos. Otol Head Neck Surg 1990;102:391-401.)

inward, with a bulb-like enlargement adjacent to the middle ear. It is not until the seventh fetal month that the cord canalizes, beginning medially to form the tympanic membrane and extending laterally to join with the primary meatus to form the completed external auditory meatus. The external and middle ears, although capable of transmitting sound to the inner ear, are not yet of adult form and size.

In the seventh fetal month, pneumatization of the temporal bone begins. At birth, the eustachian tube inflates; the fetal mesoderm tissue in the middle ear and antrum continues to resorb until the epithelium lies close to the periosteum, and pneumatization of the temporal bone proceeds.

The external auditory meatus, entirely cartilaginous at birth (except for the narrow incomplete ring of the tympanic bone), deepens by growth of the tympanic bone to form the adult osseous meatus. Except for some pneumatization of the petrous apex, which may continue into adult life, the external and middle ears finally attain adult form and size in late childhood (in contrast to the inner ear, which becomes adult in fetal life). It is generally accepted that the first branchial arch furnishes the anterior part of the auricle; the second arch provides the structures of the remaining external ear. The embryology of the external ear is also discussed in Chapter 85.

The maxilla, palatine bone, and zygoma develop from the maxillary process of the first branchial arch, whereas the mandible forms from the mandibular process. Meckel cartilage, the primary jaw of lower vertebrates, represents the temporary skeleton of the first pharyngeal arch; the two symmetric cartilaginous bars describe a parabolic arch that serves as a model and guide in the early morphogenesis of the mandible.

Three main regions of Meckel cartilage should be considered: the distal portion, which becomes incorporated into the anterior part of the body of the mandible; a middle portion, which gives rise to the sphenomandibular ligament and contributes to the mylohyoid groove of the mandible; and the proximal or intratympanic portion, which differentiates into the malleus, the incus, and the anterior malleolar ligament.

The embryology of the face is discussed in more detail in Chapter 85.

PATHOLOGY

Skeletal Tissue

A fundamental characteristic of the syndrome is the variable manifestation of the pathologic findings.

The deformity in CFM usually has the three major features of auricular, mandibular, and maxillary hypoplasia. The hypoplasia, however, can also involve adjacent anatomic structures: the zygoma, the pterygoid processes of the sphenoid bone, the temporal bone (the middle ear; the mastoid process is small and acellular), the frontal bone, the facial nerve, the muscles of mastication, the parotid, the cutaneous and subcutaneous tissues, the tongue, the soft palate, the pharynx, and the floor of the nose.

Whereas the jaw and ear deformities are the most conspicuous in the majority of patients, the first and second branchial arches and the structures derived from them are intimately interlinked with the chondrocranium and membranous bones of the skull; associated deformities of the temporal bone and other cranial bones are inevitable. In extreme forms of the dysplasia, extensive craniofacial involvement is evident (Fig. 91-4). As Pruzansky[43] stated, maldevelopment in one area may trigger a "domino effect," with involvement of the entire craniofacial skeleton—microphthalmos, orbital dystopia, and orbitofacial clefts.

The most conspicuous deformity of unilateral CFM is the hypoplasia of the mandible on the affected side. The ramus is hypoplastic or virtually absent, and the body of the mandible curves upward to join the vertically reduced ramus. The chin is deviated to the affected side. On the "normal" or "less affected" side, the body of the mandible is also characterized by abnormalities in the skeletal and soft tissue anatomy. The body of the "normal" mandible shows an increased horizontal dimension and an increase in the gonial angle.[44] The increase in length of soft and hard tissue structures on the less affected side may represent compensatory growth, secondary to the growth deficiency on the affected side.

Ramus and condyle malformations vary from minimal hypoplasia of the condyle to its complete absence in association with hypoplasia or agenesis of the ramus (Fig. 91-5). In all patients, condylar anomalies can be demonstrated, and this finding may be pathognomonic of the syndrome. As a consequence, the spatial relationships of the distorted or deficient anatomic parts, as well as the associated neuromuscular components, become of paramount importance in the diagnosis and planning of appropriate treatment.

The posterior wall of the glenoid fossa is partially formed by the tympanic portion of the temporal bone, which provides the bony portion of the external auditory canal in the normally developed ear. When there is hypoplasia of the temporal bone, the posterior wall of the glenoid fossa cannot be identified. The infratemporal surface is flat, and the hypoplastic ramus is often hinged on this flat surface at a point anterior to the contralateral "unaffected" temporomandibular joint.

Mandibular growth deficiency usually is closely related to the degree of hypoplasia of the condyle. In the more severe conditions, there is considerable disparity in condylar growth between the affected and contralateral sides. The cant of the occlusal plane (higher on the affected side) is caused by the short, hypoplastic ramus and by hypoplasia of the ipsilateral

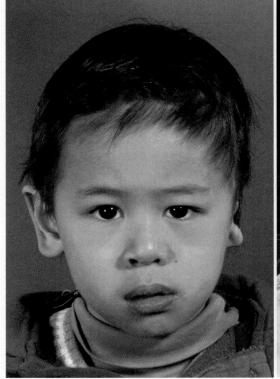

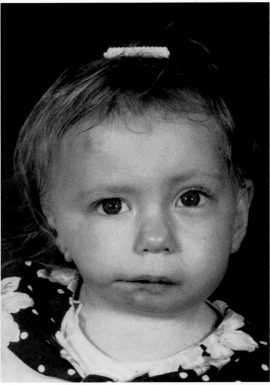

A

B

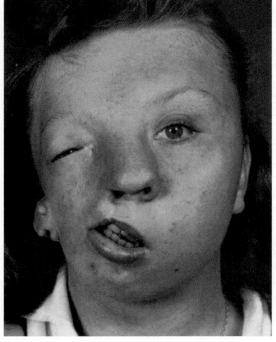

C

FIGURE 91-4. Variable clinical manifestations of unilateral craniofacial microsomia. *A,* Mild example characterized by microtia, canting of the oral commissure and alar base plane, deficiency of the affected cheek soft tissues, and deviation of the chin to the ipsilateral side. *B,* Moderate example. Note the microtia, deficient cheek soft tissue, macrostomia, canting of the oral commissure, and retruded and deviated chin. *C,* Severe example with microtia, microphthalmos, retrusion of the brow, occlusal cant, elevation of the oral commissure, and deviation of the chin.

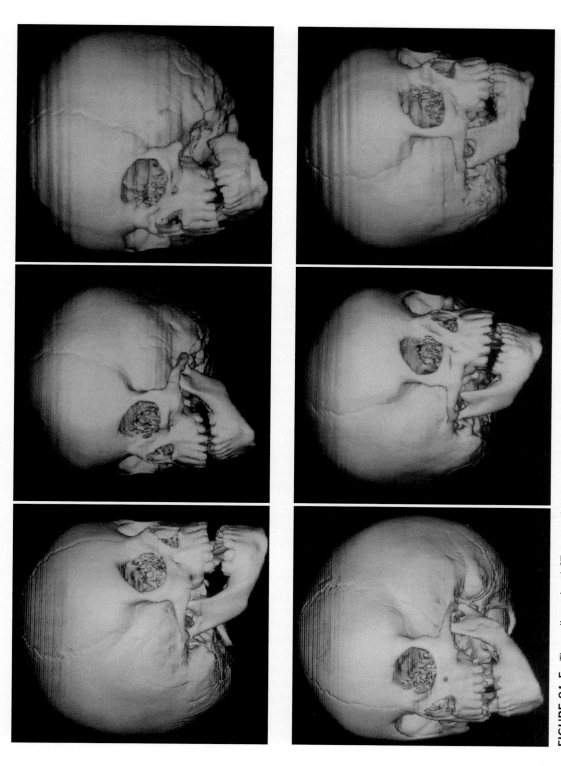

FIGURE 91-5. Three-dimensional CT scans of three unilateral craniofacial microsomia cases demonstrating increasing severity from left to right. The affected side of each case is on the top panel, with the corresponding normal contralateral side on the lower panel. The three cases correspond to the Pruzansky classification of mandibular deformity described later in the chapter: class I (*left*), class II (*center*), class III (*right*).

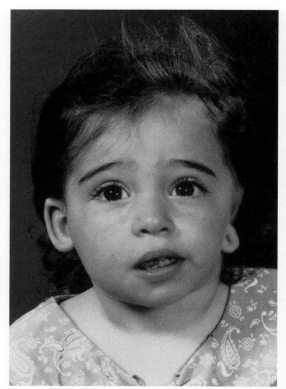

FIGURE 91-6. Patient with left-sided craniofacial microsomia demonstrating the characteristic occlusal cant upward on the affected side with associated cheek hypoplasia and ear anomaly.

maxillary dentoalveolar process (Fig. 91-6). The floor of the maxillary sinus and of the nose on the affected side is canted at a higher level. In some patients, it was noted that the base of the skull was elevated on an inclined plane similar to the inclined occlusal plane. Anteroposterior and superoinferior dentoalveolar and skeletal dimensions are reduced on the affected side. Crowded dentition, with a characteristic tilt of the anterior maxillary and mandibular occlusal planes upward on the affected side, is often noted.

Craniofacial bones other than the mandible or maxilla can be involved, especially the tympanic and mastoid portions of the temporal bone; the petrous portion usually is remarkably spared. The styloid process is frequently smaller and shorter on the affected side. The mastoid process can have a flattened appearance, and there can be partial or complete lack of pneumatization of the mastoid air cells (Fig. 91-7).

The zygoma can be underdeveloped in all its dimensions, with flattening of the malar eminence. A decrease in the span of the zygomatic arch results in a decrease in the length of the canthal-tragal line on the affected side.

Disparities in the vertical axis of the orbit can be seen, with or without evidence of microphthalmos (Fig. 91-8). Often in this situation, there is flattening of the ipsilateral frontal bone—an appearance of plagiocephaly without radiographic evidence of coronal synostosis.

Nonskeletal (Soft) Tissue

An area of research is the relationship between the soft tissue and skeletal dysmorphology of CFM. One theory is that they are independent manifestations of the same genetic or environmental event. Another possibility is that one is primarily involved, whereas the other is only a secondary event.

The "functional matrix" theory, promoted by Moss,[45] attributes the overall growth and development of the head to the development of the soft tissue matrix and functional spaces. The matrix is composed of cells, tissues, organs, and air volumes that serve a functional role. The associated "hard" tissues, such as bone and cartilage, serve to protect and support the functional matrix. Their morphology is solely determined by the functional matrix. As summarized by Moss, "bones do not grow, they are grown."[45] This theory has been supported by animal research examining the effect of transposition of muscles of mastication on bone morphology.[46-48] Investigation of the effect of soft tissue on bone shape in humans with unilateral CFM has been limited to computed tomographic analysis. Results of these studies do suggest that changes in muscles of mastication can elicit a postnatal change in bone morphology but that the opposite—bone changes affecting muscle—does not take place (Fig. 91-9).[49-51] If the functional matrix theory is validated, future treatment of CFM may be limited to early manipulation of the soft tissue matrix to elicit a secondary effect on the bone.

MUSCLES OF MASTICATION

Muscle function, especially that of the lateral pterygoid muscle, is impaired in many patients with CFM. The right muscle is responsible for the lateral movement of the mandible to the left side, whereas the left muscle controls movement to the right. Both sides act synergistically in executing protrusive opening movements. In patients with CFM, a severe limitation of protrusive and lateral movements due to hypoplasia of the lateral pterygoid muscle is observed.

The impact of this factor is apparent both on the developing musculature and on the morphologic character of the attached bone. An alteration in mandibular movements (opening, lateral, and protrusive) comparable with the degree of mandibular deficiency is often noted.

When the patient opens the mouth, the deviation toward the affected side is produced not only by the

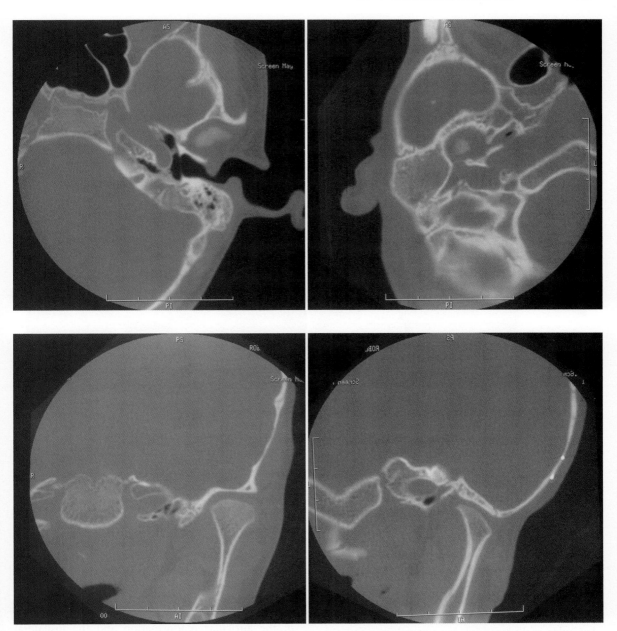

FIGURE 91-7. CT scan images of condylar and temporal abnormalities in unilateral craniofacial microsomia compared with the contralateral side. *Upper,* Axial cuts through the temporal bone at the level of the condylar head. *Upper left,* On the less affected side, normal lateral location of the glenoid fossa and pneumatization of the mastoid bone are visualized. *Upper right,* On the affected side, the glenoid fossa and condylar head are medially displaced, and there is an absence of air cells in the mastoid bone. *Lower,* Coronal cuts through the condyle and temporal bone. *Lower left,* On the less affected side, there is normal condylar morphology with level articulation with the temporal bone. *Lower right,* On the affected side, the condylar head is dysmorphic and articulates with the temporal bone at an angle.

skeletal asymmetry but also by the minimal or absent contribution of the ipsilateral medial and lateral ptery-goid muscles in countering the opposing actions of the muscles on the unaffected side. The condyle on the less affected side is displaced abnormally downward and laterally when the mandible is depressed, almost to the point of dislocating the condyle. No discernible condylar movement can be elicited on the affected side during opening and protrusive movements of the mandible. Thus, in testing for lateral pterygoid muscle

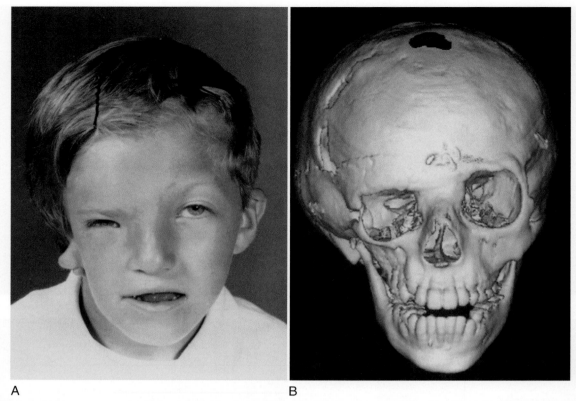

FIGURE 91-8. *A,* Craniofacial microsomia with orbital and frontal bone involvement on the right side. There is vertical orbital dystopia. *B,* The congenital fronto-orbital asymmetry persists after cranial vault remodeling.

weakness, one finds an inability to shift the jaw laterally toward the unaffected side and to deviate the midline of the chin toward the affected side during opening and during forceful protrusion.

In many cases, the coronoid process is absent, and there is reduction in the size of the temporalis muscle. The associated masseter and medial pterygoid muscles are also grossly deficient.

EAR

Auricular malformations are a usual manifestation of the syndrome. Meurman[84] proposed a classification of the auricular anomalies based on the studies of Marx (1926): grade I, distinctly smaller malformed auricles with most of the characteristic components; grade II, vertical remnant of cartilage and skin with a small anterior hook and complete atresia of the canal; and grade III, an almost entirely absent auricle except for only a small remnant, such as a deformed lobule. This grading scale forms the basis of describing ear anomalies in more recent classification systems (Fig. 91-10).

In a comprehensive study, Caldarelli et al, using air and bone conduction audiometry and temporal bone tomography, evaluated 57 patients with CFM.[51a] It was observed that the degree of Meurman auricular deformity does not correlate exactly with hearing function. The type of hearing loss, although usually assumed to be conductive in origin, can be determined only by audiometry. Tomography, not auricular morphology, is the only indicator of middle ear structure. The unaffected ear may also harbor abnormalities in structure and function and should be evaluated. There was, however, a direct relationship between the severity of the auricular malformation and the ipsilateral mandibular deformity.

NERVOUS SYSTEM

A wide variety of cerebral anomalies exist in CFM and may include ipsilateral cerebral hypoplasia,[52] hypoplasia of the corpus callosum,[53] hydrocephalus of the communicating type[52,53] and obstructive type,[54] intracranial lipoma,[55,56] and hypoplasia and impression of the brainstem and cerebellum.[52,57] Other associated abnormalities include cognitive delay,[58] epilepsy, and encephalographic findings suggestive of epilepsy.[52,59]

Cranial nerve abnormalities are frequent in CFM and can range from arhinencephaly of the bilateral

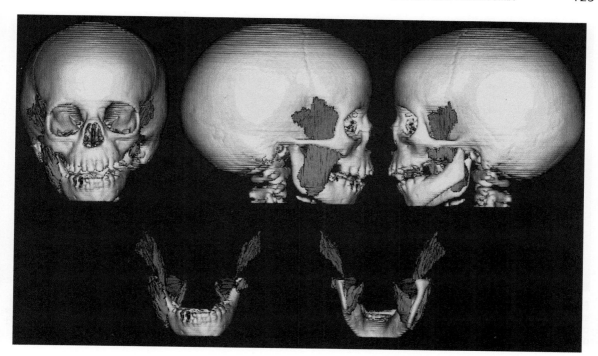

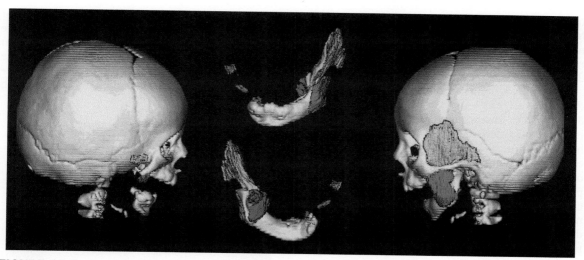

FIGURE 91-9. *Top panel,* Images of a child with unilateral (left) craniofacial microsomia and grade I Pruzansky mandible. The images show composites of the osseous surface and segmented masticatory musculature derived from CT data. *Bottom panel,* Images of a child with unilateral (right) craniofacial microsomia and grade III Pruzansky mandible. Images show composites of the osseous surface and segmented masticatory musculature derived from CT data. (Courtesy of Drs. Alex Kane and Jeffrey Marsh, Washington University, St. Louis.)

type[53] and unilateral type[56] to unilateral agenesis and hypoplasia of the optic nerve with secondary changes in the lateral geniculate body and visual cortex,[60] congenital ophthalmoplegia and Duane retraction syndrome,[61] hypoplasia of the trochlear and abducens nuclei and nerves,[60] congenital trigeminal anesthesia,[62] and aplasia of the trigeminal nerve and motor and sensory nucleus.[56] The most common cranial nerve anomaly is facial paralysis secondary to agenesis of the facial nerve in the temporal bone[63] or hypoplasia of the intracranial portion of the facial nerve and facial nucleus in the brainstem.[56] Congenital hearing loss may be due to a malformed inner ear,[60] hypoplasia of the cochlear nerve and brainstem auditory nuclei, or hypoplasia and impaired function of cranial nerves IX through XII.[57,64] Any cranial nerve can be clinically

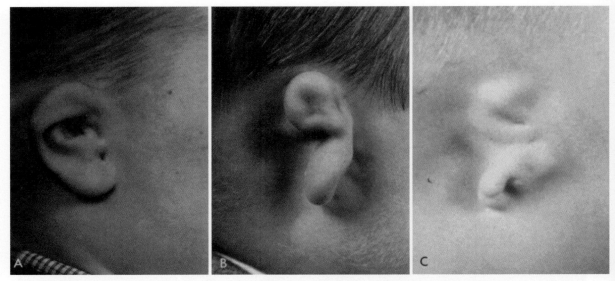

FIGURE 91-10. Example of the three grades of auricular anomalies in the Meurman classification.[10] *A,* Grade I: small malformed ear with most components present. *B,* Grade II: vertical remnant of skin and cartilage. There is atresia of the external auditory meatus. *C,* Grade III: the auricle is almost entirely absent except for a misplaced lobule and diminutive skin and cartilage remnants.

involved in patients with CFM, and it is likely that hypoplasia or agenesis of a portion of the entire cranial nerve trunk and corresponding brainstem nuclei represents the pathoanatomic substrate of the clinical dysfunction.

Electromyographic abnormalities have been described in the literature. Grabb[2] measured diminished or low-normal motor conduction velocity of the facial nerves, usually unilateral, in several of his patients. Another study by Aleksic et al[56] described electromyographic abnormalities ranging from absence of the muscle to long polyphasic potential with incomplete interference pattern on active innervation. No cases of fibrillation potentials have yet been documented. The interpretation of the electrodiagnostic data was hampered by the past history of surgical procedures in the region of the mandible and auricle.

SKIN AND SUBCUTANEOUS TISSUE

The deficiency of soft tissues on the affected side in CFM is evident from the reduced distance between the mastoid process and the oral commissure or lateral canthus of the eye. The skin and subcutaneous tissue show varying degrees of atrophy, particularly in the parotid-masseteric and auriculomastoid areas. Hypoplasia or aplasia of the parotid gland, previously described by Entin,[64a] can place the branches of the facial nerve in a superficial and surgically vulnerable position.

In the series of patients described by Grabb,[2] 10% had malformations of the eyes and eyelids or palate. Transverse facial clefting, ranging from macrostomia

to a full-thickness defect of the cheek, can be present (Fig. 91-11).[65] The clefts probably result from a failure of the maxillary and mandibular processes to fuse. In embryonic development, the lateral commissure of the oral fissure is initially situated at the point of bifurcation of the maxillary and mandibular processes. With

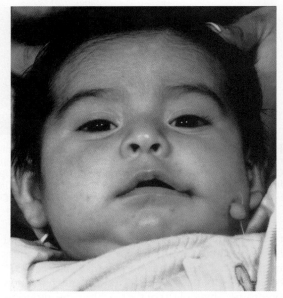

FIGURE 91-11. Transverse facial cleft in a patient with left unilateral craniofacial microsomia. The soft tissue cleft is manifested by the left macrostomia. The soft tissue deficiency extends toward the tragal region.

TABLE 91-1 ✦ PRIMARY AND ASSOCIATED ANOMALIES OF CRANIOFACIAL MICROSOMIA

	Principal Anomalies	Associated Anomalies	
Mandibular	Mandibular hypoplasia (89%-100%) Malformed glenoid fossa (24%-27%)	*Craniofacial* Velopharyngeal insufficiency (35%-55%)	*General* Vertebral/rib defects (16%-60%) Cervical spine anomalies (24%-42%)
Ear	Microtia (66%-99%) Preauricular tags (34%-61%) Conductive hearing loss (50%-66%) Middle ear (ossicle) defects	Palatal deviation (39%-50%) Orbital dystopia (15%-43%) Ocular motility disorders (19%-22%) Epibulbar dermoids (4%-35%) Cranial base anomalies (9%-30%)	Scoliosis (11%-26%) Cardiac anomalies (4%-33%) Pigmentation changes (13%-14%) Extremity defects (3%-21%)
Midfacial	Maxillary hypoplasia Zygomatic hypoplasia Occlusal canting	Cleft lip and/or palate (15%-22%) Eyelid defects (12%-25%) Hypodontia/dental hypoplasia (8%-25%)	Central nervous system defects (5%-18%) Genitourinary defects (4%-15%) Pulmonary anomalies (1%-15%)
Soft tissue	Masticatory muscles hypoplasia (85%-95%) Macrostomia (17%-62%) VII nerve palsy (10%-45%)	Lacrimal drainage abnormalities (11%-14%) Frontal plagiocephaly (10%-12%) Sensorineural hearing loss (6%-16%) Preauricular sinus (6%-9%) Parotid gland hypoplasia Other cranial nerve defects (e.g., V, IX, XII)	Gastrointestinal defects (2%-12%)

The prevalence rates were summarized from 19 reports in the literature from 1983 to 1996. Studies based on selected samples were omitted to minimize selection bias. It was recognized by the authors that the prevalence rate may be falsely elevated because the reporting tertiary centers may have a referral bias of more severely affected patients.

Adapted from Cousley RR, Calvert ML: Current concepts in the understanding and management of hemifacial microsomia. Br J Plast Surg 1997;50:536-551.

fusion of these and development of the muscles of mastication, the original broad mouth is reduced in size. In addition, the parotid glands, originally near the embryonic oral commissure, grow laterally toward the developing ear, but the parotid duct papillae remain in their more medial position.[65]

Extracraniofacial Anatomy

Horgan et al[12] reviewed 121 cases of CFM and reported that 67 patients (55%) had at least one extracraniofacial anomaly, with some having up to seven malformations. They also identified a relationship between the presence of these malformations and the severity of the craniofacial bone and soft tissue involvement. The spectrum and incidence of associated malformations are listed in Table 91-1.

Natural History

There are two schools of thought about the natural history of CFM without operation. One asserts that the severity of skeletal deformity is not progressive, with growth of the affected side paralleling that of the nonaffected side.[66,67] The other school of thought is that CFM is a progressive anomaly, with inhibited growth on the affected side resulting in increasing facial asymmetry with age.[68-74] The natural history of the soft tissue changes in CFM is not known.

Rune et al[67] examined the facial growth of 11 patients with unoperated unilateral CFM by use of metallic implants and roentgen stereophotogrammetry. They reported a mild increase in occlusal cant in five patients and stable or improving occlusal cant in the remaining six. The authors concluded that asymmetry of the jaws does not increase with time; however, only one patient in their study group had reached skeletal maturity at the time of the study. More recently, Polley et al[66] retrospectively examined longitudinal posteroanterior cephalograms of 26 patients with unoperated unilateral CFM. The patients were divided into three groups on the basis of Pruzansky grading of their mandibular severity. Both vertical and horizontal asymmetries were analyzed by a combination of angular and linear measurements. They reported that growth on the affected side paralleled that on the unaffected side, regardless of grade of severity or side that was affected.

Kearns et al[68] interpreted the significant changes in gonial height difference and in intergonial angle reported in the Polley paper to indicate a progressive vertical asymmetry that is correlated with the severity of mandibular deformity. This reinterpretation was consistent with their findings when they retrospectively examined 67 patients with unoperated unilateral CFM by horizontal angular analysis of posteroanterior cephalograms. They divided the patients into two groups based on the Pruzansky classification: group I, Pruzansky I and IIa; group II, Pruzansky IIb and III. They found no significant changes in group I but significant changes in all measurements in group II.

If the true natural history of CFM is progression, early surgical intervention may be indicated in an attempt to minimize the deformity.[69,70,76,77] If, instead, CFM remains relatively stable, one could argue that surgery can be deferred to minimize the need for revisionary surgery.[66,78]

CLINICAL SPECTRUM
Differential Diagnosis

The differential diagnosis of facial asymmetry includes temporomandibular joint ankylosis, Romberg syndrome, postirradiation deformity, condylar hyperplasia, and facial hemihypertrophy. Treacher Collins syndrome or severe orbitofacial clefts can also be confused with bilateral CFM; however, the deformed ramus and condyle so characteristic of CFM are not present. Postnatal trauma or infection that affects the condylar cartilage can result in decreased mandibular growth, with a secondary effect on the growth of the surrounding ipsilateral craniofacial skeleton.[79,80] Unlike the postnatal deformities, CFM is characterized by deficient soft tissue and external ear malformations on the affected side as well as more widespread involvement of the bone, including the temporal bone, mastoid, and skull base. Minimal diagnostic criteria

for CFM have been suggested by Cousley and Calvert[30] as (1) ipsilateral mandibular *and* ear defects or (2) asymmetric mandibular *or* ear defects in association with either (a) two or more indirectly associated anomalies or (b) a positive family history of CFM. Indirectly associated anomalies were defined as those "not normally related either in terms of developmental fields or function."

Unilateral Versus Bilateral

It is difficult to determine the true ratio of unilateral to bilateral CFM. Patients diagnosed with unilateral involvement often have subtle abnormalities of the ear, mandible, or orbit on the contralateral side. Grabb[2] reported 12 bilateral cases in his series of 102 (12%), Meurman[84] reported 8 in 74 (11%), and Converse[65] reported 15 in a series of 280 (5%). In contrast, on a review of 294 oculoauriculovertebral patients, 98 (33%) had some form of bilateral involvement, and the ear involvement was symmetric in 34 of these.[8] Similarly, Mulliken reported 34 cases (28%) with bilateral involvement among 121 cases of CFM.[70] This higher ratio of bilateral involvement on more recent reviews may be due to an increased appreciation of subtle contralateral soft tissue anomalies by the examining physician (Fig. 91-12).

Classification Systems

Multiple classification systems have been described for CFM, rendering comparison of clinical experiences confusing. An ideal classification system would be one

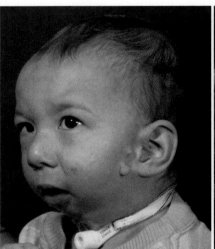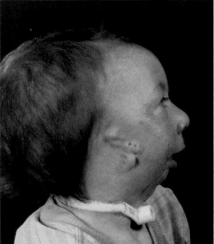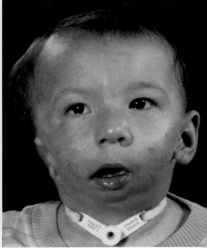

FIGURE 91-12. Patient with bilateral craniofacial microsomia of the Goldenhar variant. The right side of the face is more severely affected with a Meurman III ear deformity, epibulbar dermoid, cheek soft tissue deficiency, and micrognathia. The left side of the face is less affected; however, mandibular abnormality is evident along with a pretragal cartilaginous rest and skin tag.

that describes accurately and reliably all anatomic components of CFM and the associated severity to facilitate communication between health professionals, to allow comparison of clinical experiences, and to formulate classification-based comprehensive treatment plans. No classification system has yet achieved this ideal; each has its strengths and weaknesses.[81,82]

In 1963, Longacre et al[83] divided 44 cases of first and second branchial arch syndrome into unilateral or bilateral on the basis of external ear involvement; they further subdivided into absent, slight, moderate, or severe on the basis of the degree of facial deformity. Two years later, Grabb[2] categorized 102 patients into one of six groups based on the combination of external ear, middle ear, mandible, maxilla, zygoma, temporal bone, and oral involvement. He emphasized in his paper that the syndrome is "a spectrum of facial malformations which blend into one another, and, there are no bold lines which delineate any of these six groups."

Pruzansky[43] reported a grading system of progressive mandibular deficiency: grade I (minimal hypoplasia of the mandible), grade II (functioning but deformed temporomandibular joint with anteriorly and medially displaced condyle), or grade III (absence of the ramus and glenoid fossa) (Fig. 91-13). This classification was later modified by Kaban, Padwa, and Mulliken[99] (Table 91-2). With this system and a modification of the three-grade auricular malformation classification of Meurman,[84] Pruzansky

divided his patients into nine groups. In a later report, his group continued to support this classification scheme but recognized the limitation of describing the variable CFM population solely on the basis of jaw and ear malformations.[85] The variability of anatomic involvement in CFM had been recognized by Converse 10 years earlier, when he and his colleagues appreciated the involvement of the soft tissue and muscles of mastication.[86] In their division of 15 bilateral CFM patients into four groups, the first three groups were based on ear and mandible findings, whereas the fourth included facial soft tissue and bone involvement.[65]

From a review of 17 surgically treated CFM patients, Edgerton and Marsh[71] described four clinical groups based on the dominant pattern of dysplasia: I, mandibular; II, craniofacial soft tissues; III, auricular; and IV, composite deformity. They stated that treatment of the first three groups required only a decision as to the proper age to commence the reconstruction, whereas the fourth group, with composite deformity, dictated the establishment of a logical sequence of reconstructive steps based on anatomic, physiologic, and psychosocial considerations.[71]

The comprehensive phenotypic classification system, described by Tenconi and Hall[86a] and based on 67 patients with CFM, was one of the first to incorporate the ocular and extracranial findings in CFM, such as ocular dermoids, microphthalmos, limb deficiencies, and vertebral, heart, or renal

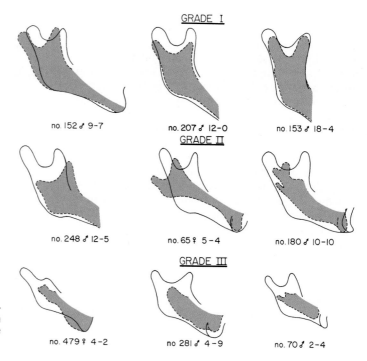

FIGURE 91-13. Classification of mandibular anomalies. See text for details. (From Pruzansky S: Not all dwarfed mandibles are alike. Birth Defects 1969;5:120.)

TABLE 91-2 ✦ PRUZANSKY CLASSIFICATION OF MANDIBULAR DEFORMITY WITH KABAN, PADWA, AND MULLIKEN MODIFICATION

Type I

All mandibular and temporomandibular joint components are present and normal in shape but hypoplastic to a variable degree.

Type IIa

The mandibular ramus, condyle, and temporomandibular joint are present but hypoplastic and abnormal in shape.

Type IIb

The mandibular ramus is hypoplastic and markedly abnormal in form and location, being medial and anterior. There is no articulation with the temporal bone.

Type III

The mandibular ramus, condyle, and temporomandibular joint are absent. The lateral pterygoid muscle and temporalis, if present, are not attached to the mandibular remnant.

Adapted from Kaban LB, Padwa BL, Mulliken JB: Surgical correction of mandibular hypoplasia in hemifacial microsomia: the case for treatment in early childhood. J Oral Maxillofac Surg 1998;56:628-638.

abnormalities. Type I was hemifacial microsomia, divided into classic, microphthalmic, bilateral asymmetric, and complex types; type II was hemifacial microsomia, limb deficiency type; type III was hemifacial microsomia, frontonasal type; and type IV was hemifacial microsomia, Goldenhar type, divided into type A (unilateral) and type B (bilateral).

Munro and Lauritzen[87,88] described a five-part surgical-anatomic classification scheme divided according to the skeletal deformity but based on treatment considerations. The classification is determined by whether the skeleton is complete (type I) or incomplete (types II to V), whether the occlusal plane is level (type Ia) or tilted (types Ib to V), and whether the orbit is involved (types IV and V). The classification forms the basis of a treatment plan for the bone abnormalities of the face (Fig. 91-14).

David et al[98] devised an alphanumeric (SAT) coding classification in the spirit of the TMN classification system of malignant tumors (Table 91-3). The SAT classification system grades skeletal (S), auricle (A),

and soft tissue (T) anomalies on an increasing numeric scale of severity. S_1, S_2, and S_3 skeletal deformities are similar to the three grades of mandibular hypoplasia described by Pruzansky,[43] with S_4 and S_5 representing mandible changes with orbital involvement. A_0 describes a normal ear, and A_1, A_2, and A_3 are increasing degrees of malformation. T_1, T_2, and T_3 are mild, moderate, and major soft tissue defects, respectively.

The OMENS classification of CFM, described by Vento, LaBrie, and Mulliken in 1991,[89] also uses alphanumeric codes to classify patients by the severity of malformation of different anatomic components (Table 91-4). Similar to the SAT classification, it grades ear anomalies (E in OMENS, A in SAT) in four grades from 0 to 3 and soft tissue defects (S in OMENS, and T in SAT) in three grades. Unlike in the SAT classification, however, the skeletal component is broken down into four orbital (O) and four mandibular (M) grades of deformity. The mandibular grading

TABLE 91-3 ✦ SAT CLASSIFICATION

Skeletal

S_1 Small mandible with normal shape
S_2 Condyle, ramus, and sigmoid notch identifiable but grossly distorted; mandible strikingly different in size and shape from normal
S_3 Mandible severely malformed and strikingly different in size and shape from normal
S_4 S_3 mandible plus orbital involvement with gross posterior recession of lateral and inferior orbital rims
S_5 S_4 defects plus orbital dystopia and frequently hypoplasia and asymmetric neurocranium with a flat temporal fossa

Auricle

A_0 Normal
A_1 Small, malformed auricle retaining characteristic features
A_2 Rudimentary auricle with hook at cranial end corresponding to the helix
A_3 Malformed lobule with rest of pinna absent

Soft Tissue

T_1 Minimal contour defect with no cranial nerve involvement
T_2 Moderate defect
T_3 Major defect with obvious facial scoliosis, possible severe hypoplasia of cranial nerves, parotid gland, and muscles of mastication; eye involvement; cleft of face or lips

Adapted from David DJ, Mahatumarat C, Cooter RD: Hemifacial microsomia: a multisystem classification. Plast Reconstr Surg 1987;80:525-535.

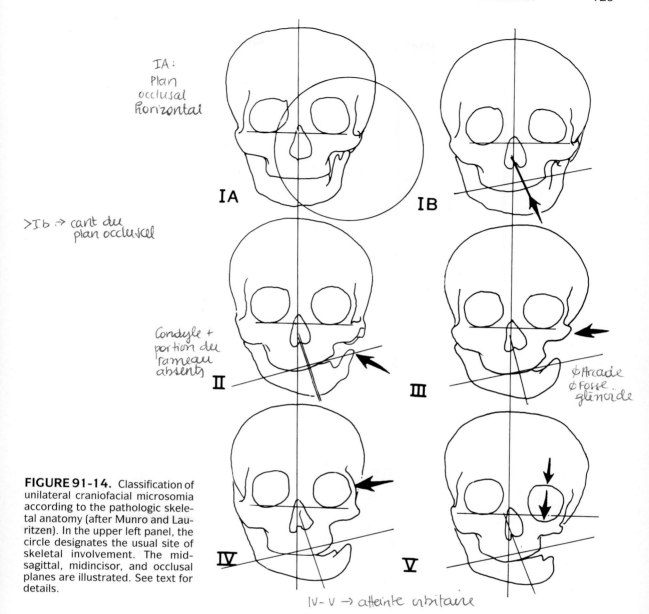

IA:
Plan
occlusal
horizontal

>Ib → cant du
plan occlusal

Condyle +
portion du
rameau
absents

φ Arcade
φ Fosse
glénoïde

IV - V → atteinte orbitaire

FIGURE 91-14. Classification of unilateral craniofacial microsomia according to the pathologic skeletal anatomy (after Munro and Lauritzen). In the upper left panel, the circle designates the usual site of skeletal involvement. The midsagittal, midincisor, and occlusal planes are illustrated. See text for details.

system includes the subdivision of Pruzansky type II into IIa and IIb, as first proposed by Kaban and associates.[77] Facial nerve involvement is also addressed as the N in OMENS. Both SAT and OMENS systems can be used to describe separately each side in a patient with bilateral CFM.

In comparison studies of the various CFM classification systems, OMENS has been regarded as one of the most complete while still being relatively easy to use.[81,82] Suggested modifications include adding a suffix to the acronym, such as a plus sign[12] (OMENS⁺) or an asterisk[82] (OMENS*), to indicate those patients

with severe extracranial manifestations. It has also been suggested that ear tags and conductive deafness be included in the ear category.[82]

DIAGNOSTIC STUDIES
Cephalometric Analysis

Despite the popularity of computed tomography in imaging the craniofacial skeleton, cephalograms remain useful in repeated examination of the facial bones, such as during the activation phase of distraction

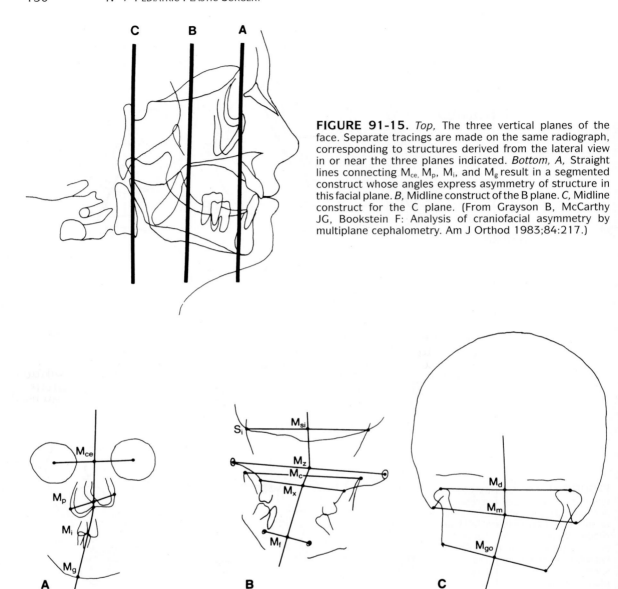

FIGURE 91-15. *Top,* The three vertical planes of the face. Separate tracings are made on the same radiograph, corresponding to structures derived from the lateral view in or near the three planes indicated. *Bottom, A,* Straight lines connecting M_{ce}, M_p, M_i, and M_g result in a segmented construct whose angles express asymmetry of structure in this facial plane. *B,* Midline construct of the B plane. *C,* Midline construct for the C plane. (From Grayson B, McCarthy JG, Bookstein F: Analysis of craniofacial asymmetry by multiplane cephalometry. Am J Orthod 1983;84:217.)

osteogenesis, and in determining and documenting the skeletal midline.

In the standard cephalometric technique, the ear rods of the cephalostat are inserted in the external auditory meatus, and the patient's head is placed in the Frankfort horizontal or natural head position. The patient with CFM usually has one ear positioned inferior and anterior to the other. If the malpositioned ear is used in this technique, the head is incorrectly oriented to the x-ray beam and the film. The technician should project an imaginary line from the normal ear, perpendicular to the midsagittal plane and passing to the opposite side of the head. The x-y coordinates of

this point, in millimeters, should be recorded directly on the cephalogram for future reference. Clinical determination of the midsagittal plane can be made by tipping the head down and observing the gross shape of the calvaria from above.

The classic lateral cephalogram provides information on maxillomandibular relationship as well as the deviation of the bone and soft tissue profile from documented norms.[90] The posteroanterior and basilar cephalograms are equally important in assessing patients with CFM in that they allow documentation of the facial midline and the degree of facial asymmetry in three dimensions.

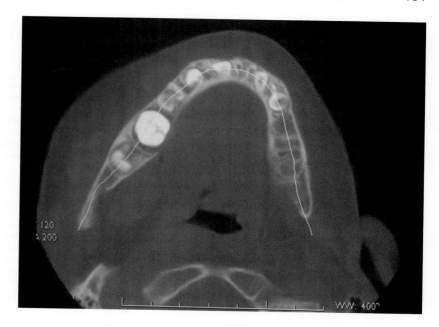

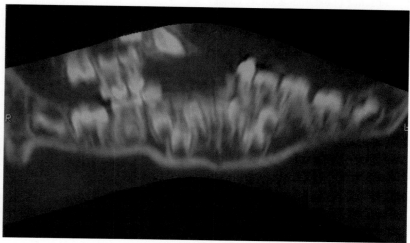

FIGURE 91-16. CT multiplanar reformation (CT/MPR) or DentaScan imaging of a unilateral craniofacial microsomia mandible with primary dentition. The tooth follicles of the secondary dentition can be visualized to aid in planning osteotomies and pin placement. *Upper,* Axial CT scan through mandibular occlusion. *Lower,* Reformatted DentaScan. Note the tooth follicles in the rami.

Grayson et al[44] described the technique of multiplane cephalometry. With lateral, coronal, and basilar radiographs, skeletal landmarks can be identified in three coronal and three axial planes and used to construct an estimation of the midline for each plane. These midlines are compared with the midsagittal plane, which is determined by relatively stable bilateral structures such as the occipital condyles, the center of the foramen magnum, and the medial axis of the spheno-occipital synchondrosis.[91] By use of this technique, a phenomenon termed warping can be observed within the craniofacial microsomic skeleton (Fig. 91-15). The midline constructs deviate progressively laterally as one passes anteriorly from the skull base to the piriform rim in the coronal plane and inferiorly from the orbits to the mandible in the axial plane.

Computed Tomography

Computed tomography (CT) has become a fundamental diagnostic and evaluation tool for all patients with CFM. Unlike cephalography, CT can image both bone and soft tissue, and it does not have the problem of superimposition of skeletal landmarks. Axial and coronal cuts provide detailed information on the bone and soft tissue asymmetry and the severity of malformation throughout the entire craniofacial skeleton. For the young patient who cannot be evaluated with conventional cephalographic imaging because of lack of cooperation, a CT scan performed under sedation or general anesthesia has provided information for early treatment planning that was previously unavailable (Fig. 91-16).

TABLE 91-4 ✦ OMENS CLASSIFICATION

Orbit

O_0	Normal orbit size and position
O_1	Abnormal size
O_2	Abnormal position
O_3	Abnormal size and position

Mandible

M_0	Normal mandible
M_1	Mandible and glenoid fossa are small ("mini-mandible")
M_2	Mandibular ramus short and abnormally shaped
M_{2A}	Glenoid in acceptable position
M_{2B}	Temporomandibular joint medially displaced
M_3	Complete absence of ramus, glenoid fossa, and temporomandibular joint

Ear

E_0	Normal
E_1	Mild hypoplasia and cupping
E_2	Absence of external auditory canal
E_3	Malpositioned lobule with absent auricle

Nerve

$N_0{}^7$	No facial nerve involvement
$N_1{}^7$	Upper facial nerve involvement
$N_2{}^7$	Lower facial nerve involvement
$N_3{}^7$	All branches affected

Soft Tissue

S_0	No soft tissue deformity
S_1	Minimal (mild) tissue deformity
S_2	Moderate tissue deformity (between the two extremes)
S_3	Major (severe) subcutaneous and muscular deficiency

Adapted from Vento AR, LaBrie RA, Mulliken JB: The O.M.E.N.S. classification of hemifacial microsomia. Cleft Palate Craniofac J 1991;28:68-76, discussion 77.

Because data derived from the CT scan are computer based, programs can be written to present the information in any number of formats. Three-dimensional presentation of CT images provides a visual summary of the underlying skeleton, which can be viewed and analyzed at any angle.[92-94] Another useful manipulation of CT data is multiplanar reformation (CT/MPR), or DentaScan, which processes axial CT scan information to obtain true cross-sectional images and panoramic views of the mandible and maxilla similar to a Panorex (see Fig. 91-16).[95-97] This is invaluable in imaging tooth follicles in relation to available bone stock in the immature patient who is too young for conventional dental imaging and in whom mandibular surgery is planned.

REFERENCES

1. Francois JJ, Haustrate L: Anomalies colobomateuses du globe oculaire et syndrome du premier arc. Ann Ocul 1954;187:340-368.
2. Grabb WC: The first and second branchial arch syndrome. Plast Reconstr Surg 1965;36:485-508.
3. Ross RB: Lateral facial dysplasia (first and second branchial arch syndrome, hemifacial microsomia). Birth Defects 1975;11:51-59.
4. Gorlin RJ, Pindborg JJ, Cohen MM: Syndromes of the Head and Neck, 2nd ed. New York, McGraw-Hill, 1976.
5. Goldenhar M: Associations malformatives de l'oeil et de l'oreille, en particulier le syndrome dermoide epibulbaire-appendices auricullaires-fistula auris congenita et ses relations avec la dystose mandibulo-faciale. J Genet Hum 1952;1:243-282.
6. Converse JM, Coccaro PJ, Becker MH, et al: Clinical aspects of craniofacial microsomia. In Converse JM, McCarthy JG, Woodsmith D, eds: Symposium on Diagnosis and Treatment of Craniofacial Anomalies. St. Louis, CV Mosby, 1979:461-475.
7. Feingold M, Baum J: Goldenhar's syndrome. Am J Dis Child 1978;132:136-138.
8. Rollnick BR, Kaye CI, Nagatoshi K, et al: Oculoauriculovertebral dysplasia and variants: phenotypic characteristics of 294 patients. Am J Med Genet 1987;26:361-375.
9. Gorlin RJ, Cohen MM, Levin LS: Syndromes of the Head and Neck, 3rd ed. New York, Oxford University Press, 1990.
10. Cohen MM Jr, Rollnick BR, Kaye CI: Oculoauriculovertebral spectrum: an updated critique. Cleft Palate J 1989;26:276-286.
11. Munro IR: A description of craniofacial anomalies: the mechanism and rationale of surgery. In Eder R, ed: Craniofacial Anomalies: Psychological Perspectives. New York, Springer-Verlag, 1995:3-21.
12. Horgan JE, Padwa BL, LaBrie RA, et al: OMENS-Plus: analysis of craniofacial and extracraniofacial anomalies in hemifacial microsomia. Cleft Palate Craniofac J 1995;32:405-412.
13. Bergstrom L, Baker BB: Syndromes associated with congenital facial paralysis. Otolaryngol Head Neck Surg 1981;89:336-342.
14. Ewart-Toland A, Yankowitz J, Winder A, et al: Oculoauriculovertebral abnormalities in children of diabetic mothers. Am J Med Genet 2000;90:303-309.
15. Jacobsson C, Granstrom G: Clinical appearance of spontaneous and induced first and second branchial arch syndromes. Scand J Plast Reconstr Surg Hand Surg 1997;31:125-136.
16. Jacobsson C: Teratological studies on craniofacial malformations. Swed Dent J Suppl 1997;121:3-84.
17. Poswillo D: Hemorrhage in development of the face. Birth Defects 1975;11:61-81.
18. Kaye CI, Martin AO, Rollnick BR, et al: Oculoauriculovertebral anomaly: segregation analysis [see comments]. Am J Med Genet 1992;43:913-917.
19. Singer SL, Haan E, Slee J, et al: Familial hemifacial microsomia due to autosomal dominant inheritance. Case reports. Aust Dent J 1994;39:287-291.
20. Glineur R, Louryan S, Lemaitre A, et al: Cranio-facial dysmorphism: experimental study in the mouse, clinical applications. Surg Radiol Anat 1999;21:41-47.
21. Escobar LF, Liechty EA: Late gestational vascular disruptions inducing craniofacial anomalies: a fetal lamb model. J Craniofac Genet Dev Biol 1998;18:159-163.
22. Poswillo D: The pathogenesis of the first and second branchial arch syndrome. Oral Surg Oral Med Oral Pathol 1973;35:302-328.
23. Sulik KK: Craniofacial defects from genetic and teratogen-induced deficiencies in presomite embryos. Birth Defects 1984;20:79-98.

24. Naora H, Kimura M, Otani H, et al: Transgenic mouse model of hemifacial microsomia: cloning and characterization of insertional mutation region on chromosome 10. Genomics 1994;23:515-519.

25. Otani H, Tanaka O, Naora H, et al: Microtia as an autosomal dominant mutation in a transgenic mouse line: a possible animal model of branchial arch anomalies. Anat Anz 1991;172:1-9.

26. McInerney AM, Donnai D, Calvert M, et al: Multiple etiologies for hemifacial microsomia. ASHG Abstracts 1999;1882.

27. Mansour AM, Wang F, Henkind P, et al: Ocular findings in the facioauriculovertebral sequence (Goldenhar-Gorlin syndrome). Am J Ophthalmol 1985;100:555-559.

28. Bestelmeyer U, Weerda H, Siegert R, et al: Familial occurrence of oculoauriculovertebral dysplasia and Franceschetti syndrome [in German]. HNO 1996;44:452-455.

29. Rollnick BR, Kaye CI: Hemifacial microsomia and variants: pedigree data. Am J Med Genet 1983;15:233-253.

30. Cousley RR, Calvert ML: Current concepts in the understanding and management of hemifacial microsomia. Br J Plast Surg 1997;50:536-551.

31. Satokata I, Maas R: Msx1 deficient mice exhibit cleft palate and abnormalities of craniofacial and tooth development [see comments]. Nat Genet 1994;6:348-356.

32. Letterio JJ, Geiser AG, Kulkarni AB, et al: Maternal rescue of transforming growth factor-beta 1 null mice. Science 1994;264:1936-1938.

33. Hall JG: Genomic imprinting: review and relevance to human diseases [see comments]. Am J Hum Genet 1990;46:857-873.

34. Hall JG: Human diseases and genomic imprinting. Results Probl Cell Differ 1999;25:119-132.

35. Wilson GN, Barr M Jr: Trisomy 9 mosaicism: another etiology for the manifestations of Goldenhar syndrome. J Craniofac Genet Dev Biol 1983;3:313-316.

36. Kurnit DM, Layton WM, Matthysse S: Genetics, chance, and morphogenesis. Am J Hum Genet 1987;41:979-995.

37. Keusch CF, Mulliken JB, Kaplan LC: Craniofacial anomalies in twins. Plast Reconstr Surg 1991;87:16-23.

38. Ryan CA, Finer NN, Ives E: Discordance of signs in monozygotic twins concordant for the Goldenhar anomaly. Am J Med Genet 1988;29:755-761.

39. Boles DJ, Bodurtha J, Nance WE: Goldenhar complex in discordant monozygotic twins: a case report and review of the literature. Am J Med Genet 1987;28:103-109.

40. Perez Alvarez F, Martinez Santana S, Sin Opi JM, et al: Asymmetrical otocraniofacial syndrome (hemifacial microsomy) in discordant monozygotic twins. Otologic aspects [in Spanish]. An Esp Pediatr 1984;21:769-773.

41. Satoh K, Shibata Y, Tokushige H, et al: A mirror image of the first and second branchial arch syndrome associated with cleft lip and palate in monozygotic twins. Br J Plast Surg 1995;48:601-605.

42. Smithells RW: The pathogenesis of the first and second branchial arch syndrome. Lancet 1963;1:1095.

43. Pruzansky S: Not all dwarfed mandibles are alike. Birth Defects 1969;5:120.

44. Grayson BH, McCarthy JG, Bookstein F: Analysis of craniofacial asymmetry by multiplane cephalometry. Am J Orthod 1983;84:217-224.

45. Moss ML: Growth and development of the craniofacial complex: an epigenetic viewpoint. In Goodrich JT, Hall CD, eds: Craniofacial Anomalies: Growth and Development from a Surgical Perspective. New York, Thieme, 1995:1-7.

46. Nanda SK, Merow WW, Sassouni V: Repositioning of the masseter muscle and its effect on skeletal form and structure. Angle Orthod 1967;37:304-308.

47. Hohl TH: Masticatory muscle transposition in primates: effects on craniofacial growth. J Maxillofac Surg 1983;11:149-156.

48. Boyd TG, Castelli WA, Huelke DF: Removal of the temporalis muscle from its origin: effects on the size and shape of the coronoid process. J Dent Res 1967;46:997-1001.

49. Kane AA, Lo LJ, Christensen GE, et al: Relationship between bone and muscles of mastication in hemifacial microsomia. Plast Reconstr Surg 1997;99:990-997, discussion 998-999.

50. Marsh JL, Baca D, Vannier MW: Facial musculoskeletal asymmetry in hemifacial microsomia. Cleft Palate J 1989;26:292-302.

51. Vargervik K, Miller AJ: Neuromuscular patterns in hemifacial microsomia. Am J Orthod 1984;86:33-42.

51a. Caldarelli DD, Hutchinson JG Jr, Pruzansky S, Valvassori GE: A comparison of microtia and temporal bone anomalies in hemifacial microsomia and mandibulofacial dysostosis. Cleft Palate J 1980;17:103.

52. Aleksic S, Budzilovich G, Reuben R, et al: Unilateral arhinencephaly in Goldenhar-Gorlin syndrome. Dev Med Child Neurol 1975;17:498-504.

53. Timm G: Morphologie des Auges bei Missbildungen Syndrome. Klin Monatsbl Augenheilkd 1960;137:557.

54. Hermann J, Opitz JM: A dominantly inherited first arch syndrome. First Conference on Clinical Delineation of Birth Defects. Part II. Malformation Syndromes. In Bergsma D, ed: Birth Defects, Original Article Series, vol 2. New York, National Foundation-March of Dimes. Baltimore, Williams & Wilkins, 1969.

55. Gaupp R, Janz J: Zur Kasuistik der Balkenlipome. Nervenarzt 1942;15:58.

56. Aleksic S, Budzilovich G, Reuben R, et al: Congenital trigeminal neuropathy in oculoauriculovertebral dysplasia- hemifacial microsomia (Goldenhar-Gorlin syndrome). J Neurol Neurosurg Psychiatry 1975;38:1033-1035.

57. Gosain AK, McCarthy JG, Pinto RS: Cervicovertebral anomalies and basilar impression in Goldenhar syndrome. Plast Reconstr Surg 1994;93:498-506.

58. Gorlin RJ, Jue KL, Jacobsen U, et al: Oculoauriculovertebral dysplasia. J Pediatr 1963;63:991.

59. Franceschetti A, Klein D, Brocher JEW: La dysostose mandibulofaciale dans la cadre des syndromes du premier arc branchial. Schweiz Med Wochenschr 1959;89:478.

60. Aleksic S, Budzilovich G, Choy A, et al: Congenital ophthalmoplegia in oculoauriculovertebral dysplasia- hemifacial microsomia (Goldenhar-Gorlin syndrome). A clinicopathologic study and review of the literature. Neurology 1976;26:638-644.

61. Bowen DI, Collum LM, Rees DO: Clinical aspects of oculoauriculo-vertebral dysplasia. Br J Ophthalmol 1971;55:145-154.

62. Sugar HS: An unusual example of the oculo-auriculo-vertebral dysplasia syndrome of Goldenhar. J Pediatr Ophthalmol 1967;4:9.

63. Bellucci RJ: Congenital auricular malformations. Indications, contraindications, and timing of middle ear surgery. Ann Otol Rhinol Laryngol 1972;81:659-663.

64. Berkman MD, Feingold M: Oculoauriculovertebral dysplasia (Goldenhar's syndrome). Oral Surg Oral Med Oral Pathol 1968;25:408-417.

64a. Entin MA: Reconstruction in congenital deformity of the temporomandibular component. Plast Reconstr Surg 1958;241:461.

65. Converse JM, Wood-Smith D, McCarthy JG, et al: Bilateral facial microsomia. Diagnosis, classification, treatment. Plast Reconstr Surg 1974;54:413-423.

66. Polley JW, Figueroa AA, Liou EJ, et al: Longitudinal analysis of mandibular asymmetry in hemifacial microsomia. Plast Reconstr Surg 1997;99:328-339.

67. Rune B, Selvik G, Sarnas KV, et al: Growth in hemifacial microsomia studied with the aid of roentgen stereophotogrammetry and metallic implants. Cleft Palate J 1981;18:128-146.

68. Kearns GJ, Padwa BL, Mulliken JB, et al: Progression of facial asymmetry in hemifacial microsomia. Plast Reconstr Surg 2000;105:492-498.

69. Kaban LB, Mulliken JB, Murray JE: Three-dimensional approach to analysis and treatment of hemifacial microsomia. Cleft Palate J 1981;18:90-99.

70. Mulliken JB, Kaban LB: Analysis and treatment of hemifacial microsomia in childhood. Clin Plast Surg 1987;14:91-100.

71. Edgerton MT, Marsh JL: Surgical treatment of hemifacial microsomia (first and second branchial arch syndrome). Plast Reconstr Surg 1977;59:653-666.

72. Kaplan RG: Induced condylar growth in a patient with hemifacial microsomia [see comments]. Angle Orthod 1989;59: 85-90.

73. Knowles CC: Cephalometric treatment planning and analysis of maxillary growth following bone grafting in hemifacial microsomia. Dent Pract Dent Rec 1966;17:28-38.

74. Stringer DE, Steed DL, Johnson RP, et al: Correction of hemifacial microsomia. J Oral Surg 1981;39:35-39.

75. Rune B, Sarnas KV, Selvik G, et al: Roentgen stereometry with the aid of metallic implants in hemifacial microsomia. Am J Orthod 1983;84:231-247.

76. Murray JE, Kaban LB, Mulliken JB: Analysis and treatment of hemifacial microsomia. Plast Reconstr Surg 1984;74:186-199.

77. Kaban LB, Moses MH, Mulliken JB: Surgical correction of hemifacial microsomia in the growing child. Plast Reconstr Surg 1988;82:9-19.

78. Vargervik K: Sequence and timing of treatment phases in hemifacial microsomia. In Harvold EP, Vargervik K, Chierici G, eds: Treatment of Hemifacial Microsomia. New York, Alan R. Liss, 1983.

79. Brodie AG: Contribution of the mandibular condyle to the growth of the face. In Sarnat BG, ed: The Temporomandibular Joint. Springfield, Ill, Charles C Thomas, 1964:77.

80. Sarnat BG, Engel MB: A serial study of mandibular growth after removal of the condyle in the *Macaca* rhesus monkey. Plast Reconstr Surg 1951;7:364.

81. Rodgers SF, Eppley BL, Nelson CL, et al: Hemifacial microsomia: assessment of classification systems. J Craniofac Surg 1991;2:114-126.

82. Cousley RR: A comparison of two classification systems for hemifacial microsomia. Br J Oral Maxillofac Surg 1993;31:78-82.

83. Longacre JJ, deStefano GA, Holmstrand KE: The surgical management of first and second branchial arch syndromes. Plast Reconstr Surg 1963;31:507-520.

84. Meurman Y: Congenital microtia and meatal atresia. Arch Otolaryngol 1957;66:443-463.

85. Figueroa AA, Pruzansky S: The external ear, mandible and other components of hemifacial microsomia. J Maxillofac Surg 1982;10:200-211.

86. Converse JM, Coccaro PJ, Becker M, et al: On hemifacial microsomia. The first and second branchial arch syndrome. Plast Reconstr Surg 1973;51:268-279.

86a. Tanconi R, Hall BD: Hemifacial microsomias: phenotypic classification, clinical implications and genetic aspects. In Harvold EP, Vargervik K, Chierici G, eds: Treatment of Hemifacial Microsomia. New York, Alan R. Liss, 1983:39-49.

87. Lauritzen C, Munro IR, Ross RB: Classification and treatment of hemifacial microsomia. Scand J Plast Reconstr Surg 1985;19:33-39.

88. Munro IR: Treatment of craniofacial microsomia. Clin Plast Surg 1987;14:177-186.

89. Vento AR, LaBrie RA, Mulliken JB: The O.M.E.N.S. classification of hemifacial microsomia. Cleft Palate Craniofac J 1991;28:68-76, discussion 77.

90. Schendel SA: Cephalometrics and orthognathic surgery. In Bell WH, ed: Modern Practice in Orthognathic and Reconstructive Surgery. Philadelphia, WB Saunders, 1992:84-99.

91. Grayson BH, LaBatto FA, Kolber AB, et al: Basilar multiplane cephalometric analysis. Am J Orthod 1985;88:503-516.

92. Whyte AM, Hourihan MD, Earley MJ, et al: Radiological assessment of hemifacial microsomia by three-dimensional computed tomography. Dentomaxillofac Radiol 1990;19:119-125.

93. Ono I, Ohura T, Narumi E, et al: Three-dimensional analysis of craniofacial bones using three-dimensional computer tomography. J Craniomaxillofac Surg 1992;20:49-60.

94. Kusnoto B, Figueroa AA, Polley JW: A longitudinal three-dimensional evaluation of the growth pattern in hemifacial microsomia treated by mandibular distraction osteogenesis: a preliminary report. J Craniofac Surg 1999;10:480-486.

95. Casselman JW, Deryckere F, Robert Y, et al: Denta Scan: programme of x-ray computed tomographic reconstruction used for the anatomical evaluation of the mandible and maxilla in preoperative assessment of dental implants [in French]. Ann Radiol (Paris) 1990;33:408-417.

96. Casselman JW, Deryckere F, Hermans R, et al: Denta Scan: CT software program used in the anatomic evaluation of the mandible and maxilla in the perspective of endosseous implant surgery. Rofo Fortschr Geb Rontgenstr Neuen Bildgeb Verfahr 1991;155:4-10.

97. King JM, Caldarelli DD, Petasnick JP: DentaScan: a new diagnostic method for evaluating mandibular and maxillary pathology. Laryngoscope 1992;102:379-387.

98. David DJ, Mahatumarat C, Cooter RD: Hemifacial microsomia: a multisystem classification. Plast Reconstr Surg 1987;80:525-535.

99. Kaban LB, Padwa BL, Mulliken JB: Surgical correction of mandibular hypoplasia in hemifacial microsomia: the case for treatment in early childhood. J Oral Maxillofac Surg 1998;56:628-638.

Nonsyndromic Craniosynostosis

Jeffrey L. Marsh, MD ✦ Judith M. Gurley, MD ✦ Alex A. Kane, MD

The term *craniosynostosis* denotes pathologic partial or complete absence of one or more cranial sutures. Although it is often referred to as premature fusion of cranial sutures, this is a misleading definition because it implies that timely fusion of cranial sutures is a normal event. Only the metopic suture fuses in normal individuals; the remaining sutures alter ("mature") in gross and microscopic form during childhood but remain patent.[1]

Some individuals with craniosynostosis also have dysmorphism of one or more of the following anatomic regions: the midface, the lower face, the axial skeleton, the hands, and the feet.[2] Specific constellations of craniosynostosis and other dysmorphisms are known as the craniosynostosis syndromes. Individuals who have craniosynostosis without other dysmorphisms are said to have nonsyndromic craniosynostosis. Until the past decade, individuals were assigned eponymous syndromic designations based on physical findings and inheritance patterns. The identification of specific codon DNA errors associated with one or more of the eponymous syndromes has made classification more specific.[3] Interestingly, some individuals with nonsyndromic craniosynostosis have been found to have the codon errors usually associated with syndromic craniosynostosis.[4] Some have argued that this overlap makes the differentiation between syndromic and nonsyndromic craniosynostosis moot. Because the term *syndrome* is unambiguous, meaning "the aggregate of signs and symptoms associated with any morbid process, and constituting together the picture of the disease,"[5] the separation of patients having craniosynostosis into those who have associated signs and symptoms and those who do not remains clinically useful. This chapter discusses the types of craniosynostosis that are nonsyndromic.

Craniosynostosis was recognized as a pathologic entity in the mid-19th century. Its etiology and pathogenesis have been speculated on since. Whereas some genetic errors, proteins, tissue interface interactions, and mechanical factors have been associated with craniosynostosis during the past decade,[3,6,7] what fundamentally differentiates an abnormally fusing suture from a normal suture remains elusive. The pathoetiology of craniosynostosis is incompletely understood. Observation of humans with craniosynostosis,[8] with and without surgical intervention, and the results of animal experimentation, with both heritable actual craniosynostosis[9,10] and induced sutural fusion in otherwise normal animals,[11] have documented craniofacial and soft tissue dysmorphism that is secondary to and specific for the synostotic sutures. Whether craniosynostosis has a primary, genetically determined dysmorphology is unclear. Some of the biochemical differences between synostotic and normal sutures have begun to be delineated in the past decade. These primarily involve growth factors.[12] Furthermore, identification of the genome codon errors for most of the craniosynostosis syndromes and their localization to the region coding for fibroblast growth factor strongly suggest a biochemical error in connective tissue development or growth.[3] The direct path of cause and effect from altered amino acid sequence to craniofacial dysmorphism remains to be illuminated.[13] A further unresolved confounding variable is the relationship between craniosynostosis and the intracranial contents. The embryonic brain precedes development of the embryonic skull.[14] That neural anomalies can affect cranial sutural status and shape

is evident from consideration of the premature synostosis of microcephaly due to inadequate brain
expansion and the persistence of widely patent sutures
in hydrocephalus due to excessive expansion of
intracranial volume. Topographic brain anomalies
and central nervous system dysfunctions have been
observed in association with craniosynostosis.[15,16]
Whether these findings reflect primary neural abnormality that in turn induces craniosynostosis or secondary neural damage due to synostosis is unresolved.

Surgical management of craniosynostosis began in
the late 19th century with an operation that has come
to be known as strip craniectomy: removal of the synostosed suture. The hypotheses underlying this procedure included the following: that failure to remove
the synostosis would lead to dire consequences, including hydrocephalus, blindness, mental retardation, and
premature death; that removal of the synostosis would
allow normal cranial growth and development; and
that maintenance of the suturectomy site as a
nonossified zone into childhood was necessary for
normal cranial growth and development. By the
1960s, it had become clear that "dire consequences"
rarely occurred secondary to craniosynostosis, with
the possible exception of syndromic individuals with
synostosis of multiple sutures. Furthermore, the failure
of strip craniectomy and extended strip craniectomy
(an attempt to overcome the limitations of strip
craniectomy) to normalize cranial and facial dysmorphisms began to be documented as early as the
1950s. Finally, no correlation could be made between
attempts to prevent reossification within synostosis
zones (repetitive strip craniectomies, application of
alloplastic materials to bone edges, and placement of
toxic chemicals on the dural periosteum) and favorable outcome in regard to cranial and facial morphologic features. For all of these reasons, the primary
goal of surgery for craniosynostosis shifted from
extirpation of the synostosis zone to calvarial and superior orbital normalization. This approach has dominated surgery for craniosynostosis during the past
quarter century. Two newer surgical technologies,
endoscopic surgery[17,18] and bone distraction,[19-21] have
been adapted for treatment of craniosynostosis. A
standard extended strip craniectomy performed
with endoscopic assistance, combined with post-
extirpative calvarial molding helmet therapy, has been
advocated as a less morbid management for craniosynostosis. The hypothesis underlying this approach
is that the well-known inadequate morphologic results
from extended strip craniectomy alone can be overcome by postsurgical helmeting. Whether this
approach is any more beneficial than the inadequate
procedure of synostosis extirpation alone remains to
be documented objectively. Postsurgical displacement
of dysmorphic bones by either external or internal bone
distraction devices after strip craniectomy has been

transferred from the animal laboratory to human
application. The hypothesis underlying this approach
is that dysmorphic bone displaced during days rather
than minutes can normalize. Whether slowly displaced
un-remodeled bone can normalize, whereas it is
known that intraoperatively displaced dysmorphic
bone cannot, also remains to be documented.

In addition to the extent and nature of surgical intervention, the timing of intervention is a much-debated
topic with little substantive evidence. Some surgeons
believe that limited operations (e.g., strip craniectomy
or extended strip craniectomy) are effective in
"younger" infants.[22] There is debate among the proponents of this opinion about the maximum age at
which such limited interventions are useful, ranging
from weeks to months of life. Other surgeons believe
that craniosynostosis surgery should be delayed until
the cranial bones become quite hard, after 10 to 12
months of age, to minimize the need for revision
surgery.[23] Still others have documented changes in
the endocranial base toward normalization in infants
whose craniosynostosis was operated on before 6
months of age but not in those operated on later.[24,25]
The degree to which the endocranial base is normalized seems to be related to the degree of normalcy
achieved in head shape and the amount of mini-
mization of secondary facial dysmorphism. A further
confounding variable affecting the decisions for timing
and extent of intervention is that of possible deleterious effect of the synostosis on the developing brain.[26]
Whereas low-grade increased intracranial pressure
in individuals with nonsyndromic craniosynostosis
has been documented by multiple centers,[27-30] the
significance of these findings is unclear. Preliminary
positron emission tomographic scan data suggest that
release of calvarial constraint due to single-suture synostosis is beneficial for brain metabolism.[31] Although
evaluation of infants and young children with nonsyndromic craniosynostoses has failed to demonstrate
consistent neuropsychological defects,[32-34] testing of
older children has documented discrete cognitive or
behavioral impairments for sagittal and metopic synostosis.[15,35] The absence of significant numbers of individuals who have not undergone surgical repair of
nonsyndromic craniosynostosis precludes meaningful determination of the optimal technique and timing
of surgery. However, there exists the impression in some
craniofacial centers that the neuropsychological dysfunctions are unrelated to intervention.[36]

Outcome assessment of craniosynostosis surgery
has lagged well behind introduction of surgical techniques.[37] The largest reported series have tended to
focus on operative and perioperative morbidity rather
than on structural and functional growth and development.[38-43] Those few studies that have addressed craniofacial growth or neuropsychological function are
limited by small numbers, short length of follow-up,

and grouping of craniosynostosis with other craniofacial anomalies. Several groups are currently attempting to analyze outcomes of specific sutural synostoses from birth to adolescence with respect to both structure and function. Most of the few reports on appearance outcome are limited in that assessments were performed by the care providers or their trainees, with the major outcome criterion being the need for revisional surgery.[40] Others have assumed that the incidence of revisional surgery is inversely related to normalcy of outcome, without validation of this hypothesis.[44] Whereas some authors express firm opinions about both the extent and the timing of surgical intervention, few data exist to substantiate claims of superiority of one approach over another. Furthermore, in individuals not having undergone surgical intervention, the natural history of nonsyndromic craniosynostoses with regard to appearance, neuropsychological function, and socialization from birth through adolescence is largely unreported. The scarcity of such data prevents rigorous assessment of the benefits of any intervention.

An additional confounder in processing published data about craniosynostosis is inconsistent use of nomenclature. The relationship between dysmorphic skull shape and specific sutural synostosis was thought to be exclusive from the mid-19th to the mid-20th centuries. It is now well appreciated that similar head shapes may be caused by different patterns of craniosynostosis or nonsynostotic causes (Table 92-1). For this reason, we have advocated that abnormal head shapes be described as either nonsynostotic or synostotic.

The cause, if known, of nonsynostotic cranial dysmorphism is stated as a modifier. The affected sutures are stated for synostotic cranial dysmorphism with the additional modifier of an identified genetic error. Unfortunately, authors still persist in using ambiguous terminology, such as plagiocephaly, without clearly delineating whether they mean it to be an exclusive synonym for unilateral coronal synostosis or an inclusive term for all causes of plagiocephaly. Another ill-considered recommendation was the separation of plagiocephaly into the diagnostic categories "anterior"[45] and "posterior"[46] when sophisticated imaging techniques had already been established to clarify the occasional patient with sutural status ambiguity on routine skull radiographs. In this chapter, each affected suture is discussed independently because this is the only unambiguous means of presenting the information.

MANAGEMENT OF CLEFT PALATE AND CRANIOFACIAL DEFORMITIES

The management of individuals with nonsyndromic craniosynostosis has rested on a basic assumption in regard to surgical intervention for these patients, namely, normalization of craniofacial appearance requires release of the fused sutural constraint and intraoperative correction of associated calvarial and superior-orbital deformities.[47] Care should be provided within the context of a multidisciplinary craniofacial team[8] with standardized annual or biennial evaluations from infancy through late adolescence.

✳ T1

TABLE 92-1 ✦ HEAD SHAPES DUE TO CRANIOSYNOSTOSIS OR NONSYNOSTOTIC CAUSES

Name	Literal Translation	Traditional Associated Suture	Causal Synostosis	Nonsynostotic Causes
Scaphocephaly	Boat head	Sagittal	Sagittal	Deformation secondary to prematurity, neurologic impairment, intentional head binding
Trigonocephaly	Triangle head	Metopic	Metopic Multiple	
Plagiocephaly	Twisted head	Unilateral coronal	Unilateral coronal Unilateral lambdoid Multiple	Deformation secondary to sleep position, torticollis
Brachycephaly	Short head	Bilateral coronal	Bilateral coronal Multiple	Deformation secondary to sleep position, intentional head binding
Acrocephaly	Peak head	Multiple	Multiple	Deformation secondary to intentional head binding
Oxycephaly	Pointed head	Multiple	Multiple	Deformation secondary to intentional head binding
Turricephaly	Tower head	Multiple	Multiple	Deformation secondary to intentional head binding
Kleeblattschädel	Cloverleaf skull	Multiple	Multiple	

NUMBER OF PATIENTS/YEAR BY AFFECTED SUTURE(S)

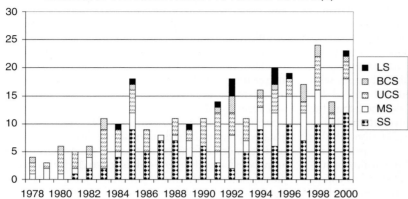

FIGURE 92-1. Number of new patients evaluated for nonsyndromic craniosynostosis per year at the Cleft Palate and Craniofacial Deformities Institute, St. Louis Children's Hospital, from 1978 to 2000. Although there are variations in affected sutures from year to year, the general distribution remains consistent. LS, lambdoid synostosis; BCS, bilateral coronal synostosis; UCS, unilateral coronal synostosis; MS, metopic synostosis; SS, sagittal synostosis.

To provide a frame of reference for the frequency with which craniosynostosis is evaluated, it is useful to briefly examine clinical activity for a particular clinic in total. At the authors' center, 5872 patients were enrolled between 1978 and 2001 for evaluation and management of congenital craniofacial deformities; 45% had cleft lip with or without cleft palate but no other craniofacial anomalies, and 55% had other craniofacial diagnoses. Of the noncleft diagnoses, the largest group was positional cranial deformation (47%), which became dominant in the mid-1990s. Craniosynostosis accounted for 30% of the remainder, with 80% of these nonsyndromic and 20% syndromic. The distribution of the nonsyndromic synostoses by affected suture was as follows: sagittal, 36%; unilateral coronal, 26%; metopic, 19%; bilateral coronal, 8%; other multiple, 7%; and lambdoid, 4% (Fig. 92-1).

General Treatment Comments

Whereas the details of surgical intervention are specific to the affected sutures, the general scheme of evaluation, treatment, and follow-up is uniform. Patients should be evaluated on referral; the nature of the evaluation depends on the age at referral. If possible, infants younger than 12 months are evaluated by a craniofacial plastic surgeon, pediatric neurosurgeon, pediatric ophthalmologist, and pediatric psychologist. Patients presenting at 12 months of age or older are evaluated by a full craniofacial team (Table 92-2). Head imaging studies, computed tomographic (CT) scans, and magnetic resonance imaging should be obtained for all patients to delineate the aberrant anatomy and individualize surgical planning. Ophthalmologic screening should be an integral part of the evaluation of all patients with craniosynostosis because of the high incidence of abnormal findings (most frequently amblyopia, strabismus, and hyperopia). Abnormal eye findings accompany unilateral synostoses more frequently than bilateral synostoses. In the authors' experience, this has broken down as follows: unilateral coronal, 82%; unilateral lambdoid, 67%; bilateral coronal, 50%; bilateral lambdoid, 50%; sagittal, 46%; and metopic, 38%.

The timing of surgery also depends on the age at referral. Infants evaluated before 6 months of age should be scheduled for elective release of the synostotic sutures and calvarial recontouring between 3 and 6 months of age. This timing is considered optimal because of the high probability of passive postoperative endocranial remodeling, the likelihood of reossification of calvariectomy defects, the malleability of the calvarial bone, and the favorable effect on minimizing facial dysmorphism specifically in unilateral coronal synostosis. When a patient presents with untreated craniosynostosis after the age of 6 months, surgery should be scheduled as soon as it can be arranged. Most patients

TABLE 92-2 ✦ CRANIOFACIAL TEAM DISCIPLINES AT THE CLEFT PALATE AND CRANIOFACIAL DEFORMITIES INSTITUTE, ST. LOUIS CHILDREN'S HOSPITAL

Audiology
Craniofacial plastic surgery
Genetics
Neurosurgery
Nursing
Pediatric dentistry
Prosthodontics
Psychology
Ophthalmology
Oral-maxillofacial surgery
Orthodontics
Otolaryngology
Speech-language pathology

are referred in the "ideal" window before 6 months of age (Fig. 92-2).

Technical details of the operation change markedly in children older than 12 months for a number of reasons: the calvarial bone is no longer easily molded by the surgeon's fingers or light instruments; calvarial defects cannot be expected to predictably reossify; the endocranial base will not alter; and facial dysmorphism will usually persist or progress. Whereas these changes are specific to the affected sutures, they generally include a more extensive calvariectomy and remodeling, greater segmentation of the calvaria to assist remodeling, avoidance of calvariectomy defects by use of split cranioplasty and interdigitation calvarial expansion techniques, and more rigid osseous fixation.

Although the timing of surgery and the technique of surgery have remained relatively constant, there have been two relatively recent substantive changes in preferred technique. The first was a major change in fixation of remodeled calvarial segments in the late 1990s. Before that time, interosseous fixation was achieved with biodegradable sutures (4-0 polyglactin), and advanced bones (superolateral orbital rims) were stabilized with autogenous full-thickness calvarial interposition grafts by the tenon-in-mortise technique.[47,48] This technique was effective for all patients except those with bilateral coronal synostosis, in whom the advancement at the nasion often failed to persist long term.[49] For this reason, a single extrapericranial titanium facial fixation plate was used to strut the nasion

advancement. However, the use of metallic plates as the primary means of interosseous fixation in infants was never adopted by the authors. Although the combination of biodegradable suture and bone grafts is effective, it is a tedious process. For this reason, when biodegradable plates and screws became available for osseous fixation in infants, the authors adopted them as the preferred means of fixation.[50] Resorption has been somewhat erratic, seeming to range from months to years on the basis of visibility and palpability in the same patient.

The second change in preferred technique was retropositioning of the calvariectomy defect from the region of the coronal sutures to a location posterior to the coronal meridian of the skull. This change was motivated by the frequent observation of a constriction behind the frontal prominence in the region of the temples. Whereas some have attributed this constriction to hypoplasia of the temporalis muscles either due to the anomaly or as a consequence of surgical mobilization, we did not notice any difference in temporalis mass on preoperative and postoperative CT scans. The constriction often occurs in the region of the intentional calvariectomy, at the site of the coronal sutures. Once the perioperative edema resolves, depression of the scalp can be observed in this area when the infant is sleeping or resting quietly, much as a normally patent anterior fontanel depresses slightly in similar conditions. It is hypothesized that the brain does not expand into the calvariectomy gap and that reossification, through the periosteal dura, follows the

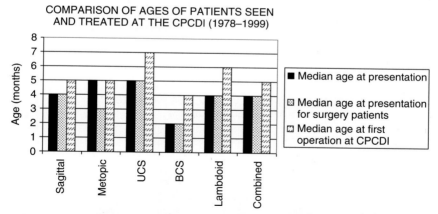

FIGURE 92-2. Age at presentation to the Cleft Palate and Craniofacial Deformities Institute (CPCDI) as a function of affected sutures and whether surgery was performed. The range in age at presentation suggests that infants with bilateral coronal synostosis appear more dysmorphic to their primary care providers than do those with the other synostoses. Infants with unilateral coronal synostosis may be referred later than the infants with other synostoses because their dysmorphism may be misinterpreted as either an ophthalmologic or positional deformational problem. The discrete discrepancy in age at referral between all patients with metopic synostosis and those who receive surgery may reflect the difference between those with overt dysmorphic features and those with an incidental radiologic finding. BCS, bilateral coronal synostosis; UCS, unilateral coronal synostosis.

slight recession. To compensate, the calvariectomy gap should be displaced posteriorly, well under the hair-bearing scalp, by dividing the mobilized parietotemporal bones coronally and then moving the ventral segment to abut the dorsal edge of the frontal bone, where it is fixed (Fig. 92-3). This modification is suitable for all patients with synostoses except those for whom a prone position is used to optimize occipital reconstruction—lambdoid and sagittal bullet (occipital prominence).

Follow-up should be standardized for all patients with craniosynostoses regardless of the affected suture and whether the patient has a surgical procedure performed. Patients should have a full evaluation[8] annually from 1 to 4 years of age and then biennially through 14 years. Re-evaluation should then be carried out at 17 years for female patients and at 20 years for male patients. As of 1999, at the authors' center, 47% of patients with nonsyndromic craniosynostosis remained in active follow-up (Fig. 92-4). The remainder had either graduated from the program or terminated because of departure from the geographic area, incompatible insurance coverage, or parental desire or were "lost to follow-up."

Many centers do not provide orthodontic services, so patients often receive their orthodontics elsewhere. Dental models and standard dental radiographs (periapicals, panoramics, and cephalograms) should be obtained from the treating orthodontists for study and treatment planning.

Sagittal Synostosis

Sagittal synostosis is the most frequently occurring of the nonsyndromic synostoses. The dominance of males over females is approximately 73%.[38,51]

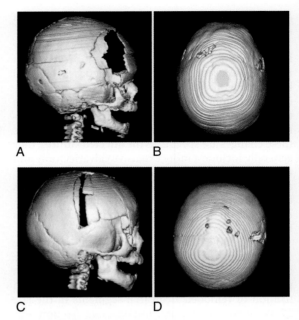

FIGURE 92-3. Change in site of intentional calvariectomy defect for unilateral coronal, bilateral coronal, and metopic synostosis operations in infants younger than 12 months. (All osseous images are three-dimensional CT scan osseous reformations.) *A,* The original calvariectomy defect was at the site of the patent or synostosed coronal sutures. *B,* One year postoperatively, the calvarial contour is irregular with frontotemporal concavities. *C,* More recently, the defect has been retropositioned to the coronal meridian of the skull to avoid frontotemporal narrowing. *D,* One year postoperatively, the calvarial contour is smooth without frontotemporal concavity. (From Perlyn CA, Marsh JL, Vannier MW, et al: The craniofacial anomalies archive at St. Louis Children's Hospital: 20 years of craniofacial imaging experience. Plast Reconstr Surg 2001;108:1862-1870.)

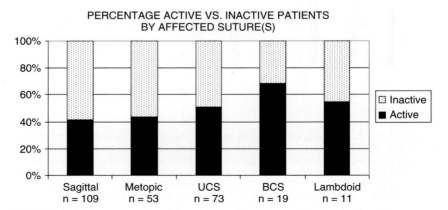

FIGURE 92-4. Percentage of active versus inactive patients by affected suture. Uncertainty about midface and lower face deformity with growth may account for the higher percentage of active patients with unilateral coronal synostosis (UCS) and bilateral coronal synostosis (BCS).

The crania of individuals with sagittal synostosis resemble each other with a long, narrow shape that reminded the 19th century classifiers of a boat, that is, scaphocephaly (Fig. 92-5). Fusion of the sagittal suture impairs expansion of skull width, which seems to be compensated for by excessive skull length. The magnitude of this disproportion can be expressed quantitatively as the cranial index (biparietal diameter/anteroposterior diameter × 100). The cranial index is a useful shorthand measure of the degree of calvarial deviation from normalcy in that it is easily assessed, is reproducible, and has published normative values by age. Whereas the cranial index has been used effectively to assess outcome from different treatment protocols for sagittal synostosis,[52-58] it assesses only the major dysmorphic feature of the condition. Additional compensations (Fig. 92-6) for the limitation of lateral cranial expansion occur in the frontal bones with bossing (excessive ventral projection and rectangularization of the normal curvilinear forehead), in the temporal squamosa with lateral bulging, in the occiput with central projection (bulleting due to similarity to the projectile's shape), and in the interorbital bones with increased width (telecanthus or orbital hypertelorism). The endocranial base dysmorphism of sagittal synostosis includes expansion of the anterior and posterior fossae compared with normal subjects. In some patients with sagittal synostosis, the patent coronal sutures seem to be a constricting ring between the expanded anterior and

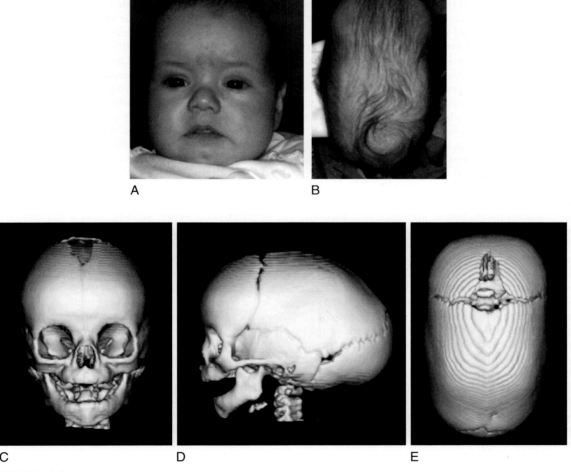

A   B

C   D   E

FIGURE 92-5. Scaphocephaly—the surface (A and B) and osseous (C to E) dysmorphology of sagittal synostosis in a 3-month-old girl. The head is narrow in width and elongated front to back. The forehead is "boxy" because of protrusion of the frontal bones laterally (bossing).

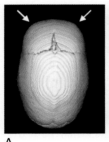
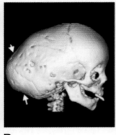
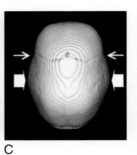

A   B   C

FIGURE 92-6. Several secondary calvarial dysmorphisms can be observed in sagittal synostosis. *A,* Frontal bossing *(arrows).* *B,* Occipital protuberance or "bullet." There may be a band-like constriction *(arrows)* ventral to the protrusion. *C,* There can be marked coronal constriction *(line arrows)* and temporal bulging *(block arrows).*

middle cranial fossae. The factors that may be responsible for these variations in secondary dysmorphic features are unknown, and attempts to subcategorize them have been unfruitful.

Infants younger than 12 months with sagittal synostosis are usually recommended for surgical treatment. Because the final magnitude of the dysmorphism is not predictable and there is the possibility of low-grade increased intracranial pressure and symptomatic headache in untreated individuals, the operation is optimally performed between 3 and 6 months of age. Individuals older than 12 months should be assessed for extent of dysmorphism and neurologic symptoms. If the scaphocephaly and frontal bossing are overt or there are signs and symptoms of possible neurologic impairment without other discernible cause, it is best to proceed with subtotal calvarial reconstruction. If the dysmorphic change is subtle and there are no suggestive neurologic signs and symptoms, the individual should be observed over time.

Because of dissatisfaction with the inconsistency of cranial shape outcome with extended sagittal strip craniectomy, the preferable approach to sagittal synostosis has usually been subtotal calvariectomy with calvarial reconstruction (Figs. 92-7 and 92-8), leaving calvariectomy gaps in infants younger than 12 months but not in those older than 12 months. Operative position depends on the subcategory of the dysmorphism. If the occipital prominence (bullet) is the most striking feature, the patient is placed prone for the surgery. The calvaria is removed by the neurosurgeon from the coronal sutures to below the occipital prominence. The craniofacial plastic surgeon then cuts the removed calvaria into fragments to reconstruct the right and left occipital and right and left parietotemporal skull; no surgery is performed on the frontal bones. If the occipital bullet is not the dominant dysmorphic feature, the patient is placed in the supine position for surgery. The calvaria is removed by the neurosurgeon from 1 cm above the superior orbital rims to as close to the occipital prominence as is comfortable for that surgeon. The craniofacial plastic surgeon then cuts the removed calvaria into

fragments to reconstruct the right and left frontal, right and left parietotemporal, and right and left occipital skull. Whereas the calvariectomy for these patients is more extensive than that for those who are prone, the caudal extent of the occipital unroofing is less than that achieved when the patient is prone.

In the early 1990s, extended strip craniectomy was performed exclusively at the authors' center because of the neurosurgeon's preference. This cohort of patients having undergone differing procedures within the same general care system provided the authors with a unique opportunity of assessing the effect of two interventions (Fig. 92-9). As reported,[52,56] subtotal calvarial remodeling is more effective both immediately postoperatively and 1 year postoperatively in normalizing the cranial index than is extended strip craniectomy. Furthermore, the extended strip craniectomy, whether the patients were operated on before or after 4 months of age, did not affect the cranial index result (4 months was chosen as the separator because there were insufficient numbers of patients operated on at earlier dates to make a younger separator meaningful). As these two populations age, any significant neuropsychological functional differences will be noted and reported.

Investigators have rigorously attempted to assess the outcome of patients with sagittal synostosis. Two features can attract unfavorable attention in an individual with untreated or poorly treated sagittal synostosis: head shape and forehead configuration. Some surgeons argue that normalization of the cranium should not be an objective of sagittal synostosis surgery because hair camouflages the deficiency. Blinded assessors, both medical professionals and laypersons, have been shown to be unable to discern documented differences in skull width-to-length ratios in older children with full heads of dry hair.[59] However, the frequency with which parents or children purposefully avoid certain hairstyles or swimming in public because of scaphocephaly has not been assessed. The most characteristic dysmorphic feature of sagittal synostosis, the elongated narrow head, has been

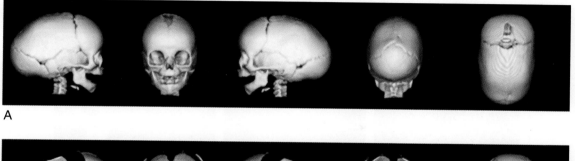

A

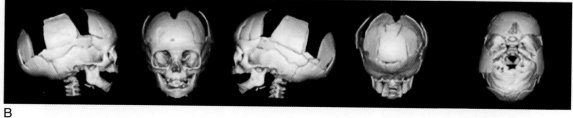

B

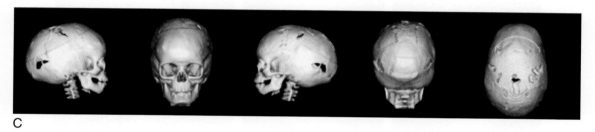

C

FIGURE 92-7. Subtotal calvarial reconstruction: preferred surgical procedure for sagittal synostosis. *A,* Preoperative appearance of a 3-month-old girl (same patient as in Figures 92-5 and 92-8). *B,* One-week perioperative views. Anterior, posterior, and midsagittal calvariectomy defects are present. The frontal curvature has been remodeled to reduce the lateral prominences ("boxiness"). The frontal, lateral, and occipital widths have been increased. *C,* One year postoperatively. The anteroposterior and bitemporal diameters of the skull are normally proportioned (cranial index of 76 versus 55 preoperatively). The endocranial base has remodeled toward normal compared with the preoperative configuration.

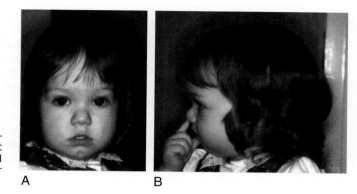

FIGURE 92-8. *A* and *B,* Postoperative appearance of the patient in Figures 92-5 and 92-7 at 1 year, 5 months of age. Hair makes critical assessment of calvarial shape difficult in older individuals.

A   B

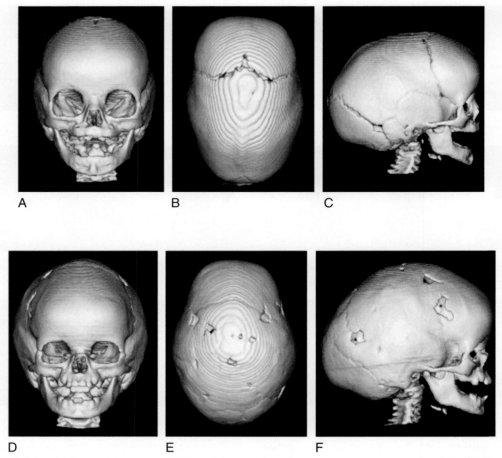

A   B   C

D   E   F

FIGURE 92-9. Extended strip craniectomy with barrel stave cuts perpendicular to the midsagittal calvariectomy. *A* to *C*, Preoperative appearance of a 3-month-old girl. *D* to *F*, One year postoperatively. Comparison of these images with those in Figure 92-6 shows greater persistence of the untreated dysmorphic features of sagittal synostosis with extended strip craniectomy than with subtotal calvarial reconstruction. Although the cranial index increased from 65 to 72, the occipital deformation and coronal constriction remain. These deformities would be camouflaged by a full head of hair, giving a fallacious appearance of normalcy.

quantitatively assessed by the cranial index. Several authors have documented the inadequacy of strip craniectomy even when it is "extended" to include additional calvariectomy and parietotemporal outfracturing compared with subtotal calvariectomy in normalizing the cranial index.[52,55,56]

Unable to refute these findings, proponents of more limited operations argue that the cranial index is not an adequate determinant of outcome for sagittal synostosis, yet they do not propose an alternative criterion. It has been documented quantitatively that late calvarial recontouring for sagittal synostosis does not affect the aberrant width-to-length ratio of the cranial base. Thus, whereas frontal bossing, biparietal narrowing, and occipital protrusion can be reversed

surgically in older individuals, the scaphocephaly of the cranial base cannot. Not only does this mean that the basic head shape remains scaphocephalic, excessively narrow and long, but it has implications for facial growth as well. It has been documented that untreated sagittal synostosis produces a dysmorphic appearance of the face presumably through the aberrant cranial base.[60,61] Furthermore, it has been demonstrated that calvarial surgery in infancy can positively affect the endocranial base (i.e., decrease dysmorphic appearance toward normalcy).[25] Therefore, it can be hypothesized that those individuals with sagittal synostosis who have increased normalization of their endocranial base dysmorphism after calvarial surgery should have concomitant increased normalization of their face as well. This hypothesis is currently being tested. With respect to neuropsychological function, it had been assumed that individuals with sagittal synostosis were indistinguishable from those without synostosis. This has been reported to be true for infants and young children.[33,34] The authors have noted, however, an unusually high frequency of speech and language disorders in older children with sagittal synostosis that seems to be independent of whether these patients underwent calvarial surgery in infancy. In the authors' population, 48% of patients with sagittal synostosis who underwent speech and language screening had impairments that required speech and language therapy. Additional data are needed to validate these observations and to determine whether other neuropsychological defects are associated with sagittal synostosis that can be detected only by focused testing in older individuals.

Unilateral Coronal Synostosis

Unilateral coronal synostosis is the second most frequently occurring nonsyndromic synostosis. The dominance of females over males is 68%.[38,62] Unilateral coronal synostosis is notable because of its repercussions for midface and lower face growth. Unlike with the other nonsyndromic craniosynostoses, individuals with untreated or inadequately treated unilateral coronal synostosis have progressive stigmatizing facial deformity (Fig. 92-10).

The descriptive term assigned to the calvarial dysmorphic feature of unilateral coronal synostosis, plagiocephaly, is a source of confusion in the literature because some authors have used it as an exclusive synonym for unilateral coronal synostosis while others have used it as an inclusive descriptor for all forms of the asymmetric head. Plagiocephaly, the roots of which mean "twisted head," can be used to describe the calvarial dysmorphic feature associated with either of the unilateral craniosynostoses (coronal or lambdoid), the asymmetric multiple synostoses, and the positional skull deformation associated most commonly with back sleeping.[63] In spite of this, the plagiocephaly of unilateral coronal synostosis is distinctive to a knowledgeable observer: the frontal region is more deformed than the occiput, with recession of the brow ipsilateral to the synostosis and protrusion, or bossing, contralaterally; there is reciprocal but less marked protrusion of the occiput ipsilaterally and flattening of the occiput contralaterally (Fig. 92-11). Because the midsagittal plane is not a barrier to the dysmorphologic process of unilateral coronal synostosis, *ipsilateral* is used to indicate the side of the synostosed coronal suture and *contralateral* the patent opposite coronal suture. "Affected" versus "unaffected" and "abnormal" versus ""normal" are not useful terms in describing the dysmorphology of unilateral craniosynostosis.

The most useful craniofacial features for clinical identification of unilateral coronal synostosis are those of the face rather than the skull. The major facial dysmorphism consists of right-left asymmetries and

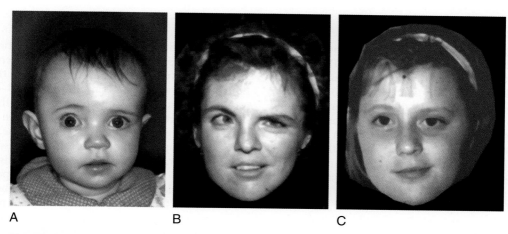

A   B   C

FIGURE 92-10. Facial dysmorphism of unilateral coronal synostosis. *A,* A 10-month-old with untreated right unilateral coronal synostosis. The ipsilateral eyebrow is elevated and the contralateral depressed. The ipsilateral palpebral fissure is excessively opened. The nasal tip is deviated contralateral to the synostosis, as is the chin. The ipsilateral hemiface is "expanded," whereas the contralateral is "compressed." *B,* A 27-year-old with untreated right unilateral coronal synostosis. The same findings as in the infant are present with accentuation of the orbital region asymmetry. *C,* A child at 9 years, 5 months of age after strip craniectomy at 11 months of age for left unilateral coronal synostosis. (Note: the photograph has been reversed right to left to facilitate comparison with other images.) Her appearance does not differ from that of either the untreated infant or the adult.

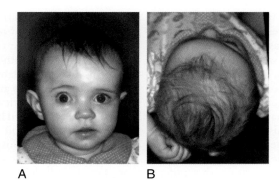

A   B

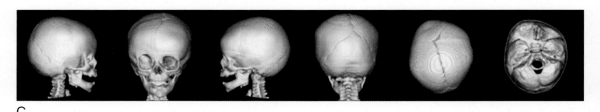

C

FIGURE 92-11. Plagiocephaly secondary to unilateral coronal synostosis: the surface (*A* and *B*) and osseous *(C)* dysmorphology of right unilateral coronal synostosis in a 10-month-old girl. The facial features described in Figure 92-10*A* reflect the orbital elongation ipsilateral to the synostosis, the deviation of the nasal bones, and the maxillary and mandibular asymmetry seen on the osseous CT reformations. The bird's-eye views document the ipsilateral frontal recession and contralateral protrusion (bossing) in both surface and osseous images. The endocranial base image *(far right)* documents deviation of the anterior cranial fossa midline toward the synostosis with compression of the ipsilateral anterior cranial fossa and expansion of the contralateral. Unlike the sutural patterns in sagittal, metopic, and bilateral coronal synostosis that retain the rectilinearity of normalcy, the patent metopic and sagittal sutures accompanying unilateral coronal synostosis *(second to right)* are deviated off the ideal midsagittal plane, resembling the endocranial base midline deviation.

deviation of true anatomic midline structures from the ideal midsagittal plane (see Fig. 92-10). The right-left asymmetries include the brows, the eyes, the cheeks, and the lower face. The midline deviations include the nose, lips, and chin. These soft tissue asymmetries and deviations mirror the underlying osseous dysmorphology[64,65] (see Fig. 92-11). However, in spite of the overt facial dysmorphism associated with unilateral coronal synostosis, it seems to be recognized later than the other synostoses by referring physicians (see Fig. 92-2).

Unlike with sagittal and metopic synostoses, for which the management should be individualized on the basis of the severity of the dysmorphic features and the age of the patient, release of the synostosed suture with fronto-orbital reconstruction is recommended for all patients with unilateral coronal synostosis. As for the other synostoses, the preferred age at operation is between 3 and 6 months to facilitate handling of the calvaria and to optimize the potential for endocranial base normalization.[25] Infants up to 12 months of age should receive bifrontal

craniotomy with bilateral frontal reconstruction and ipsilateral superolateral orbital advancement and caudal displacement[48] (details of this are in the following paragraph). Children between 1 and 4 years of age usually also have some modification of the contralateral superolateral orbital rims, elevation of the superior rim, and mesial displacement of the lateral rim, depending on the degree of dysmorphism. The entire ipsilateral lateral orbital wall may be displaced laterally as well. After 4 years of age but before puberty, serious consideration should be given to subcranial Le Fort III midface mobilization to correct the midline shift and occlusal cant when they are marked in the hope of eliminating the need for orthognathic surgery at dentoskeletal maturity. Patients presenting with untreated or inadequately treated unilateral coronal synostosis in late mixed or adult dentition undergo bilateral fronto-orbital reconstruction followed by definitive orthognathic two-jaw surgery in conjunction with preoperative and postoperative orthodontics. Although these operations can be performed synchronously, it is preferable to separate the transcranial

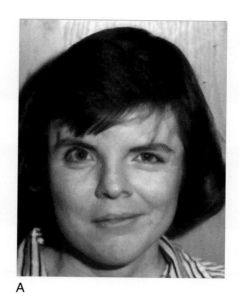

A

FIGURE 92-12. Late reconstruction of residual unilateral coronal synostosis dysmorphism. *A,* Photograph of the patient in Figure 92-10*B* at 29 years of age, 1 year after bilateral frontal bone reconstruction, reconstruction of the left supraorbital rim, left temporal fossa alloplastic augmentation, and left brow lift. The patient elected camouflage of the frontal-orbital region rather than anatomic orbital, midface, and mandibular reconstruction. *B,* Preoperative photograph of the patient in Figure 92-10*C. C,* At 18 years of age, after secondary frontal cranioplasty including autogenous rib reconstruction of a postsurgical left frontal defect and left orbital repositioning performed at 10 years of age. Reduction of the left zygoma was performed at 11 years of age. After presurgical orthodontics, maxilla and mandible osteotomies were performed elsewhere at 17 years of age to center her midface and lower face. (Note: the photographs have been reversed right to left to match the photograph in Figure 92-10.)

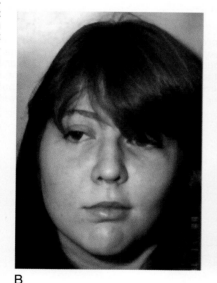

B

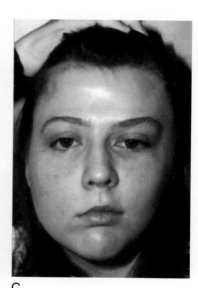

C

portion from the orthognathic to minimize morbidity. Some adults elect lesser camouflage procedures, such as centering rhinoplasty and genioplasty. Although these may not effectively destigmatize the dysmorphic facies in the opinion of others, they can be satisfactory for the patient who has chosen them purposefully to minimize the extent of intervention, time commitment, and risk (Fig. 92-12).

Our standard approach to unilateral coronal synostosis in infants has been bifrontal craniotomy with mobilization of the ipsilateral superolateral orbital rim[48] (Figs. 92-13 and 92-14). The patient is positioned supine. After a bilateral coronal scalp flap is reflected, the neurosurgeon performs the craniotomy at midcranium and 1 cm above the superior orbital rims. (Previously, the craniotomy was performed at the site of the synostosed and patent coronal sutures. However, this often led to a visible unsatisfactory frontotemporal recession.) Care is taken during the placement of the burr holes and division of the pericranium not

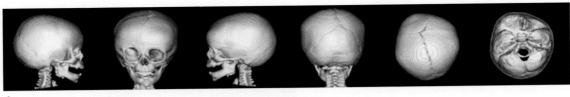

A

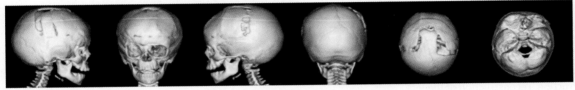

B

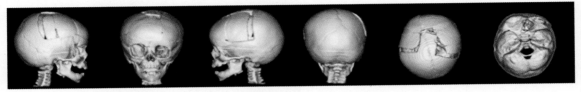

C

FIGURE 92-13. Preferred surgical procedure for unilateral coronal synostosis in infancy. Images are three-dimensional CT osseous reformations. *A,* Preoperative views, 10-month-old girl. *B,* One-week perioperative views. Frontal and temporoparietal symmetry has been achieved intraoperatively. The calvariectomy defect is posterior to the coronal meridian of the skull to avoid iatrogenic frontotemporal hollowing. The right superior orbital rim was not displaced sufficiently caudally to achieve symmetry with the left. *C,* One year postoperatively. The residual orbital asymmetry is reflected in the remaining brow asymmetry, although it is improved compared with the preoperative condition (Fig. 92-11).

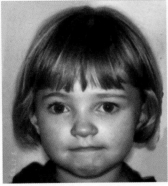

A

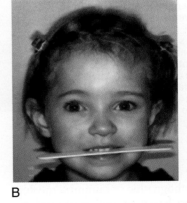

B

FIGURE 92-14. *A and B,* Postoperative appearance of the patient in Figures 92-11 and 92-13 at 3 years, 2 months of age. The patient is photographed in her "natural" state and then with hair reflected to clearly display the forehead and brows and with a tongue blade to demonstrate any cant of the occlusal plane. The forehead is symmetric, but there is minor residual brow and palpebral fissure asymmetry. Reference to the underlying skeleton (Fig. 92-13) permits the surgeon to understand the cause of these asymmetries and to plan technical modifications for unilateral coronal synostosis surgery in subsequent patients. (In this patient, more caudal repositioning of the right supraorbital rim would have been ideal.)

to violate the pterion or transect the temporalis muscle. (Preservation of the pterion was essential for placement of the tenon-in-mortise calvarial grafts used to stabilize the superolateral orbital rim advancement before the introduction of biodegradable fixation.) The craniofacial plastic surgeon continues the dissection subperiosteally over the superior, lateral, and cephalad medial rims of the ipsilateral orbit, elevating the periorbita sufficiently to allow safe osteotomies of the nasion, ventral orbital roof, and lateral orbital wall. The ipsilateral temporalis muscle is dissected sufficiently off its origins to allow safe osteotomy of the lateral orbital wall. The superolateral orbital rim is then cut free with a reciprocating saw. The rim is molded into a normal curvature with the Tessier bone bending forceps, and the caudal portions of its medial and lateral aspects are resected, usually 5 mm but measured on the CT osseous reformations to achieve symmetry of orbital height. The dura is stripped from the middle fossa immediately posterior to the pterion so that a lazy L cut can be made in the temporal squamosa, allowing it to be straightened and outfractured. The remodeled superolateral orbital rim is then advanced at the pterion and displaced caudally; it is fixed to the remodeled and repositioned temporal squamosa with a single long biodegradable plate. The Tessier bone bending forceps is used to infracture and recontour the contralateral caudal frontal bone, which remains attached to the contralateral orbit, to achieve symmetry of the bandeau (the superior orbital rims and caudal frontal bones). The frontal bones are divided into as many segments as is necessary and recontoured to achieve a symmetric forehead, usually two in infants and four or more in older individuals. In younger infants, the Tessier bone bending forceps and digital pressure are sufficient for the recontouring, at times inducing greenstick fracture lines; in older patients, kerfing osteotomies are made with either the heavy scissors or the reciprocating saw, depending on bone hardness. The remodeled frontal bones are then fixed to the bandeau with biodegradable plates. A 2-cm calvariectomy defect, from one temporal squamosa to the other, is left in infants younger than 12 months; the frontal bones are not fixed posteriorly in such infants. In older patients, a solid calvaria is reconstructed by circumferential biodegradable fixation with expanded interdigitation to compensate for the ipsilateral anterior fossa expansion. The scalp is closed in two layers over nonsuction drains.

That excision alone of a fused coronal suture fails to correct either the calvarial or orbital deformity of unilateral coronal synostosis was recognized by some neurosurgeons as early as the 1950s. As the indications for craniosynostosis surgery began to shift from prevention of dire neurologic and ophthalmologic consequences to craniofacial normalization, both neurosurgeons and nascent craniofacial surgeons extended their operations to include remodeling and repositioning of both the frontal and superolateral orbital bones.[39,66-68] By the 1980s, these calvarial-orbital procedures had become standard. Qualitative assessment of outcome based on photographic assessment of the need for revisional surgery has been used to compare unilateral frontal craniotomy with bifrontal craniotomy.[69] Nonstandardized photographs, hair-obscuring forehead contour, and intramural raters involved in the patient's care compromise the interpretation of the findings. Whereas the effects of fronto-orbital operations on objective measurements of the endocranial base[25] and of the orbit[70] have been reported up to 1 year postoperatively, long-term effects have yet to be documented. A major limitation in assessing outcome for any of the craniosynostoses is the absence of documentation of the unaltered natural history. Quantitative in vivo skeletal measurements have been reported for a small set of individuals, ranging in age from early childhood to adulthood, with untreated unilateral coronal synostosis.[65] These data can serve as a frame of reference for long-term outcome studies of surgically treated unilateral coronal synostosis. Complex facial asymmetry including the mandible[71] is the dominant dysmorphic feature of untreated or poorly treated unilateral coronal synostosis once a full head of hair has grown. Cranio-orbital surgery in infancy can minimize or even prevent the midface and lower face dysmorphism of untreated unilateral coronal synostosis (Fig. 92-15). Nonetheless, some dentoskeletal abnormalities persist. Occlusal assessment of 14 patients with unilateral coronal synostosis younger than 12 months operated on by the senior author with the described technique was performed between the ages of 9 and 16 years (mean, 12.5 years). All patients had symmetric molar Angle classifications: class I, 36%; class II, 45%; class III, 18%. No patient had anterior or posterior open bites. One patient had an anterior crossbite, and three had posterior crossbites. The occlusal plane was canted cephalad 1 to 11 mm (mean, 4.5 mm) contralateral to the synostosis in two thirds of the patients. The maxillary dental midline was shifted (mean, 2.8 mm) with respect to the ideal midsagittal line of the face in half of the patients, usually contralaterally. The mandibular dental midline was shifted less frequently (one third of the patients), also usually contralaterally. Quantification of the craniofacial skeletal changes from infancy to dentoskeletal maturity, by longitudinal high-resolution thin-slice CT scan digital data, is in progress at the authors' center.

Bilateral Coronal Synostosis

Bilateral coronal synostosis does occur as a nonsyndromic craniosynostosis, although it is more commonly associated with the syndromic craniosynostoses.

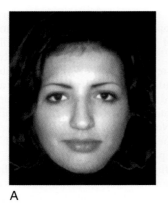
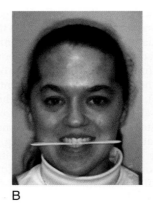
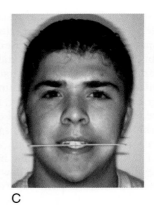

A   B   C

FIGURE 92-15. Long-term postoperative appearance of patients with unilateral coronal synostosis operated on in infancy by the authors' preferred method. None of these patients had secondary orbital, nasal, or orthognathic surgery. *A,* At 16 years, 11 months of age, right unilateral coronal synostosis—one operation at 6 months of age. *B,* At 16 years, 1 month of age, left unilateral coronal synostosis—one operation at 3 months of age. (Note: the photograph has been reversed right to left to facilitate comparisons among patients.) *C,* At 17 years, 4 months of age, right unilateral coronal synostosis—fronto-orbital surgery at 4 months of age, with autogenous cranioplasty for residual calvarial defects at 3 years of age and hydroxyapatite cranioplasty at 16 years. (Hair is reflected to fully display the forehead; the tongue blade is used to demonstrate the presence or absence of occlusal cant.) Comparison of these patients with those in Figure 92-10 documents the change in facial as well as calvarial dysmorphism secondary to an effective operation in infancy.

Some individuals with nonsyndromic bilateral coronal synostosis have identifiable DNA errors that are also associated with the phenotypes of syndromic craniosynostoses.[72,73] As additional genetic errors associated with craniosynostosis are identified and become more easily detectable, the debate of whether bilateral coronal synostosis can occur as a nongenetic event will be resolved. As with unilateral coronal synostosis, the majority of patients with bilateral coronal synostosis are female (79%).[73]

The crania of individuals with bilateral coronal synostosis have a decreased anteroposterior diameter and an increased temporoparietal width that has been labeled brachycephaly ("short head") (Fig. 92-16). In some individuals, the vertical height of the skull increases, giving the head a tower (turricephaly) or peaked (acrocephaly) appearance, although these configurations usually occur in syndromic multiply synostotic individuals. The facies of bilateral coronal synostosis are characteristic as well (see Fig. 92-16). The forehead is usually high with cephalad prominence (bossing) that protrudes beyond the brow recession and is excessively broad. There is superior exorbitism due to retropositioning of the superior orbital rims. The relationship of the inferior orbital rim to the globe is usually normal, unlike in patients with syndromic bilateral coronal synostosis, because of unimpaired maxillary size and ventral development. There may or may not be orbital hypertelorism as documented by increased bony interorbital or interpupillary distances. The nasal dorsum is usually low, and this can give an illusion of orbital hypertelorism when the bony interorbital distance is actually within normal limits.

The most challenging aspect of surgical fronto-orbital reconstruction for bilateral coronal synostosis is achieving and maintaining adequate advancement of the brow. This has led some surgeons to advocate delaying the operation until the calvarial bone is quite hard, after 9 months of age.[74] Such delayed release of the constraint to normocephalic calvarial expansion precludes normalization of the endocranial base (Fig. 92-17). To optimize normalization of the endocranial base and, in turn, the facial skeleton, it is preferable to perform surgery for bilateral coronal synostosis between 3 and 6 months of age.[75,76] Several techniques have been used to ensure adequate brow advancement[49,77] (Fig. 92-18). Until the early 1990s, calvarial grafts were often used as a strut at the nasion and placed on the endocranial surface of the reconstructed bandeau (superolateral orbits and caudal frontal bones) to reinforce it. Some advocated placement of a single titanium microplate between the nasion and the advanced bandeau, ventral to the pericranium so that it would not lie intracranially as reossification occurred. However, the preferable method is the use of resorbable plates and screws for bandeau fixation across the midline and to each temporal squamosa. The amount of ventral displacement of the bandeau is determined from both quantitative preoperative planning, by use of the lateral orbital projection reformation from the preoperative CT scan, and the intraoperative relationship achieved between the corneal

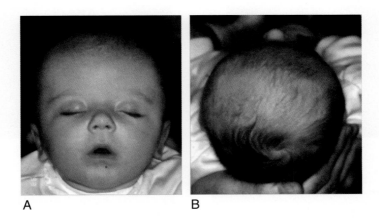

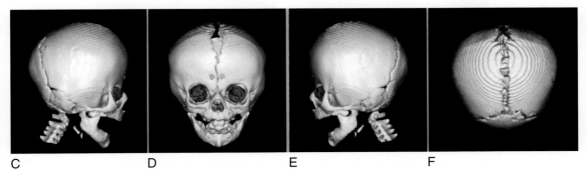

FIGURE 92-16. Brachycephaly secondary to bilateral coronal synostosis: the surface (*A* and *B*) and osseous (*C* to *F*) dysmorphology of bilateral coronal synostosis in a 2-month-old girl. The head is broad in width and short in anteroposterior dimension. The synostosed coronal sutures impair the ventral movement of the superior orbital rims and caudal frontal bones. This produces a flat, broad forehead with protruding eyes. The "unroofing" of the superior globes by the retruded superior orbital rims is evident on the globe-opacified osseous reformations.

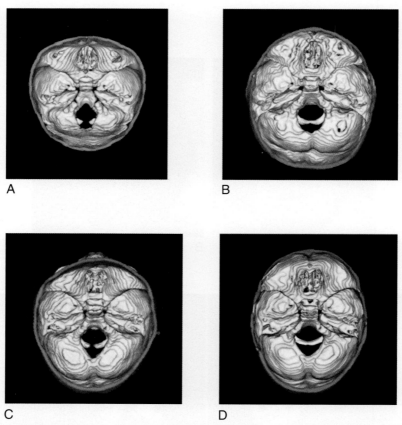

FIGURE 92-17. Effect of age at cranio-orbital surgery for bilateral coronal synostosis on endocranial base morphology. *A,* Girl with bilateral coronal synostosis operated on at 4 months of age. The preoperative anterior cranial fossa is foreshortened and widened, and the temporal fossae and the posterior fossa are compressed in the occiput. *B,* The same patient 1 year postoperatively; the configuration and proportions of the anterior, middle, and posterior fossae resemble a normal skull. *C,* Girl with bilateral coronal synostosis operated on at 13 months of age. The preoperative endocranial base resembles that of the 4-month-old with bilateral coronal synostosis illustrated in *A* with exaggerated elongation of the posterior fossa. *D,* One year postoperatively, the anterior fossa maintains the ventral enlargement of the fronto-orbital surgery. There is no change in the configuration or proportions of the middle and posterior fossae.

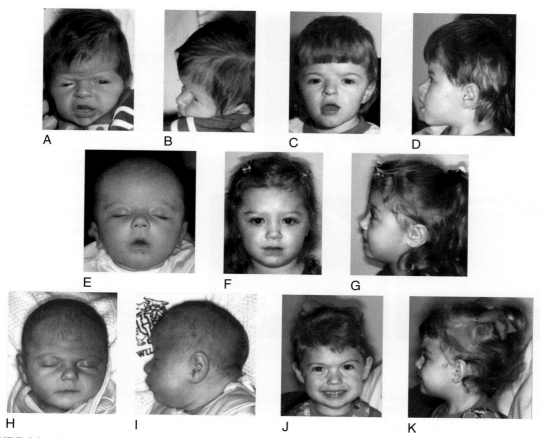

FIGURE 92-18. Effect of type of fixation at the nasion for bilateral coronal synostosis on brow projection. *A* to *D*, Boy with bilateral coronal synostosis operated on at 3 months of age (1986) with autologous calvarial graft strut at nasion: *A* and *B*, preoperative appearance of 1-month-old; *C* and *D*, 2 years postoperatively—a flat, broad, retruded forehead persists. *E* to *G*, Girl with bilateral coronal synostosis operated on at 4 months of age (1993) with titanium plate at nasion: *E*, preoperative appearance of 2-month-old; *F* and *G*, 3 years postoperatively—the forehead and frontonasal configurations are better than those of the patient seen in *A* to *D* but still somewhat flat. (Note: this is the same patient as in Figures 92-16 and 92-20.) *H* to *K*, Girl with bilateral coronal synostosis operated on at 4 months of age (1997) with biodegradable plate at nasion: *H* and *I*, preoperative appearance of 1-month-old; *J* and *K*, 2 years postoperatively—the forehead, brow, and frontonasal configurations appear more normal.

plane and the brow so that the brow is ventral to the corneal plane at midglobe[70] (Fig. 92-19).

The preferred technique for bilateral coronal synostosis is generally bilateral execution of the procedure described earlier for the ipsilateral side of patients having unilateral coronal synostosis (Fig. 92-20; see also Fig. 92-13B). Unlike in unilateral coronal synostosis, the superior orbital rims are recontoured and moved mesially, for an "interorbital" distance of 20 mm. Whereas this maneuver does not change the actual interorbital distance, it can be effective camouflage for grade I orbital hypertelorism. Incorporation of temporal squamosal flattening and retropositioning of the intentional calvarial defect, in infants younger than 12 months, can improve the aesthetic outcome in bilateral coronal synostosis as for patients with unilateral coronal and metopic

synostosis. Delayed reconstruction of the nasal dorsum, with use of an autogenous costochondral graft, between 4 and 6 years of age is recommended for those patients with bilateral coronal synostosis who do not have adequate nasal dorsal projection before beginning primary school. If the patient has overt orbital hypertelorism (grade II or grade III) or ocular dysfunction secondary to the hypertelorism, bilateral orbital mesial repositioning should be performed between 4 and 6 years of age. Midface growth should be monitored. If a class III dentoskeletal relationship develops, maxillary advancement with or without mandibular setback should be performed in the mid to late teens unless airway or psychosocial issues mandated earlier intervention.

In the year 2000, 29 patients with nonsyndromic bilateral coronal synostosis were compared with 89

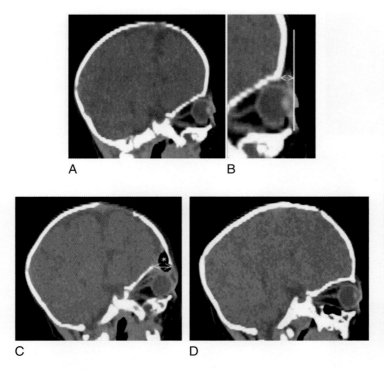

FIGURE 92-19. Planning and assessment of brow advancement with longitudinal orbital CT reformation. *A,* The preoperative longitudinal orbital image demonstrates retrusion of the brow with respect to the globe. *B,* A line is drawn from the inferior orbital rim tangent to the cornea to determine the ideal position for the superior orbital rim. The distance *(double-arrowed line)* between the superior orbital rim and that line is the minimum necessary advancement of the brow. *C,* The perioperative reformation documents the operative brow advancement. The orbital roof is discontinuous with the osseous gap, documenting the amount of advancement *(double-arrowed line).* A small amount of intracranial air *(asterisk)* persists. *D,* The 1-year postoperative reformation. The orbital roof has reossified with normal configuration, and the caudal frontal bone advancement has remained tangent to the inferior orbital rim. (From Marsh JL, Gado M: The longitudinal orbital CT projection: a versatile image for orbital assessment. Plast Reconstr Surg 1983;71: 308-317.)

patients with syndromic bilateral coronal synostosis.[76] None of the nonsyndromic patients received nasal dorsum augmentation in contrast to 17% of the syndromic patients. Hypertelorism correction was similar; 10% of the nonsyndromic and 11% of the syndromic patients underwent this procedure. None of the nonsyndromic patients required or is expected to require midface advancement, in contrast to 69% of the syndromic patients who have already had such an operation. Of nonsyndromic patients, 19% received secondary calvarial reconstruction, primarily for residual dysmorphic appearance but also for persistent nonreossified calvarial defects, versus 37% of syndromic patients. This rate is lower than the 55% reported by Wagner et al.[78] Lack of specific details of their operative technique precludes direct comparison.

Metopic Synostosis

Metopic synostosis is the third most frequently occurring of the nonsyndromic synostoses.[79] However, metopic synostosis has been reported as the most common craniosynostosis noted in newborns.[79] Patients with metopic synostosis are considered the most at risk for cognitive or behavioral impairment[15,35] because of a greater frequency of central nervous system anomalies and chromosome defects detectable on routine karyotyping than for other nonsyndromic synostoses. The majority of patients with metopic synostosis are male (72%).[80]

The crania of individuals with metopic synostosis are unique, with a midfrontal keel, bifrontotemporal narrowing, and parietal-occipital protrusion that give the head a triangular shape (trigonocephaly) when it is viewed from above (Fig. 92-21). It is appropriate to describe metopic synostosis as premature fusion because the metopic is the only calvarial suture that normally fuses in humans. Metopic fusion is associated with a distinctive facies due to excessive narrowing of the interorbital space: orbital hypotelorism, epicanthal folds, superiorly converging lateral orbital walls, and low nasal dorsum. To the unsophisticated observer, the epicanthal folds are the most obvious dysmorphic feature and are often incorrectly interpreted as indicative of either increased interorbital distance (orbital hypertelorism) or extraocular muscle dysfunction (strabismus) (Fig. 92-22).

There is some difference of opinion among surgeons about the indications for surgery and the objectives of the operation. Two factors confounding the decision for surgery are radiographic metopic fusion without dysmorphism and metopic keel without additional dysmorphic features. There are infants without any cranial or facial dysmorphism who undergo screening skull radiographs because of small head circumference and who are then identified as having fusion of their metopic suture. For these infants, it is helpful to assess their developmental level. If they are normal, observation of head circumference and neurologic development by the pediatrician is

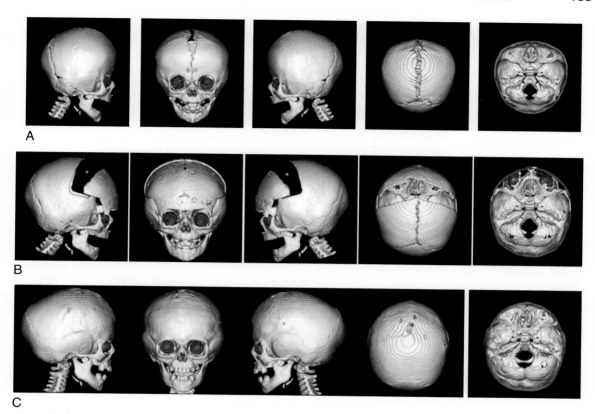

FIGURE 92-20. Preferred surgical procedure for bilateral coronal synostosis in infancy (same patient as in Figure 92-16). *A,* Preoperative appearance of 2-month-old girl. *B,* One-week perioperative views. The frontal bones and supraorbital bandeau have been recontoured, reconstructed, and advanced; the double arrow indicates the ventral enlargement of the anterior cranial fossa–roof of orbit, which exposes the superior orbital contents *(asterisk).* A single extrapericranial titanium plate struts the nasion *(arrow).* The remainder of the fixation is resorbable suture. The calvariectomy defect is posterior to the coronal synostoses to prevent temporal depression. *C,* One year postoperatively. The calvariectomy defects have reossified. The frontonasal and lateral orbital connection between the bandeau and the upper face is reossified. The endocranial image *(far right)* documents reossification of the ventral anterior fossa and roof of orbits with preservation of the surgical advancement documented in the perioperative endocranial image.

recommended. If they are not normal, a pediatric neurologic work-up is recommended. In either instance, it is not advisable to perform surgery.

With respect to frontal keel, it has been appreciated since the 1960s that isolated frontal keel can remodel and become insignificant without intervention. If the infant has a frontal keel without bifrontal narrowing and an abnormal facies, the patient should be observed. Parents should be informed that if the keel does not flatten by 3 years of age and they wish it to be removed, it can be burred down. If the infant has bifrontal narrowing and abnormal facies, then surgery can be performed to reconstruct the forehead and superolateral orbits. In either instance, the children are screened for developmental level, karyotype abnormalities, and central nervous system anomalies to better advise parents about long-term expectations (see Fig. 92-2).

The major issue with respect to the objectives of surgery is whether to treat the hypotelorism. Unlike hypertelorism, which can preclude normal binocular stereoscopic vision without orbital repositioning surgery, hypotelorism does not cause visual aberrations that require orbital repositioning for treatment. That is not to say that some patients with metopic synostosis do not have associated ophthalmologic findings; rather, it is to say that there is no ophthalmologic reason for surgical widening of the interorbital space. With respect to facial dysmorphism, hypotelorism does not particularly stigmatize, again in contrast to most patients with hypertelorism. The major dysmorphic facial feature of metopic synostosis is prominent epicanthal folds. In most patients, the folds are spontaneously effaced by 6 years of age because of growth of the previously low nasal dorsum (Fig. 92-23). Most patients do not require surgical

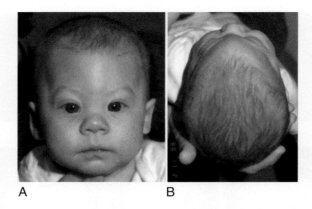

A   B

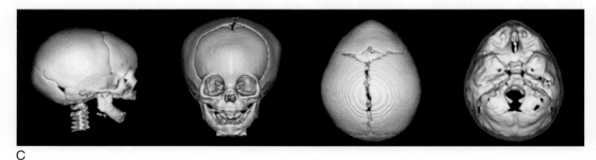

C

FIGURE 92-21. Trigonocephaly secondary to metopic synostosis: the surface (A and B) and osseous (C) dysmorphology of metopic synostosis in a 3-month-old boy. The synostosed metopic suture is apparent on the frontal photograph as a midsagittal light reflex and on the bird's-eye image as a projection or "keel." Bifrontotemporal narrowing gives the upper face a pinched look that is compounded by the mesial angulation of the superior lateral orbital rims. The combination of orbital hypotelorism, low nasal dorsum, and epicanthal folds creates the illusion of extraocular muscle dysfunction. The endocranial CT reformation documents compression of the anterior fossa.

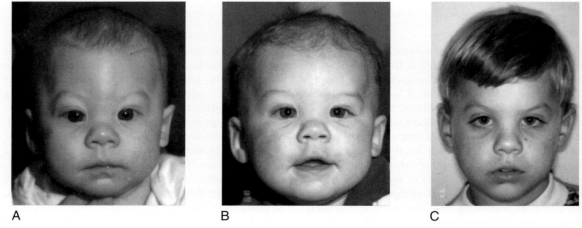

A   B   C

FIGURE 92-22. The effect of cranio-orbital surgery and aging on the upper face appearance (same patient as in Figure 92-21). A, At 3 months of age. B, At 7 months of age (3 months after fronto-orbital reconstruction). The frontal keel and bifrontotemporal narrowing have been resolved. There has been no change in the intermedial canthal appearance. The interpupillary distance is 42 mm (15th percentile for age). C, At 5 years, 1 month of age. The epicanthal folds are still present but to a lesser degree with visibility of the medial sclera but not of the medial caruncles. The interpupillary distance is 45 mm (15th percentile for age).

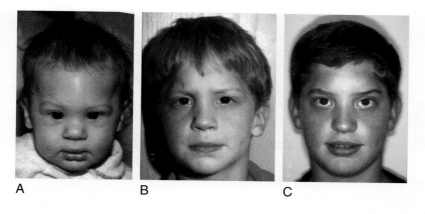

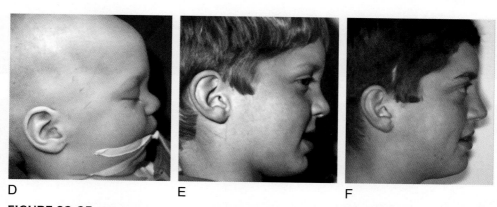

FIGURE 92-23. The effect of cranio-orbital surgery and nasal growth on epicanthal folds. *A* and *D,* At 3 months of age, 1 month before fronto-orbital surgery for metopic synostosis. There are bilateral epicanthal folds with coverage of the caruncles and medial sclera. The interpupillary distance is 37 mm (10th percentile for age). No additional craniofacial surgery was performed after the synostosis procedure at 4 months of age. *B* and *E,* At 5 years, 6 months of age. The medial sclera is now visible bilaterally, but the caruncles are still obscured. The interpupillary distance is 46 mm (10th percentile for age). *C* and *F,* At 13 years, 10 months of age. The medial caruncles are now visible as well. The interpupillary distance is 66 mm (>97th percentile for age). The nasal dorsum has developed with age, effacing the epicanthal folds.

correction of persistent epicanthal folds or nasal dorsum augmentation.

The standard approach to metopic synostosis in infants has been bifrontal craniotomy with bilateral recontouring, lateral advancement, and lateral displacement of the superior orbital rims[47] (Figs. 92-24 and 92-25). The initial phase of the operation is the same as that described for unilateral coronal synostosis except that the superior orbital and temporal fossa dissections and osteotomies are performed bilaterally in all patients with metopic synostosis. The bandeau (caudal 1 cm of frontal bones and superiormost orbital rims) is then divided in the midline through the thick bone of the metopic fusion. The contour of the superior orbital rims is normalized with the Tessier bone bending forceps. The axial width between the most

inferior aspects of the lateral orbital walls, as they join the inferior orbital rims, is measured, as is the axial width at the most superior aspects, as they join the superior orbital rims. The superior width is subtracted from the inferior width, and the difference is the amount of separation between the mesial ends of the right and left bandeau segments (Fig. 92-26). A portion of the craniectomy is harvested as an interposition bone graft and secured to the two bandeau segments by biodegradable rigid fixation. The frontal bones are divided through the frontal keel, rotated to optimize forehead contour, and subsegmented as necessary, then recontoured to achieve a symmetric forehead. The remodeled frontal bones are then fixed to the bandeau with biodegradable plates. A 2-cm calvariectomy defect, from one temporal squamosa to

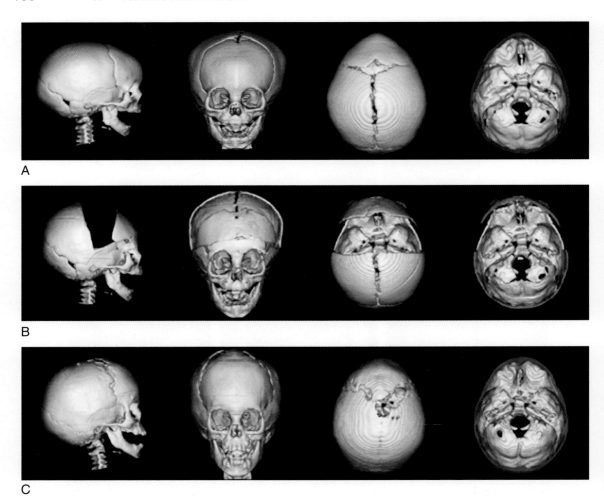

FIGURE 92-24. Preferred surgical procedure for metopic synostosis in infancy (same patient as in Figure 92-21). *A,* Preoperative views of 3-month-old boy. *B,* One-week perioperative views. The bandeau (superolateral orbital rims and caudal frontal bones) has been divided through the fused metopic suture to facilitate recontouring. The two bandeau segments would currently be separated to achieve the age-appropriate distance between the lateral orbital walls with an autogenous calvarial graft interposed between them at the nasion for osseous continuity (see Figure 92-25). In addition, the calvariectomy defect would be half as wide to minimize iatrogenic frontotemporal recession. *C,* One-year postoperative views. The nasofrontal junction and lateral orbital walls have reossified with diminished superior convergence of the lateral walls. There has been no significant endocranial base change beyond that achieved intraoperatively. This is characteristic for metopic synostosis.

the other, is left in infants younger than 12 months; the frontal bones are not fixed posteriorly in such infants. In older patients, a solid calvaria is reconstructed by circumferential biodegradable fixation with expanded interdigitation to compensate for the ipsilateral anterior fossa expansion. The scalp is closed in two layers over nonsuction drains.

A few outcome reports regarding metopic synostosis have been presented and published. Whereas some have asserted that orbital hypotelorism is ameliorated with time after fronto-orbital surgery,[81] this is not the usual experience. The difference in opinion seems to

result from use of raw data rather than data corrected to percentile for age; although it is true that the absolute values for interpupillary and bony interorbital distances do increase in patients with metopic synostosis over time, the percentiles for these distances do not, remaining at the low end of or below the normal range. An unexpectedly high incidence of cognitive and behavioral impairments in older children with metopic synostosis has been reported.[15] More neuropsychological data and correlation with central nervous system anomalies are required to determine the cause and significance of these preliminary findings.

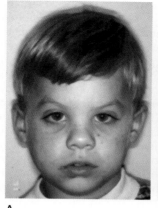
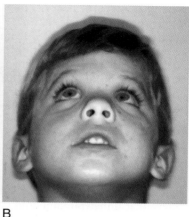

FIGURE 92-25. *A* and *B,* Postoperative appearance of the patient in Figures 92-21, 92-22, and 92-24 at 5 years, 1 month of age. The forehead is smooth with an even transition across the frontotemporal region without iatrogenic concavity.

A   B

Lambdoid Synostosis

Lambdoid synostosis is the least common of the nonsyndromic synostoses. Reports of marked increases of lambdoid synostosis in the mid-1990s seem to be errors of interpretation of routine skull radiographs reading false-positives for patients with deformational plagiocephaly.[82-84] The skewing of the posterior cranium moves the unfused lambdoid suture out of the perpendicular plane to the x-ray beam into one approaching parallel, thereby blurring the visualization of the suture. CT scanning perpendicular to the suture can clarify this imaging artifact. Whereas lambdoid synostosis usually occurs unilaterally, it does also

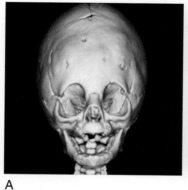
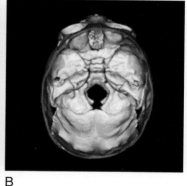

A   B

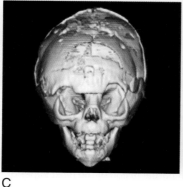
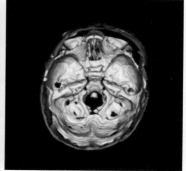

FIGURE 92-26. The current technique of bandeau widening. *A* and *B,* Preoperative views of 4-month-old girl with metopic and bilateral coronal synostoses. *C* and *D,* One-week perioperative views. A 10-mm autogenous calvarial interposition graft was placed between the remodeled and laterally displaced superolateral orbital rims. Whereas this does not affect the bony interorbital distance or the interpupillary distance (i.e., it does not correct hypotelorism), it does remedy the superior convergence of the lateral orbital walls. This maneuver assists the normalization of upper facial appearance.

C   D

occur bilaterally. The majority of patients with lambdoid synostosis are male (82%).[84]

The crania of individuals with unilateral lambdoid synostosis are asymmetric, fitting the descriptive term *plagiocephaly*.[63] Unlike in unilateral coronal synostosis, the most common craniosynostotic cause of plagiocephaly in which the primary dysmorphism is frontal, the primary dysmorphism in unilateral lambdoid synostosis is in the occiput (Fig. 92-27). There is reciprocal flattening and bossing of the frontal region to a much lesser degree. The combination of frontal dominance and pathognomonic facial dysmorphism can clinically separate unilateral coronal synostosis from other causes of plagiocephaly. A few authors believe that unilateral lambdoid synostosis can reliably be differentiated by physical examination alone[85] from deformational plagiocephaly, the most common cause of plagiocephaly in the United States during the past decade.[86] Excessive caudal protrusion of one mastoid with minimalization of the other does seem to be a pathognomonic physical examination and radiographic sign for unilateral lambdoid synostosis. Unfortunately, not all histologically proven instances of unilateral lambdoid synostosis have this sign (Fig. 92-28). For this reason, routine four-view skull radiographs of all patients with plagiocephaly should be obtained to identify the subset with poor visualization or nonvisualization of one or both lambdoid sutures. This subset undergoes thin-slice, high-resolution CT scanning to unambiguously separate those who have true lambdoid synostosis.[87] When lambdoid synostosis is identified, surgery is recommended.

Patients with lambdoid synostosis, whether unilateral or bilateral, should be placed in the prone position for surgery (Figs. 92-29 and 92-30). The neurosurgeon performs a bilateral occipital-parietal craniotomy, for unilateral as well as for bilateral lambdoid synostosis, as far caudally as is comfortable for that surgeon. The dura having been reflected, the remaining caudal occiput is cut vertically in barrel stave fashion to allow greenstick outfracturing and recontouring with the bone bending forceps. The plastic craniofacial surgeon segments the craniectomy bone into as many pieces as is necessary for reshaping, trying to preserve maximum bone size and to minimize fragmentation. If the patient is younger than 12 months, the caudal calvaria is reconstructed and rigidly fixed to the in situ recontoured inferiormost occiput with biodegradable plates and screws, and a 2-cm coronal craniectomy defect is left ventrally. If the patient is older than 12 months, a "complete" calvaria is reconstructed and rigidly fixed with use of interdigitation expansion as necessary.

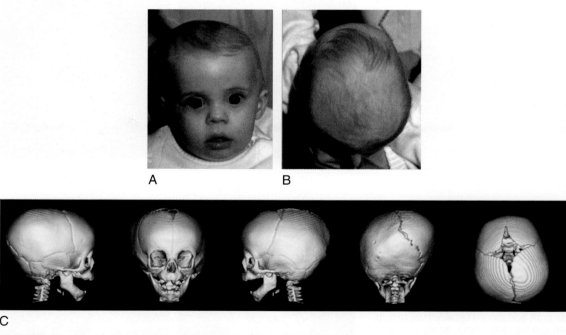

A   B

C

FIGURE 92-27. Plagiocephaly secondary to unilateral lambdoid synostosis: the surface (*A* and *B*) and osseous (*C*) dysmorphology of unilateral left lambdoid synostosis in a 6-month-old boy. The frontal photograph shows asymmetry of the brows and orbits with nasal and chin deviation off of the midsagittal line of the face. Orbital symmetry can be appreciated in the frontal osseous reformation. The bird's-eye photograph shows mild plagiocephaly primarily affecting the occiput, which is more evident in the osseous reformation. The asymmetry is most marked in the rear osseous reformation with partial fusion of the most superior portion of the left lambdoid suture. The left mastoid projects more caudally than the right.

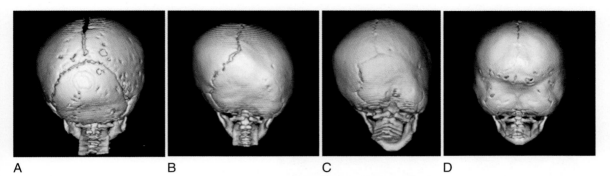

FIGURE 92-28. Spectrum of posterior calvarial configurations in lambdoid synostosis. *A* to *C*, The variation in osseous dysmorphology of unilateral lambdoid synostosis is presented in three infants. (Note: the images from infants with left lambdoid synostosis have been reversed right to left, "flipped," to facilitate comparisons.) The degree of occipital asymmetry and mastoid caudal projection varies from slight (*A*, right lambdoid synostosis) to marked (*C*, left lambdoid synostosis). *D*, An infant with bilateral lambdoid synostosis has symmetric dysmorphism with marked midocciput grooving and bilateral supramastoid constriction.

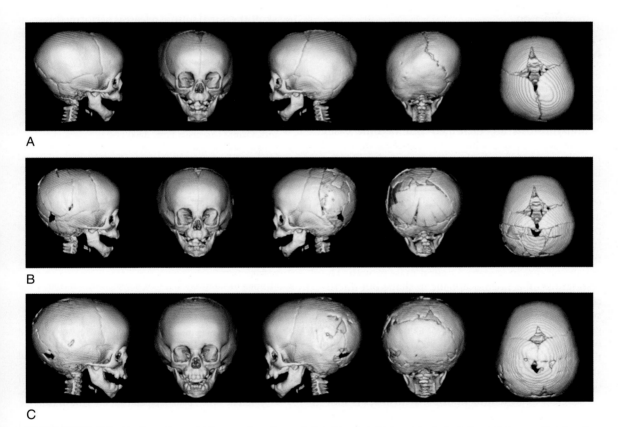

FIGURE 92-29. Preferred surgical procedure for unilateral lambdoid synostosis in infancy (same patient as in Figure 92-27). *A*, Preoperative appearance of a 6-month-old boy with left unilateral lambdoid synostosis. *B*, One week perioperatively. The majority of the occiput has been resected inferiorly at the level of the transverse sinuses, remodeled, and then reconstructed with the calvariectomy defect ipsilateral to the lambdoid synostosis. *C*, One year postoperatively. The cranium is essentially symmetric in all views with minor residual mastoid asymmetry.

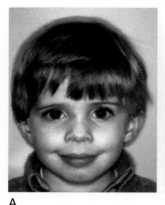 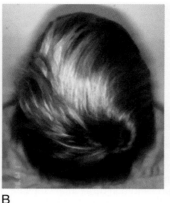

A   B

FIGURE 92-30. *A* and *B*, Postoperative appearance of the patient in Figures 92-27 and 92-29 at 4 years, 3 months of age. The face and calvaria are symmetric.

No reports of long-term outcome in lambdoid synostosis have been published with respect to either craniofacial morphologic features or central nervous system function.

Multiple Suture Synostoses

Synostosis of multiple sutures, similar to bilateral coronal synostosis, does occur in nonsyndromic individuals but is more commonly a feature of syndromic craniosynostosis. As more genetic errors associated with craniosynostosis are identified and become easily detectable, it seems probable that the cause of most if not all instances of multiple craniosynostosis will prove to be genetic errors.

The crania of individuals with multiple suture synostoses do not have a distinctive dysmorphic appearance; the abnormal shape depends on the specific pattern of sutural synostoses. Pansynostosis denotes fusion of all calvarial sutures. Nonsyndromic pansynostosis results from inadequate intracranial volume expansion due to impaired neural mass growth. The resultant skull is normocephalic in shape but microcephalic in dimensions. There is no role for cranial surgery in such patients. In contrast, the actively growing but constrained brain in syndromic pansynostosis produces ballooning of the cranial vertex and the temporal squamosas, which results in a distinctive shape resembling a three-leafed clover (Kleeblattschädel).

Surgical treatment of multiple synostoses is individualized on the basis of the affected sutures and the resultant dysmorphism. The techniques described previously are incorporated to achieve the desired result. This often requires two operations, one prone and one supine, to achieve total calvarial release and reconstruction, including superior orbital reconstruction. The positioning for the first operation is determined by the extent of calvarial constraint; that portion of the skull most deformed with respect to

osseous thinning and gyral-sulcal modeling is treated first. In such patients, the second operation is performed 3 months after the first. In those patients with cloverleaf skull, the initial sutural release is performed as soon after birth as the neonate is stabilized to minimize irreversible central nervous system damage as well as craniofacial dysmorphism.

REFERENCES

1. Cohen MM: Sutural biology. In Cohen MM, MacLean RE, eds: Craniosynostosis: Diagnosis, Evaluation, and Management. New York, Oxford University Press, 2000:11-23.
2. Cohen MM: Syndromes with craniosynostosis. In Cohen MM, MacLean RE, eds: Craniosynostosis: Diagnosis, Evaluation, and Management. New York, Oxford University Press, 2000:309-440.
3. Wilkie AO: Molecular genetics of craniosynostosis. In Lin KY, Ogle RC, Jane JA, eds: Craniofacial Surgery: Science and Surgical Technique. Philadelphia, WB Saunders, 2001:41-54.
4. Gripp KW, McDonald-McGinn DM, Gaudenz K, et al: Identification of a genetic cause for isolated unilateral coronal synostosis: a unique mutation in the fibroblast growth receptor 3. J Pediatr 1998;132:714-716.
5. Stedman's Medical Dictionary, 22nd ed. Baltimore, Williams & Wilkins, 1972.
6. Mehrara BJ, Longaker MT: New developments in craniofacial surgery research. Cleft Palate Craniofac J 1999;36:377-387.
7. Pashley DH, Borke JL, Yu J: Biomechanics and craniofacial morphogenesis. In Cohen MM, MacLean RE, eds: Craniosynostosis: Diagnosis, Evaluation, and Management. New York, Oxford University Press, 2000:84-100.
8. Marsh JL, Vannier MW: Comprehensive Care for Craniofacial Deformities. St. Louis, CV Mosby, 1985.
9. Mooney MP, Siegel MI, Burrows AM, et al: A rabbit model of human familial, nonsyndromic unicoronal suture synostosis. I. Synostotic onset, pathology, and sutural growth patterns. Childs Nerv Syst 1998;14:236-246.
10. Mooney MP, Siegel MI, Burrows AM, et al: A rabbit model of human familial, nonsyndromic unicoronal suture synostosis. II. Intracranial contents, intracranial volume, and intracranial pressure. Childs Nerv Syst 1998;14:247-255.
11. Babler WJ, Persing JA: Experimental alteration of cranial suture growth: effects on the neurocranium, basicranium, and midface. Prog Clin Biol Res 1982;101:333-345.
12. Carinci P, Becchetti E, Bodo M: Role of the extracellular matrix and growth factors in skull morphogenesis and in the pathogenesis of craniosynostosis. Int J Dev Biol 2000;44:715-723.

13. Opperman LA: Cranial sutures as intramembranous bone growth sites. Dev Dyn 2000;219:472-485.

14. Sperber GH: Craniofacial Development. Hamilton, Ontario, BC Decker, 2001.

15. Sidoti EJ Jr, Marsh JL, Marty-Grames L, Noetzel MJ: Long-term studies of metopic synostosis: frequency of cognitive impairment and behavioral disturbances. Plast Reconstr Surg 1996;97:276-281.

16. Aldridge K, Marsh JL, Perlyn CA, Richtsmeier JA: Quantification of Central Nervous System Dysmorphology in Isolated Craniosynostosis. Minneapolis, Minn, American Cleft Palate-Craniofacial Association, 2001:61.

17. Jimenez DF, Barone CM: Endoscopic craniectomy for early surgical correction of sagittal craniosynostosis. J Neurosurg 1998;88:77-81.

18. Barone CM, Jimenez DF: Endoscopic craniectomy for early correction of craniosynostosis. Plast Reconstr Surg 1999;104:1965-1973.

19. Losken HW, Mooney MP, Zoldos J, et al: Internal calvarial bone distraction in rabbits with delayed-onset coronal suture synostosis. Plast Reconstr Surg 1998;102:1109-1119.

20. Kobayashi S, Honda T, Saitoh A, Kashiwa K: Unilateral coronal synostosis treated by internal forehead distraction. J Craniofac Surg 1999;10:467-471.

21. Nadal E, Dogliotti PL, Rodriguez JC, Zuccaro G: Craniofacial distraction osteogenesis en bloc. J Craniofac Surg 2000;11:246-251.

22. Shillito J Jr: A plea for early operation for craniosynostosis. Surg Neurol 1992;37:182-188.

23. Posnick JC: Unilateral coronal synostosis (anterior plagiocephaly): current clinical perspectives. Ann Plast Surg 1996;36:430-447.

24. DeLeon VB, Zumpano MP, Richtsmeier JT: The effect of neurocranial surgery on basicranial morphology in isolated sagittal craniosynostosis. Cleft Palate Craniofac J 2001;38:134-146.

25. Perlyn CA, Marsh JL, Pilgram TK, Kane A: Plasticity of the endocranial base in nonsyndromic craniosynostosis. Plast Reconstr Surg 2001;108:294-301.

26. Camfield PR, Camfield CS, Cohen MM: Neurological aspects of craniosynostosis. In Cohen MM, MacLean RE, eds: Craniosynostosis: Diagnosis, Evaluation, and Management. New York, Oxford University Press, 2000:177-183.

27. Renier D, Sainte-Rose C, Marchac D: Intracranial pressure in craniostenosis. J Neurosurg 1982;57:370-377.

28. Thompson DN, Malcolm GP, Jones BM, et al: Intracranial pressure in single-suture craniosynostosis. Pediatr Neurosurg 1995;22:235-240.

29. Gault DT, Renier D, Marchac D, Jones BM: Intracranial pressure and intracranial volume in children with craniosynostosis. Plast Reconstr Surg 1992;90:377-381.

30. Cohen SR, Persing JA: Intracranial pressure in single-suture craniosynostosis. Cleft Palate Craniofac J 1998;35:194-196.

31. David LR, Genecov DG, Camastra AA, et al: Positron emission tomography studies confirm the need for early surgical intervention in patients with single-suture craniosynostosis. J Craniofac Surg 1999;10:38-42.

32. Kapp-Simon KA, Figueroa A, Jocher CA, Schafer M: Longitudinal assessment of mental development in infants with nonsyndromic craniosynostosis with and without cranial release and reconstruction. Plast Reconstr Surg 1993;92:831-839.

33. Arnaud E, Renier D, Marchac D: Prognosis for mental function in scaphocephaly. J Neurosurg 1995;83:476-479.

34. Kapp-Simon KA: Mental development and learning disorders in children with single suture craniosynostosis. Cleft Palate Craniofac J 1998;35:197-203.

35. Bottero L, Lajeunie E, Arnaud E, et al: Functional outcome after surgery for trigonocephaly. Plast Reconstr Surg 1998;102:952-958.

36. Hayward R, Jones B, Evans R: Functional outcome after surgery for trigonocephaly. Plast Reconstr Surg 1999;104:582-583.

37. Marsh JL: Craniofacial surgery research for craniosynostosis. In Cohen MM, MacLean RE, eds: Craniosynostosis: Diagnosis, Evaluation, and Management. New York, Oxford University Press, 2000:292-308.

38. Shillito JJ, Matson DD: Craniosynostosis. A review of 519 surgical patients. Pediatrics 1968;41:829-853.

39. Anderson FM: Treatment of coronal and metopic synostosis: 107 cases. Neurosurgery 1981;8:143-149.

40. Whitaker LA, Bartlett SP, Schut L, Bruce D: Craniosynostosis: an analysis of the timing, treatment, and complications in 164 consecutive patients. Plast Reconstr Surg 1987;80:195-212.

41. McCarthy JG, Glasberg SB, Cutting CB, et al: Twenty-year experience with early surgery for craniosynostosis. I. Isolated craniofacial synostosis—results and unsolved problems. Plast Reconstr Surg 1995;96:272-283.

42. Sloan GM, Wells KC, Raffel C, McComb JG: Surgical treatment of craniosynostosis: outcome analysis of 250 consecutive patients. Pediatrics 1997;100:E2.

43. Breugem CC, van R Zeeman BJ: Retrospective study of nonsyndromic craniosynostosis treated over a 10-year period. J Craniofac Surg 1999;10:140-143.

44. Williams JK, Cohen SR, Burstein FD, et al: A longitudinal, statistical study of reoperation rates in craniosynostosis. Plast Reconstr Surg 1997;100:305-310.

45. Bruneteau RJ, Mulliken JB: Frontal plagiocephaly: synostotic, compensational, or deformational. Plast Reconstr Surg 1992;89:21-31.

46. Mulliken JB, Vander Woude DL, Hansen M, et al: Analysis of posterior plagiocephaly: deformational versus synostotic. Plast Reconstr Surg 1999;103:371-380.

47. Marsh JL, Schwartz HG: The surgical correction of coronal and metopic craniosynostoses. J Neurosurg 1983;59:245-251.

48. Hardesty RA, Marsh JL, Vannier MW: Unicoronal synostosis. A surgical intervention. Neurosurg Clin North Am 1991;2:641-653.

49. Lo LJ, Marsh JL, Yoon J, Vannier MW: Stability of fronto-orbital advancement in nonsyndromic bilateral coronal synostosis: a quantitative three-dimensional computed tomographic study. Plast Reconstr Surg 199698:393-405.

50. Kurpad SN, Goldstein JA, Cohen AR: Bioresorbable fixation for congenital pediatric craniofacial surgery: a 2-year follow-up. Pediatr Neurosurg 2000;33:306-310.

51. Hunter AGW, Rudd NL: Craniosynostosis. I. Sagittal synostosis: its genetics and associated clinical findings in 214 patients who lacked involvement of the coronal suture(s). Teratology 1977;15:301-310.

52. Panchal J, Marsh JL, Park TS, et al: Sagittal craniosynostosis outcome assessment for two methods and timings of intervention. Plast Reconstr Surg 1999;103:1574-1584.

53. Friede H, Lauritzen C, Figueroa AA: Roentgencephalometric follow-up after early osteotomies in patients with scaphocephaly. J Craniofac Surg 1996;7:96-101.

54. Posnick JC, Lin KY, Chen P, Armstrong D: Sagittal synostosis: quantitative assessment of presenting deformity and surgical results based on CT scans. Plast Reconstr Surg 1993;92:1015-1024.

55. Kaiser G: Sagittal synostosis—its clinical significance and the results of three different methods of craniectomy. Childs Nerv Syst 1988;4:223-230.

56. Marsh JL, Jenny A, Galic M, et al: Surgical management of sagittal synostosis. A quantitative evaluation of two techniques. Neurosurg Clin North Am 1991;2:629-640.

57. Krasnicanova H, Zemkova D, Skodova I: Longitudinal follow-up of children after surgical treatment of scaphocephaly. Acta Chir Plast 1996;38:50-53.

58. Albright AL, Towbin RB, Shultz BL: Long-term outcome after sagittal synostosis operations. Pediatr Neurosurg 1996;25:78-82.

59. Panchal J, Marsh JL, Park TS, et al: Photographic assessment of head shape following sagittal synostosis surgery. Plast Reconstr Surg 1999;103:1585-1591.

60. Kohn LA, Vannier MW, Marsh JL, Cheverud JM: Effect of premature sagittal suture closure on craniofacial morphology in a prehistoric male Hopi. Cleft Palate Craniofac J 1994;31:385-396.

61. Richtsmeier JT, Grausz HM, Morris GR, et al: Growth of the cranial base in craniosynostosis. Cleft Palate Craniofac J 1991;28:55-67.

62. Hunter AG, Rudd NL: Craniosynostosis. II. Coronal synostosis: its familial characteristics and associated clinical findings in 109 patients lacking bilateral polysyndactyly or syndactyly. Teratology 1977;15:301-309.

63. Lo LJ, Marsh JL, Pilgram TK, Vannier MW: Plagiocephaly: differential diagnosis based on endocranial morphology. Plast Reconstr Surg 1996;97:282-291.

64. Marsh JL, Gado MH, Vannier MW, Stevens WG: Osseous anatomy of unilateral coronal synostosis. Cleft Palate J 1986;23:87-100.

65. Kane AA, Kim YO, Eaton A, et al: Quantification of osseous facial dysmorphology in untreated unilateral coronal synostosis. Plast Reconstr Surg 2000;106:251-258.

66. Raimondi AJ, Gutierrez FA: A new surgical approach to the treatment of coronal synostosis. J Neurosurg 1977;46:210-214.

67. Hoffman H, Mohr G: Lateral canthal advancement of the supraorbital margin: a new corrective technique in the treatment of coronal synostosis. J Neurosurg 1976;45:376-381.

68. Marchac D: Radical forehead remodeling for craniostenosis. Plast Reconstr Surg 1978;61:823-835.

69. Bartlett SP, Whitaker LA, Marchac D: The operative treatment of isolated craniofacial dysostosis (plagiocephaly): a comparison of the unilateral and bilateral techniques. Plast Reconstr Surg 1990;85:677-683.

70. Lo LJ, Marsh JL, Kane AA, Vannier MW: Orbital dysmorphology in unilateral coronal synostosis. Cleft Palate Craniofac J 1996;33:190-197.

71. Kane AA, Lo LJ, Vannier MW, Marsh JL: Mandibular dysmorphology in unicoronal synostosis and plagiocephaly without synostosis. Cleft Palate Craniofac J 1996;33:418-423.

72. Robin NH: Molecular genetic advances in understanding craniosynostosis. Plast Reconstr Surg 1999;103:1060-1070.

73. Mulliken JB, Steinberger D, Kunze S, Muller U: Molecular diagnosis of bilateral coronal synostosis. Plast Reconstr Surg 1999;104:1603-1615.

74. Posnick JC, Ruiz RL: The craniofacial dysostosis syndromes: current surgical thinking and future directions. Cleft Palate Craniofac J 2000;37:433.

75. Marsh JL, Vannier MW: Cranial base changes following surgical treatment of craniosynostosis. Cleft Palate J 1986;23(suppl 1):9-18.

76. Marsh JL, Kaufman B: Bilateral coronal craniosynostosis. In Lin KY, Ogle RC, Jane JA, eds: Craniofacial Surgery: Science and Surgical Technique. Philadelphia, WB Saunders, 2001:218-224.

77. Trott J, David D, Mixter R: Self-stabilizing osteotomy for frontal bar advancement. Plast Reconstr Surg 1986;78:246-248.

78. Wagner JD, Cohen SR, Maher H, et al: Critical analysis of results of craniofacial surgery for nonsyndromic bicoronal synostosis. J Craniofac Surg 1995;6:32-37.

79. Shuper A, Merlob P, Grunebaum M, Reisner SH: The incidence of isolated craniosynostosis in the newborn infant. Am J Dis Child 1985;139:85-86.

80. Lajeunie E, Le Merrer M, Marchac D, Renier D: Syndromal and nonsyndromal primary trigonocephaly: analysis of a series of 237 patients. Am J Med Genet 1998;75:211-215.

81. Fearon JA, Kolar JC, Munro IR: Trigonocephaly-associated hypotelorism: is treatment necessary? Plast Reconstr Surg 1996;97:503-509.

82. Jones BM, Hayward R, Evans R, Britto J: Occipital plagiocephaly: an epidemic of craniosynostosis? [editorial]. BMJ 1997;315:693-694.

83. Cohen MM: The problem of epidemics of craniosynostosis and misdiagnosis. In Cohen MM, MacLean RE, eds: Craniosynostosis: Diagnosis, Evaluation, and Management. New York, Oxford University Press, 2000:115-116.

84. Ellenbogen RG, Gruss JS, Cunningham ML: Update on craniofacial surgery: the differential diagnosis of lambdoid synostosis/posterior plagiocephaly. Clin Neurosurg 2000;47:303-318.

85. Huang MH, Gruss JS, Clarren SK, et al: The differential diagnosis of posterior plagiocephaly: true lambdoid synostosis versus positional molding. Plast Reconstr Surg 1996;98:765-774.

86. Kane AA, Mitchell LE, Craven KP, Marsh JL: Observations on a recent increase in plagiocephaly without synostosis. Pediatrics 1996;97:877-885.

87. Menard RM, David DJ: Unilateral lambdoid synostosis: morphological characteristics. J Craniofac Surg 1998;9:240-246.

Unilateral Cheiloplasty

M. Samuel Noordhoff, MD ✦ Philip Kuo-Ting Chen, MD

Central and foremost, the multidisciplinary approach is essential to the satisfactory treatment of the cleft patient.[1] This includes plastic surgeons, orthodontists, speech pathologists, pedodontists, prosthodontists, otolaryngologists, social workers, psychologists, and ophthalmologists as well as a photographer. In addition, the center's coordinator serves to coordinate all these specialties for the benefit of the patient as well as for gathering and recording vital information. All of these contribute to the care of the cleft person from infancy to adulthood, a time when lasting friendships

and care contribute to the psychological, aesthetic, functional, and spiritual development of the person.

THE CLEFT PROBLEM: DYSMORPHOLOGY

Prenatal Diagnosis

Ultrasound examination for the diagnosis of prenatal anomalies and problems related to the fetus is common in many countries. This means of prenatal diagnosis is helpful in identification of serious problems of the fetus as well as of the cleft lip or palate. Prenatal diagnosis of cleft lip is usually made in the second or third trimester. The detection rate has increased in recent years.[2] A prenatal diagnosis of the cleft lip anomaly is made in approximately half of the new clefts seen in the Chang Gung Craniofacial Center. Statistics from the Department of Health in Taiwan revealed that there was one cleft lip/palate or cleft palate in every 438.5 live births in 1994. The incidence decreased to one in every 781 births in 1996, a decrease of almost 50%. The stillbirth incidence of cleft lip/palate and cleft palate was 18.89 in every 1000 stillbirths in 1994, and this increased to 31.51 in every 1000 stillbirths in 1996, an increase of 67%. This seems to indicate that there is an increased diagnosis of clefts in the prenatal period and that these fetuses are aborted. The clinical experience in the Chang Gung Craniofacial Center supports these statistics. When the cleft fetuses had other associated malformations, the detection rate for cleft lip was higher.[3-5] With the advancement of three-dimensional ultrasonography, visualization of the cleft lip has become more convenient and accurate.[6,7] The three-dimensional volume imaging is helpful for prenatal counseling because the parents can visualize the face of the fetus clearly.[6,7] Prenatal diagnosis is related to the development of the fetal cleft lip surgery; fetal surgery results in less scarring and can be endoscopically performed.[8] Fetal surgery has as yet been adopted only in rare cases and is not an acceptable procedure.

It is important for the surgeon to take time and to provide information to prospective parents who are faced with a prenatal diagnosis of their cleft lip/palate fetus. In addition to professional counselors, cleft lip patients or parents of children with a cleft lip/palate can explain how they have become normal functioning persons in society.

Genetics

The genetics of orofacial clefting are only partially understood but are of great importance in counseling of affected families. It is generally believed that isolated cleft palate is a genetic entity distinct from unilateral cleft lip with or without cleft palate.[9-11] This conclusion has followed from both epidemiologic studies and the fact that embryologic events leading to cleft lip/palate and cleft palate occur at somewhat different times (3 to 7 weeks versus 5 to 12 weeks). It has long been assumed that both genetic and environmental (epigenetic) factors play important roles in the etiopathology of clefts, and this is supported by the varying incidence of clefting with ethnicity, geographic location, and socioeconomic conditions.[12-14] Twin studies have clearly demonstrated a genetic basis for cleft lip/palate, with a 43% pairwise concordance

TABLE 93-1 ✦ INCIDENCE OF CLEFT LIP/PALATE

Race/Ethnicity	Incidence per 1000 Births
Amerindian	3.6
Japanese	2.1
Chinese	1.7
White	1.0
African American	0.3

Data from Wyszynski DF, Beaty TH, Maestri NE: Genetics of nonsyndromic oral clefts revisited. Cleft Palate Craniofac J 1996;33:406-417; and Vieira AR, Orioli IM: Candidate genes for nonsyndromic cleft lip and palate. ASDC J Dent Child 2001;68:272-279, 229.

rate in monozygotic twins versus a 5% concordance in dizygotic twins.[9,15,16]

The incidence of cleft lip/palate in white newborns is approximately 1 in 1000 (Table 93-1); isolated cleft palate occurs in about 0.5 in 1000. Annual reports in Taiwan indicate an incidence range of 0.81 to 1.62 per 1000 for cleft lip with or without cleft palate and 0.47 to 0.66 per 1000 for isolated cleft palate. The incidence of cleft palate alone is significantly less than that of cleft lip/palate, occurring one-third to one-half as often.[12] Whereas there are more than 250 syndromes associated with orofacial clefting,[13] it is generally considered that most cases occur as an isolated abnormality, so-called nonsyndromic cleft lip/palate.[12] Given the incomplete understanding of the genetics of orofacial clefting and the imprecision in employing nonsyndromic versus syndromic nomenclature, estimates vary about the frequency with which other malformations occur in children with clefts. In a large review of their center's experience, Rollnick and Pruzansky[17] identified other malformations in 35% of cleft lip/palate patients and 54% of cleft palate patients. Cleft lip/palate has an unequal gender distribution, favoring boys over girls, whereas this relationship is reversed in cleft palate.[18] Cleft lip/palate affects the left side more often.[19,20]

Unaffected (i.e., noncleft) parents who have one child with cleft lip/palate have an estimated recurrence risk of 4%, which rises to 9% with two affected children. If one parent is affected, the risk of having a child with cleft lip/palate is also 4%, increasing to 17% if there is already both an affected parent and an affected child.[21] As the degree of familial relationship increases, recurrence risk decreases; first-, second-, and third-degree relatives have 4%, 0.7%, and 0.3% risk, respectively.[22] Recurrence risk increases with the severity of the cleft.[23]

The most appropriate genetic model for the inheritance pattern of nonsyndromic cleft lip/palate is a matter of considerable debate, and consensus has not been achieved. Classically, Fogh-Anderson proposed the idea that cleft lip/palate was transmitted by a gene of variable penetrance that could act dominantly or recessively, depending on the individual.[9,22] Multifactorial and multifactorial/threshold models have been widely advanced[24] and have predominated; others believe there is little evidence to support the concept of transmission as a discontinuous threshold trait.[12] In the past decade, the prevailing method of genetic analysis of cleft lip/palate has been by allelic association, whereby "candidate" genes are selected on the basis of functional properties, expression pattern, chromosome location, or mouse homologues.[24] Numerous studies of this type have found significant association to the transforming growth factor-α (TGFA),[25] transforming growth factor-$\beta3$ (TGFB3),[26] retinoic acid receptor-α (RARA),[27] homeobox gene MSX1,[26] and BCL3 proto-oncogene[28] loci. Although such studies are useful, their results must be interpreted with caution; it is not clear whether the ever-increasing implicated loci are truly representative of a large number of genes involved in the etiology of cleft lip/palate or whether this type of analysis has the ability to produce false-positive results.[22,24] The subtleties of the interplay between genes and environment in cleft lip/palate are yet to be uncovered, and new tools such as sophisticated linkage disequilibrium approaches may be needed to unravel these complexities.[22,24]

Classification of the Cleft

Veau[29] suggested that all clefts be classified into four groups: group 1, cleft of the soft palate only; group 2, cleft of soft and hard palate; group 3, unilateral cleft of lip and palate; and group 4, bilateral cleft lip and palate. The simple classification has ignored the clefts of primary palate only and failed to separate the incomplete from the complete clefts of lip and palate.

Kernahan[30] reported the Y classification. The upper limbs represent right and left sides of the primary palate, that is, the lip, the alveolus, and the hard palate anterior to the incisive foramen. The lower limb represents the hard and soft palate posterior to the incisive foramen. The limitation of the Kernahan Y classification is that clefts of the secondary palate cannot be classified into right or left sides. The Y classification was modified (Fig. 93-1) into a better numeric system that allows a more accurate recording of all left or right clefts of the primary and secondary palate and is easily adapted to the computer.[31,32] In the modified Y classification, each right or left limb is assigned a number, 1 to 5 or 11 to 15 for the primary palate and 6 to 9 or 16 to 19 for the secondary palate, with 10 being a submucous cleft palate.

All clefts are also recorded by letter codes. The first letter is the side of cleft (R, right; L, left), the second letter is the location of the cleft (P, primary palate; S, secondary palate posterior to incisive foramen), and the third letter represents the degree of cleft (C, complete; I, incomplete). This classification is simpler

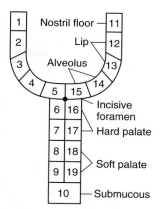

FIGURE 93-1. A double Y uses numbers to classify clefts. Clefts of the primary palate anterior to the incisive foramen are numbered 1 to 5 and 11 to 15. Clefts of the secondary palate posterior to the incisive foramen are numbered 6 to 9 and 16 to 19. Any number combination is used to describe the type of cleft. (From Bardach J, Morris HL, eds: Multidisciplinary Management of Cleft Lip and Palate. Philadelphia, WB Saunders, 1990:23.)

for communication and sorting compared with the modified Y, but it is not as accurate. The letter coding is as follows: RPC, right primary complete; RSC, right secondary complete; LPC, left primary complete; LSC, left secondary complete; RPI, right primary incomplete; RSI, right secondary incomplete; LPI, left primary incomplete; and LSI, left secondary incomplete.

All clefts in the illustrations of patients in this chapter are classified according to the letter method and the modified Y numeric method. The letter method is more accurate in classifying partial clefts. Any combination of numbers can readily record the finer degrees of partial clefts and is easily adaptable to the computer. A classification of 6423 clefts in the Chang Gung Craniofacial Center from 1976 to 1998 revealed that 41% were left sided, 20% were right sided, 17% were bilateral, and 22% were of the palate only. Examples of classification are shown in Figures 93-2 to 93-4.

Diversity of the Cleft Pathology

Deficiencies of soft tissue, cartilage, and bone in cleft patients are difficult to evaluate accurately. There is an obvious difference in the availability of soft tissue (skin and muscle) of the left incomplete cleft of the primary palate (LPI, 13-14; Fig. 93-2A), the right incomplete cleft of the primary palate (RPI, 2-4; Fig. 93-3A), the left complete cleft of the primary and secondary palate (LPC, LSC, 11-19; Fig. 93-4A), and the median facial dysplasia patient[33] in Figure 93-5A. The surgeon can make an overall impression of cleft

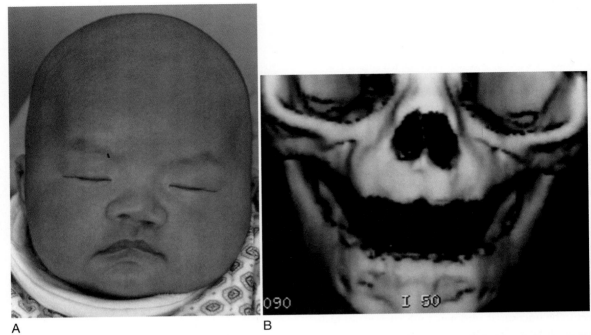

A   B

FIGURE 93-2. *A,* A 1-month-old Chinese boy with a left occult cleft of the primary palate (left primary incomplete; LPI, 13-14). There is muscle separation and minimal elevation of the cleft-side Cupid's bow and a depressed left ala due to deficient bone in the piriform area, as seen on the computed tomographic scan *(B)*.

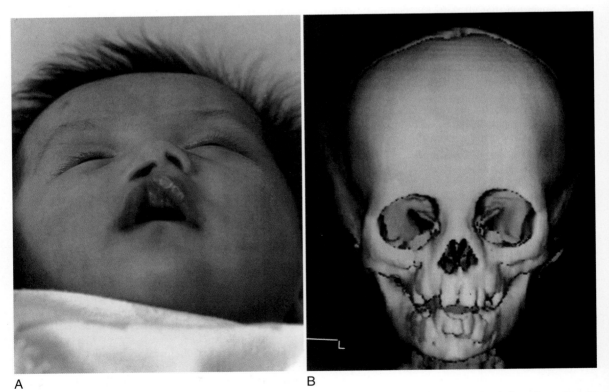

A   B

FIGURE 93-3. *A,* A 2-month-old Chinese girl with a right incomplete cleft of the primary palate (right primary incomplete; RPI, 2-4). There is marked distortion and flattening of the right alar cartilage. *B,* The computed tomographic scan discloses deficient bone in the right maxilla and piriform area.

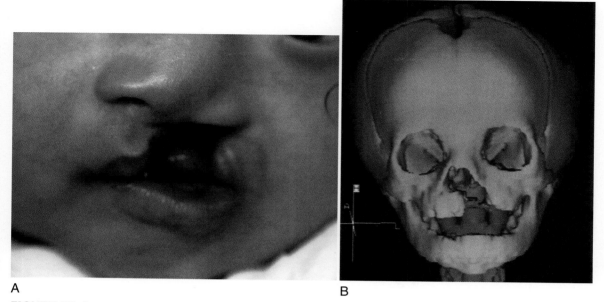

FIGURE 93-4. *A,* Preoperative view at 1 month of a Chinese girl with a left complete cleft of the primary and secondary palate (left primary and left secondary complete; LPC, LSC, 11-19). *B,* The computed tomographic scan showed deficient bone in the cleft alveolus and piriform area.

width, alar cartilage distortion, soft tissue deficiencies including the thickness and amount of orbicularis muscle, and underlying bony framework. Although impressions are useful, they cannot be quantitatively recorded.

Linear lip measurements of anthropometric marks provide a means of evaluating lip deficiencies. The quality and deficiency of the alar cartilage are impossible to evaluate accurately without a "cadaver-like" dissection. Deficiencies of bone can be recorded with three-dimensional computed tomographic scans, an accurate method of evaluating bone deficiencies but not practical in all patients.[34] The computed tomographic scans (see Figs. 93-2B, 93-3B, 93-4B, and 93-5B) show a wide spectrum of bone deficiency that is present in the piriform area and cleft maxilla. There is evident piriform deficiency in the occult cleft of Figure 93-2B. There is a progressive deficiency of bone in the piriform area and maxilla as shown in Figures 93-3B, 93-4B, and 93-5B. These patients demonstrate a wide variety of bone, cartilage, and soft tissue deficiencies. This helps support the concept that all clefts are different, and the potential for normal growth probably varies considerably from patient to patient in part because of these deficiencies.

Three-dimensional Measurements

Although the features of unilateral cleft lip nasal deformity have been well described, the characteristics of the three-dimensional relationship have not been

quantitated. A study of 3-month-old infants with complete unilateral cleft lip and palate was done before surgery with three-dimensional computed tomographic scan measurements.[34] There was no nasal or alveolar molding in this group of 12 patients. Four soft tissue surface landmarks were obtained, including sellion, subnasale, and subalare on the cleft and noncleft sides. The osseous landmarks of sella, nasion, anterior nasal spine, and posterior piriform aperture were identified as well. Three-dimensional linear and angle measurements among the landmarks were performed. The sellion was used as the face midline for comparison between the cleft and noncleft sides (Fig. 93-6).

The results showed that the subnasale point was anterior to sellion and deviated to the noncleft side. The cleft-side subalare point was more medial, posterior, and inferior than the noncleft-side subalare point, and the posterior piriform aperture point on the cleft-side piriform margin was more lateral, posterior, and inferior than on the noncleft side. These discrepancies were not constantly observed. However, four findings were observed without exception ($P < .01$): (1) the subnasale was deviated to the noncleft side, (2) the cleft-side alar base was more posterior than the noncleft-side alar base, (3) the noncleft-side alar base was farther from the midline than the cleft-side alar base, and (4) the cleft-side piriform margin was more posterior than the noncleft-side piriform margin. Another significant finding was that the angle of the sella–nasion–anterior nasal spine was

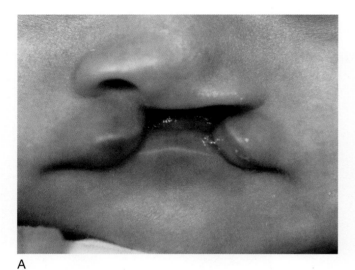

A

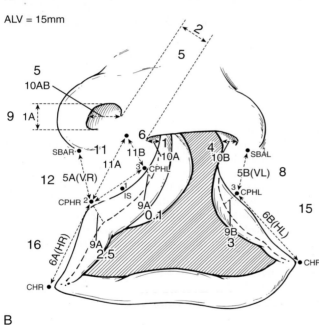

ALV = 15mm

B

FIGURE 93-5. *A,* A 3-month-old Chinese girl with a left complete cleft of the primary and secondary palate and a right complete cleft of the secondary palate (left primary and secondary complete, right secondary complete; LPC, LSC, RSC, 11-19, 6-9). This is a median facial dysplasia patient demonstrating a severe cleft deformity. (From Noordhoff MS, Huang CS, Lo LJ: Median facial dysplasia in unilateral and bilateral cleft lip and palate: a subgroup of median cerebrofacial malformations. Plast Reconstr Surg 1993;91:996-1005; discussion 1006-1007). *B,* Measurements in millimeters made at the time of surgery.

increased with the increased alveolar cleft width. These features characterize the nasal deformity in complete unilateral cleft lip and palate that has not been operated on. This three-dimensional evaluation identifies significant abnormalities of the cleft facial bones.

LIP MEASUREMENTS AND MARKINGS

Simple measurements with a caliper of important anthropometric points provide an inexpensive and accurate assessment of soft tissue deficiencies.[35]

Measurements, on the basis of the anthropometric marks (Fig. 93-7), are made at the time of surgery and recorded (Fig. 93-5C).

Cupid's Bow and Vermilion

The points of the Cupid's bow (CPHR, IS, CPHL) are marked on the epidermis-vermilion junction line, the white skin roll, as identified by Millard.[36] The vermilion-mucosa junction line, the red line,[37] is also marked. This clearly defines the intervening vermilion and also helps identify the deficient vermilion beneath the cleft-side Cupid's bow. Other points

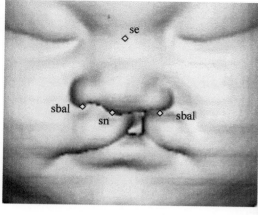

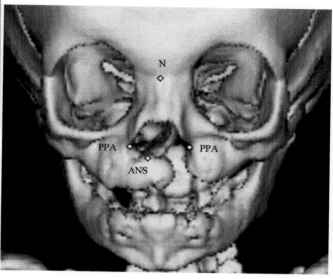

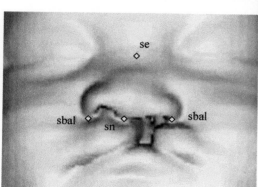

FIGURE 93-6. Three-dimensional computed tomographic scan of 3-month-old infant with a left complete cleft of the primary and secondary palate (left primary and secondary complete; LPC, LSC, 11-19). sbal, subalare; se, sellion; sn, subnasale; N, nasion; ANS, anterior nasal spine; PPA, posterior piriform aperture; S, sella. (From Fisher DM, Lo LJ, Chen YR, et al: Three-dimensional computed tomographic analysis of the primary nasal deformity in 3-month-old infants with complete unilateral cleft lip and palate. Plast Reconstr Surg 1999;103:1826-1834.)

marked are the base of the ala (SBAR, SBAL) and the commissure (CHR, CHL) (Fig. 93-7A).

Identification of the Base of the Cleft-side Philtral Column

The base of the cleft-side philtral column (CPHL') is a definite anatomic point but difficult to identify. The red line always converges and meets the white skin roll medially. There is frequently a distinct point where the white skin roll changes directions and makes a slight curve about 3 to 4 mm before it meets the red line.[38,39] The base of the cleft-side philtral column is where the white skin roll changes directions and where the vermilion first becomes widest, usually 3 to 4 mm lateral to the converging red line and white skin roll. This is an important anatomic point for the cleft-side philtral column and should seldom be moved (Fig. 93-7A).

EVALUATION AND IDENTIFICATION OF TISSUE DEFICIENCIES

Pool[39] noted areas of vital concern to the surgeon: the amount of tissue medial to the base of the ala and the vertical height of the lateral lip. In addition, the horizontal length of the lateral lip and the epidermal extension from the columella onto the premaxilla are important.

Lateral Lip Deficiencies or Excess

All other measurements for complete (Fig. 93-7A) and incomplete (93-7B) clefts are recorded at the time of surgery for evaluation and a record of the cleft deformity. The most important measurements for the surgeon to evaluate are the vertical length (VR, VL) and the horizontal length (HR, HL) (Fig. 93-7C). The measurements of the patient in Figure 93-5A are applied

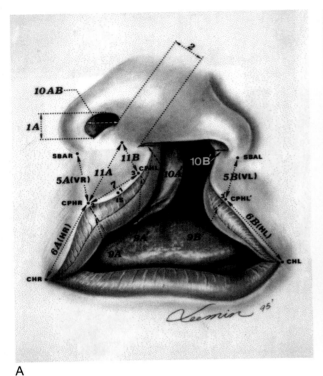

A

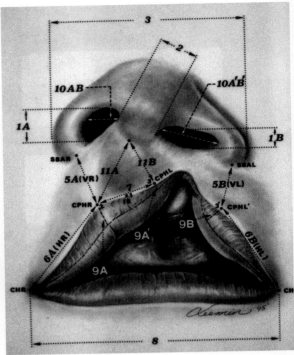

B

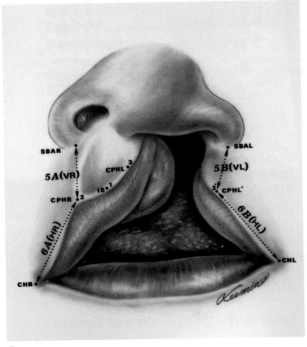

C

FIGURE 93-7. *A,* Unilateral complete cleft with anthropometric markings for measurements: CHR, CHL, commissure; HR, HL, right and left horizontal length; VR, VL, right and left vertical length; CPHR, noncleft-side philtral column; CPHL, cleft-side Cupid's bow; IS, central Cupid's bow; CPHL′, cleft-side philtral column; SBAR, SBAL, right and left base of ala. *B,* Similar markings for the incomplete cleft lip. *C,* Unilateral complete cleft with anthropometric markings showing the most important measurements of vertical length (VR, VL) and horizontal length (HR, HL). (From Noordhoff MS, Chen YR, Chen KT, et al: The surgical technique for the complete unilateral cleft lip–nasal deformity. Operative Techniques Plast Reconstr Surg 1995;2:167-174.)

to Figure 93-7C as an example: VR, 12 mm; VL, 8 mm; HR, 16 mm; and HL, 15 mm. It is apparent that the cleft-side lip is short in the vertical dimension by 4 mm and in the horizontal dimension by 1 mm. The short lateral length (HL) can be lengthened by moving point CPHL′ medially, but this would give an even shorter vertical length (VL). Vertical length is more important aesthetically compared with the horizontal length. Therefore, vertical length is seldom sacrificed for horizontal length. Thus, moving point CPHL′ medially would be a poor choice. The short vertical length can be increased by moving point CPHL′ laterally, but this would result in an even shorter horizontal length that is already short. Extending the upper rotation-advancement incision around the ala can also increase the short vertical length. However, extending the incision around the ala results in an unacceptable scar and should be avoided if at all possible. It is stressed that point CPHL′ is an anatomic point[37-39] similar to other anatomic points. If moved at all, it is not moved until all incisions, muscle dissection, and reconstruction are completed. The reason for this is that an increased vertical length of up to 4 mm can be achieved by adequate muscle dissection and redraping of the skin over the muscle, thus eliminating the need of perialar incisions.[38] Kernahan[40] also noted that release of the muscle from the skin and redraping of the skin over the muscle would increase the vertical length of the lip. In incomplete clefts, it is not uncommon to have the cleft-side vertical length of the lip longer than the noncleft side.[38,39] It is important to recognize this problem to prevent having a long lateral lip that is difficult to correct in a secondary procedure.

Columella and Nostril Floor Skin

If the columella is narrow and if there is deficient skin lateral to the base of the columella, use of C flap tissue to elongate the columella could result in a small nostril. In addition, it is advocated that increased vertical length of the advancement flap can be obtained by use of vestibular skin.[41] The disadvantage of vestibular skin is that it often includes hair follicles, which are unattractive. Also, when there is deficient skin lateral to the base of the columella, the use of vestibular skin for increasing length of the advancement flap would result in a small nostril. Careful evaluation of skin lateral to the columella and medial to the alar base is important to prevent a small nostril.

Deficient Vermilion Beneath the Cleft-side Cupid's Bow

The vermilion beneath the cleft-side Cupid's bow is deficient compared with the counterpart vermilion width on the noncleft side (Fig. 93-7A). Inadequate reconstruction of this deficient vermilion will result

in free border deformities as seen in a straight-line lip closure. The vermilion medial to the base of the philtral column at point CPHL′ fits into the deficient vermilion beneath the Cupid's bow (Fig. 93-7A).

HISTORICAL SURGICAL ASPECTS

The earliest account of a cleft lip operation was recorded in the *Chin Annals* of China. The time of the operation was dated 390 AD.[42] Surgery at that time was probably simply cutting and approximating of the cleft edges. Ambroise Paré (1564) is usually credited with describing a cleft operation by freshening the cleft edge and holding the edges together with a needle secured by a figure-of-eight thread. Early closures were essentially a straight-line closure of Rose[43] (Fig. 93-8A) and Thompson.[44] Mirault[45] in 1844 is generally credited as the first to use a lower lip flap from the lateral segment across the lower margin of the cleft (Fig. 93-8B). Blair[46] and Brown,[47] in 1945, modified this approach, leaving essentially a straight repair without a Cupid's bow. Jalaguier[48] in 1880 used a triangular flap from the lateral lip that was similar to the Hagedorn technique.[49] Hagedorn[49] was the first to design a Cupid's bow using a lateral quadrilateral lip flap. The recognition that there was a Cupid's bow present in the cleft lip was a major change in cleft surgery. This led to a modification by LeMesurier[50] in 1949 (Fig. 93-8C). The Tennison[51] method (Fig. 93-8D) was the start of a more sophisticated repair with actual preservation and positioning of the Cupid's bow. Randall[52] popularized this method. In 1955, Millard presented his rotation-advancement method, and this was first published in 1957,[53] followed by another historical presentation in 1958 (Fig. 93-8E).[54] Since then, the two most popular types of repairs have been the Tennison and Millard techniques with many modifications. The evolution of Millard's early presentation in 1957 to his most recent report in 1999[55] spans a lifetime of change and innovation.

OVERALL CLEFT TREATMENT PLAN: CHANG GUNG CRANIOFACIAL CENTER
Treatment Before Surgery

A genetic diagnosis and evaluation for other systemic conditions should be done at the time a prenatal diagnosis of the cleft is made. The newborn cleft baby should have a pediatric evaluation; parents are counseled about feeding and given information for subsequent care and treatment. Early treatment with presurgical orthopedics and nasal molding is started at 2 weeks or earlier whenever possible. After completion of the nasoalveolar molding, usually at 3 to 4 months, a surgical correction of the cleft lip and nose is done (Fig. 93-9A).

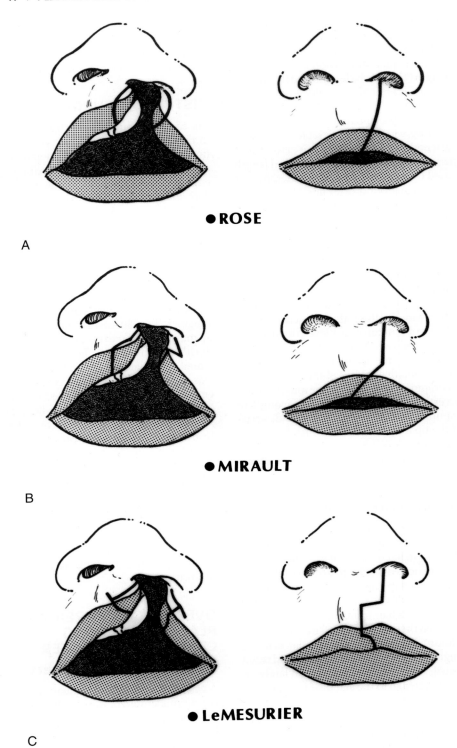

●ROSE

A

●MIRAULT

B

●LeMESURIER

C

FIGURE 93-8. *A*, Rose cheiloplasty. *B*, Mirault cheiloplasty. *C*, LeMesurier cheiloplasty.

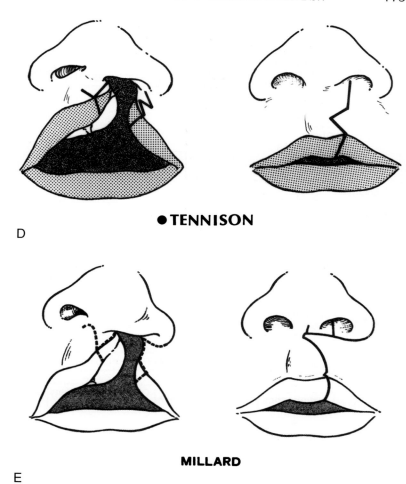

● TENNISON

D

MILLARD

E

FIGURE 93-8, cont'd. *D,* Tennison cheiloplasty. *E,* Millard rotation-advancement cheiloplasty.

The Surgical Approach

There are several different treatment plans leading to the surgical correction of the deformity (Fig. 93-9*B*). With effective presurgical nasoalveolar molding, a definitive cheiloplasty is done at the age of 3 to 5 months when the alveolus is approximated. A gingivoperiosteoplasty can be done, if desired, in association with a definitive cheiloplasty when there is edge-to-edge approximation of the alveolus. Whenever presurgical orthopedics is not available or if the child is older than 3 months, a definitive cheiloplasty with nasal correction is done because presurgical orthopedics is usually not effective after 3 months. If there is a wide cleft (>10 mm) and an associated tissue deficiency, an initial nasolabial adhesion cheiloplasty is done at 3 months followed by a definitive cheiloplasty at about 9 months.

Treatment After Cheiloplasty

A two-flap palatoplasty is done at 11 to 12 months. In most instances, a complete closure of all operative areas is achieved along with a radical repositioning of the levator musculature as recommended by Sommerlad.[56] Timing of alveolar bone grafting relates to the eruption of the central incisor and canine. It is determined by the orthodontist. This is usually at the age of 7 to 11 years. Alveolar bone grafting is sometimes unnecessary after a gingivoperiosteoplasty; however, there may be a need for additional bone in the piriform area. Speech evaluation starts at the age of 2½ years. Early intervention for velopharyngeal insufficiency is done as soon as possible on the basis of speech evaluation, nasopharyngoscopy, and videofluoroscopy (see Fig. 93-9*A*).

With continued improvement in the primary nasal reconstruction, secondary correction of nasal

CLEFT TREATMENT PLAN

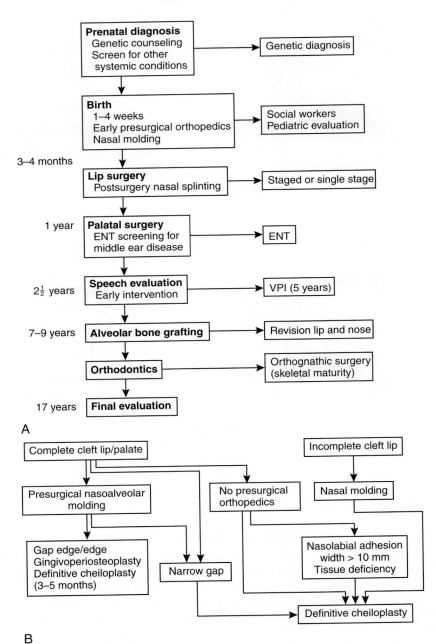

FIGURE 93-9. Cleft treatment plan. *A,* Overall plan. *B,* Surgical algorithm.

deformities can usually be delayed until after reconstruction of the bony base by alveolar bone grafting. However, if there is a significant nasal or lip deformity or psychological reasons that warrant correction, it is done at 5 years of age, before schooling.

Orthodontic treatment in the primary dentition is not done except for functional problems that can be corrected in a short time. Orthodontic treatment in the mixed dentition is done to correct anterior crossbite or to align deviated incisors before alveolar bone grafting. Continuous orthodontic treatment in the mixed dentition is avoided. For most patients, a fixed orthodontic appliance is used to improve dental occlusion in the permanent dentition. Orthognathic surgery is done for maxillary hypoplasia associated with malocclusion at the time of skeletal maturity. Some patients with maxillary hypoplasia are possible candidates for distraction osteogenesis at an earlier age for both psychological and functional improvement.[57,58]

PRESURGICAL ALVEOLAR AND NASOALVEOLAR MOLDING

There is a wide variation in the facilities and expertise for performing cleft surgery throughout the world. In many areas, the facilities, personnel, and finances are inadequate for comprehensive treatment. It would be impossible to deliver a complicated presurgical orthopedic regimen in many areas. Therefore, presurgical care of the cleft infant may vary from nothing to a more complicated method such as nasoalveolar molding. However, some simple methods can be used to provide good care to the cleft child. It is important to begin the following techniques as soon after birth

as possible, preferably within the first 2 weeks after birth.

Alveolar Molding: External Taping With or Without Dental Plate

The external taping (nonsurgical lip adhesion) is the simplest technique for both presurgical molding of the maxillary halves and approximation of the alveolus. A strip of Micropore tape is placed across the cleft to approximate the upper lips. The objective of the tape is to simulate effects of an adhesion cheiloplasty and reposition the maxillary segments into proper alignment.[59] The external taping transfers the tension caused by the approximation of the cleft lip into an inward molding force on the premaxillary alveolus of the greater segment, gradually approximating the separated alveolus (Fig. 93-10A).

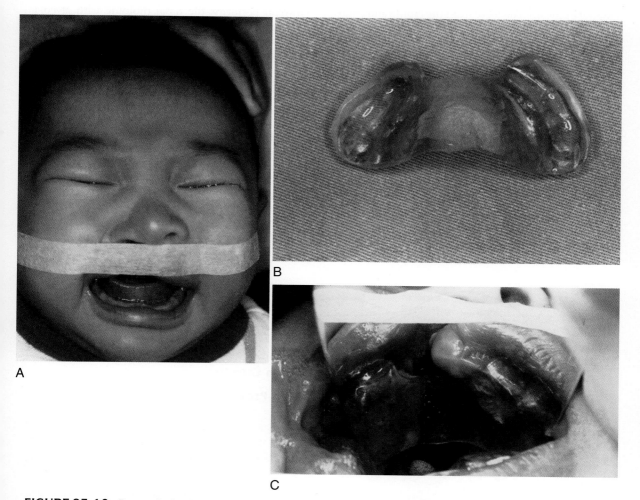

FIGURE 93-10. Presurgical orthopedics with external tape and dental plate. *A,* Micropore tape across lip and cheek. *B,* Dental plate. *C,* Dental plate in place to keep the tongue out of the cleft and to reposition the cleft maxilla and alveolus.

A dental plate used in conjunction with the external taping keeps the tongue out of the cleft and prevents uncontrolled collapse of the dental arches (Fig. 93-10*B* and *C*).[31] The central forces of the tongue pushing into the cleft and lateral muscle pull contribute to the cleft deformity (Fig. 93-11). The dental plate is gradually ground out on its inner surface for controlled movement of the maxillary segments into their proper position. The addition of a simple dental plate with adjustment and Micropore taping of the lip preoperatively is beneficial, molding the alveolus into a better position.

Nasoalveolar Molding

LIOU METHOD

This technique is a modification of the external taping. It uses a molding bulb attached to the dental plate as an outrigger to mold the nose along with the external taping of the lip. The force from the taping and counterforce from the molding bulb provide the force necessary to bring the alveolus into proper position. The nasal molding and arch realignment are done at the same time, taking approximately 3 months.

The first step is to approximate the cleft lip and separated nostril by finger manipulation. This manual lip positioning reveals the actual form, size, and shape of the nostril for proper positioning of the outrigger dental bulb that is attached to the dental plate.[60] The dental plate is made from the dental casts. The nasal projection is made of a 0.028-inch stainless steel wire with one end imbedded in the buccal flange of the dental plate. The other end of the nasal projection wire has a soft resin material to form a molding bulb. Under manual lip adhesion, the depressed nasal dome

elevates and the columella on the cleft side becomes longer, revealing the exact site where the molding bulb on the dental plate needs to be positioned. The lip is held in the proper position while the external Micropore tape is applied, and the dental plate is secured with dental adhesive.

The alveolar molding and nasal molding are performed at the same time. Overstretching of the nasal cartilage on the cleft side should be avoided by simultaneous gradual movement of the maxilla. Nasal projection and the dental plate are modified or adjusted every 1 to 2 weeks until arch and nose are properly positioned. It is important that the nasal cartilage on the cleft side rest on the supporting molding bulb; a too aggressive upward overstretching will result in a large nostril or possible skin and cartilage necrosis (Fig. 93-12).

GRAYSON METHOD[61]

Grayson performs the nasal molding with alveolar approximation, emphasizing complete approximation of the alveolus and avoiding overstretching of the nasal cartilage. The molding device is a dental plate with one forward and downward resin projection holding the dental plate and one forward and upward wire, or resin extension, for nasal molding. The nasal projection is added only if the alveolar cleft has been reduced to less than 6 mm. Micropore tape and orthodontic elastics hold the dental plate without need of a denture adhesive.

Gradually adding soft resin on the inner surface of the buccal flange and grinding out the palatal surface of the dental plate approximate the alveolar cleft. The premaxillary alveolus of the greater segment is molded and bent inward while the posterior dental arches are

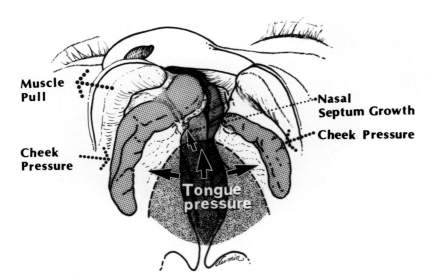

FIGURE 93-11. The forces that exert an influence on the cleft alveolus are the central tongue force, pushing the cleft laterally, and the tongue in the cleft alveolus, preventing approximation. Anteriorly, the muscle pulls laterally and the cheek pressure pushes posteriorly on the palate. A dental plate keeps the tongue out of the cleft, and Micropore tape will have an adhesion effect on the cleft by pulling the muscles together.

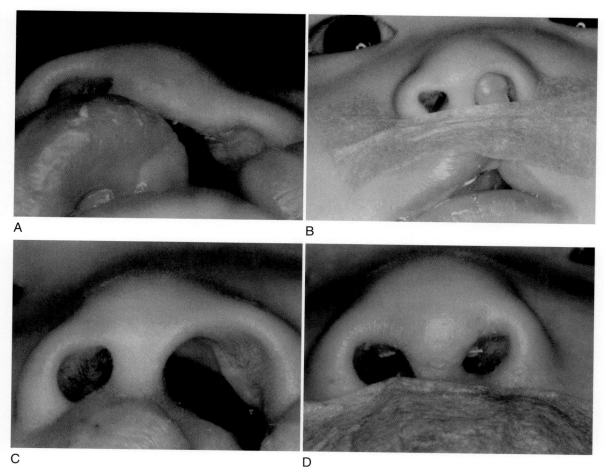

FIGURE 93-12. Presurgical nasoalveolar molding, Liou technique. Left complete cleft of primary and secondary palate (left primary and secondary complete; LPC, LSC, 11-19). *A,* Alveolus at 2 weeks before molding. *B,* During molding with dental plate and attached soft acrylic bulb in place. *C,* Presurgical view after molding at 3 months. *D,* Postsurgical result at 2 weeks.

held by the dental plate. The nasal projection is added and adjusted underneath the deformed cartilage. Soft resin is added to the molding bulbs as indicated. There are two molding bulbs on the top of the nasal projection. One molding bulb faces upward for molding of the nasal dome and nasal cartilage, and another molding bulb projects forward for supporting the nostril rim. This technique should be started within the first 2 weeks after birth; careful monitoring is required every 1 to 2 weeks for a period of 3 to 6 months to complete it (Fig. 93-13).

Discussion of Presurgical Orthopedics

McNeil[62,63] first initiated the use of a dental plate and extraoral forces for maxillary alignment. Brogan[64,65] and Hotz[66,67] have made presurgical orthopedics an

integral part of their cleft protocol. Presurgical orthopedics was used in 22 of 32 cleft lip and palate centers represented at the Zurich symposium *Early Treatment of Cleft Lip and Palate* in 1984[68] and in 40 of 45 British cleft teams in 1990.[69] Brogan[64] stated that the primary objective of presurgical orthopedics is to correct the skeletal deformities of the cleft maxilla before surgery. Keeping the tongue out of the cleft and replacing the pull of the separated lip muscle by tape traction across the lip accomplish this purpose (see Fig. 93-11). According to McComb,[70] presurgical orthopedics facilitates primary repair of the lip and decreases the need for secondary revisions. Such a conclusion is not universally accepted. Huddart[71] and Ross[72] noted no improvement of dental alignment on the permanent dentition. Winters[73] states there is general agreement that a narrow cleft is easier to repair, but it has not been proved that it facilitates nose and lip repair.

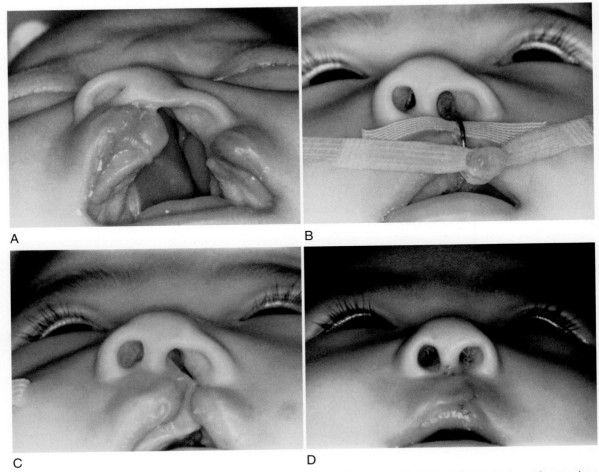

A

B

C

D

FIGURE 93-13. Nasoalveolar molding, Grayson technique (left unilateral complete cleft of primary and secondary palate; LPC, LSC, 11-19). *A,* Position of alveolus before nasoalveolar molding at 2 weeks. *B,* During nasal molding. *C,* After nasal molding before surgery at 4 months. *D,* One week postoperatively.

Regardless of no improvement of facial growth or dentition,[72,74] presurgical orthopedics provides a better bony framework with a narrower cleft. Most surgeons, given a choice, would like a closely approximated cleft alveolus at the time of surgery. It is also noted that there is a statistically significant increased narrowing of the cleft when the infant sleeps on the side compared with sleeping on the back.[75]

Passive Molding with a Dental Plate and Traction. Passive gentle molding of the maxilla and alveolus by use of Micropore tape as an adhesive force attached to the lip and cheek along with a dental plate provides a simple mechanism for molding the maxilla into a proper position with narrowing of the cleft. In some centers, the molding plate remains after cheiloplasty. However, more commonly, it is not used because of patient or parent cooperation. This method seems more physiologic and similar to normal muscle tension with a gradual force during 3 months to achieve a satisfactory repositioning of the maxillary halves and alveolus.

Passive Molding with a Dental Plate Only. Hotz[66,76] advocates a more gradual passive molding of the dental arch by use of a dental plate without extraoral pressure. It takes approximately 6 months to achieve satisfactory repositioning of the maxilla. In addition to the dental plate, there is a posterior extension between the soft palate to keep the tongue in proper position.

Aggressive Forced Molding of the Maxilla with a Fixed Appliance. Latham and Millard[55,77,78] advocate a more aggressive forceful correction of the maxillary segments. It takes 3 to 5 weeks of active movement of the maxillary segments to achieve approximation of the alveolus. The Latham method uses a fixed prosthesis with pins for fixation of the prosthesis on the palate. The prosthesis is inserted under anesthesia for expansion and positioning of the maxillary halves and alveolus. The pin retainer does not have any adverse effects on the dentition.[79] It applies a stronger force to move the maxillary segments forcibly into proper position in a short time.

PASSIVE NASOALVEOLAR MOLDING. The next stage in the evolution of the treatment of the cleft nose was the combination of presurgical orthopedics and nasal molding.[61,80] This is accomplished by the addition of soft acrylic extensions from the dental plate or the use of wire outrigger types of bulbs. With a widely separated alveolus, there is a risk of overcorrection and stretching of tissue and cartilage, resulting in a large nostril. Bennun[81] stressed the importance of starting this technique within 2 weeks of birth and noted excellent results without an excessively large nostril. Presurgical orthopedics with alveolar molding and nasal molding facilitates nasal reconstruction.[61,80-83] Careful attention to avoid overstretching of the lower lateral cartilage and soft tissue will prevent a large nostril. A large nostril will become smaller over time. The addition of presurgical nasoalveolar molding with gingivoperiosteoplasty[61] or without associated gingivoperiosteoplasty[81] promises to be a method of improving the primary surgical result.

During the perinatal period, maternal estrogen rises,[84] which triggers an increase in hyaluronic acid. The fetus acquires the estrogen through the placenta. The hyaluronic acid interacts with cartilage proteoglycans, increasing cartilage, ligament, and connective tissue elasticity by breaking down the intercellular matrix.[85] Approximately 6 weeks after birth, the baby's estrogen level begins to fall off, and the cartilage becomes less plastic. It is important to start any presurgical molding of the maxilla or nasal cartilages as soon after birth as possible to have the hormonal advantage of cartilage plasticity.

THE CLEFT ALVEOLUS
Primary Bone Grafting

There have been efforts to close the alveolar cleft with bone as a part of the primary surgical procedure. Primary bone grafting with cancellous bone is detrimental to growth.[86,87] Onlay rib grafts as described by Rosenstein[88] did not produce growth disturbances.[89] The poor results with primary autogenous bone have frightened many surgeons away from any kind of surgical procedure in this area. However, secondary bone grafting with cancellous bone has proved to be a useful procedure between the ages of 8 and 11 years. This grafting shows no growth problems and good results.[90,91] The failure of primary bone grafting has led to the finding of other procedures that could close

the alveolus, such as periosteoplasty and gingivoperiosteoplasty.

Periosteoplasty

Skoog[92,93] initiated the use of periosteoplasty to close the cleft alveolus with a rotation flap of periosteum overlying the maxilla. Bone formation was noted in about 50% of the patients with no significant growth disturbance.[94,95] Rintala[96] used a similar technique and noted bone formation in 64% of the patients; however, this bone formation was inadequate, requiring secondary alveolar bone grafts in 72% of the complete clefts.

Gingivoperiosteoplasty

Millard[55,97,98] strongly advocated use of the Latham appliance[77,78] for the presurgical alignment of the alveolar segments and maxilla into an edge-to-edge position, enabling the performance of a gingivoperiosteoplasty. The rationale for this is to effect bone union of the alveolus, thus stabilizing the arch and providing a platform for reconstruction of the lip and nose and support of tooth eruption. Others have used this method.[99-101] Millard[55] noted no adverse effect on growth up to the age of 9 years; others have noted no detrimental impact at 5 years.[99,102,103] There is a general concept that gingivoperiosteoplasty does not interfere with growth because it does not involve the vomerine growth centers.[103] Yet in none of the evaluations is there any study of the results after mixed dentition or at dentoskeletal maturity. Henkel[104] evaluated dental casts and lateral head radiographs of 55 patients who received a gingivoperiosteoplasty and compared them with a group who had similar procedures but no gingivoperiosteoplasty. The same surgeon and orthodontist managed all these patients. Three-dimensional growth disturbances were noted. In the unilateral group, 42% of the gingivoperiosteoplasty patients and 5% of the control group had an open bite. The length of the upper jaw was shorter in the gingivoperiosteoplasty group, and there was a higher posterior crossbite. The conclusion was that treatment with the Latham device and gingivoperiosteoplasty disturbs facial growth. An alternative approach to primary gingivoperiosteoplasty is a delayed procedure.[105] Samuel Berkowitz, in a personal communication, stated that "the surgeon-orthodontist should not commit themselves to a treatment plan at birth that reduces their ability to perform future corrective treatment depending on the developing facial pattern." Gingivoperiosteoplasty remains a controversial method of treatment.

Grayson[61] believes that a gradual alignment of the maxillary halves may represent a more physiologic repositioning of the maxilla, which is achieved during a period of 3 months. At 3 months, when there is approximation of the alveolus, a one-stage cheiloplasty and gingivoperiosteoplasty are performed. Presurgical nasal molding has become a part of the presurgical treatment—the presurgical nasoalveolar orthopedic regimen.

SURGICAL APPROACH: UNILATERAL CHEILOPLASTY

Adhesion Cheiloplasty: Two-Stage Repair

The use of the adhesion cheiloplasty was first credited to Johanson.[106] The adhesion cheiloplasty is used as a routine part of the primary repair at some centers,[55,100,107-109] whereas it is used selectively at other centers when the cleft is wide with an associated tissue deficiency.[38,110,111] A number of techniques are used. They vary from a simple type of lip adhesion[112,113] or a nasolabial adhesion, in which there is a more definitive nasal correction as described by Mulliken,[100] to a similar type of nasolabial adhesion used at the Chang Gung Center. The incidence of dehiscence varies from 2% to 22%.[100,112,114] In 1986, 37% of Chang Gung's primary clefts had a nasolabial adhesion cheiloplasty without presurgical orthodontia. From 1990 to 1996, 8% to 11% of complete clefts had a nasolabial adhesion. Following more effective presurgical orthopedics, nasolabial adhesions decreased to 4% in 1997 and 1% in 1999. The dehiscence rate decreased from 2% in 1980 to 0% in the last 2 years. Factors contributing to a decreased incidence are more experienced cleft surgeons, improved presurgical orthopedics, and changing the sleep position from the supine to the prone or side position, thus decreasing cleft width.[75]

THE ADVANTAGES AND DISADVANTAGES OF A TWO-STAGE NASOLABIAL ADHESION CHEILOPLASTY

The advantages of a two-stage cheiloplasty are frequently stated to be narrowing of the cleft, decreased tension across the maxilla, easier correction of the nasal deformity because of a better bony framework on which the nose can be reconstructed, and development of more muscle or elongation of a short lip before definitive cheiloplasty.[115] If a preliminary nasolabial adhesion is warranted, it should produce better results with fewer secondary revisions and less disturbance of growth than a single-stage cheiloplasty.

In an evaluation of a two-stage procedure, Mulliken[100] reported that 75% required nasal revision and 21% a revision of the lip in a recently operated-on group. In a description of a group of 38 consecutive complete unilateral clefts, patients who were older than 14 years at the time of follow-up, Cohen[116] noted that 29% of the group had undergone an adhesion cheiloplasty and that the nose and lip and the entire group of

patients had 1.3 secondary operations. There was no reference to a difference in the adhesion group compared with the nonadhesion group. There are too many variables to determine whether an initial two-stage procedure or one-stage cheiloplasty gives a better result. In both instances, there will be a need for secondary procedures. This question relates to the surgeon's confidence in the ability to correct the problem, the timing of the procedure, and the desires of the patient or family.

Tension could possibly be decreased in a two-stage procedure, but even with an adhesion cheiloplasty, there is a muscular sling that causes increased tension, which molds the maxillary segments into position in a more gentle fashion.[96] Bardach[117] demonstrated that there was increased tension across the maxilla in infants that lasted as long as 2 years. In experiments on beagles, there was increased pressure after lip repair, which caused growth disturbances.[118] Also, in the same experimental model, lip repair with extensive soft tissue dissection caused increased growth disturbances compared with those who had only lip repair.[119] However, in a group of bilateral clefts with and without muscle reconstruction, there was no significant difference in growth in these two groups.[120] Tension from muscle approximation in the bilateral cleft would certainly be greater than in a unilateral repair.[120] Kapucu,[121,122] on the other hand, noted a significant growth disturbance in clefts that had a lip repair and that palatoplasty had no evident effect on growth. Any extensive undermining could contribute to increased tension during wound healing and scar maturation, increasing the possibility of growth disturbances. There is no evidence to support the theory that a staged repair is better than a one-stage repair because of less tension. Obtaining a better nostril with a two-stage procedure is questioned because in one study,[100] 75% of the patients required a nasal revision of some type after two operations, a nasolabial adhesion and definitive cheiloplasty. In the future, presurgical orthopedics with nasal molding may have an advantage in decreasing the number of secondary procedures.

The biggest disadvantage of an adhesion cheiloplasty is that even with no dissection of the muscle, the operative area is firm with scar tissue, secondary to the healing process. This makes dissection and mobilization of the tissues more difficult than in a one-stage procedure where there is no scarring. There is a suggestion that after lip adhesion, there is an increase in the vertical length and more muscle, thus making the subsequent cheiloplasty easier and delivering a better result. A 10% increase in vertical height after nasolabial adhesions is reported with the conclusion that the relatively small increase in vertical length is an insufficient reason for advocating a preliminary adhesion cheiloplasty.[123] The increase in height is more likely due to muscle stretch and hypertrophy rather than an increase of muscle fibers.

NASOLABIAL ADHESION CHEILOPLASTY: SURGICAL TECHNIQUE

INDICATIONS. An adhesion cheiloplasty is done in less than 1% of all clefts after the use of nasoalveolar molding in the Chang Gung Craniofacial Center. Current indications for a nasolabial adhesion cheiloplasty are (1) a cleft more than 10 mm wide with an associated discrepancy of 4 to 5 mm or more in the vertical cleft length between SBAR-CPHR and SBAL-CPHL', (2) a complete cleft of the primary palate in which there is a prominent protruding premaxilla resulting in a long vertical discrepancy between the premaxilla alveolus and maxilla, and (3) older children with wide clefts and no presurgical orthodontia. Cleft tissue deficiencies are more important than cleft width as a criterion in decision-making for a nasolabial adhesion cheiloplasty.

MARKINGS. Standard markings and measurements for an adhesion cheiloplasty are similar to those of the complete unilateral clefts. However, vital landmarks CPHL and CPHL' and the vermilion medial to the base of the cleft-side philtral column CPHL' must not be violated (see Fig. 93-7A).

ELEVATION AND INSERTION OF C FLAP MUCOSA. An incision is made on the free edge of skin and mucosa and extended posteriorly at the junction of columella skin and septum. All skin overlying the premaxilla is preserved. The mucosal C flap, based on the premaxilla, is incised and elevated. It is rotated and inserted behind the columella. This allows mobilization of the medial lip. There is no dissection of muscle (Fig. 93-14, *inset*). The turbinate (T) flap is elevated, and the buccal mucosal flap is marked out for elevation in Figure 93-14.

LATERAL LIP INCISIONS. The buccal mucosal flap and T flap are elevated based on vestibular skin (Fig. 93-15). The free edge of the lateral lip is opened, preserving the vermilion medial to CPHL' on the lateral lip (Fig. 93-15, *upper inset*). There is no muscle dissection. The fibrous attachments between the lower

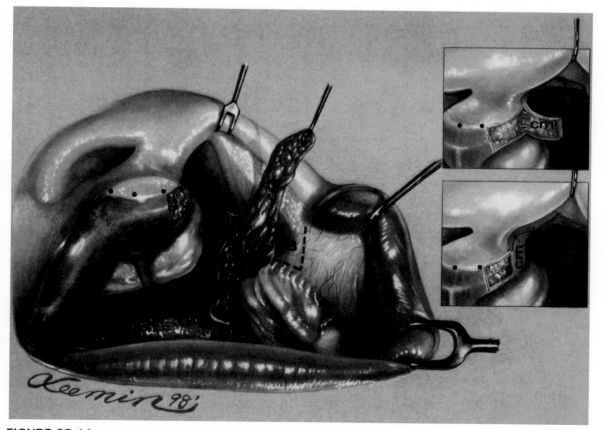

FIGURE 93-14. Nasoalveolar adhesion. *Insets,* The incisions are on the skin border elevating a mucosal flap, cm, that is inserted along the skin columella-septal line behind the columella. The turbinate flap (T) is elevated, and the buccal mucosal flap (B) based on vestibular skin is marked for incision, varying the length according to the width of the cleft.

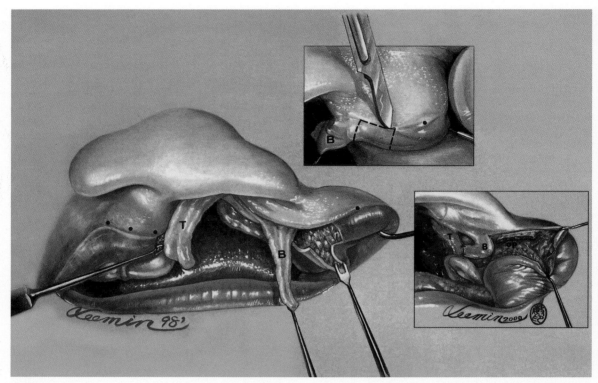

FIGURE 93-15. Nasoalveolar adhesion. The turbinate (T) and buccal mucosal (B) flaps are elevated. *Upper inset,* The free edge of the lip is incised from the converging points of the red line and white skin roll to the base of the buccal flap, preserving the lateral lip vermilion and exposing the muscle. *Lower inset,* The turbinate flap (T) is rotated into the piriform area, and the free edge of the folded mucosal flap (B) is attached to the inferior edge of the turbinate flap.

lateral cartilage (LLC) and piriform rim are released for mobilization of the LLC superiorly.

ELEVATION OF THE LLC AND PIRIFORM LINING WITH T FLAP. With traction on a suspension suture through the dome of the upper lateral cartilage (ULC), the LLC is advanced and sutured to the ULC (Fig. 93-15, *lower inset*). The T flap is rotated and sutured to the piriform rim. The buccal mucosal flap is folded on itself and sutured to the edge of the T flap (Fig. 93-15, *lower inset*).

NOSTRIL FLOOR AND MUCOSAL CLOSURE. The leading edge of the folded buccal flap (Fig. 93-15, *lower inset*) is advanced and sutured to the periosteum of the premaxilla (Fig. 93-16). The buccal lip mucosa is advanced and sutured to the bridging mucosal flap and to the periosteum and mucosa of the premaxilla (Fig. 93-16, *upper inset*).

MUSCLE AND SKIN CLOSURE. Several interrupted horizontal sutures are placed in the muscle, and the skin is closed (Fig. 93-16, *insets*). There is no dissection of the LLC between the skin and the dome of the LLC and no dissection over the maxilla.

DEFINITIVE CHEILOPLASTY AFTER ADHESION. The rotation-advancement is more of a straight-line type of incision from the cleft side of the Cupid's bow to the base of the columella. The C flap is usually brought lateral and the advancement flap incised and rotated medially (Fig. 93-17). Because there has been resurfacing of the piriform area with mucosal flaps at the initial procedure, no dissection is needed over the maxilla. The LLC is released from the overlying skin through the base of the ala if necessary. Muscle, triangular flap augmentation of the deficient vermilion, and skin are closed, followed by a nasal conformer. An example of a two-stage cheiloplasty is shown in Figure 93-18.

Principles of Surgery: Unilateral Cheiloplasty

SURGICAL PRINCIPLES

The following principles are basic to the correction of the cleft deformity:

- Understanding of the embryologic development and anatomy

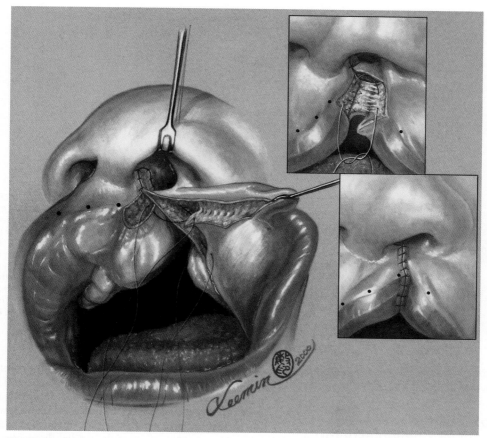

FIGURE 93-16. Nasoalveolar adhesion. The leading edge of the folded mucosal flap is sutured to the periosteum of the premaxilla and the edge of the mucosal C flap. *Insets,* The posterior mucosa is closed, followed by several muscle sutures without muscle dissection, followed by skin closure.

- Understanding of the nature of the deformity to be corrected
- Awareness of the different surgical procedures and their limitations
- Use of an atraumatic surgical technique with delicate handling of tissues, sharp dissection, and careful hemostasis
- Limited dissection to avoid surgical trauma to adjacent tissues
- Knowledge of the healing process
- Lifeboat: an alternative plan for complications or unexpected difficulties at the time of surgery
- Understanding and awareness of the problems related to anesthesia, preoperative care, and postoperative care

KEY SURGICAL CONCEPTS

In addition to the basic principles that are applicable to any surgical procedure, some key concepts apply to the surgical technique. The key concepts of the surgical technique in the unilateral cheiloplasty are as follows:

- No dissection over the maxilla
- Rotation of the Cupid's bow without "back-cuts"
- Reconstruction of deficient vermilion beneath the cleft-side Cupid's bow
- Muscle release and reconstruction to simulate the philtral column
- Complete mucosal closure of all areas by use of inferior turbinate and mucosal flaps that allow repositioning of the LLC and correction of mucosal deficiency in the piriform area
- Advancement and fixation of the LLC at its base and to the ULC, the medial crura, and the skin
- Short upper limb advancement flap, limiting scars around the ala and nostril floor
- Definition of the alar groove
- Postoperative splinting of the nostril with a silicone conformer to limit the effects of wound contracture

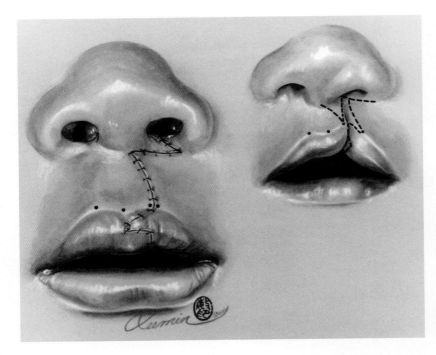

FIGURE 93-17. Incision lines for the rotation-advancement flap. The two flaps are incised, and muscle is dissected for a distance of 2 to 4 mm. The two flaps are interdigitated with closure of mucosa, muscle, and skin. No dissection is necessary in the piriform or maxillary area. Release of the LLC is done through the base of the ala when indicated to achieve nostril symmetry.

- Postoperative wound care with supportive Micropore tape across the scar and lip massage

Surgical Technique: Rotation-Advancement Cheiloplasty for Complete Clefts

Adequate endotracheal anesthesia and monitoring of the patient are mandatory to minimize morbidity and mortalities. Of utmost importance is the fixation of the endotracheal tube, which is secured in the nasopharynx and mouth with a moist, tightly packed sponge and to the lower lip with tape. This also prevents aspiration of blood or mucus during the procedure. Immediate postoperative monitoring of vital signs and airway is imperative.

MEDIAL INCISIONS AND THE C FLAP

The basic points for markings are shown in Figure 93-7A. The rotation incision line is marked as a curving line from the columella-lip crease to CPHL (Fig. 93-19). This incision must not extend beyond the noncleft-side philtral column, or the lip will become too long. Also, the incision across the free border of the lip at CPHL should be at right angles to the axis of the white skin roll to facilitate subsequent lip closure.

The C flap incisions are made on a line that extends from point CPHL along the junction of skin and mucosa to the most lateral point of skin overlying the premaxilla. The incision on the premaxilla extends superiorly at the junction of the columella skin and septal mucosa for a distance of 0.5 cm. This allows mobilization of the C flap and columella complex. Relaxing incisions on the mucosal C flap allow its mobilization later across the cleft to the cleft-side maxilla for reconstruction of the nostril floor. The muscle is freed from the skin in the subdermal plane for a distance of 2 to 3 mm (Fig. 93-20).

ADEQUACY OF ROTATION

Placement of a hook in the nostril rim with simultaneous traction on the free border of the lip will determine if the rotation is adequate, that is, both sides of the Cupid's bow at the same level (Fig. 93-21). If the rotation is inadequate, a horizontal extension of the incision is done up to but not across the noncleft-side philtral column. Incision across the noncleft-side philtral column will result in a long lip. If this fails to achieve adequate rotation, nothing further is done until after muscle repositioning. A back-cut as advocated by Millard[124] leaves a wide defect at the apex of the rotation incision that must be closed with the C flap or the advancement flap. This area is always the tightest and most difficult area of skin closure. Therefore, to avoid a difficult, tight skin closure, a back-cut is avoided (Fig. 93-22).

OVERROTATION OF THE CUPID'S BOW

If the rotation is inadvertently excessive at surgery, suturing and shortening of the muscle at that time are

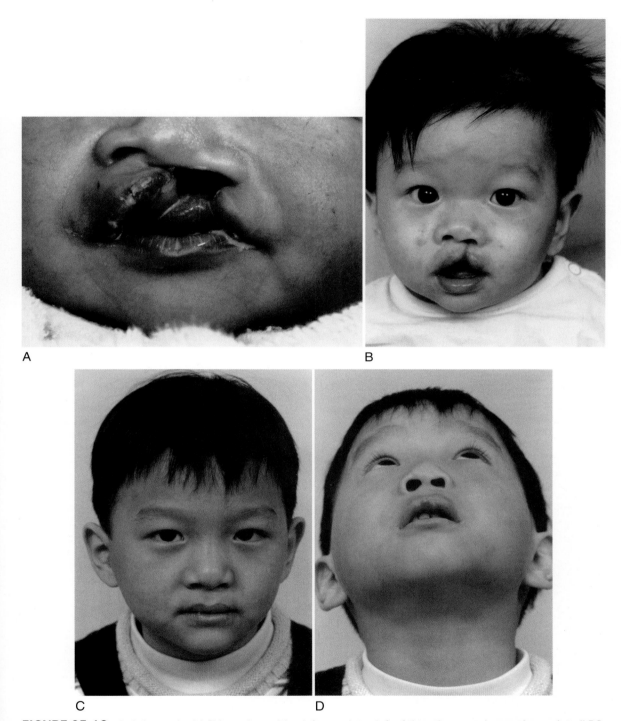

FIGURE 93-18. *A,* A 1-month-old Chinese boy with a left complete cleft of the primary and secondary palate (LPC, LSC, 11-19). Presurgical orthopedics was unsuccessful. The alveolar cleft was 10 mm wide, and there was associated vertical shortness of the lateral lip. *B,* Postoperative view after a nasoalveolar adhesion cheiloplasty at 7 months, when a definitive cheiloplasty was done. *C* and *D,* Postoperative views at 5 years.

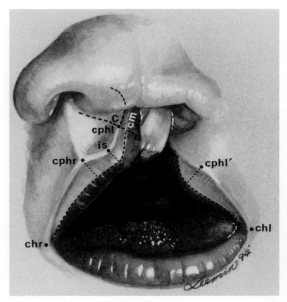

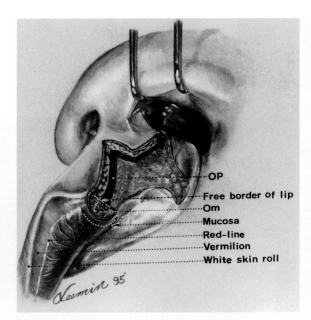

FIGURE 93-19. Preoperative marking: cphr, is, cphl, cphl', chr, and chl as described in Figure 93-7*A*. The C flap (c) and C flap mucosa (cm) are marked. The dotted line on the lip is the red line, which is the junction between vermilion and mucosa. Incision lines are shown on the lip extending from point cphl lateral to the columella on the skin edge overlying the premaxilla extending superiorly along the junction line of columella skin and septal cartilage mucosa. The cleft-side base of the philtral column is also marked (cphl').

FIGURE 93-20. The free border of the lip after incision. Note the orbicularis marginalis muscle covered by vermilion and mucosa and bordered by the white skin roll. The vermilion is deficient beneath the cleft-side Cupid's bow. Om, orbicularis marginalis muscle; OP, orbicularis peripheralis muscle.

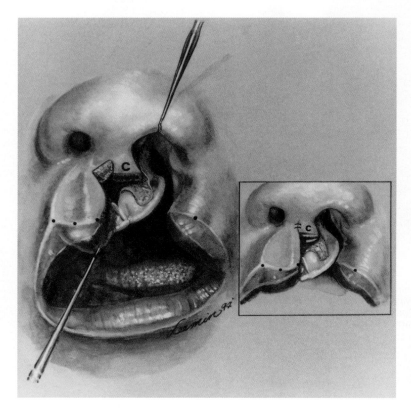

FIGURE 93-21. Traction on the rim of the nostril will disclose in what direction the C flap will be placed, laterally or medially, as in the inset. (From Noordhoff MS, Chen YR, Chen KT, et al: The surgical technique for the complete unilateral cleft lip–nasal deformity. Operative Techniques Plast Reconstr Surg 1995;2:167-174.)

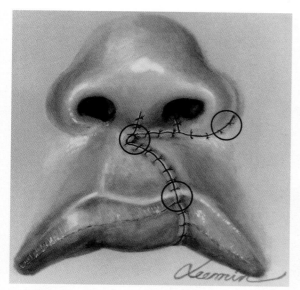

FIGURE 93-22. Three areas of concern. A straight-line closure of the lip does not reconstruct the deficient vermilion beneath the Cupid's bow, leaving a stepped-off appearance of the red line. A back-cut at the apex of the rotation incision leaves a broad area that is difficult to close with the advancement flap. Incisions around the alar base produce an unacceptable scar and are to be avoided.

necessary. Extreme caution is mandatory to prevent overrotation of the Cupid's bow, resulting in a vertically long lip that is difficult to correct in a secondary procedure.

POSITIONING OF THE C FLAP

souvent utilisé pour le plancher nasal

With traction on the rim of the nostril and the free border of the lip at point CPHL, the C flap will rotate into the columella or go laterally. It will also define adequacy of rotation (see Fig. 93-21). The C flap is placed where it "wants to go," into the columella or laterally; however, whenever there is a vertically short lateral lip of more than 4 mm, the C flap must be brought laterally to a point just beneath the ala. This allows rotation of the ala inward, thus preventing a "turned-out nasal sill." It will also slightly increase the vertical height of a vertically short lateral lip.

LATERAL LIP INCISIONS

The turbinate flap is marked. The L flap[125] is marked based on the maxilla, extending on the free border of the lip to the point where the red line and white skin roll converge, preserving the vermilion on the lateral lip (Fig. 93-23, *lower inset*). The skin incision line on the free border of the lip extends from point CPHL' to the maxilla and the inferior edge of the turbinate flap (Fig. 93-23, *lower inset*). The turbinate and L flaps are elevated (Fig. 93-23).

THE ORBICULARIS MARGINALIS FLAP

The orbicularis marginalis (OM) flap is incised along the free border of the lip to include the orbicularis marginalis muscle, the vermilion medial to point CPHL', and the corresponding mucosa posteriorly (Fig. 93-23, *top inset*). The OM flap is elevated to its base beneath the philtral column (CPHL') in such a way that the volume of muscle at its base CPHL' is similar to the volume of muscle at the opposite point CPHR on the noncleft side of the lip. The OM flap is cut squarely and not beveled.

ELEVATION OF THE INFERIOR TURBINATE FLAP AND RELEASE OF THE LOWER LATERAL CARTILAGE

The incision line on the inferior turbinate extends from the piriform rim inward on the upper and lower edges of the inferior turbinate for a distance of 1.5 cm, where a transverse cut is made (Fig. 93-23). The inferior turbinate flap (T) is elevated in a retrograde fashion based on the vestibular skin. After elevation of the L and T flaps, the attachments of the LLC to the rim of the maxilla and ULC are released, allowing easy mobilization of the LLC and the lateral lip without dissection over the maxilla. Even in wide clefts, mobilization of the lip and cartilage is easily accomplished without a dissection over the maxilla.

ORBICULARIS PERIPHERALIS MUSCLE DISSECTION AND RELEASE

The lateral lip mucosa is incised and dissected free for only 2 to 3 mm. Excessive dissection contributes to scarring and should be avoided. The orbicularis peripheralis muscle is bunched up as a disorganized mass of fibers with numerous dermal insertions.[126] By use of a blunt-nosed tenotomy scissors, the orbicularis peripheralis muscle is dissected along the edge of the dermis to a line extending from the base of the ala to the base of the philtral column CPHL'. The dissection is continued on a subdermal plane superiorly under and around the base of the ala (Fig. 93-24). This releases the abnormal insertions of the paranasal muscles including the transverse portion of the nasalis muscle, the depressor septi, and the levator muscles of the upper lip and ala.[100,127,128] Release of the muscle from the overlying skin and ala allows the tethered, bunched-up muscle to be stretched, effectively elongating the lateral lip. The skin will also stretch in a similar manner, gaining increased vertical length.

THE VERMILION TRIANGULAR FLAP

The vermilion flap is marked and incised on the OM flap while the OM flap is held under tension. A No. 11 blade is laid on the incision line, drawing the knife across to ensure an accurate cut. This results in a clean, accurate incision. After the vermilion flap is incised, an inci-

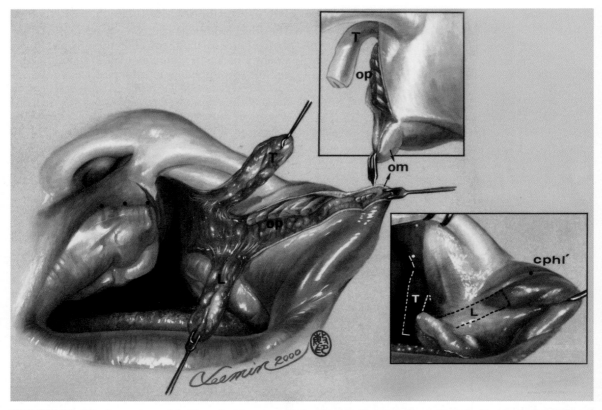

FIGURE 93-23. *Lower inset,* Markings for the mucosal flap L, based on maxilla and inferior turbinate flap T. The L flap based on the maxilla extends to the converging red line and white skin roll, leaving the vermilion between this point and cphr' available for reconstruction of the deficient vermilion beneath the cleft side of the Cupid's bow. *Top inset,* The incision along the skin edge from cphl' to the base of the inferior turbinate and elevation of the OM flap on the lateral lip. The main figure shows the completed dissection with an elevated turbinate (T) and mucosal flap (L) based on the maxilla and the released OM flap and its covering vermilion.

sion is made along the red line of the lip beneath the Cupid's bow opposite point cphl, thus opening the lip for eventual insertion of the OM vermilion flap after muscle approximation (Fig. 93-25).

CORRECTION OF PIRIFORM MUCOSAL DEFICIENCY

The LLC is repositioned superiorly with a traction suture through the dome and at its leading edge, rotating it inward. At the same time, the LLC is fixed to the ULC with interrupted polydioxanone sutures (Fig. 93-26). The T flap based on vestibular skin is rotated and sutured to the piriform rim with interrupted 5-0 polydioxanone sutures similar to the way Millard[98] uses the L flap to correct mucosal deficiency. The T flap corrects mucosal deficiency and allows repositioning of the LLC and ala without restriction.

NOSTRIL FLOOR RECONSTRUCTION

The L flap is rotated medially behind the columella and attached to the periosteum of the premaxilla and

the distal edge of the T flap with interrupted 5-0 poly-dioxanone sutures. The C flap mucosa is rotated laterally and inferiorly. It is attached to the maxilla and the lower edge of the L flap (see Fig. 93-26). This gives good mucosal coverage of the nostril floor without tension. The vestibular skin with attached ala is advanced over the mucosal bridge to the uppermost point of the C flap incision behind the columella (see Fig. 93-26, *inset*). The upper free edge of the vestibular skin flap and bridging L flap edges are closed with interrupted absorbable sutures. This gives a good two-layer closure of the nostril floor and effectively corrects the tissue deficiency in this area. The vestibular skin is advanced as far as necessary to achieve a normal nostril size (see Fig. 93-26, *inset*). This also advances and rotates the ala inward into a position comparable to the opposite side. Final positioning and closure of the nostril floor are done after muscle approximation. At this point, if the configuration of the nostril and alar cartilage is good, no further dissection of the LLC is necessary. If the configuration is not good, the LLC is released from the skin with a

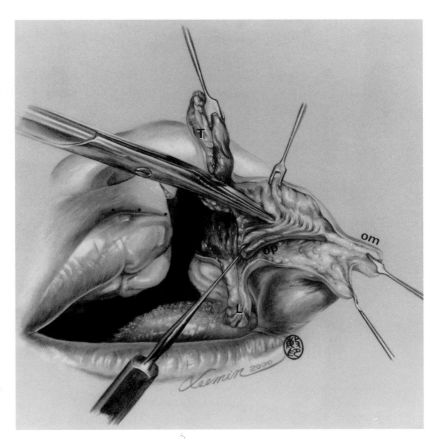

FIGURE 93-24. The orbicularis peripheralis muscle (OP) is released in a subdermal plane. The abnormally inserted fibers of the nasalis, depressor septi, and levator muscles are released from the base of the ala.

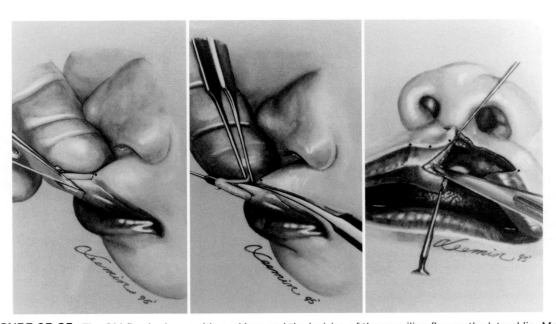

FIGURE 93-25. The OM flap is shown with markings and the incision of the vermilion flap on the lateral lip. Medially, the lip is opened on the red line beneath the Cupid's bow.

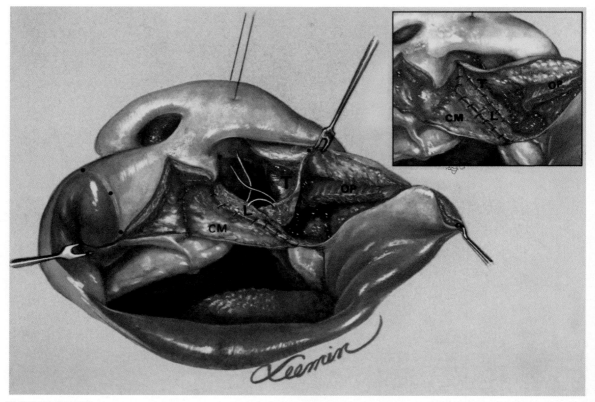

FIGURE 93-26. The LLC is freed from its fibrous attachments to the maxilla and ULC. There is no dissection over the maxilla. The LLC is elevated with a traction suture and fixed to the ULC in an elevated position. The turbinate flap (T) is rotated into the piriform area. The nostril floor is reconstructed with the L flap behind the columella, and the C flap mucosa is sutured lateral to the maxilla. *Inset* shows completion of nostril floor reconstruction with advancement of the vestibular skin rotating the alar base inward. There is good mucosal closure with no open areas for secondary healing and scar contracture. OP, orbicularis peripheralis muscle.

blunt-nosed tenotomy scissors from the base of the ala (Fig. 93-27).

MUSCLE RECONSTRUCTION

The muscle is approximated with a 5-0 polydioxanone key suture placed in the center of the muscle, opposite points CPHL and CPHL′. With continued traction on the free edge of the lip at CPHL, remaining interrupted muscle sutures are placed from the free border to nostril. These sutures are placed in such a way that the lateral muscle is slightly elevated above the medial muscle to simulate a philtral column (Fig. 93-28, *inset*). Whenever the muscle is thin and deficient, a simple direct closure is done. The final 5-0 polydioxanone sutures in the upper aspect of muscle closure are placed to attach the perialar nasalis muscle and depressor septi to the apex of the muscle beneath the columella. These muscles are thin and delicate and are not dissected out as individual muscles but rather advanced and sutured as a group medially (see Fig. 93-28).

CLOSURE OF THE FREE BORDER OF THE LIP AND MUCOSA

Points CPHL and CPHL′ are approximated with a fine 7-0 absorbable polydioxanone suture. The excess mucosa opposite points CPHL and CPHL′ on the free border of the lip is trimmed. The medial free border mucosa is also trimmed so the two edges fit together without excessive tissue. The vermilion triangular flap should fit into the medial opening beneath the Cupid's bow. Careful attention to excise excessive mucosa and muscle accurately is important (Fig. 93-29, *insets*). "You get what you see," and the most common error is to leave too much muscle or mucosa on the free border. With this technique, there is seldom any muscle deficiency or notching on the free border of the lip. Incisions on the free border are closed with interrupted 7-0 polydioxanone sutures and a continuous 7-0 suture on the vermilion.

The lateral lip buccal mucosa is trimmed and closed with interrupted fine absorbable sutures. The upper

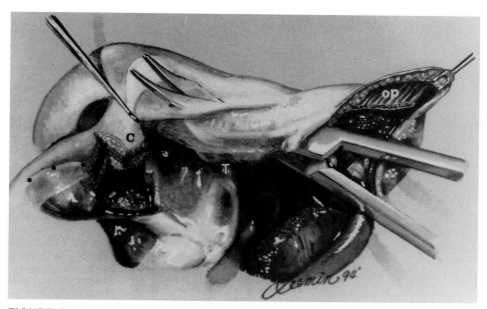

FIGURE 93-27. Release of the LLC from the overlying skin with a blunt-nosed tenotomy scissors.

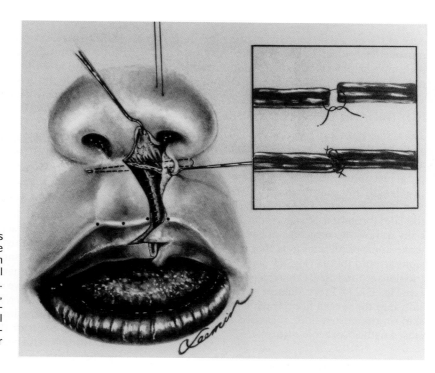

FIGURE 93-28. Orbicularis peripheralis muscle closure (optional alar base traction suture). *Inset,* Elevation of lateral muscle higher than medial muscle. (From Noordhoff MS, Chen YR, Chen KT, et al: The surgical technique for the complete unilateral cleft lip–nasal deformity. Operative Techniques Plast Reconstr Surg 1995;2:167-174.)

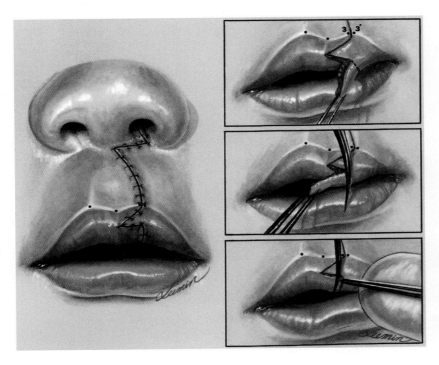

FIGURE 93-29. *Insets,* The free border of the lip is closed by inserting the triangular vermilion flap medially under slight tension and trimming the excess mucosa. The skin is closed without incisions extending around the base of the ala.

edge of the buccal lip mucosa is sutured to the C flap mucosa that bridges the alveolar gap. This gives a complete mucosal closure without tension. Careful closure of the lip mucosa gives the lip a nice pout.

NOSTRIL AND LIP SKIN CLOSURE

The C flap muscle, when usable, is placed laterally to augment the nostril floor. If the cleft is wide and the ala turns out slightly, the C flap is placed laterally to a point just under the ala to give a slight increase in vertical length and to prevent an outward flaring of the alar base. No lateral horizontal skin incisions for the lateral rotation-advancement flap are made initially, as now the surgeon can better visualize how to make appropriate incisions that will eliminate incisions around the ala (Fig. 93-30; see also Fig. 93-29). Incisions around the ala are avoided and seldom needed (see Fig. 93-23). Every attempt is made to fit the incision into the nostril floor, leaving a nasal sill. Excess skin on the nostril floor is excised as necessary and closed with absorbable sutures.

ADEQUACY OF ROTATION

It is important at this point to make any necessary minor adjustments. The cleft side of the Cupid's bow must be adequately rotated. If it is slightly elevated, a small hook is used to place the Cupid's bow under tension. A short transverse incision is made above the white

skin roll to release the Cupid's bow into its proper position. An appropriately sized small triangular skin flap, 1 to 2 mm in width, is incised from the lateral lip and rotated into the defect above the white skin roll to fill the defect, where it is held with fine 7-0 polydioxanone sutures (Fig. 93-31, *inset*).

DESIGN OF THE ALAR-FACIAL GROOVE AND SKIN FIXATION OF THE LOWER LATERAL CARTILAGE

Dissection between the skin and LLC releases the fibrous attachments between the skin and the LLC.[129] Placement of alar transfixion sutures reattaches the LLC to the skin. Traction is placed on the LLC suspension suture during placement of these 5-0 polydioxanone monofilament absorbable sutures. Grasping of the inner and outer aspect of the ala at the alar-facial groove with a forceps facilitates placement of these sutures. By use of the forceps, the suture is passed from the inside to the outer surface of the skin at the point of the forceps on the alar groove. The suture is returned through the outer suture hole and back into the inner aspect of the vestibular skin, where it is tied as a mattress subcuticular suture. Two other sutures are usually required. The remaining sutures catch the leading edge of the LLC, pass through the skin in the alar-facial groove and back again into the skin just inside the alar rim, and are tied (Fig. 93-32). These sutures help close the dead

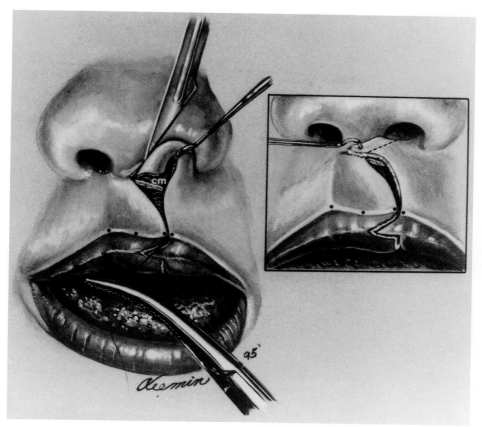

FIGURE 93-30. No upper rotation-advancement skin incisions are made until after muscle approximation. The skin is moved back and forth until the approximate incision can be determined to prevent unsightly perialar scars. This is done in both incomplete and complete clefts.

space after cartilage dissection and define the alar-skin groove, eliminate prominent vestibular webbing, and support the LLC. The fixation of the LLC is now complete—first to the base of the ULC, at the genua, and finally to the skin. On occasion, there is an overhang of skin on the nostril rim, which is excised as a crescent and closed with a continuous fine absorbable 7-0 polydioxanone suture.

PHILTRAL COLUMN

The philtral column is an elusive problem in reconstruction of the muscle. The lateral muscle is sutured so that it is elevated above the noncleft-side muscle. This technique is seldom effective in reconstructing a good philtral column. First of all, good muscle bulk is needed with a tight approximation. However, the muscle is often underdeveloped, precluding a good result. A good philtral column is dependent on a tight muscle closure and loose skin draped over the muscle without tension.

Nasal Repair

With the addition of nasoalveolar molding, there is less need for extensive dissection of the LLC to achieve a good configuration and appearance of the nostril. More extensive careful dissection of the LLC does not interfere with subsequent growth. The surgeon needs to evaluate the deformity at this time and decide whether further surgery on the LLC is indicated. Whenever the nostril does not have a good configuration after reconstruction of the nostril floor and advancement of the ala, a release of the LLC from the overlying skin with a blunt-nosed tenotomy scissors is done through the base of the ala (see Fig. 93-27). The patient shown in Figure 93-33 had this technique used in the primary procedure for nasal correction along with the described surgical technique and presurgical alveolar molding with a dental plate and Micropore tape.

An alternative procedure is indicated whenever the medial crura are separated at the dome. The LLC

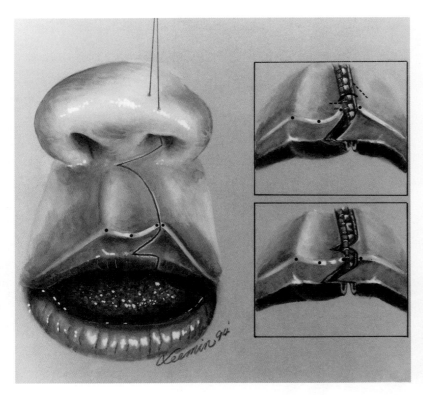

FIGURE 93-31. The skin closure is depicted to show inadequate rotation and peaking of the Cupid's bow. A horizontal incision is made above CPHL on the cleft side of the Cupid's bow to rotate it down. An appropriately sized triangular flap from the lateral lip skin is inserted into this defect to correct the deformity.

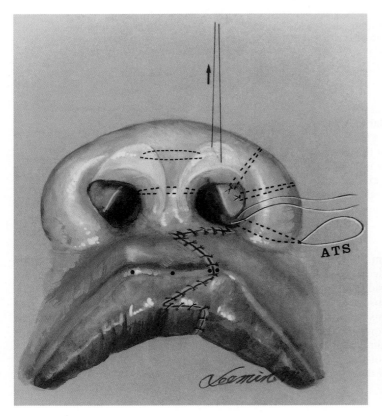

FIGURE 93-32. Alar transfixion sutures (ATS) of 5-0 absorbable monofilament are placed with traction on the LLC. One suture is placed in the vestibular skin. The remaining sutures catch the leading edge of the LLC, pass through the alar-facial groove and back near the rim of the ala, and are tied on the inner side. Notching of the skin disappears within 1 to 2 weeks. (From Noordhoff MS, Chen YR, Chen KT, et al: The surgical technique for the complete unilateral cleft lip–nasal deformity. Operative Techniques Plast Reconstr Surg 1995;2:167-174.)

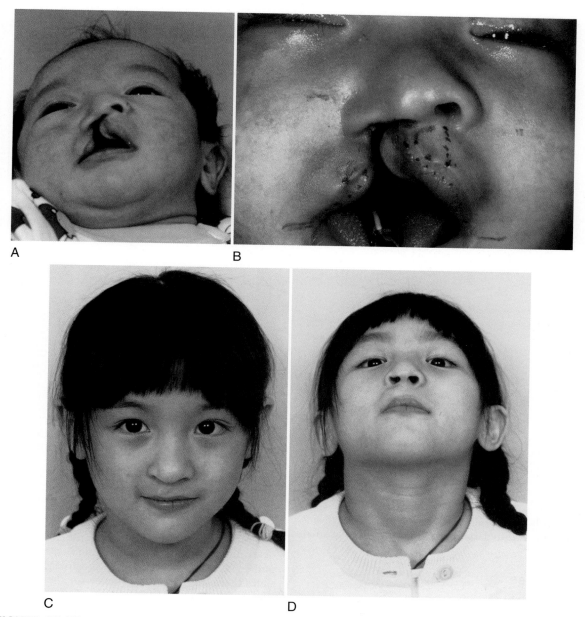

FIGURE 93-33. *A,* Right complete cleft of the primary and secondary palate in a 1-month-old Chinese girl (RPC, RSC, 1-9). *B,* Operative markings at 3 months; note the anatomic base of the cleft-side philtral column. The patient had presurgical orthopedics with Micropore tape and a dental plate. *C* and *D,* Postoperative views at the age of 5 years.

can be dissected by an inner rim infracartilaginous incision. The fat between the domes of the LLC is dissected from between the crura. The crura are reapproximated and held with a 5-0 absorbable suture. The genua of the LLC are now approximated without the intervening fat for a better configuration. The small incisions are closed with a fine absorbable suture (Fig. 93-34).

The nose should sit by itself supported by the approximation of lip musculature. Overcorrection with extensive dissection of the LLC[130] is unnecessary to achieve a satisfactory result and can cause a small nostril and nostril stenosis. With use of the current technique, there were no postoperative problems of nostril stenosis requiring correction. A slightly small nostril at the time of surgery can be corrected by progressive splint-

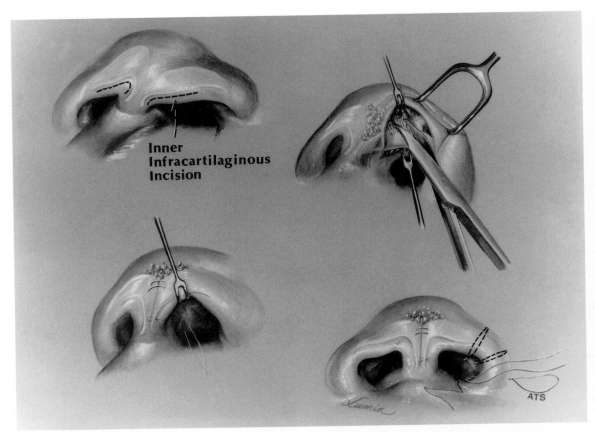

FIGURE 93-34. An inner infracartilaginous rim incision exposes the leading edge of the LLC. The fat between the medial crura is removed. The medial crura are approximated under direct vision with a monofilament absorbable suture.

ing with a silicone nasal conformer. If anything, having a slightly larger nostril is better than a small nostril.[131,132]

Alar Base

The most important factor in achieving alar symmetry is the release of the abnormally attached paranasal muscles. In reconstructing the nostril floor, the alar base is advanced farther to its proper width compared with the normal side. The alar-facial groove is further accentuated by the approximation of the lip musculature.

Extensive subperiosteal undermining is often recommended to achieve adequate correction and symmetry.[93,133-136] Delaire[135] attests that subperiosteal dissection contributes to increased bone formation. Augmentation of the nasal floor with Surgicel in the primary repair was not beneficial in achieving a better aesthetic result.[137] Subperiosteal dissection is unnecessary for adequate mobilization of tissue and of questionable value in stimulating bone formation.

Alar Cartilage

The most difficult problem of all in the cleft lip/nose deformity is the long-term satisfactory repositioning of the LLC to achieve a symmetric nostril. Mulliken[100] states there is a perverse tendency for the genua to slump with time, and permanent elevation of the alar cartilage is almost never seen. Problems related to this are immature and deficient cartilage, fibrofatty tissue between the genua, and adequate support of the cartilage. The genua of the LLC are loosely approximated with fibrous tissue, along with attachments to the ULC, the rim of the maxilla,[138] and fibrous attachments to the skin.[129] It is therefore important to reconstruct these key anatomic points of support to achieve a satisfactory result. The released LLC is reattached in an elevated position to the base of the ULC. Further support is obtained with alar transfixion sutures between cartilage and skin. The fibrofatty tissue is dissected free from between the opposing genua, thus allowing their approximation and support with an absorbable transfixion suture. It is possible that presurgical molding of the LLC may help solve this problem. However, long-term evaluation is currently not available in centers using this approach. An evaluation of the patients who had presurgical cartilage molding also showed a tendency of some relapse over time.

Muscle Reconstruction

Reconstruction of the orbicularis oris muscle is vital to achieve a good appearance for the patient.[139] Developmentally in the cleft embryo, there is a failure of adequate ectomesenchyme penetration migrating along the natural cleavage planes between the mesoderm, ectoderm, and endoderm.[140] This was clearly illustrated by Stark,[141,142] who also noticed a decrease in the numbers of muscle fibers. This is also apparent clinically where the surgeon notes a "poor thin" or "good thick" muscle for repair. Cleft muscle fibers are hypoplastic[126] and have mitochondrial abnormalities.[143] Details of the muscle anatomy are described by Fara,[144] who noted superficial retractor and deep constrictor components and recommended the separate reconstruction of these muscles at the time of surgery. Kernahan[145] noted the bunching up of the muscle in a random disoriented manner with no separate muscle layers. More important, after dissection, the muscle fibers tend to stretch and reorient after lip approximation and release of the fibers. This results in a vertical lengthening of lip that includes muscle and skin.[146]

Release of the lateral orbicularis peripheralis muscle from its skin attachments in a subdermal plane allows stretching and elongation of the muscle when it is approximated to the medial orbicularis peripheralis muscle. The skin is redraped over the muscle. Advocates of the straight-line repair[134] are depending on this principle for lip elongation. By use of the technique of muscle release in a one-stage rotation, cheiloplasty can achieve an increase of up to 4 mm in the vertical length of the lip (see Fig. 93-5C). For this reason, it is important to avoid making any upper incisions of the advancement flap skin until after the muscle is approximated. Appropriate skin incisions are made after muscle approximation to eliminate undesirable incisions around the alar base. Interdigitating or dissection of individual muscle fibers is not done because it is technically difficult and could cause more fibrosis and scarring and a poor result.

It is important to release the abnormally inserted paranasal muscles in the cleft lip that normally attach to the nasal spine.[128] These muscles must be released from the ala along with the facial muscles for the ala to be repositioned without influence of muscle attachment. Joos[147] recommends that these muscles be reattached to the nasal spine. The muscles are small and thin, making isolation and reattachment difficult without tearing the muscle and destroying it. In contrast, dissection and mobilization of the muscles around the alar base and orbicularis peripheralis muscles as a unit or sheet allows easier medial reattachment in a more normal position.

Adjustments at Cheiloplasty

Making the necessary minor adjustments to achieve a satisfactory result is the enjoyment and challenge of cleft surgery. Every cleft is different and always needs minor adjustments. The following are some points that need to be considered and evaluated. Changes are made at the time of surgery when indicated.

LONG VERTICAL LENGTH OF THE CLEFT-SIDE LIP

The anatomic base of the philtral column CPHL′ is usually left where it should be as defined anatomically in the identification of the base of the cleft-side philtral column. The point could be moved medially to shorten the lip, but the problem with this is that the white skin roll frequently becomes indistinct or has a turned-down appearance, and there is less vermilion for reconstruction of deficient vermilion beneath the Cupid's bow. A vertically long lateral lip is avoided first by being aware of the problem during surgical measurement. Second, overrotation of the Cupid's bow must be carefully avoided. In reconstructing the muscle, the first key suture is placed in the muscle opposite points CPHL and CPHL′. After this, the muscle is advanced superiorly, leaving the excess muscle under the nostril or excising it. The skin is then redraped over the shortened muscle to effectively shorten the vertical length of the lip. A long vertical length is uncommon in complete clefts, but it is a frequent problem in incomplete clefts of the primary palate. A horizontal incision is avoided by proper excision of excess skin in the nostril floor.

SHORT VERTICAL LENGTH OF THE CLEFT-SIDE LIP

This is a common problem in most complete clefts. First of all, after adequate release of the orbicularis muscle and approximation of the muscle, the vertical length can be increased 3 to 4 mm. If the lip is still short in its vertical dimension, point CPHL′ can be moved laterally 1 to 2 mm, but only after muscle approximation. This also shortens the horizontal lateral lip length and would be avoided if the lateral lip is also short horizontally; however, horizontal length is always sacrificed when necessary to achieve vertical length. Placement of the C flap tip laterally, just under the ala, is beneficial because it turns the ala inward and will increase the vertical length slightly. Last, a perialar incision can be made; however, this is done as a last resort.

LONG HORIZONTAL LENGTH OF THE CLEFT-SIDE LIP

This is a relatively simple problem. Point CPHL' can be moved as far as necessary laterally to shorten the horizontal lip length.

SHORT HORIZONTAL LENGTH OF THE CLEFT-SIDE LIP

This is an almost impossible problem to solve. Point CPHL' can be moved medially, but that will shorten the vertical length of the lip. Vertical length takes precedence over lateral lip shortness, and vertical length is usually always short, so this should not be done. The alternative is to make everything else very good. After muscle dissection, release, and approximation, the horizontal length of the cleft-side lip will usually increase several millimeters, and a short horizontal length does not look bad compared with a shortened vertical length with peaking of the Cupid's bow.

LONG VERTICAL LENGTH ON THE NONCLEFT SIDE

The vertical length is usually longer on the noncleft side than on the cleft side. Any vertical length over 10 mm of the noncleft-side lip is long and difficult to manage. It is really impossible to correct because the distance from SBAR to CPHR is made up of muscle, mucosa, and skin. To shorten this would entail excising a portion of a full-thickness segment of the lip, and that is not feasible. The Cupid's bow must not be overrotated, and the opposite cleft-side lip needs to be reconstructed to fit the noncleft side as well as possible.

FREE BORDER OF THE LIP—EXCESS OR DEFICIENCY

Whenever the cleft-side lateral lip is too thick on its free margin, a horizontal wedge of orbicularis marginalis with mucosa is excised and closed with a continuous absorbable fine suture. If the lateral lip is too thin or deficient, the mucosa can be released, but this seldom corrects the problem. This needs to be corrected as a secondary procedure with use of temporoparietal fascia to fill out the free border of the lip.

NOSTRIL FLOOR

Preoperative measurement will disclose tissue deficiencies lateral to the base of the columella and medial to the ala. Whenever there is deficient epidermal tissue in these areas, extension of the advancement flap with use of vestibular skin would result in a small nostril.

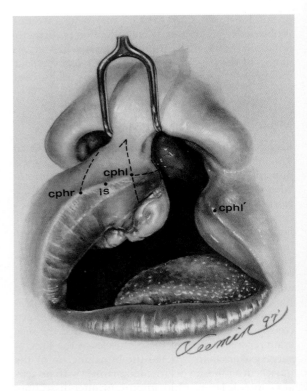

FIGURE 93-35. Mohler's technique—incision lines.

Mohler Repair

The Mohler[148,149] method of unilateral cheiloplasty (Figs. 93-35 to 93-38) is an excellent technique and can be used in most clefts, including incomplete clefts. It is very useful in staged reconstruction of the bilateral asymmetric cleft lip. The Mohler rotation incision should not be used when there is a narrow columella and minimal tissue lateral to the base of the columella. Another possible contraindication is when there is a very short vertical length of the lateral lip between SBAL and point CPHL'. In this situation, the C flap should be brought lateral to a point just under the ala to allow the ala to be rotated inward and to prevent alar flaring.

MARKINGS AND INCISIONS

The columella is fixed and elevated with a wide double hook. The back-cut type of incision starts slightly to the noncleft side of the columella at the columella-lip crease. It extends superiorly for 3 to 4 mm and then down to the cleft side of the Cupid's bow (cphl-3) to match the vertical length of the noncleft-side philtral column. The incision across the free border of the lip must be at right angles to the axis of the free border of the lip (see Fig. 93-35).

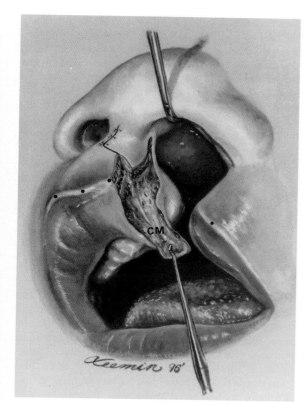

FIGURE 93-36. Incision and rotation of C flap into columella and elevation of mucosal C flap.

C FLAP INCISIONS

C flap incisions are made as previously described. The C flap is rotated inward to fill in the defect and to elongate the columella. It is sutured with fine 7-0 polydioxanone sutures (see Fig. 93-36). The muscle is freed from the overlying skin for a distance of 2 to 3 mm (see Fig. 93-36).

LATERAL INCISIONS

The lateral lip, orbicularis marginalis, orbicularis peripheralis, vermilion flap, and mucosal (T and L flap) incisions are made, and muscle dissection and dissection of the LLC are done as previously described (see Figs. 93-23 to 93-25).

RECONSTRUCTION

All of the flaps are repositioned and sutured (see Fig. 93-37) similar to the repositioned flaps already described (see Figs. 93-26 and 93-27). The free border of the lip is closed (see Fig. 93-29, *insets*), and the alar transfixion sutures are placed (see Fig. 93-32). Essentially, the technique is similar in all aspects to rotation-advancement with the exception of the medial incisions on the lip and columella (see Fig. 93-38).

The advantage of the Mohler technique is that the cleft-side philtral column is placed in a more ideal anatomic position. Also, the lateral advancement skin flap does not need to be advanced as far medially (see

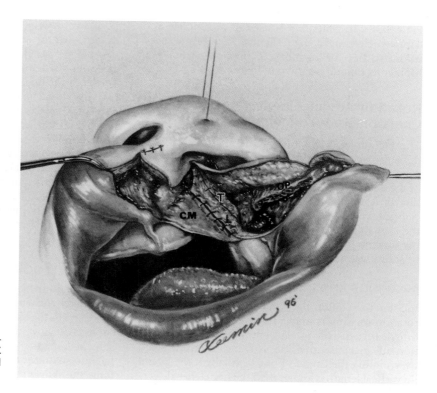

FIGURE 93-37. Mucosal closure after repositioning of the LLC similar to that in Figures 93-16 and 93-24 to 93-28.

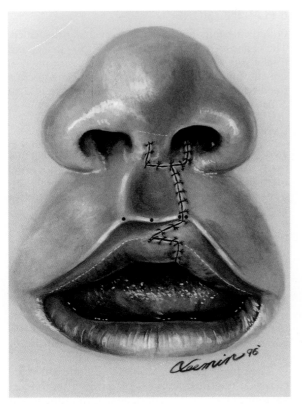

FIGURE 93-38. Complete wound closure with columella elongation; note the laterally positioned philtral column.

Fig. 93-38). In general, it is used in incomplete and complete clefts and is an excellent procedure in a staged reconstruction of asymmetric bilateral clefts. The Mohler technique is shown in Figure 93-39.

Rotation-Advancement Cheiloplasty for Incomplete Clefts

The incomplete cleft lip is sometimes surprisingly difficult to reconstruct. Also, the expectations for a good result are higher. It is important to make measurements of the deformity. The most critical measurements are the vertical height SBAR-CPHL and SBAL-CPHL'. If the cleft-side vertical height is longer than the noncleft side, the cleft side must be shortened. It is important for the surgeon to be aware of this problem so the lip can be shortened in the primary procedure.

MARKINGS AND INCISIONS

Incision lines follow the skin border (Fig. 93-40). The rotation incision is made, followed by release of the muscle for a distance of 3 to 4 mm on the medial rotation-advancement incision. It is important to avoid overrotating the Cupid's bow, especially if the lateral lip vertical length is longer than the noncleft-side vertical length. The OM flap is elevated, and the orbicu-

laris peripheralis muscle is dissected off the maxilla to the base of the ala (Fig. 93-41). The muscle is released from the skin in a subdermal plane from the base of the ala to the base of the philtral column. The dissection of the muscle is continued under and around the base of the ala to release the perialar facial muscles from the base of the ala as previously described (Fig. 93-42).

The alar base is elevated with a small hook to expose the fibrous attachment of the LLC to the piriform rim. The fibrous attachments between LLC and piriform rim are incised under direct vision. This allows the mobilization of the LLC (Fig. 93-42, *inset*). The incision of the vermilion flap on the lateral lip and the fish mouth opening of the lip on the red line beneath the Cupid's bow (see Fig. 93-29, *inset*) complete the dissection.

RECONSTRUCTION

The ala is elevated with an alar suspension suture. The key muscle suture is placed opposite points CPHL and CPHL', and the orbicularis peripheralis muscle is approximated in a fashion similar to that described in the unilateral complete cleft (see Fig. 93-28). A temporary 5-0 polydioxanone suture is placed but not tied from the para-alar facial muscles, nasalis muscle, and depressor septi muscles to the nasal spine and medial musculature. It is tied after closure of the orbicularis peripheralis muscle. If the nostril has a good configuration, nothing is done to the LLC. If not, the LLC is released from the skin (see Fig. 93-27), or if there is fibrofatty tissue between the medial crura, it is removed as indicated through the infracartilaginous incisions (see Fig. 93-34). The white skin roll is approximated at points CPHL and CPHL' (see Fig. 93-30). The free border of the lip is closed (see Fig. 93-29, *inset*).

If the lateral lip is too long, the muscle is advanced, allowing the excessive muscle to be trimmed or placed underneath the nostril floor and ala. This gives additional support to the ala. The free border of the lip and mucosa are closed as previously described. Adequacy of rotation is evaluated; if it is inadequate (see Fig. 93-31), a small triangular flap of skin from the lateral lip is inserted medially to correct the problem (see Fig. 93-31, *inset*). The medial C flap musculature is released and inserted laterally beneath the ala for further support.

NOSTRIL FLOOR AND SKIN CLOSURE

No upper limb incision was made on the advancement flap, thereby leaving redundant skin in the nostril floor. By delaying the skin incision on the nasal floor, the surgeon can now, in a freehand manner, incise the excess skin, keeping the scars short and letting the incision fall into anatomic lines. Also, when the lateral lip is too long, the skin is shortened as needed. Each situation is different, but it is readily apparent where to incise

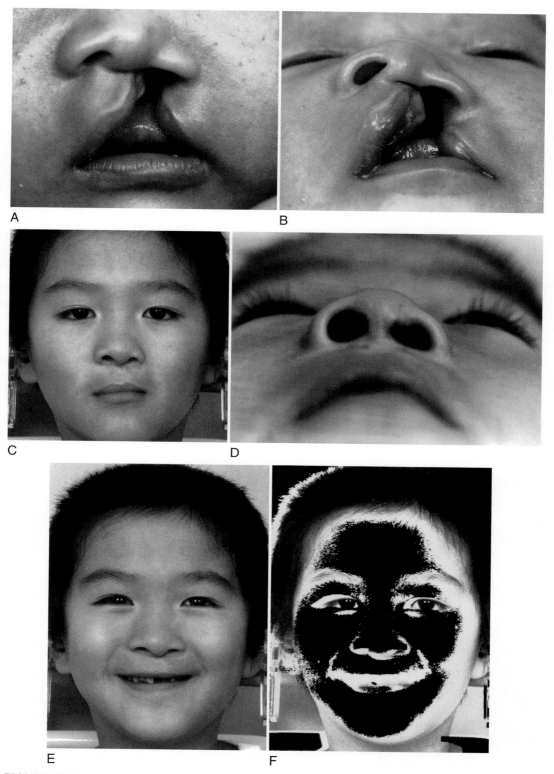

FIGURE 93-39. *A* and *B,* Left complete cleft of the primary and secondary palate at age 1 month (LPC, LSC, 11-19). A Mohler cheiloplasty was done at the age of 3 months. *C* and *D,* Postoperative views at 5 years. *E,* Patient with full smile. *F,* Smile analysis showing relatively good symmetry in both the nose and lip movement.

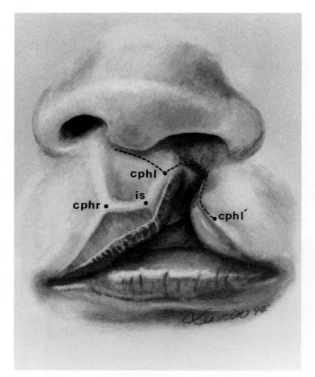

FIGURE 93-40. Markings for incision lines with incision made along the free edge of the skin.

the skin so it will drape over the underlying muscle with no incisions around the ala. The excessive skin on the nostril floor is excised to give a symmetric, appropriately sized nostril (see Fig. 93-30, *inset*). Alar transfixion sutures are placed (see Fig. 93-32), and a silicone nostril conformer is placed (Fig. 93-43).

Tennison Repair

The technique for the Tennison repair is well described by Bardach[150,151] and Randall[52,110] (see Fig. 93-8*D*). Indications for the Tennison cheiloplasty are a wide cleft and high peaking of the Cupid's bow or a vertical deficiency of more than 4 mm between points CPHR and CPHL. Another advantage is that the Tennison cheiloplasty seems to have less hypertrophic scarring. The Tennison cheiloplasty is a good technique that has stood the test of time. Surgeons familiar with this technique can achieve satisfactory results (see Fig. 93-8*D*).

COMPARISON OF REPAIRS. In the Chang Gung Craniofacial Center of four surgeons repairing more than 50 new clefts yearly, one surgeon uses the Tennison repair part of the time. The others use only the standard rotation-advancement cheiloplasty or the Mohler adaptation. The nasoalveolar adhesion cheiloplasty is used in 1% of all clefts after nasoalveolar molding. With presurgical orthopedics of Micropore

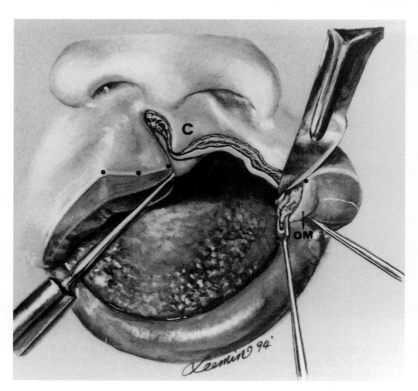

FIGURE 93-41. Elevation of the OM flap from the free edge of the lip to the base of the philtral column, CPHL'.

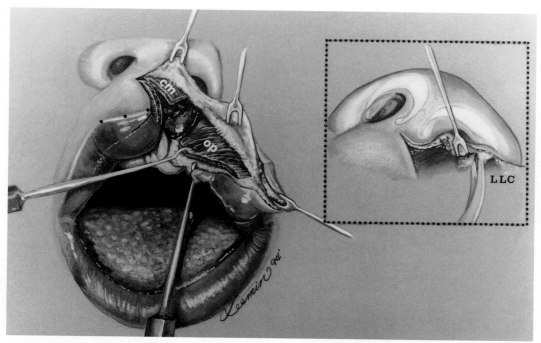

FIGURE 93-42. Release of the orbicularis peripheralis muscle (op) and the muscles around the alar base. *Inset* shows release of the fibrous attachments of the LLC to the piriform rim.

tape and dental plate, an adhesion cheiloplasty was used in 4% of cases. Surgeons tend to became comfortable with a particular type of repair and use it exclusively because of fewer patients or their training. The value of the techniques presented is that certain aspects of the technique can be adapted to any type of cheiloplasty.

POSTOPERATIVE CARE

Immediate postoperative care is monitored in the recovery room. The mother is allowed to enter the recovery room to hold the baby and is given instructions about maintaining the airway. The anesthesiologist approves release of the baby to the ward. The mother and a nursing aide accompany the patient. A nursing specialist gives further instructions about the airway and subsequent care of the infant. Instructions are given for clearing any mucus in the mouth or upper airway. This is done by patting the baby's back periodically after surgery and after feeding. Breast-feeding before and after surgery is encouraged. A soft nipple with good flow is used with bottle feeding. Feeding is started as soon as the baby desires, making sure there is adequate intake the first 24 hours. No arm restrictions are used because they make the baby more irritable.

Wound care is important. The wound is cleaned of any blood or mucus by a normal saline–soaked swab every 2 to 6 hours as necessary. Antibiotic ointment is placed on the suture line after it is cleaned to keep the suture line from drying out or crusting. Ice-cold normal saline sponges placed on the wound seem to reduce pain and swelling. The nasal conformer is placed in the nostril at the time of surgery and is cleaned when the lip is cleaned. The infant and mother are discharged home the day after surgery and seen in the outpatient department in 5 days. At that time, skin sutures are removed with use of oral chloral hydrate as a sedative. The wound is supported with Micropore tape. The patient is usually seen in another week and then periodically until the wound is satisfactory with no evidence of a hypertrophic scar. Postsurgical massage of the lip is usually encouraged to prevent hypertrophic scarring and to hasten wound maturity. A nasal conformer is used for 6 months to 1 year if possible. Success in use of the nasal conformer depends on good cooperation of the parents.

Postsurgical Nasal Molding

Postsurgical molding was first used in 1969 by Osada[152] and Skoog.[93] Osada used a silicone conformer and Skoog an acrylic prosthesis. Friede,[153] using an acrylic conformer, noted improvement in nasal contour. The silicone conformer was subsequently used routinely in many centers to support the LLC during the healing phase, limiting the possibility of contracture and nasal

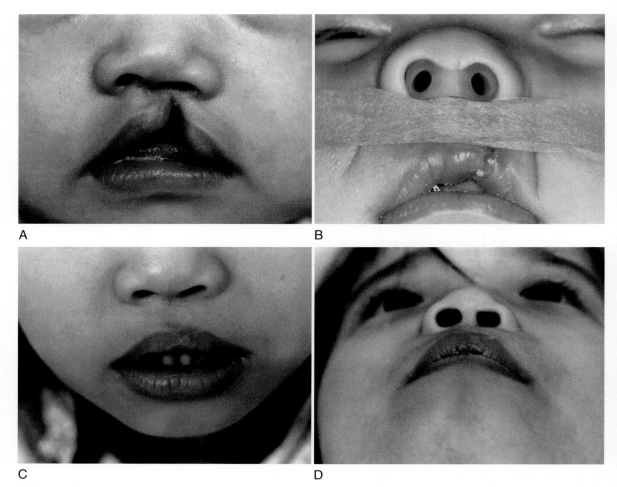

A

B

C

D

FIGURE 93-43. *A,* A 3-month-old Chinese boy with a right incomplete cleft of the primary palate (RPI, 2-3). The cleft-side lip was 3 mm longer than on the noncleft side and was shortened at the initial operation at the age of 3 months. *B,* Immediate postoperative view with nasal conformer. *C* and *D,* Postoperative views at 1 year.

stenosis.[38,101,154,155] The silicone conformer is a logical treatment because nasal wounds tend to be circumferential and more likely to contract.

Matsuo[156,157] first reported presurgical molding in the unilateral incomplete cleft with a Simonart band. At 6 weeks of age, a silicone conformer is inserted into the patient's nostril to improve its shape and contour. It remains there until surgery at the age of 3 months. The conformer is continued full time for 3 months postoperatively and at night up to the age of 12 months (Fig. 93-43*B*). The deformed nasal cartilage is more easily molded while it is still plastic enough to be manipulated.[157]

POSTOPERATIVE COMPLICATIONS

One hundred randomly selected cheiloplasty patients in a 1-year period (1995) were evaluated for postop-

erative complications. There were no instances of wound dehiscence. There were three patients who had a partial separation of the nasal floor that healed without problems or need of subsequent correction. There was a 2% incidence of wound infection that cleared without problems. There was a stitch abscess in 9% and hypertrophic scar in 3% of the patients. There were no instances of bleeding, and there was one prolonged hospitalization of more than 3 days for a urinary tract infection.

POSTOPERATIVE EVALUATION
Function

The postoperative evaluation of the reconstructed cleft lip/nose deformity is based on anatomic anthropometric marks.[35,158-163] A successful restoration of the lip should include both the anatomic alignment and the dynamic physiologic movement.[164,165] The functional movements include sucking, mastication, speech, and facial expression. A normal beautiful smile goes a long way in overcoming a slight abnormality or scar. Facial expressions including the smile are of clinical importance and one of the critical points as judged by patients for the success of lip surgery.[166,167] The upper lip as well as the nasolabial fold plays an important role in making a pleasing, natural smile.[168]

The smile is initiated by raising the upper lip with contraction of the levator labii superioris muscles originating in the nasolabial fold. A full smile involves further raising of the upper lip and nasolabial fold superiorly by the levator labii superioris originating at the infraorbital region, the zygomaticus major, and the superior fibers of the buccinator. The smile is a complicated movement that is difficult to analyze. Smile aesthetics are enhanced by (1) "symmetric" horizontal movement of the upper lip, nasolabial fold, eyelids, and other orofacial muscles, (2) "harmony" of vertical movement between the curvature of the lower lip and the curvature of the incisal edges of the maxillary teeth, and (3) a "good" display of teeth, dentoalveolar process, gingival smile line, and interlabial gap.[167,168] The description of a smile and its beauty is illusive.

Objective evaluation of facial movement has been analyzed by two-dimensional images (e.g., extraoral photography, video camera) or by three-dimensional images (e.g., laser scanning, video-based tracking system). Three-dimensional methods are far more expensive to operate and are unpopular in most craniofacial centers.[166,169,170] Although distortion might be introduced into a two-dimensional image from a three-dimensional object, extraoral photography remains a widely used two-dimensional method to document the face before and after surgical treatment. Image-processing hardware and software are becoming more common and relatively inexpensive.[171]

Digitized two-dimensional photography with a cephalostat head-holding device and desktop computer software* can provide images representing the moving part of the lip. A digital camera† mounted on a tripod at a constant relationship of 125 cm with standard illumination provides standardization for documentation. A sequence of photographs taken at rest (see Fig. 93-40C) with a progressively increasing smile (see Fig. 93-40E and F) are recorded. The digital images are transferred into a computer with pixel subtraction performed by use of Photoshop to see the differential lip movements between rest and smiling positions. The moving part of the lip is illustrated as positive dark spots, the static part as negative white spots (see Fig.

93-40F). The symmetric horizontal and vertical lip movements are clearly elicited by comparing the shape and size of white spots on the left and right sides. The asymmetric or abnormal smile can be accurately assessed with this computer-assisted image-subtraction objective method.

The subtraction two-dimensional image technique provides a readily interpretable, objectively analyzed picture of the functional impairments of the lip for study and evaluation. By this method of functional evaluation, surgical procedures can be evaluated preoperatively and postoperatively to improve surgical techniques. The subtraction two-dimensional image technique offers a practical way to assess the static alignment and dynamic functional movement of the lip.

Aesthetic Assessment

A total of 77 patients with a complete cleft of the lip operated on in 1996 were evaluated by four experienced plastic surgeons to determine whether secondary procedures were needed. The evaluation was made on a 5-point basis:

5. Significant deformity, or just a "bad" result definitely requiring surgery, preferably before schooling.
4. Revision needed after alveolar bone graft.
3. Needs minor revision anytime.
2. Minor deformity; revision possible if requested by parents or child—no immediate concern.
1. No further surgery indicated.

The primary interest in this evaluation was to determine how many patients would need revision. No revision of the nose or lip was indicated in 24% of the children. Thirty-six percent of the patients required a nasal correction. Ten percent needed a lip correction only, and 28% required both a nasal and lip revision. One patient had a significantly poor result that was secondary to hypertrophic scarring. The most common problem was some excess fullness of the free border of the lip. Another lip deformity that needed correction was inadequate rotation of the Cupid's bow. There were no infrasill depressions and vestibular webbing that needed correction. The residual nasal deformity was noted in 64% of patients, and most of these were minimal deformities with nostril hooding or inadequate support of the LLC. This is corrected after alveolar bone grafting when it is minimal; if it is indicated, it is done before schooling at the age of 5 years.

Satisfaction of the Patient

Eighty-five percent of 157 patients who had a secondary nasal correction were satisfied. Continued

*Adobe Photoshop 5.0, Adobe Systems Inc., Mountain View, CA 94043.
†Olympus 2500L, Olympus Optical Co., Tokyo, Japan.

support, including psychological evaluation and speech therapy, is an integral part of the total program for rehabilitation of the cleft person. It requires a multidisciplinary cooperative effort to rehabilitate the cleft person. These aspects of the care and treatment of the cleft person are as vital to the success as the surgical procedure, but they are not in the scope of this discussion. Included in this multidisciplinary approach are education of the parents and discussions between social worker, psychologist, and schoolteachers when indicated.

CORRECTION OF UNSATISFACTORY RESULTS

It is unlikely that any surgeon has a complete success rate without the need for revisions. Major revisions are unlikely, but minor revisions may change a good result into an excellent result. Minor revisions are usually made at the age of 5 years before schooling and with the cooperation of the child. The following are some of the more common minor changes that may need to be addressed.

Peaking of Cupid's Bow

Adequate rotation of the Cupid's bow is probably the most important aspect in achieving a good aesthetic result. Inadequate rotation of the Cupid's bow is corrected at the initial primary procedure by making a horizontal incision just above point CPHL as far as needed to achieve adequate rotation (see Fig. 93-31). An appropriately adequate triangular flap of skin is incised above the base of the lateral advancement flap and inserted into the medial defect to correct the deformity.[38] The white skin roll should not be violated and used as a part of this flap because it is a special type of tissue.[172] Direct approximation of the white skin roll achieves a more normal appearance. There are a number of descriptions for the skin flap in this area, and it is difficult to determine just where they differ.[38,100,173-177] The same technique is used for a secondary correction of an inadequately rotated Cupid's bow (see Fig. 93-31). The objection to use of a small triangular flap above the white skin roll is that it disrupts the philtral column. This is not a problem, and the small 1- to 2-mm triangular flaps heal well without disrupting the philtral column.

Lateral Lip

Excessive rotation of the Cupid's bow, which results in a long lip, is extremely difficult to correct and should be avoided in the primary cheiloplasty. Recognizing a vertically long lateral lip at the time measurements are made and shortening the lip in the initial procedure can prevent this problem. Secondary shortening of a long lip is difficult and requires excision of skin, muscle, and mucosa. The lip muscle must then be fixed to the septal cartilage to prevent drifting and elongation postoperatively.

Secondary correction of a vertically short lateral lip as measured from point SBAL and CPHL′ is difficult, and every effort must be made initially to correct this problem. Any correction will entail a complete opening of the lip and further advancement and rotation of the perialar skin and muscle from the cheek region to a position beneath the ala for elongation of the vertical lip height. At the initial surgery, vertical shortness of the lip is corrected at the expense of horizontal length, which has been described.

Horizontal Shortness of the Lateral Lip

This cannot be corrected. The nature of the deformity in some instances precludes a less than optimal result, and it is important to note this at the time of surgery so the postoperative result can be evaluated in terms of the deformity.[178] The only other possible solution is an Abbe flap, which is rarely used. If used, it should be placed centrally.

Vermilion Deficiency

With use of the triangular vermilion flap from the lateral lip, vermilion deficiencies are rare and seldom need correction (see Figs. 93-29, 93-30, 93-32, *inset*). The problem of the free border deformities after placement of the vermilion flap centrally is not vermilion deficiency but usually failure to trim the muscle or mucosa adequately at the initial surgical procedure. As a secondary procedure, any excess mucosa or muscle is easily excised as indicated.

The free border of the lip consists of orbicularis marginalis muscle, which is covered with vermilion and mucosa (see Fig. 93-20). Failure to reconstruct the vermilion adequately by a straight-line closure of the free border of the lip results in a characteristic deformity (see Fig. 93-22). The vermilion is deficient beneath the cleft side of the Cupid's bow, and the red line is interrupted with a step-off appearance instead of a paralleling red line and white skin roll. Deformities of the free border of the lip are usually described as vermilion deformities in the literature without regard to whether the deformity is a vermilion deficiency (Fig. 93-44), muscle separation, or excess or tight mucosa. Bardach[179] noted that the most common deformity of the lip is notching (Fig. 93-45). These deformities can be prevented in the primary cheiloplasty with use of the vermilion flap. It is impossible to replace lost vermilion because it is a special epithelium.[172] It is important to correct this problem in the initial procedure.

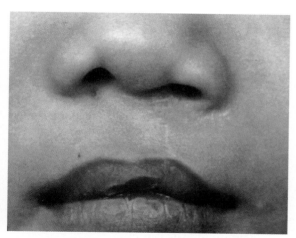

FIGURE 93-44. Free border of the lip deformity with only vermilion deficiency; note the dry mucosa.

Lateral Lip Deficiency

If the lateral lip is thin without a full free border of the orbicularis marginalis muscle, it can be augmented with temporoparietal fascia.[180]

Wide Nostril

As a general rule, it is better to have a nostril that is too large rather than too small.[132] If the nostril is small postoperatively, it can be improved by splinting with a progressively larger silicone conformer. A wide nostril is corrected by a V-Y advancement of the alar base, which should be fixed with an absorbable retention suture between the alar base and the nasal spine.

Hooding Effect in the Soft Triangle on the Nostril Rim

The hooding effect in the soft triangle is corrected by proper repositioning of the LLC. If this is still inadequate, a semilunar excision of the redundant skin in the soft triangle is done. In secondary procedures, this excision should be done only after repositioning of the LLCs.

Inadequate Correction of the Lower Lateral Cartilage

It is impossible to obtain a satisfactory appearance of the nostril in all instances. This is due to cartilage deficiencies, fibrofatty tissue between the medial crura, and weakness of the alar cartilages. At the primary procedure, fibrofatty tissue should be dissected free and the genua fixed to each other with a transfixion suture when indicated. If the alar cartilage slumps after the initial surgery, it is easily corrected with a secondary

open tip rhinoplasty and additional tip support with cartilage strut after the age of 5 years.[1]

Turned-out Alar Base

The flaring out of the alar base gives the nose an unattractive appearance. This is prevented at the time of surgery by making sure that the vestibular floor skin is advanced far enough inside the nose behind the columella. Also, adequate release of the abnormally inserted muscles around the alar base and reconstruction into a normal position support the ala. Secondary correction of this deformity is much more difficult than correction of a wide nostril. It is done in a way similar to correcting a wide nostril. The para-alar muscles tend to cause the ala to drift laterally and inferiorly. The paranasal muscles must be released from the alar base, followed by rotation of the ala inward and a V-Y closure of the nostril floor. A retention suture between the nasal spine and alar base supports the alar base.

Vestibular Webbing

If the LLC is released from the overlying skin, the fibrous attachments going from the LLC to the nasolabial fold area have been severed.[129] These insertions between the LLC and the skin need to be reattached. This is accomplished by alar transfixion sutures, which minimize the vestibular fold, support the LLC, and help define the alar groove. Skin dimpling from the sutures disappears 2 weeks after surgery. Another means of fixation of the skin is with bolster sutures.[181] This deformity is usually associated with distortion of the LLC and corrected at the same time as the rhinoplasty.

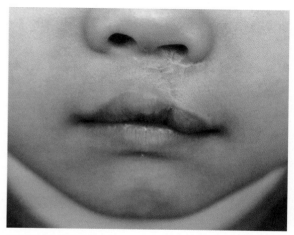

FIGURE 93-45. Free border of the lip deformity with notching (inappropriate muscle closure) and associated vermilion deficiency.

Infrasill Depression

A depression along the upper limb of the advancement flap can occur. This is rare in the technique described. It can be prevented by avoiding inappropriate excision of dermis on the free edge of the advancement flap. Good muscle approximation is also imperative. If correction is needed, it can be done by adequate muscle approximation, insertion of a dermal graft, or fat injection.

SOFT PALATE REPAIR AT TIME OF CLEFT LIP REPAIR

It is frequently reported that early repair of the soft palate induces narrowing of the remaining palatal cleft and thus facilitates later hard palate closure. In a comparative study of closure of cleft lip with or without simultaneous soft palate repair, the addition of simple posterior palatoplasty did not further narrow the cleft or influence palatal arch development. In animal studies, Bardach has shown that simultaneous palatoplasty and cheiloplasty have an adverse effect on growth.[182-184]

RHINOPLASTY

Correction of the nasal deformity in cleft lip patients is a challenging problem to every surgeon. The deformity is notorious for its resistance to surgical correction because it involves all the components of the nose, including coverage, support, and lining, and it is difficult to correct all these problems in a single operation. Primary nasal reconstruction is done in the initial repair. Previous reports on the long-term primary nasal correction do not show any adverse effect on growth.[185,186]

In considering secondary nasal correction, a balanced skeletal base is the key factor for achieving a satisfactory result. Whenever possible, the hypoplastic maxilla with an asymmetric base for the nose must be corrected before a rhinoplasty is performed. This requires a combined evaluation and discussion between the orthodontist and plastic surgeon. Evaluations by lay persons and plastic surgeons are equally important in determining surgical intervention.[163] With the technique of distraction osteogenesis,[57,58] the skeletal deformity can be corrected at an earlier age. Minor degrees of an asymmetric alar base can be corrected orthodontically, but the more severe discrepancy between the greater and lesser segments can only be corrected surgically with orthognathic surgery or distraction osteogenesis.

Alveolar bone grafting, including bone placed into the cleft and piriform area for alar base support, repairs the alveolar cleft. This surgery is done around the time of eruption of the permanent central incisor or canine tooth. In some instances, patients will refuse orthognathic surgery; in these situations, a corrective rhinoplasty is still indicated to improve facial features and the psychological impact of an unsatisfactory aesthetic appearance.

An open tip rhinoplasty[1] is used to correct the nasal deformity in most patients. The procedure can provide undistorted exposure to the cartilages and bony framework. The pathologic deformities are addressed in a systematic approach and precise fashion by a combination of several rhinoplasty procedures and also considering the patient's age. The following points are important to achieve a good correction:

- Symmetric dissection of covering skin
- Adequate release of any deficient mucosal lining with different techniques, including a Potter VY-plasty[187] of the LLC, vestibular triangular flap, and inferior turbinate flap
- Adequate mobilization of the deformed LLC with release of the interdomal ligaments, longitudinal fibers between the LLC and ULC, and lateral attachment to the piriform rim
- Use of a strong cartilaginous septal columellar strut
- Correction of columellar deficiency and careful reshaping of the nostril hood
- Alar transfixion sutures for support
- Septal plasty when indicated

At present, a satisfactory result is obtained in almost all cases.

SUMMARY

The treatment of the cleft lip/palate patient continues to evolve with, it is hoped, better results in all areas—functional, aesthetic, and psychological-spiritual. The current general overall concept is that passive movement of the maxillary arches is more physiologic than a rapid forced movement. Early presurgical orthopedics with nasal conformer is a useful addition to the treatment of the cleft infant. It achieves the benefits of repositioning the maxillary segments to a close approximation, making it easier for the surgeon, and helps mold the nasal cartilages to achieve a potentially better nasal symmetry.[81] However, the long-term effects of this nasal molding are lacking. The long-term effects of primary nasal cartilage surgery are good.[181,185] On this basis, the addition of nasal molding should not be detrimental but an advantage because there is less need for the surgical manipulation of the LLC to achieve a satisfactory result.

Gingivoperiosteoplasty is performed in the Chang Gung Craniofacial Center but in limited numbers. The expense and time involved pose a significant financial problem for most families, including time off work and travel expenses during the time required to mobilize the maxillary arches into a touch position for gingivoperiosteoplasty. It requires a dedicated, experienced orthodontist. The addition of the gingivoperiosteoplasty to the primary procedure is still controversial. There are no reports of results after mixed dentition. In the most extensive study,[188] it was considered a questionable procedure. Bone formation was considered adequate in 60% of a small group of patients[189]; however, there is still probably a need for additional bone placed in the piriform area to achieve a satisfactory aesthetic result.

The caregiver may be limited to simpler methods of treatment by necessity of availability of supportive care, as in developing countries. At the Chang Gung Craniofacial Center, these choices are given to the parents with explanation of the cost and time involved to make them a part of the decision process. Every attempt is made to meet financial costs of the indigent patient through financial support from foundations. Regardless, there is no surgeon who can obtain a 100% satisfactory result because of inherent growth problems, the great variance of tissue deficiencies (cartilage, bone, and soft tissue), and the degree of cooperation of parents and patients.

The care and treatment of the cleft lip/palate person represent a lifetime commitment and continue to be a challenge for all involved.

Acknowledgments

Contributions to this chapter were made by medical illustrator Lee-Min Lee and by the following members of the Chang Gung Craniofacial Center: Daniel C.S. Huang, DDS, PhD; Lun-Jou Lo, MD; Kai-Fong Hung, MD; Eric J.W. Liou, DDS, MS; and Wen-Yuan Lin, DDS. Alex Kane, MD, Assistant Professor, Washington University School of Medicine, Division of Plastic Surgery, St. Louis Children's Hospital, contributed as well. The nursing specialists are also appreciated for their dedicated care of our patients, as are the coordinators of the Craniofacial Center for their dedication to record keeping and education of parents. Finally, we are grateful to the patients and parents who give our work meaning.

REFERENCES

1. Chen KT, Noordhoff MS: Open tip rhinoplasty. Ann Plast Surg 1992;28:119-130.
2. Stoll C, Alembik Y, Dott B, Roth MP: Associated malformations in cases with oral clefts. Cleft Palate Craniofac J 2000;37:41-47.
3. Stoll C, Dott B, Alembik Y, Roth M: Evaluation of prenatal diagnosis of cleft lip/palate by foetal ultrasonographic examination. Ann Genet 2000;43:11-14.
4. Lopoo JB, Hedrick MH, Chasen S, et al: Natural history of fetuses with cleft lip. Plast Reconstr Surg 1999;103:34-38.
5. Hafner E, Sterniste W, Scholler J, et al: Prenatal diagnosis of facial malformations. Prenat Diagn 1997;17:51-58.
6. Devonald KJ, Ellwood DA, Griffiths KA, et al: Volume imaging: three-dimensional appreciation of the fetal head and face. J Ultrasound Med 1995;14:919-925.
7. Pretorius DH, House M, Nelson TR, Hollenbach KA: Evaluation of normal and abnormal lips in fetuses: comparison between three- and two-dimensional sonography. AJR Am J Roentgenol 1995;165:1233-1237.
8. Oberg KC, Robles AE, Ducsay C, et al: Endoscopic excision and repair of simulated bilateral cleft lips in fetal lambs [see comments]. Plast Reconstr Surg 1998;102:1-9.
9. Fogh-Andersen P: Inheritance of Harelip and Cleft Palate. Copenhagen, Nyt Nordisk Forlag, 1942.
10. Fraser FC: The William Allan Memorial Award Address: evolution of a palatable multifactorial threshold model. Am J Hum Genet 1980;32:796-813.
11. McKusick VA: OMIM: Online Mendelian Inheritance in Man. McKusick-Nathans Institute for Genetic Medicine, Johns Hopkins University and National Center for Biotechnology Information, National Library of Medicine.
12. Spritz RA: The genetics and epigenetics of orofacial clefts. Curr Opin Pediatr 2001;13:556-560.
13. Jones MC: Facial clefting. Etiology and developmental pathogenesis. Clin Plast Surg 1993;20:599-606.
14. Vieira AR, Orioli IM: Candidate genes for nonsyndromic cleft lip and palate. ASDC J Dent Child 2001;68:272-279, 229.
15. Christensen K, Fogh-Andersen P: Cleft lip (± cleft palate) in Danish twins, 1970-1990. Am J Med Genet 1993;47:910-916.
16. Lin YC, Lo LJ, Noordhoff MS, Chen YR: Cleft of the lip and palate in twins. Changgeng Yi Xue Za Zhi 1999;22:61-67.
17. Rollnick BR, Pruzansky S: Genetic services at a center for craniofacial anomalies. Cleft Palate J 1981;18:304-313.
18. Derijcke A, Eerens A, Carels C: The incidence of oral clefts: a review. Br J Oral Maxillofac Surg 1996;34:488-494.
19. Czeizel A: Studies of cleft lip and cleft palate in east European populations. Prog Clin Biol Res 1980;46:249-296.
20. Tolarova M: Orofacial clefts in Czechoslovakia. Incidence, genetics and prevention of cleft lip and palate over a 19-year period. Scand J Plast Reconstr Surg Hand Surg 1987;21:19-25.
21. Curtis E, Fraser FC, Warburton D: Congenital cleft lip and palate: risk figures for counseling. Am J Dis Child 1961;102:853-857.
22. Wyszynski DF, Beaty TH, Maestri NE: Genetics of nonsyndromic oral clefts revisited. Cleft Palate Craniofac J 1996;33:406-417.
23. Melnick M, Bixler D, Fogh-Andersen P, Conneally PM: Cleft lip ± cleft palate: an overview of the literature and an analysis of Danish cases born between 1941 and 1968. Am J Med Genet 1980;6:83-97.
24. Prescott NJ, Winter RM, Malcolm S: Nonsyndromic cleft lip and palate: complex genetics and environmental effects. Ann Hum Genet 2001;65:505-515.
25. Ardinger HH, Buetow KH, Bell GI, et al: Association of genetic variation of the transforming growth factor-alpha gene with cleft lip and palate. Am J Hum Genet 1989;45:348-353.
26. Lidral AC, Romitti PA, Basart AM, et al: Association of MSX1 and TGFB3 with nonsyndromic clefting in humans. Am J Hum Genet 1998;63:557-568.
27. Chenevix-Trench G, Jones K, Green AC, et al: Cleft lip with or without cleft palate: associations with transforming growth factor alpha and retinoic acid receptor loci. Am J Hum Genet 1992;51:1377-1385.
28. Wyszynski DF, Maestri N, McIntosh I, et al: Evidence for an association between markers on chromosome 19q and nonsyndromic cleft lip with or without cleft palate in two groups of multiplex families. Hum Genet 1997;99:22-26.
29. Veau V: Division Palatine. Paris, Masson, 1931.
30. Kernahan DA: The striped Y—a symbolic classification for cleft lip and palate. Plast Reconstr Surg 1971;47:469-470.
31. Noordhoff MS, Huang CS, Wu J: Multidisciplinary management of cleft lip and palate in Taiwan. In Bardach J, Morris HL, eds: Multidisciplinary Management of Cleft Lip and Palate. Philadelphia, WB Saunders, 1990:18-26.
32. Noordhoff MS: Response to Kernahan's commentary on symbolic representation of cleft lip and palate by Friedman et al (1991) [letter]. Cleft Palate Craniofac J 1992;29:96.
33. Noordhoff MS, Huang CS, Lo LJ: Median facial dysplasia in unilateral and bilateral cleft lip and palate: a subgroup of median cerebrofacial malformations. Plast Reconstr Surg 1993;91:996-1005, discussion 1006-1007.

34. Fisher DM, Lo LJ, Chen YR, Noordhoff MS: Three-dimensional computed tomographic analysis of the primary nasal deformity in 3-month-old infants with complete unilateral cleft lip and palate. Plast Reconstr Surg 1999;103:1826-1834.

35. Farkas LG, Hajnis K, Posnick JC: Anthropometric and anthroposcopic findings of the nasal and facial region in cleft patients before and after primary lip and palate repair. Cleft Palate Craniofac J 1993;30:1-12.

36. Millard DR Jr: The unilateral deformity. In Millard DR Jr, ed: Cleft Craft—The Evolution of Its Surgery, vol I. Boston, Little, Brown, 1976.

37. Noordhoff MS: Reconstruction of vermilion in unilateral and bilateral cleft lips. Plast Reconstr Surg 1984;73:52-61.

38. Noordhoff MS, Chen YR, Chen KT, et al: The surgical technique for the complete unilateral cleft lip—nasal deformity. Operative Techniques Plast Reconstr Surg 1995;2:167-174.

39. Pool R: The configurations of the unilateral cleft lip, with reference to the rotation advancement repair. Plast Reconstr Surg 1966;37:558-565.

40. Kernahan DA, Bauer BS: Functional cleft lip repair: a sequential, layered closure with orbicularis muscle realignment. Plast Reconstr Surg 1983;72:459-467.

41. Millard DR Jr: Rotation-advancement principle in cleft lip closure. Cleft Palate J 1964;1:246-252.

42. Boo-Chai K: Ancient Chinese text on a cleft lip. Plast Reconstr Surg 1966;38:89.

43. Rose W: On Harelip and Cleft Palate. London, H. K. Lewis, 1891.

44. Thompson JE: An artistic and mathematically accurate method of repairing the defects in cases of harelip. Surg Gynecol Obstet 1912;14:498.

45. Mirault G: Deux lettres sur l'operation du bec-de-lievre. J Chir Paris 1844;2:257.

46. Blair VP, Brown JB: Mirault operation for single harelip. Surg Gynecol Obstet 1930;51:81.

47. Brown JB, McDowell F: Simplified design for repair of single cleft lips. Surg Gynecol Obstet 1945;80:12-26.

48. Jalaguier: A propos de la staphylorrhaphie. Bull Mem Soc Chir Paris 1922.

49. Hagedorn WH: A modification of the harelip operation. The classic reprint. Plast Reconstr Surg 1884;58:89-91.

50. LeMesurier AB: A method of cutting and suturing the lip in the treatment of complete unilateral clefts. Plast Reconstr Surg 1949;4:1-12.

51. Tennison CW: The repair of the unilateral cleft lip by the stencil method. Plast Reconstr Surg 1952;9:11.

52. Randall P: A triangular flap operation for the primary repair of unilateral clefts of the lip. Plast Reconstr Surg 1959;23:331-347.

53. Millard DR Jr: The primary camouflage of the unilateral harelook. In Skoog T, Ivy R, eds: Transactions of the International Society of Plastic Surgeons, First Congress, Stockholm, 1955. Baltimore, Williams & Wilkins, 1957:160-166.

54. Millard DR Jr: A radical rotation in single harelip. Am J Surg 1958;95:318-322.

55. Millard DR, Latham R, Huifen X, et al: Cleft lip and palate treated by presurgical orthopedics, gingivoperiosteoplasty, and lip adhesion (POPLA) compared with previous lip adhesion method: a preliminary study of serial dental casts. Plast Reconstr Surg 1999;103:1630-1644.

56. Sommerlad BC, Henley M, Birch M, et al: Cleft palate re-repair—a clinical and radiographic study of 32 consecutive cases. Br J Plast Surg 1994;47:406-410.

57. Polley JW, Figueroa AA: Rigid external distraction: its application in cleft maxillary deformities. Plast Reconstr Surg 1998;102:1360-1372, discussion 1373-1374.

58. Figueroa AA, Polley JW, Ko EW: Maxillary distraction for the management of cleft maxillary hypoplasia with a rigid external distraction system. Semin Orthod 1999;5:46-51.

59. Pool R, Farnworth TK: Preoperative lip taping in the cleft lip. Ann Plast Surg 1994 32:243-249.

60. Liou E, Chen K, Huang CS: A modified technique in presurgical columella lengthening in bilateral cleft lip and palate patients. Fourth Asian Pacific Cleft Lip and Palate Conference, Fukuoka, Japan, 1999.

61. Grayson BH, Santiago PE, Brecht LE, Cutting CB: Presurgical nasoalveolar molding in infants with cleft lip and palate. Cleft Palate Craniofac J 1999;36:486-498.

62. McNeil C: Orthodontic procedures in the treatment of congenital cleft plate. Dent Rec 1950;70:126.

63. McNeil C: Congenital oral deformities. Br Dent J 1956;101:191.

64. Brogan WF: Cleft lip and palate. The state of the art. Ann R Australas Coll Dent Surg 1986;9:172-184.

65. Brogan WF: Effect of presurgical infant orthopedics on facial esthetics in complete bilateral cleft lip and palate [letter; comment]. Cleft Palate Craniofac J 1994;31:410-411.

66. Hotz MM, Gnoinski WM: Effects of early maxillary orthopaedics in coordination with delayed surgery for cleft lip and palate. J Maxillofac Surg 1979;7:201-210.

67. Hotz MM, Gnoinski WM, Nussbaumer H, Kistler E: Early maxillary orthopedics in CLP cases: guidelines for surgery. Cleft Palate J 1978;15:405-411.

68. Hotz M, Gnoinski W, Perko M, et al: Early Treatment of Cleft Lip and Palate. Toronto, Hans Huber, 1986.

69. Asher-McDade C, Shaw WC: Current cleft lip and palate management in the United Kingdom. Br J Plast Surg 1990;43:318-321.

70. McComb H: Primary correction of unilateral cleft lip nasal deformity: a 10-year review. Plast Reconstr Surg 1985;75:791-799.

71. Huddart AJ, North JF, Davis MEH: Observations on the treatment of cleft lip and palate. Dent Pract 1966;16:265.

72. Ross RB: The clinical implications of facial growth in cleft lip and palate. Cleft Palate J 1970;7:37-47.

73. Winters JC, Hurwitz DJ: Presurgical orthopedics in the surgical management of unilateral cleft lip and palate. Plast Reconstr Surg 1995;95:755-764.

74. Mazaheri M, Harding RL, Cooper JA, et al: Changes in arch form and dimensions of cleft patients. Am J Orthod 1971;60:19-32.

75. Huang CS, Cheng HC, Chen YR, Noordhoff MS: Maxillary dental arch affected by different sleep positions in unilateral complete cleft lip and palate infants. Cleft Palate Craniofac J 1994;31:179-184.

76. Hotz M, Gnoinski W: Comprehensive care of cleft lip and palate children at Zurich University: a preliminary report. Am J Orthod 1976;70:481-504.

77. Latham RA: Orthopedic advancement of the cleft maxillary segment: a preliminary report. Cleft Palate J 1980;17:227-233.

78. Latham RA, Kusy RP, Georgiade NG: An extraorally activated expansion appliance for cleft palate infants. Cleft Palate J 1976;13:253-261.

79. Jorgensen RJ, Salinas CF, Hirsch H: The pin retained palatal prosthesis and its influence on the dentition. J Dent Res 1979;58:1570.

80. Cutting C, Grayson B, Brecht L, et al: Presurgical columellar elongation and primary retrograde nasal reconstruction in one-stage bilateral cleft lip and nose repair [see comments]. Plast Reconstr Surg 1998;101:630-639.

81. Bennun RD, Perandones C, Sepliarsky VA, et al: Nonsurgical correction of nasal deformity in unilateral complete cleft lip: a 6-year follow-up. Plast Reconstr Surg 1999;104:616-630.

82. Grayson B, Santiago P, Brecht L: Presurgical orthopedics for cleft lip and palate. In Aston S, Beasley C, Thorne C, eds: Grabb and Smith's Plastic Surgery. Philadelphia, Lippincott-Raven, 1997:237-244.

83. Grayson BH, Cutting C, Wood R: Preoperative columella lengthening in bilateral cleft lip and palate [letter]. Plast Reconstr Surg 1993;92:1422-1423.

84. Kenny FM, Angsusingha K, Stinson D, Hotchkiss J: Unconjugated estrogens in the perinatal period. Pediatr Res 1973;7:826-831.

85. Hardingham TE, Muir H: The specific interaction of hyaluronic acid with cartilage proteoglycans. Biochim Biophys Acta 1972;279:401-405.

86. Friede H, Johanson B: A follow-up study of cleft children treated with primary bone grafting. 1. Orthodontic aspects. Scand J Plast Reconstr Surg 1974;8:88-103.

87. Millard DR Jr: Adaptation of the rotation-advancement principles in bilateral cleft lip. Transactions of the International Society of Plastic Surgeons, 2nd Congress, London, 1959. Edinburgh, E & S Livingstone, 1960.

88. Rosenstein S, Dado DV, Kernahan D, et al: The case for early bone grafting in cleft lip and palate: a second report. Plast Reconstr Surg 1991;87:644-654, discussion 655-656.

89. Dado DV, Rosenstein SW, Alder ME, Kernahan DA: Long-term assessment of early alveolar bone grafts using three-dimensional computer-assisted tomography: a pilot study. Plast Reconstr Surg 1997;99:1840-1845.

90. Semb G: Effect of alveolar bone grafting on maxillary growth in unilateral cleft lip and palate patients. Cleft Palate J 1988;25:288-295.

91. Abyholm F, Bergland O, Semb G: Secondary bone grafting of alveolar clefts. A surgical/orthodontic treatment enabling a nonprosthodontic rehabilitation in cleft lip and palate patients. Scand J Plast Reconstr Surg 1981;15:127-140.

92. Skoog T: The use of periosteum and Surgicel for bone restoration in congenital clefts of the maxilla. Scand J Plast Reconstr Surg 1967;1:113-130.

93. Skoog T: Repair of unilateral cleft lip deformity: maxilla, nose and lip. Scand J Plast Reconstr Surg 1969;3:109-133.

94. Hellquist R, Skoog T: The influence of primary periosteoplasty on maxillary growth and deciduous occlusion in cases of complete unilateral cleft lip and palate. A longitudinal study from infancy to the age of 5. Scand J Plast Reconstr Surg 1976;10:197-208.

95. Tomanova M, Mullerova Z: Growth of the dental arch in patients with complete unilateral cleft lip and palate after primary periosteoplasty. Acta Chir Plast 1994;36:119-123.

96. Rintala AE, Ranta R: Periosteal flaps and grafts in primary cleft repair: a follow-up study. Plast Reconstr Surg 1989;83:17-24.

97. Millard DR Jr: Embryonic rationale for the primary correction of classical congenital clefts of the lip and palate. Ann R Coll Surg Engl 1994;76:150-160.

98. Millard DR Jr, Latham RA: Improved primary surgical and dental treatment of clefts. Plast Reconstr Surg 1990;86:856-871.

99. Armstrong GT, Burk RW 3rd, Griffin DW, Howard PS: A modification of the primary nasal correction in the rotation-advancement unilateral cleft lip repair. Ann Plast Surg 1997;38:236-245.

100. Mulliken JB, Martinez-Perez D: The principle of rotation advancement for repair of unilateral complete cleft lip and nasal deformity: technical variations and analysis of results. Plast Reconstr Surg 1999;104:1247-1260.

101. Shah JS: Stenosis of the nostrils: a case report, following smallpox. Plast Reconstr Surg 1967;39:57-58.

102. Wood RJ, Grayson BH, Cutting CB: Gingivoperiosteoplasty and midfacial growth [see comments]. Cleft Palate Craniofac J 1997;34:17-20.

103. Lukash FN, Schwartz M, Grauer S, Tuminelli F: Dynamic cleft maxillary orthopedics and periosteoplasty: benefit or detriment? Ann Plast Surg 1998;40:321-326, discussion 326-327.

104. Henkel KO, Gundlach KK: Analysis of primary gingivoperiosteoplasty in alveolar cleft repair. Part I. Facial growth. J Craniomaxillofac Surg 1997;25:266-269.

105. Brusati R, Mannucci N: The early gingivoalveoloplasty. Preliminary results. Scand J Plast Reconstr Surg Hand Surg 1992;26:65-70.

106. Johanson B: Die Osteoplastik bei Spatbehandlung der Lippen-Kiefer-Gaummenspalten. Arch Klin Chir 1960;295:876.

107. Witt PD, Hardesty RA: Rotation-advancement repair of the unilateral cleft lip. One center's perspective. Clin Plast Surg 1993;20:633-645.

108. Huebener DV, Marsh JL: Alveolar molding appliances in the treatment of cleft lip and palate infants. In Bardach J, Morris HL, eds: Multidisciplinary Management of Cleft Lip and Palate. Philadelphia, WB Saunders, 1990:601-607.

109. Takahashi S: Lip adhesion operation. Jpn J Oral Surg 1970;16:68.

110. Randall P: Cleft lip. Clin Plast Surg 1975;2:215-233.

111. Rintala A, Haataja J: The effect of the lip adhesion procedure on the alveolar arch. With special reference to the type and width of the cleft and the age at operation. Scand J Plast Reconstr Surg 1979;13:301-304.

112. Randall P: A lip adhesion operation in cleft lip surgery. Plast Reconstr Surg 1965;35:371.

113. Walker JC Jr, Collito MB, Mancusi-Ungaro A, Meijer R: Physiologic considerations in cleft lip closure: the C-W technique. Plast Reconstr Surg 1966;37:552-557.

114. Lesavoy MA: Lip adhesion in unilateral and bilateral cleft lip repair. In Bardach J, Morris HL, eds: Multidisciplinary Management of Cleft Lip and Palate. Philadelphia, WB Saunders, 1990:166-173.

115. Seibert RW: The role of adhesions in cleft lip repair. J Ark Med Soc 1980;77:139.

116. Cohen SR, Corrigan M, Wilmot J, Trotman CA: Cumulative operative procedures in patients aged 14 years and older with unilateral or bilateral cleft lip and palate. Plast Reconstr Surg 1995;96:267-271.

117. Bardach J, Bakowska J, McDermott-Murray J, et al: Lip pressure changes following lip repair in infants with unilateral clefts of the lip and palate. Plast Reconstr Surg 1984;74:476-481.

118. Bardach J, Mooney MP: The relationship between lip pressure following lip repair and craniofacial growth: an experimental study in beagles. Plast Reconstr Surg 1984;73:544-555.

119. Bardach J, Kelly KM: The influence of lip repair with and without soft-tissue undermining on facial growth in beagles [see comments]. Plast Reconstr Surg 1988;82:747-759.

120. Nagase T, Januszkiewicz JS, Keall HJ, de Geus JJ: The effect of muscle repair on postoperative facial skeletal growth in children with bilateral cleft lip and palate. Scand J Plast Reconstr Surg Hand Surg 1998;32:395-405.

121. Kapucu MR, Gursu KG, Enacar A, Aras S: The effect of cleft lip repair on maxillary morphology in patients with unilateral complete cleft lip and palate. Plast Reconstr Surg 1996;97:1371-1375, discussion 1376-1378.

122. Bardach J: Discussion: the effect of cleft lip repair on maxillary morphology in patients with unilateral complete cleft lip and palate. Plast Reconstr Surg 1996;97:1376-1378.

123. VanderWoude DL, Mulliken JB: Effect of lip adhesion on labial height in two-stage repair of unilateral complete cleft lip. Plast Reconstr Surg 1997;100:567-572, discussion 573-574.

124. Millard DR Jr: Refinements in rotation advancement cleft lip technique. Plast Reconstr Surg 1964;33:26-38.

125. Millard DR Jr: How to rotate and advance in a complete cleft. In Millard DR Jr, ed: Cleft Craft—The Evolution of Its Surgery, vol I. The Unilateral Deformity. Boston, Little, Brown, 1976:449-486.

126. Dado DV, Kernahan DA: Anatomy of the orbicularis oris muscle in incomplete unilateral cleft lip based on histological examination. Ann Plast Surg 1985;15:90-98.

127. Delaire J: Theoretical principles and technique of functional closure of the lip and nasal aperture. J Maxillofac Surg 1978;6:109-116.

128. Joos U: Muscle reconstruction in primary cleft lip surgery. J Craniomaxillofac Surg 1989;17(suppl 1):8-10.

129. Wu WTL: The Oriental nose: an anatomical basis for surgery. Ann Acad Med Singapore 1992;21:176-189.

130. Pigott RW: "Alar leapfrog." A technique for repositioning the total alar cartilage at primary cleft lip repair. Clin Plast Surg 1985;12:643-658.

131. Salyer KE: Primary correction of the unilateral cleft lip nose: a 15-year experience. Plast Reconstr Surg 1986;77:558-568.

132. Salyer KE: Early and late treatment of unilateral cleft nasal deformity. Cleft Palate Craniofac J 1992;29:556-569.

133. Anderl H: Simultaneous repair of lip and nose in the unilateral cleft (a long term report). In Jackson IT, Sommerlad BC, eds: Recent Advances in Plastic Surgery. New York, Churchill Livingstone, 1985:1-11.

134. Furnas DW: Straight-line closure: a preliminary to Millard closure in unilateral cleft lips (with a history of the straight-line closure, including the Mirault misunderstanding). Clin Plast Surg 1984;11:701-737.

135. Delaire J, Precious DS, Gordeef A: The advantage of wide subperiosteal exposure in primary surgical correction of labial maxillary clefts. Scand J Plast Reconstr Surg Hand Surg 1988;22:147-151.

136. Trott JA: Synchronous open rhinoplasty and primary unilateral cleft-lip repair: Trott's technique. In Bardach J, Salyer KE, eds: Atlas of Craniofacial and Cleft Surgery, vol 2. Philadelphia, Lippincott-Raven, 1999:464-471.

137. Chen PK, Yeow VK, Noordhoff MS, Chen YR: Augmentation of the nasal floor with Surgicel in primary lip repair: a prospective study showing no efficacy. Ann Plast Surg 1999;42:149-153.

138. Janeke JB, Wright WK: Studies on the support of the nasal tip. Arch Otolaryngol 1971;93:458-464.

139. Pennisi VR, Shadish WR, Klabunde EH: Orbicularis oris muscle in cleft lip repair. Cleft Palate J 1969;6:141.

140. Moore KL, Persaud TVN: The Developing Human: Clinically Oriented Embryology. Philadelphia, WB Saunders, 1998.

141. Stark RB: Development of the face. Surg Gynecol Obstet 1973;137:403-408.

142. Stark RB, Kaplan JM: Development of the cleft lip nose. Plast Reconstr Surg 1973;51:413-415.

143. Schendel SA, Cholon A, Delaire J: Histochemical analysis of cleft palate muscle. Plast Reconstr Surg 1994;94:919-923.

144. Fara M: Anatomy and arteriography of cleft lips in stillborn children. Plast Reconstr Surg 1968;42:29.

145. Kernahan DA, Dado DV, Bauer BS: The anatomy of the orbicularis oris muscle in unilateral cleft lip based on a three-dimensional histologic reconstruction. Plast Reconstr Surg 1984;73:875-881.

146. Dado DV: Experience with the functional cleft lip repair. Plast Reconstr Surg 1990;86:872.

147. Joos U: The importance of muscular reconstruction in the treatment of cleft lip and palate. Scand J Plast Reconstr Surg Hand Surg 1987;21:109-113.

148. Mohler L: Unilateral cleft lip repair. Operative Techniques Plast Reconstr Surg 1995;2:193-199.

149. Mohler LR: Unilateral cleft lip repair. Plast Reconstr Surg 1987;80:511-517.

150. Bardach J: Unilateral cleft lip/nose repair: Bardach's technique. Operative Techniques Plast Reconstr Surg 1995;2:187-192.

151. Bardach J: Primary unilateral cleft-lip/nose repair: Bardach's technique. In Bardach J, Salyer KE, eds: Atlas of Craniofacial and Cleft Surgery, vol 2. Philadelphia, Lippincott-Raven, 1999:434-463.

152. Osada M, Hashimoto K, Akiyama T: Application of intra and extra nasal silicone prosthesis after the operation of nasal deformities. Jpn J Plast Reconstr Surg 1969;11:191.

153. Friede H, Lilja J, Johanson B: Lip-nose morphology and symmetry in unilateral cleft lip and palate patients following a two-stage lip closure. Scand J Plast Reconstr Surg 1980;14:55-64.

154. Nakajima T, Yoshimura Y, Sakakibara A: Augmentation of the nostril splint for retaining the corrected contour of the cleft lip nose. Plast Reconstr Surg 1990;85:182-186.

155. Walter C: Nasal deformities in cleft lip cases. Facial Plast Surg 1995;11:169-183.

156. Matsuo K, Hirose T: Nonsurgical correction of cleft lip nasal deformity in the early neonate. Ann Acad Med Singapore 1988;17:358-365.

157. Matsuo K, Hirose T, Otagiri T, Norose N: Repair of cleft lip with nonsurgical correction of nasal deformity in the early neonatal period. Plast Reconstr Surg 1989;83:25-31.

158. Hurwitz DJ, Ashby ER, Llull R, et al: Computer-assisted anthropometry for outcome assessment of cleft lip. Plast Reconstr Surg 1999;103:1608-1623.

159. Coghlan BA, Laitung JK, Pigott RW: A computer-aided method of measuring nasal symmetry in the cleft lip nose [published erratum appears in Br J Plast Surg 1993;46:179]. Br J Plast Surg 1993;46:13-17.

160. Cussons PD, Murison MS, Fernandez AE, Pigott RW: A panel based assessment of early versus no nasal correction of the cleft lip nose. Br J Plast Surg 1993;46:7-12.

161. Enemark H, Friede H, Paulin G, et al: Lip and nose morphology in patients with unilateral cleft lip and palate from four Scandinavian centres. Scand J Plast Reconstr Surg Hand Surg 1993;27:41-47.

162. Thomson HG, Reinders FX: A long-term appraisal of the unilateral complete cleft lip repair: one surgeon's experience. Plast Reconstr Surg 1995;96:549-563, discussion 562-563.

163. Kane AA, Pilgram TK, Moshiri M, Marsh JL: Long-term outcome of cleft lip nasal reconstruction in childhood [in process citation]. Plast Reconstr Surg 2000;105:1600-1608.

164. Park CG, Ha B: The importance of accurate repair of the orbicularis oris muscle in the correction of unilateral cleft lip. Plast Reconstr Surg 1995;96:780-788.

165. Tessier P, Tulasne JF: Secondary repair of cleft lip deformity. Clin Plast Surg 1984;11:747-760.

166. Trotman CA, Faraway JJ, Essick GK: Three-dimensional nasolabial displacement during movement in repaired cleft lip and palate patients. Plast Reconstr Surg 2000;105:1273-1283.

167. Zachrisson B: Esthetic factors involved in anterior tooth display and the smile: vertical dimension. J Clin Orthod 1998;32:432-445.

168. Peck S, Peck L, Kataja M: The gingival smile line. Angle Orthod 1992;62:91-100, discussion 101-102.

169. Gross MM, Trotman CA: A comparison of three-dimensional and two-dimensional analyses of facial motion. Angle Orthod 1996;66:189-194.

170. McCance AM, Moss JP, Fright WR, et al: Three-dimensional analysis techniques. Part 4. Three-dimensional analysis of bone and soft tissue to bone ratio of movements in 24 cleft palate patients following Le Fort I osteotomy: a preliminary report. Cleft Palate Craniofac J 1997;34:58-62.

171. Sargent EW, Fadhli OA, Cohen RS: Measurement of facial movement with computer software. Arch Otolaryngol Head Neck Surg 1998;124:313-318.

172. Mulliken JB, Pensler JM, Kozakewich HP: The anatomy of Cupid's bow in normal and cleft lip. Plast Reconstr Surg 1993;92:395-403, discussion 404.

173. Bernstein L: Modified operation for wide unilateral cleft lips. Arch Otolaryngol 1970;91:11.

174. Millard DR Jr: Extensions of the rotation-advancement principle for wide unilateral cleft lips. Plast Reconstr Surg 1968;42:535-544.

175. Onizuka T, Keyama A, Asada K, et al: Aesthetic considerations of the cleft lip operation. Aesthetic Plast Surg 1986;10:127-136.

176. Sasaki M: Repair of cleft lip. Jpn J Oral Surg 1972;18:1972.

177. Tajima S: The importance of the musculus nasalis and the use of the cleft margin flap in the repair of complete unilateral cleft lip. J Maxillofac Surg 1983;11:64-70.

178. Lewis MB: Unilateral cleft lip repair. Z-plasty. Clin Plast Surg 1993;20:647-657.

179. Bardach J, Salyer KE, Noordhoff MS: Correction of nasal deformity associated with unilateral cleft lip. In Bardach J, Salyer KE, eds: Surgical Techniques in Cleft Lip and Palate. St. Louis, Mosby–Year Book, 1991:74-112.

180. Chen PK, Noordhoff MS, Chen YR, Bendor-Samuel R: Augmentation of the free border of the lip in cleft lip patients using temporoparietal fascia. Plast Reconstr Surg 1995;95:781-788, discussion 789.

181. Salyer KE: Primary unilateral cleft-lip/nose repair. In Bardach J, Salyer KE, eds: Atlas of Craniofacial and Cleft Surgery, vol 2. Philadelphia, Lippincott-Raven, 1999:423-433.

182. Lo LJ, Huang CS, Chen YR, Noordhoff MS: Palatoalveolar outcome at 18 months following simultaneous primary cleft lip repair and posterior palatoplasty. Ann Plast Surg 1999;42:581-588.

183. Bardach J, Kelly KM, Salyer KE: A comparative study of facial growth following lip and palate repair performed in sequence and simultaneously: an experimental study in beagles. Plast Reconstr Surg 1993;91:1008-1016.

184. Bardach J, Kelly KM, Jakobsen JR: Simultaneous cleft lip and palate repair: an experimental study in beagles. Plast Reconstr Surg 1988;82:31-41.

185. McComb HK, Coghlan BA: Primary repair of the unilateral cleft lip nose: completion of a longitudinal study. Cleft Palate Craniofac J 1996;33:23-30, discussion 30-31.

186. Salyer KE: Primary unilateral cleft-lip/nose repair: Salyer's technique. In Bardach J, Salyer KE, eds: Atlas of Craniofacial and Cleft Surgery, vol 1. Philadelphia, Lippincott-Raven, 1999:423-433.

187. Potter J: Some nasal tip deformities due to alar cartilage abnormalities. Plast Reconstr Surg 1954;49:358.

188. Henkel KO, Gundlach K, Saka B: Incidence of secondary lip surgeries as a function of cleft type and severity: one center's experience. Cleft Palate Craniofac J 1998;35:310-312.

189. Santiago PE, Grayson BH, Cutting CB, et al: Reduced need for alveolar bone grafting by presurgical orthopedics and primary gingivoperiosteoplasty. Cleft Palate Craniofac J 1998;35:77-80.

Bilateral Cleft Lip Repair

COURT BALDWIN CUTTING, MD

In the last decade, there has been a revolution in the primary care of the bilateral cleft lip. As a result, this chapter bears little resemblance to that of the previous edition of this series. This is not to say that the information presented in the earlier edition is of no value. Understanding these techniques is useful in addressing common secondary deformities of bilateral cleft lip that the plastic surgeon will encounter as well as in suggesting ways of correcting unique secondary deformities. For this reason, these older techniques are discussed within a historical context. They are, however, not recommended for the treatment of the bilateral cleft lip infant who presents to the plastic surgeon for primary correction.

The new generation of bilateral cleft lip repairs places emphasis on the primary correction of the cartilaginous deformity that is present in the bilateral cleft lip and nose. Before this, bilateral cleft lip repair was focused on the skin imbalance between the prolabium and the columella. This led to a large number of repairs in which the excess skin in an overly wide prolabium was pushed up into the nasal tip to elongate the columella. Whereas the immediate outcome of these repairs was satisfactory, the long-term effect on nasal shape was not. In most cases, the nasal tip shape became progressively worse with growth. The secondary deformity that results is quite difficult to correct secondarily. The new cleft lip repairs put their emphasis on placing the lower lateral cartilages into a normal anatomic relationship. The nasal shape that results is a good deal more satisfactory. For this reason, the plastic surgeon is encouraged to adopt one of the new repairs presented in this chapter.

The bilateral cleft lip deformity is much more difficult to correct than the unilateral deformity. It is often quoted that compared with the unilateral cleft, "the

bilateral cleft is twice as difficult, and the results are half as good." With the dramatic improvements in unilateral cleft lip results in recent years, this has been a gross understatement. With the exception of the production of the scar, it is possible to produce a nearly perfect unilateral cleft lip result. The perfect bilateral cleft lip outcome is a good deal more elusive. As the newer generation of bilateral cleft lip repairs evolves, production of a normal lip and nose form in a single surgical stage may become routine.

ANATOMY AND PATHOGENESIS

It is essential to understand the pathologic anatomy of the bilateral cleft before undertaking its correction. This section discusses only elements of particular clinical relevance. The reader is referred to Chapter 87 for a more complete exposition. Bilateral clefts represent only 14% of the total number of cleft cases, possessing a double dose of the usual unilateral pathogenesis. Although the disease is usually thought to occur as a combination of environmental and polygenic inheritance, single-gene autosomal dominant inheritance patterns can be seen, such as in the Van der Woude syndrome, in which lip clefts are accompanied by lower lip pits.[1,2]

Incomplete mesodermal streaming into the primordial epithelial bilayer connecting the lateral maxillary and frontonasal processes results in clefting of the lip and primary palate.[3,4] This results in mesodermal deficiency in the region locally and produces an environment wherein normal structures become malpositioned. When the premaxilla does not connect to the lateral palatal shelves, fetal tongue thrusting and septal cartilage growth[5-8] result in unrestrained forward movement of the premaxilla with secondary bone deposition at the vomerine-premaxillary suture.[9-13] The main body of the premaxilla is positioned anteriorly under the quadrangular cartilage of the septum. In the normal case, the premaxilla is reined back under the quadrangular cartilage by its connection to the lateral palatal shelves. As it draws back, or the quadrangular cartilage grows forward, the septopremaxillary ligament is pulled into a gentle crescent between these two structures.[14-16] As the ligament calcifies, the anterior nasal spine is formed. In the bilateral cleft, this mechanism is reversed, and the anterior nasal spine is diminutive or absent. The footplates of the medial crura of the lower lateral cartilages are thereby set back slightly into a cul-de-sac between the body of the premaxilla and the quadrangular cartilage (Fig. 94-1). Given the lack of anterior thrust of the lateral maxil-

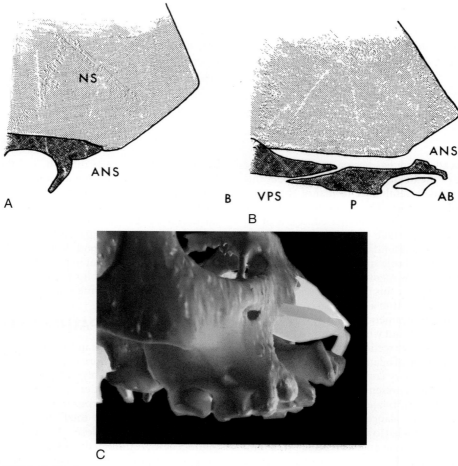

FIGURE 94-1. *A,* Normal sagittal relationships, drawn from a reconstruction, of the nasal septum (NS), basal premaxillary bone, and alveolar bone at birth. Note that the anterior nasal spine (ANS) lies posterior to the anteroinferior angle of the nasal septum. *B,* Sagittal relationships, drawn from a reconstruction, in a newborn infant with bilateral cleft lip and palate. The dentoalveolar part (AB) protrudes to lie in the same horizontal plane as the basal premaxillary bone (P), which is also protruded. Note the position of the anterior nasal spine (ANS), alveolar bone (AB), and vomeropremaxillary suture (VPS). The parts have been artificially separated to show the inferior septal border. (*A* and *B* from Latham RA: Development and structure of the premaxillary deformity in bilateral cleft lip and palate. Br J Plast Surg 1973;26:1, by permission of E & S Livingstone.) *C,* Computed tomographic three-dimensional reconstruction from the child used to construct the computer model to make the animation frames in this chapter. Note that even as the premaxilla drifts back under the cartilaginous septum with growth, the cul-de-sac between the cartilaginous septum and the body of the premaxilla remains. This cul-de-sac contains the footplates of the medial crura. (From Latham RA: Development and structure of the premaxillary deformity in bilateral cleft lip and palate. Br J Plast Surg 1973;26:1, by permission of E.S. Livingstone. Reproduced by permission of The British Association of Plastic Surgeons.)

lary shelves provided by connection with the premaxilla, as well as the mesodermal deficiency of the lateral maxilla itself, the lateral piriform aperture is posteriorly displaced.

The effect of these skeletal mispositions on the lower lateral cartilages of the nose is profound.[17-21] Rather than their normal position, the footplates of the medial crura are thrust forward while the feet of the lateral crura are drawn back. The normal junction of the medial and lateral crura (the dome) is pulled severely lateral and posterior, resulting in wide separation between the two domes (Fig. 94-2). If this abnormal position of the lower lateral cartilages is not corrected at the time of the primary repair, a severe secondary nasal deformity will be produced with growth. This is the fundamental concept that underlies the modern repair of bilateral cleft lip.

Another major problem with the bilateral cleft is the absence of muscle under the prolabium.[22-24] In the unilateral cleft, it is possible to join this central muscle element to the lateral lip muscle in such a way that a philtral column is produced. A number of surgeons suggest that the lateral lip muscles not be joined under the prolabium.[25-32] This results in a dynamic central lip with widening of the prolabial skin in the repair. It has the advantage that less lip tension is exerted on the premaxilla, possibly improving midface projection in the long term.[33-39] Repair of the muscle in the midline results in a more dynamic lip but does not mimic the normal situation. In correction of secondary deformities of bilateral cleft lip, the central lip where prolabial tissue is deficient can be successfully corrected with a midline Abbe flap. The muscle from the lateral lip elements can be everted and connected with the

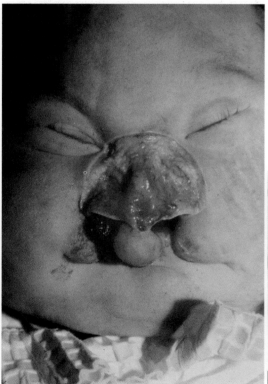
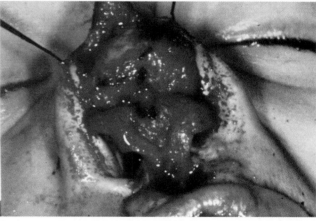

A   B

FIGURE 94-2. *A,* Photograph of a spontaneously aborted fetus with a bilateral cleft lip. The premaxilla is projected anteriorly with the footplates of the medial crura of the lower lateral cartilages. The lateral attachments of the lateral crura are tethered posteriorly to the deficient lateral maxilla. This results in the domes of the lower lateral cartilages being pulled apart during development. (Courtesy of Dr. Harold McComb.) *B,* Open secondary rhinoplasty at age 7 years in a child who did not undergo any nasal cartilage repositioning at the time of initial lip repair. Note the lack of tip projection and the broad nasal tip due to splaying of the domes of the lower lateral cartilages. (From Bardach J: Correction of secondary bilateral cleft lip and nasal deformities: Bardach's technique. In Bardach J, ed: Atlas of Craniofacial and Cleft Surgery, vol II. Philadelphia, Lippincott-Raven, 1999:611-647; and Bardach J, Salyer K: Correction of the nasal deformity associated with bilateral cleft lip. In Bardach J, Salyer K, eds: Surgical Techniques in Cleft Lip and Palate, 2nd ed. Baltimore, Mosby–Year Book, 1991:197-223.)

new central lip muscle to mimic normal anatomy. Correction of this deformity cannot be accomplished without an Abbe flap at the time of the primary procedure.

THE INCOMPLETE BILATERAL CLEFT

Methods adapted from unilateral cleft lip repair can often be applied to the incomplete bilateral cleft.[40-42] If a large Simonart band is present on one side, lip muscle can be found under the prolabial skin. This allows the muscle to be repaired in an everted fashion on both sides as described earlier. If a large Simonart band is present on one side, the nose often resembles a unilateral cleft nose deformity with a columella of normal length on the side of the Simonart band and a short columella on the more cleft side. The situation allows the surgeon to perform a standard Millard repair, which uses the C flap to elongate the short columella on the cleft side while a straight-line repair is applied to the less cleft side. In cases in which a large Simonart

band is present on both sides, a modified Millard repair can be applied on both sides in a two-stage fashion, but the results are often better if a modern bilateral cleft repair is used (Fig. 94-3).

THE PROJECTING PREMAXILLA

A severely projecting premaxilla will prevent the surgeon from achieving a satisfactory lip and nose form in a single stage. For this reason, a number of tactics are employed to bring the premaxilla back into the maxillary arch before surgery. A number of authors oppose any means of retracting the premaxilla because they think midface growth will be adversely affected.[43-45] They believe the lip should simply be repaired over the premaxilla to provide maximal projection of the structure in the teenage years. Whereas this author believes that the statement may be completely true, it is not a realistic choice if a primary lip and nose correction of high quality is to be performed. If the premaxilla is left projecting, lip repair alone is difficult, with some authors advocating lip repair in

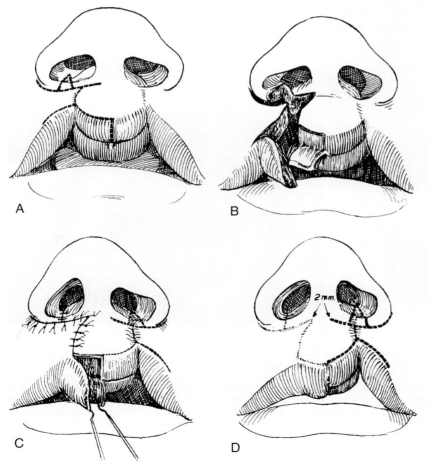

FIGURE 94-3. *A to D,* Adaptation of Millard's unilateral rotation-advancement technique used in an incomplete bilateral cleft. Most of this method is identical to that given in Chapter 93 for unilateral clefts. Note, however, that the vermilion construction under the prolabium is made with turndown flaps from the lateral lip element rather than using the prolabial mucosa for this purpose. (From Cronin T, Cronin E, Roper P, et al: Bilateral clefts. In McCarthy JG, ed: Reconstructive Plastic Surgery, vol 4. Philadelphia, WB Saunders, 1990:2653.)

two stages.[26,27,46,47] Certainly, high-quality primary nasal correction is not possible over a severely projecting premaxilla.

Resection of the projecting premaxilla is mentioned only to be condemned. Although it certainly makes primary lip repair easy, the long-term effects on dentofacial development are devastating.[48] The author has seen a number of these patients in the teenage years. Restoration requires the formation of a skin graft–lined pocket with the insertion of a partial maxillectomy prosthesis. Partial resection of the vomer stem with preservation of the body of the premaxilla would at first seem to be a better solution,[49] but the long-term effects on facial growth are undesirable. Further, the mobile premaxilla that results is not used by the patient for chewing, resulting in long-term bone hypoplasia of the structure. Section of the vomer is indicated only in secondary cases as part of premaxillary repositioning with simultaneous bilateral iliac bone grafting if an initially unretracted premaxilla has assumed an unworkable position requiring this secondary orthognathic procedure.[50] This sort of premaxillary repositioning procedure is usually required as the result of a descending premaxilla after one-stage lip repair alone. The pressure of the lip repair is often greater on the superior aspect of the projecting premaxilla than on the inferior portion. If the premaxilla has a round anterior face, the structure may be pushed inferior to the lip. The central incisor teeth may cut into the depth of the inferior gingivobuccal sulcus (Fig. 94-4).

Lip adhesion is certainly one way to handle the projecting premaxilla.[47,51] This approach, advocated by Harold McComb, has the advantage that presurgical involvement of the orthodontist or prosthodontist is not required. It has the disadvantage that lip adhesion is certainly more expensive than presurgical molding. Further, lip adhesion retracts the premaxilla in an uncontrolled way and does not mold the nose. Lip adhesion or one-stage lip repair without muscle repair can stretch the diminutive prolabium, but this can also be accomplished with presurgical molding.

Simple elastic traction is another time-honored way to retract the premaxilla. In its classic form, a bonnet is placed on the child's head with an elastic strap projecting from the earpieces stretched over the projecting prolabium and premaxilla (Fig. 94-5).[52-57] The "Liverpool strap" is another variant of this method. It consists of a broad piece of elastic tape (Elastoplast) that stretches from cheek to cheek over the prolabium and premaxilla. The problem with unguided elastic traction is that the vomer stem, which is the principal impediment to premaxillary retraction, is superior in position to the body of the premaxilla. Pressure on the premaxilla often causes it to rotate backwards such that the incisor teeth are pointed back at the tongue. Simple lip repair over the unretracted premaxilla shares this problem.

A pin-retained appliance has been used to retract the premaxilla.[13,58-63] The device consists of two custom-molded leaves that cover the lateral palatal shelves. There is a connection box at the back of this compound device that allows the width of the posterior palatal shelves to be adjusted. Given the absence of teeth, the appliance is held in with pins projecting into the bone. There is also a pin placed just behind the body of the premaxilla anterior to the premaxillary-vomerine suture. Orthodontic elastic chain is used to connect this premaxillary pin over pulleys on the back of the palatal device that are then extended anteriorly to orthodontic buttons placed on the front of the appliance (Fig. 94-6). This device will bring the

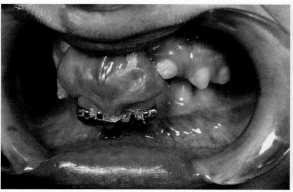 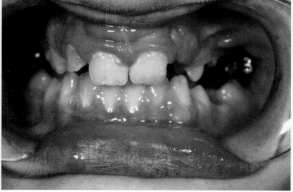

A   B

FIGURE 94-4. *A,* Child treated with lip repair alone over a projecting premaxilla that descended inferiorly below the retracting band of the lip repair, rather than the more common dorsal movement of that structure. The upper incisor teeth contact the lower buccal sulcus. *B,* After premaxillary repositioning and bilateral alveolar bone grafting.

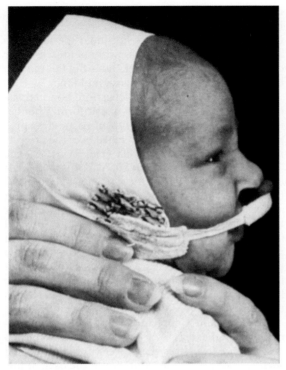

FIGURE 94-5. Elastic retraction of the premaxilla by use of a bonnet. This method is one of the earliest described for presurgical premaxillary retraction. It has the disadvantage that the premaxilla usually bends back off the vomer stem in an unpredictable way.

premaxilla and lateral palatal shelves into correct alignment in a week or two when it is applied to a 3-month-old infant with a bilateral cleft. Millard makes use of this presurgical alignment of the palatal segments to allow the performance of gingivoperiosteoplasty.[63] At present, this type of premaxillary retraction is controversial. Berkowitz[44,45,64] thinks that this rapid retraction along the premaxillary-vomerine suture causes microhematoma and synostosis leading to long-term anterior growth disturbance.

Grayson et al[65] have extended the concept of nasoalveolar molding, previously applied to unilateral clefts (Fig. 94-7), to the bilateral cleft (Fig. 94-8). Presurgical alveolar molding with a molding plate has a long history in the care of unilateral clefts.[66-68] Careful study of the long-term effects of presurgical molding plate therapy has revealed that they are not harmful, except economically, but they have not been helpful either.[69-71] None of these evaluations included gingivoperiosteoplasty in the protocol. If gingivoperiosteoplasty eliminates the need for alveolar bone grafting at age 8 years without causing significant growth restriction, alveolar molding should be re-examined. The subject of gingivoperiosteoplasty will be taken up shortly. A molding plate is basically a denture that does not fit in the direction the orthodontist wishes the alveolar segments to move. As the child feeds with the device in place, it exerts a gentle force that moves the segments in the appropriate direction. The device requires adjustment each week. At the end of

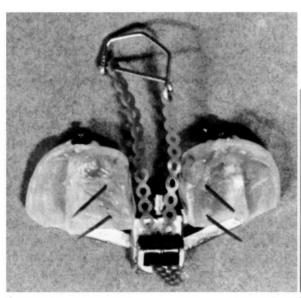

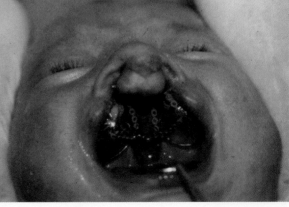

A   B

FIGURE 94-6. *A,* Latham's pin-retained device for retraction of the premaxilla. A pin is placed through the bone just behind the premaxilla. The pin is attached to elastic chains that retract the premaxilla. Posterior maxillary width can be adjusted by the screw mechanism in the back of the device. (From Cronin T, Cronin E, Roper P, et al: Bilateral clefts. In McCarthy JG, ed: Reconstructive Plastic Surgery, vol 4. Philadelphia, WB Saunders, 1990:2653.) *B,* Pin-retained device in place. The premaxilla usually retracts straight back within 2 weeks.

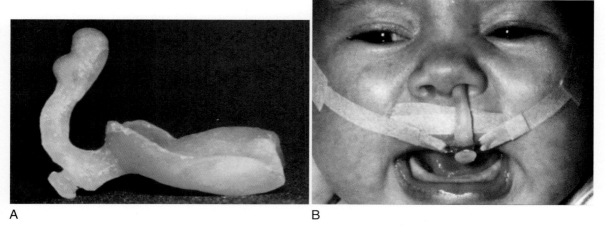

A   B

FIGURE 94-7. *A,* Grayson's unilateral nasoalveolar molding device. This is a conventional molding plate with a nasal extension to elevate the depressed dome on the cleft side. *B,* Device in place in an infant with a unilateral cleft.

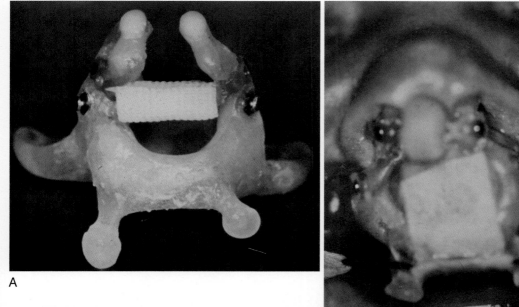

A

B

FIGURE 94-8. *A,* Grayson's bilateral version of the nasoalveolar molding device. The nasal prongs on either side are connected by a "saddle" of elastic chain that is placed over the lip-columella junction. *B,* The device in place in an infant with a complete bilateral cleft. The nasal extensions press anteriorly while the saddle retracts the lip-columella junction posteriorly. Tape is used to stretch the prolabium inferiorly to expand it if it is diminutive. The device is adjusted each week for 3 to 6 months before surgery.

3 months, the alveoli can be brought into an anatomically correct relationship. Simple molding plate therapy has generally not been successful in bilateral clefts unless it is combined with extraoral elastic traction.[72] The forces applied are not sufficient to retract the premaxilla. If nasal molding is added to the device, satisfactory premaxillary retraction can be accomplished in 3 to 6 months. As the device pushes out on the nose to elongate the columella, the nose pushes back, providing the required force for premaxillary retraction.

Nasoalveolar molding is a new concept introduced by Grayson, Brecht, et al.[65,73-78] The traditional molding plate is fitted with an extension that is designed to produce molding of the nose (see Figs. 94-7 and 94-8). Nasal molding has been used previously in situations in which the nasal floor is intact.[79-83] By extending the nasal molding device from the oral plate, it is not necessary to have a closed nasal floor. Nasal molding can bring the lower lateral cartilage up into a more normal anatomic relationship as well as tissue expand the short columella and the nasal lining to allow primary nasal reconstruction without tension and with minimal incision in the intranasal closure. In the unilateral case, a statistically significant improvement in symmetry has been observed in children having nasoalveolar molding compared with those having alveolar molding only.[84] Nasal molding in the bilateral cleft is regarded by this author as a major advance.[74,85] With use of this technique, the nasoalveolar structures may be made much more normal before surgery (Fig. 94-9). Most people focus on the columellar elongation that has been achieved. The problems with surgically elongating the short columella have preoccupied cleft surgeons for decades. In contrast to subcutaneous skin expansion, external tissue expansion of this type is not accompanied by subcutaneous fibrosis and wound contraction, causing some of the benefit of skin expansion to be lost in the long term. Long-term follow-up of these children demonstrates a columellar length that is not statistically significantly different from normal.[86,87] The tissue expansion of the nasal lining is as advantageous as the columellar elongation. It is possible to bring the domes

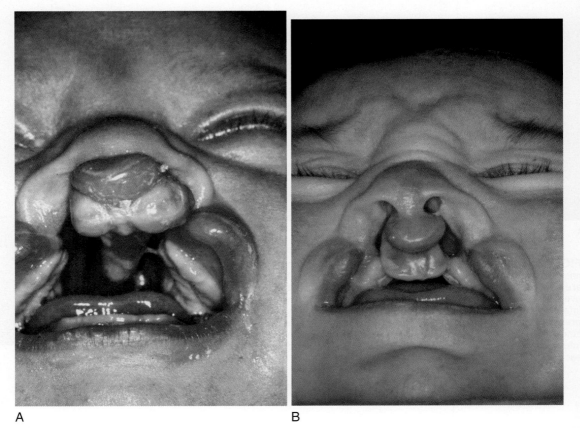

A   B

FIGURE 94-9. *A,* An infant with a bilateral cleft before treatment. *B,* Four months after nasoalveolar molding by use of the device illustrated in Figure 94-8. Note the retraction of the premaxilla, the stretching of the columella and nasal lining, and the improvement in the shape of the nasal tip.

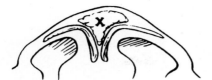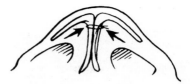

FIGURE 94-10. With the lateral separation of the domes of the lower lateral cartilages, fibrofat is deposited between them. It is essential to elevate this tissue from between the domes before attempting to suture them together in the midline with absorbable suture if relapse is to be prevented. (From Cutting C, Grayson B: The prolabial unwinding flap method for one-stage repair of bilateral cleft lip, nose, and alveolus. Plast Reconstr Surg 1993;91:37. Used by permission of the Williams & Wilkins Company.)

of the lower lateral cartilages together during primary bilateral nasal repair without tension. Lateral incisions along the piriform aperture can be minimized because of stretching of this nasal lining. The lower lateral cartilages usually are quite concave laterally. Nasal molding provides a convexity to the lateral crura that is long-lasting.

Nasoalveolar molding alone is insufficient to produce the desired nasal shape and must be combined with a coordinated surgical approach. Nasal molding cannot eliminate the soft tissue (fibrous fat) that has been deposited between the widely separated domes of the lower lateral cartilages (Fig. 94-10). It is necessary to surgically separate this fibrofatty tissue from the lower lateral cartilages and to approximate the domes in the midline. In our initial enthusiasm for nasoalveolar molding, we used molding alone. This resulted in a tip that again became broad with loss of approximately half of the columellar length due to recurrent splaying of the domes laterally.

Gingivoperiosteoplasty is currently a hotly debated topic. If the alveolar segments are aligned in an anatomic relationship owing to some type of presurgical molding, it is possible to perform a subperiosteal repair of the alveolus with minimal undermining (Fig. 94-11).[63,88,89] Gingivoperiosteoplasty without presurgical molding was originally introduced by Skoog.[90] In the absence of molding, gingivoperiosteoplasty required wide undermining over the maxilla. This caused concern about long-term facial growth.[71,79,91] Also, as the gap widens between the bone edges, it becomes less likely that bone formation will occur.[92,93] If presurgical molding is accomplished, subperiosteal elevation is limited only to the cleft edge, minimizing this risk. Primary bone grafting of the alveolus has a long history and is associated with long-term growth restriction. It is possible that the subperiosteal bone formation produced by gingivoperiosteoplasty will have a similar effect. Bone grafting carries with it a large amount of resorption of partially necrotic bone and much subperiosteal undermining to place

the graft. Gingivoperiosteoplasty after molding does not share these disadvantages. Millard states that gingivoperiosteoplasty eliminates the need for alveolar bone grafting at 8 years of age 92% of the time.[94] In our experience with the procedure, bone grafting of the alveolus is not required 60% of the time.[95,96] In our center, the premaxilla is retracted much more slowly without use of pin-retained appliances. This approach results in the gingivoperiosteoplasty being performed at 4 to 6 months of age rather than at 3 months. This short delay may account for the difference in reported success rates. Comparison of studies is difficult owing to differences in technique and in dental standards used to define success in treatment technique. Midface growth in our first group of patients at a mean of 6 and 12 years has been reported and compared with control subjects who were otherwise treated the same but did not have gingivoperiosteoplasty.[97-99] Statistically significant differences between patients having gingivoperiosteoplasty and control subjects in regard to facial growth were not observed. However, caution in interpreting these results is required because these children have not yet had their pubertal growth spurt. All control children received an Abyholm-type alveolar bone graft at age 7 to 9 years.[100] Thus, all children in both groups in the 12-year-old sample had their alveolar cleft bridged with bone. It is difficult to imagine how a difference between the two groups will emerge after the pubertal growth spurt, but this measurement requires further rigorous investigation. Using a pin-retained appliance for premaxillary retraction followed by gingivoperiosteoplasty, Millard noted a greater incidence of anterior crossbite but thought on balance with its other advantages that the protocol should be continued.[94] If gingivoperiosteoplasty results in a high number of Le Fort I advancements in the teenage years, the procedure should be abandoned. If the Le Fort I incidence were to increase only slightly, the benefits of eliminating the alveolar bone graft in the majority of patients would encourage the adoption of the technique.

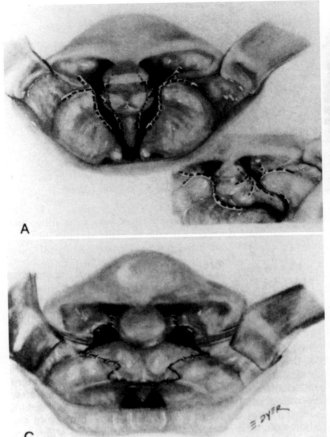

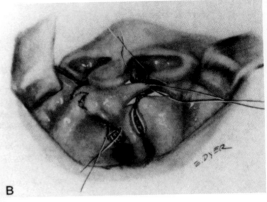

FIGURE 94-11. *A* to *C,* Millard's method for performing gingivoperiosteoplasty in the bilateral cleft. In contrast to Skoog's method,[90] this technique can be performed only after presurgical alveolar molding to align the maxillary segments. Subperiosteal elevation is done only at the cleft edges, and the alveolus and floor of nose are repaired with minimal undermining. (From Cronin T, Cronin E, Roper P, et al: Bilateral clefts. In McCarthy JG, ed: Reconstructive Plastic Surgery, vol 4. Philadelphia, WB Saunders, 1990:2653.)

THE LIP

The prolabial skin should be used to construct the full height of the central element of the lip.[26,29,32,49,101-111] In the history of the development of bilateral cleft lip repair, the prolabial skin was pushed up into the nose to form a columella, bringing the lateral lip elements together in the midline.[112] This technique produced an extremely tight lip and unsatisfactory nasal shape. Although it is not currently recommended, some have gone so far as to advocate a primary Abbe flap.[113-115] The height of the prolabial skin is usually shorter than the lateral lip elements. In some procedures, the prolabial skin was used to reconstruct only the upper portion of the central lip segments with the lateral lip elements being brought together underneath the prolabium.[116-118] This technique produced a tight lip inferiorly that was unnatural looking. For the past several decades, consensus has been reached that the prolabial skin should reach all the way down to the Cupid's bow between two vertical scars that should be used to simulate philtral columns.[102,119] This use of the prolabial skin is illustrated in all of the repairs described in this chapter. Prolabial width recommendations vary from full width to 2 mm.[120] In general, 5 mm is preferred.

The vermilion under the central lip element is usually best constructed with turndown flaps from the lateral lip elements. These turndown flaps are composed of true vermilion. By rolling out this vermilion between the thumb and forefinger before incising these flaps through and through, it is possible to provide more than enough vermilion for the purpose. This is the method that is described in all of the repairs presented in this chapter. An alternative method for central vermilion creation is to turn down the buccal mucosa that is attached to the bottom of the prolabial skin and wrap it under the repair, connecting the lateral lip elements (Fig. 94-12). Manchester[29,106,121] has demonstrated excellent results by use of this technique. With

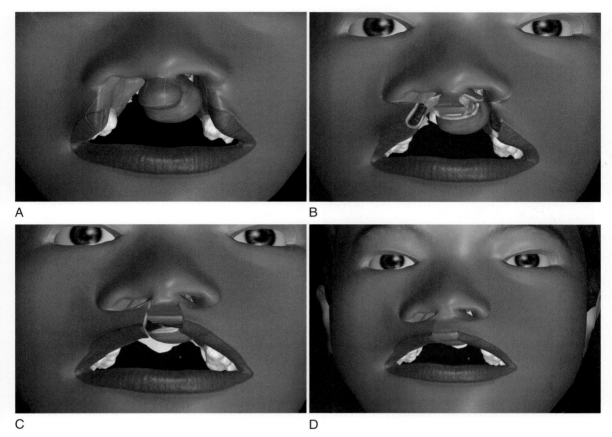

FIGURE 94-12. *A to D,* Use of the mucosa under the prolabium to construct the central vermilion of the lip. (From Cutting C, et al: Bilateral Cleft Lip [videotape]. New York, The Smile Train.)

this approach, good results are observed, but the technique often produces a central vermilion notch (Fig. 94-13). Even when the central vermilion contour is good, the character of the mucosa is different from that of the lateral lip elements. The buccal mucosa often dries out, cracks, and desquamates. Reconstruction of the central vermilion from the lateral lip elements is so reliable and easily done that it is now the technique of choice.

There continues to be controversy about how best to construct the muscle in the lip. A number of authors believe it is best not to approximate the lateral lip muscles in the midline.[26-29,31,32] They think this will produce excessive lip tension given that central muscle under the prolabium is absent in the bilateral cleft. This concept is discussed in the section on pathologic anatomy. If the premaxilla is not retracted before the lip repair, it is often difficult to repair the muscle in the midline. If the lateral lip muscle is intentionally sutured to the lateral edge of the prolabial flap, progressive contraction of the muscle with growth usually

leads to an overly wide interphiltral distance. This is sometimes done intentionally when only a tiny prolabium is present. The excessively small prolabium is common and may represent median facial dysgenesis.[122] Lip repair to this diminutive prolabium will cause it to stretch out, facilitating later secondary repair.[123] During active contraction of unapproximated lateral muscles, they can be seen to "ball up" under the lateral lip skin, producing no central lip movement at all. A number of authors repair the lateral muscles in the midline under the prolabial skin.[74,85,120,123-128] Muscle approximation is easily accomplished if the premaxilla has been presurgically retracted. It is the muscle repair that brings the alar bases into a normal position. If the muscles are not repaired, the alar bases usually drift excessively laterally. In fact, repair of the muscles in the midline is not anatomically correct. Only if nature had provided central muscle tissue under the prolabium would a truly normal lip repair be possible with use of lateral muscle elements.

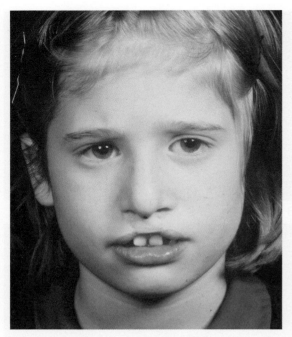

FIGURE 94-13. An extreme example of the notching that can occur in attempting to use the prolabial mucosa to form the central vermilion of the lip (see Figure 94-12). For this repair to be performed, the true vermilion tissue from the lateral lip elements is excised and cannot later be recovered. The prolabial portion of the white roll of Cupid's bow is flat or concave downward. The central mucosa often dries out, desquamates, and does not move synchronously with the lateral lip vermilion.

THE SKIN PARADIGM

For decades, bilateral cleft lip repair has been dominated by consideration of the skin imbalance between the prolabium and the columella. The columellar skin is short or absent, whereas the prolabial skin is excessively wide. This led to the perfectly reasonable design concept of using the excess prolabial width to produce columellar length. Given that blood supply to the central lip skin must be preserved, two surgical stages are usually required. A large number of procedures were based on this concept.[25,30,46,107,108,129-137] In the most popular variants of these procedures, in the first stage, the excessive prolabial width is placed under the alar bases or in the nasal floor. In a second stage, this "banked" skin is rotated superiorly to form a columella. The secondary nasal procedure was usually delayed as long as possible, with psychosocial pressures prompting repair at school age. Cleft surgeons were reluctant to perform nasal repair earlier because growth was not kind to nasal form after these repairs. The nasal tip was found to lack projection with growth, prompting

several authors to lengthen the "short" medial crura with ear cartilage grafts.[138] This problem caused Harold McComb to take a new direction, as discussed shortly.[139]

In some repairs of this type, the excessive width of the prolabium was left in the central lip. This tissue was taken up out of the lip and pushed up into the columella in a second stage. Unfortunately, this required reopening the lip. Two approaches were taken. Forked flaps could be cut from the lateral sides that were advanced into the columella. The lateral lip skin was reapproximated, producing no new lip scars, but a new vertical scar in the columella was formed.[107,108,133-135,137,140,141] Alternatively, a central V-Y advancement of the wide prolabium from the lip into the nose could be performed.[25,129] This modification did not produce a midline scar in the columella, but it did produce a new vertical scar in the lip. In both techniques, a confluence of scars was produced at the lip-columella junction.

During the evolution of currently recommended techniques, the prolabium was unwound, incorporating the circumferential prolabial artery to maintain blood supply, permitting one-stage repair.[125] Whereas the repair also incorporated anatomic repositioning of the lower lateral cartilages, the columellar skin was still recruited from the prolabium.

The classic repair of this type is the banked forked flap (Color Plate 94-1).[107,108,123,141-143] The excess width of the prolabium is taken advantage of by dividing the prolabium vertically into three parts. The central prolabial column is used to construct the midline lip skin. The two lateral forks are banked under the alar bases for later use. In a second stage, intranasal transfixion incisions extending laterally along the nasal floor to the alar base are connected as a bipedicle to the superficial V-to-Y incision between the lip and nose (Fig. 94-14). This allows rotation of the two horizontally aligned nostrils into a more vertical position, recruiting these banked forks to the production of a columella. In the diminutive prolabium, the lateral lip elements were connected to the lateral edge of the prolabium in the first stage. Subsequent stretching of the prolabium in the postoperative period allowed forks to be recruited from the central lip as described earlier.

Viewed from the perspective of maximal skin conservation, the banked forked flap is perhaps the best possible design. It is bilaterally symmetric and wastes little starting tissue. The vertical scar in the midline of the columella is a drawback. The confluence of secondary scars at the lip-columella junction is a more serious problem. The alar bases are narrowed at the time of the second procedure, resulting in tension along this horizontal scar line. As discussed in the section on pathologic anatomy, the anterior nasal spine is absent in these children. The combination of these two forces

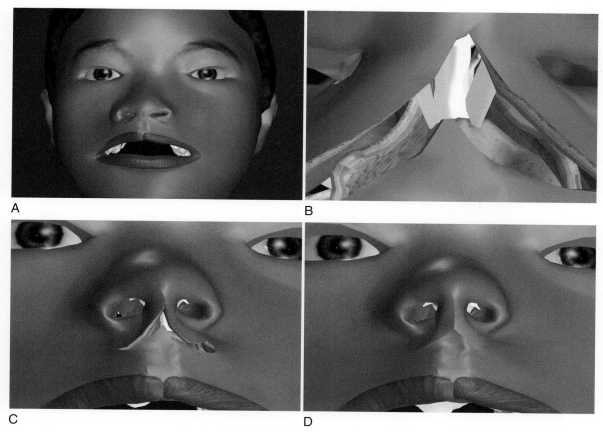

A

B

C

D

FIGURE 94-14. Second stage of the banked forked flap procedure. *A,* A continuous V-to-Y incision is made under the "banked" forked flaps. *B,* The incision is carried through into the nasal floor and up the membranous septum, elevating the forked flaps as a bipedicle on either side. *C,* The V-to-Y is advanced, narrowing the alar bases, increasing tip projection, and elongating the columella. *D,* Immediate form of the nose is much improved after closure. (From Cutting C, et al: Bilateral Cleft Lip [videotape]. New York, The Smile Train.)

often results in a sharp, retracted lip-columella angle (Fig. 94-15).

The main problem with any of the skin paradigm repairs is their secondary effect on the abnormal position of the lower lateral cartilages. If skin is pushed up from the lip or nasal floor into the base of the columella to provide length, the footplates of the medial crura are pushed out into the nasal tip. At the time the operation is done, the nasal form that results can look good (Fig. 94-16). The problem is that the abnormal position of the lower lateral cartilages has just been made worse by the procedure (Fig. 94-17). The growth of the severely abnormally positioned lower lateral cartilages in the ensuing years produces a characteristic secondary nasal deformity that is difficult to correct. In the normal situation, growth of the medial crura results in projection of the nasal tip. After advancement of the medial crura into the tip, growth of the medial crura results in progressively increasing width of the nasal tip with further separation of the domes. Because the medial crura are no longer oriented in a dorsal-caudal axis, nasal tip projection does not increase with growth. This results in the characteristic broad, flat, underprojected nasal tip commonly observed in the long-term follow-up of this repair.[144] Tertiary repair of the cartilaginous part of the deformity with open rhinoplasty and cartilage grafting is not difficult. In contrast, tertiary management of the skin envelope that results is difficult.[145] The skin envelope over the nasal tip is flat. Even if a pointed underlying cartilage framework has been constructed, draping the flat skin over it does not produce the desired skin envelope convexity. It is also commonly noted that the alar bases are deficient in fat and skin after skin paradigm repairs. If the lower lateral cartilages are in their normal position, growth of these structures stretches the alar bases. It appears that the alar base fills with fat as observed

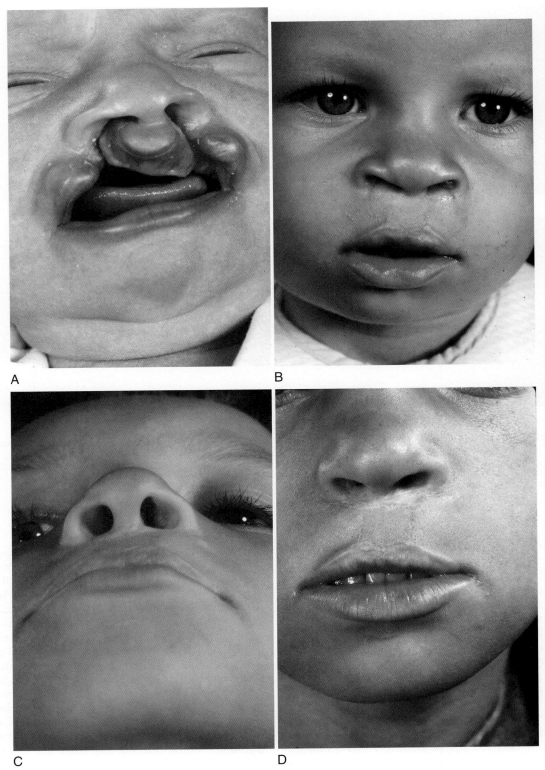

FIGURE 94-15. Long-term result of a banked forked flap. *A,* Initial deformity. *B,* Result after first stage of banked forked flap procedure. *C,* Basal view several years after second stage of the procedure with normal columella length. *D,* Front view shows an excessively broad, flat nasal tip.

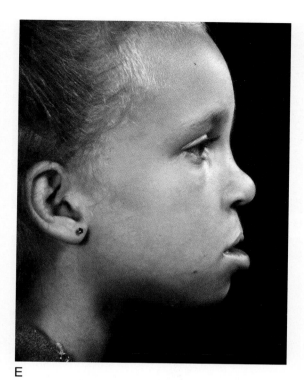

E

FIGURE 94-15, cont'd. *E,* Lateral view reveals a sharp lip-columella angle and a lack of nasal tip projection.

with internal craniofacial clefts. If the lower lateral cartilage is left laterally and inferiorly mispositioned, no stretching of the alar base occurs with growth. This malposition produces an alar base that is tiny and filled with little fat. The cartilage paradigm, unlike the skin paradigm, results in a more normal appearance to the alar bases and is now used in bilateral lip repair.

CARTILAGE PARADIGM REPAIRS

In 1990, Harold McComb[139,146] introduced a new primary bilateral repair in which the main focus is correct positioning of the lower lateral cartilages. In his many years of treating tertiary bilateral cleft patients, he concluded that achieving a satisfactory nasal form is the most difficult problem these patients face. In long-term follow-up of his unilateral cleft lip patients, primary repositioning of the lower lateral cartilage on the cleft side resulted in a much more satisfactory long-term nasal shape. His observation of unilateral cleft nasal reconstruction was confirmed by a number of authors.[18,19,147-165] In a carefully controlled experiment on immature rabbit ears, unilamellar perichondrial dissection did not adversely affect growth of cartilage surface area, although a slight warping of the ears was observed.[166] If primary repositioning of the lower lateral cartilage

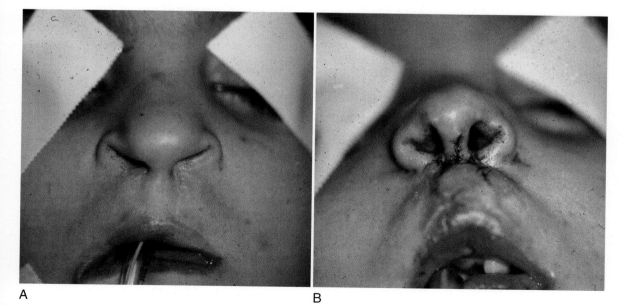

A   B

FIGURE 94-16. *A* and *B,* Intraoperative view of the second stage of the banked forked flap procedure. The alar base is narrowed and the columella is lengthened to normal proportions. Careful inspection reveals that the widely separated domes of the lower lateral cartilages remain separated. This sets up the problem with long-term nasal growth after this repair.

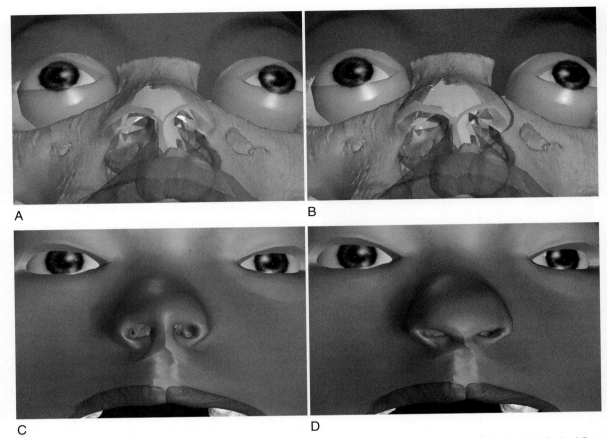

FIGURE 94-17. *A,* A transparency of Figure 94-14*D* immediately after the second stage of the banked forked flap procedure. The footplates of the medial crura have been pushed out to midcolumella; the domes remain widely separated. The proximal half of the columella is composed only of skin without cartilaginous support. The orientation of the vector of the medial crus is even more horizontal than it was before the procedure was performed. *B,* The result of simulated growth of the medial crura. Rather than medial crus growth resulting in tip projection, the tip has become increasingly broad and flat. Because there is no cartilage in the proximal half of the columella, little tip projection occurs with growth. *C,* Skin closure immediately after second-stage columellar elongation. *D,* Skin closure over the simulated growth of the lower lateral cartilages in *B.* (From Cutting C, et al: Bilateral Cleft Lip [videotape]. New York, The Smile Train.)

resulted in superior nasal form in the unilateral cleft, the same reasoning should also apply in the bilateral cleft.

McComb's new operation was performed in two steps. In the first procedure, a V-to-Y incision is performed on the nasal tip (Fig. 94-18). Nasal tip incisions had been used before for secondary cleft nasal reconstruction.[151,167] The skin and fibrofat separating the dome cartilages are elevated up away from the cartilage. The dome cartilages are then brought to the anterior midline and sutured together in a normal anatomic relationship. The V-to-Y skin incision is closed, producing an elongation of the columella. Because the main source of blood supply to the prolabial skin has been cut (external branches of the

anterior ethmoid arteries), it is not possible to repair the lip in one stage. Instead, a lip adhesion is performed at the time of this first operation. Some months later, the formal lip repair is performed with further narrowing of the alar bases.

This primary focus on correct repositioning of the lower lateral cartilages in the primary care of bilateral clefts was revolutionary. Most earlier repairs were concerned with elongation of the columellar skin as the main objective, as outlined in the preceding section. Several surgeons took up McComb's conceptual shift in emphasis and developed procedures that attempted to overcome some of the limitations of the initial McComb design. Trott and Mohan,[168] Mulliken[126,127] and Cutting[74,125,169] developed procedures based on

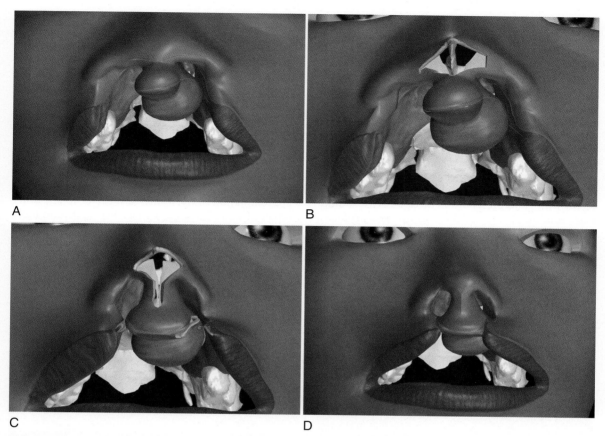

FIGURE 94-18. First stage of McComb's technique of bilateral cleft lip and nose repair. *A,* V-to-Y nasal tip incision marked. *B,* Skin and fat elevated away from the widely separated domes of the lower lateral cartilages. *C,* The domes are approximated in the midline in a normal anatomic relationship, and the lip adhesion incisions are made. *D,* Closure of the V-to-Y incision of the nasal tip elongates the columella. The lip adhesion is completed. Later, at a second stage, the formal lip repair will be performed with further narrowing of the alar bases. (From Cutting C, et al: Bilateral Cleft Lip [videotape]. New York, The Smile Train.)

McComb's concept. These repairs and the critique of this entire group complete this section.

Earlier workers addressed this concept of reapproximating the domes of the lower lateral cartilages. Bardach[170,171] performed simple closure of the lateral lip elements to the wide prolabial edges as a first stage. At 7 to 9 years of age, the columella was then lengthened by a midline V-to-Y from the prolabium into the columella extended into an open rhinoplasty. The cartilages were placed into an anatomically correct relationship at that time. Noordhoff[136] also advocated dissection of the lower lateral cartilages at the time of the initial lip repair. He described suturing the dome and cephalic scroll of the lower lateral cartilages superiorly to the upper lateral cartilages. One could argue that Noordhoff's brief description was really the first operation of this type.

Correction of the lateral vestibular web at the time of the primary nasal correction is an element that is common to all of the repairs in this group. In primary repair of the unilateral cleft lip and nose, lateralization of the intranasal vestibular web is common.[18,147,160,172] Mobilization of the tail of the lateral crus of the lower lateral cartilage in the lateral vestibular lining causes prolapse of these structures medially, resulting in nasal obstruction. Many surgeons lateralize this web by means of a bolster suture through this vestibular web coming out through the facial skin at the nasofacial groove, over a bolster again, then back. The same maneuver is now accomplished with a polydioxanone suture that passes through the vestibular web internally and is passed through the skin of the nasofacial groove externally.[144] The needle is passed through the same suture hole in the external skin, then straddles the vestibular web internally. Tying the suture down lateralizes the vestibular web and helps define the nasofacial groove. This variation is now used for both unilateral and bilateral clefts.

In 1992, Mulliken[126,127] introduced a procedure in which primary lower lateral cartilage correction was performed with bilateral lip repair in a single stage. Access to the lower lateral cartilages was achieved through nostril apex incisions and a vertical midline incision in the nasal tip (Fig. 94-19). Because a vertical incision was performed in the nasal tip, at least one of the external branches of the anterior ethmoid artery could be preserved, allowing simultaneous lip repair with good preservation of vascularity. A moderate amount of columellar elongation was produced by the nostril apex incisions. Mulliken reasoned and subsequently demonstrated that subsequent growth of the lower lateral cartilages would stretch the overlying skin and produce a more normal skin envelope without secondary surgical intervention.[127] Mulliken

now performs his operation through the nostril apex incisions alone, without the need for the vertical incision in the midline of the nasal tip.[173] This revision corrects one of the main drawbacks of the original description of his repair.

In 1993, Trott and Mohan[168,174] described a one-stage procedure that capitalizes on the open rhinoplasty concept. Nostril apex incisions are extended down the columella directly into the vertical lip incisions (Fig. 94-20). The prolabial skin flap is elevated in continuity with the cutaneous columella and nasal tip skin to provide complete exposure to the lower lateral cartilages. The exposure to the lower lateral cartilage for approximation of the domes is superior to any other repair of this type (Fig. 94-21). After repositioning of the lower lateral cartilages and suturing of the domes together in the midline, the dorsal skin is advanced down and sutured to the septal angle to provide increased nasal length. The tip and columellar skin is draped over the new cartilage construction and sutured

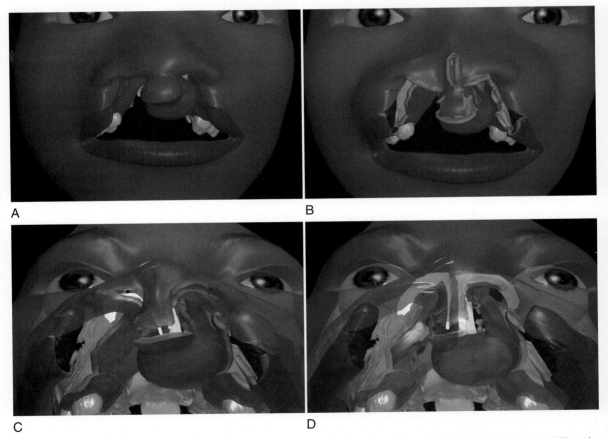

A

B

C

D

FIGURE 94-19. Mulliken's technique. *A,* Lip and nasal incisions marked. *B,* Nostril apex incisions and midline tip incisions are made to allow dissection of skin and fat from between the domes of the lower lateral cartilages. *C* and *D,* Nasal cartilages before *(C)* and after *(D)* approximation of the domes in the midline.

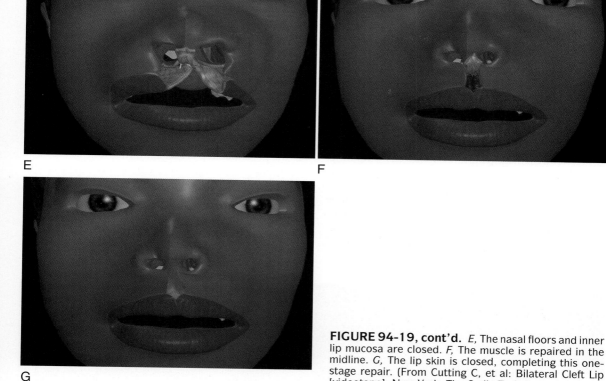

FIGURE 94-19, cont'd. *E,* The nasal floors and inner lip mucosa are closed. *F,* The muscle is repaired in the midline. *G,* The lip skin is closed, completing this one-stage repair. (From Cutting C, et al: Bilateral Cleft Lip [videotape]. New York, The Smile Train.)

in the manner of an external rhinoplasty closure. The prolabial flap is then closed to the lateral lip elements in the usual manner.

At the time of its introduction, the Trott procedure had the advantage over the Mulliken and McComb repairs in that a scar was not required in the nasal tip. Subsequently, Mulliken eliminated the nasal tip incision. The direct exposure to the lower lateral cartilages was attractive. As experience was gained with the Trott procedure in the mid-l990s, two disadvantages became apparent.[175] The external branches of the anterior ethmoid artery course down the caudal edges of the medial crura before entering the deep prolabial skin. Elevation of the prolabial flap in concert with the columellar skin divided these branches, resulting in poor blood supply to the prolabial flap. Although the prolabial skin survives, the relative ischemia of this flap is always a cause for concern. More than 65 Trott procedures have been performed by Monasterio[176] of Chile. He has learned to leave the prolabial flap wide to minimize the risk of necrosis. The other potential difficulty of the Trott procedure involves the long continuous incision from the lateral nostril apex all the way down to the Cupid's bow of the lip. In some patients, wound contracture of this scar line could have unfortunate consequences in the shape of the lip and nose.

In 1993, Cutting[125] introduced the prolabial unwinding flap. This repair unwound the prolabial skin based on the circumferential prolabial artery such that the columella could be elongated by use of columellar skin. At the same time, a retrograde approach to the nasal tip allowed the dome cartilages to be brought together in the midline to effect a one-stage lip and nose correction without the need for any incisions in the nostril apex or nasal tip. Given the asymmetric nature of the design, it was a major technical exercise to produce a symmetric result. It also had the fault that the footplates of the medial crura were advanced halfway into the columella. The error of effecting this kind of movement is chronicled in the section on the skin paradigm, and this approach is no longer advocated.

In 1998, Cutting, Grayson, et al[74,169] described a combined surgical-orthodontic approach to one-stage correction of the bilateral cleft lip and nose deformity. Grayson's approach to nasoalveolar molding in the complete bilateral cleft is described in the section on the projecting premaxilla. The details of this orthodontic technique are beyond the scope of this chapter and are described in detail elsewhere.[65,73,75,76] At the conclusion of this kind of molding, the premaxilla has been retracted, the columellar skin has been elongated, the nasal lining is expanded, the domes are brought up into a more normal position, and the lower lateral cartilages are given a convex shape (see Fig. 94-9). This molding is accomplished during a 3- to 5-month period with weekly orthodontic visits.

Nasoalveolar molding alone is not sufficient to produce the desired nasal shape. The fibrofatty tissues that have been deposited between the domes of the lower lateral cartilages cannot be removed by molding. A combined surgical approach must be taken wherein this fibrofatty tissue and skin are elevated away from the lower lateral cartilages, allowing the domes to be sutured together in the midline (see Fig. 94-10). This is done by a retrograde approach (Fig. 94-22). A through-and-through incision at the membranous septum is brought over the septal angle. This incision is continuous with a deep elevation of the prolabial flap such that the prolabium and composite chondrocutaneous columella and nasal tip can be reflected up over the nasal dorsum to allow retrograde separation of the domes of the lower lateral cartilage from the skin of the nasal tip. The dome cartilages are then approximated in the midline with polydioxanone suture as a horizontal mattress passed through the mucosa and cartilage on either side. Because the arterial branches from the external branches of the anterior ethmoid artery are not injured, the blood supply to the prolabial flap is excellent. Incisions in the nasal tip skin or at the nostril apex are not required. Long-term results of this repair are satisfactory (Fig. 94-23).

When the patient presents too late for nasoalveolar molding, or when nasal molding is not adequate,

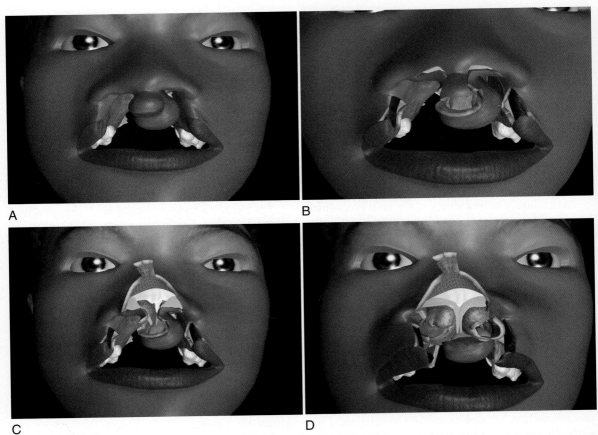

FIGURE 94-20. Trott's method of bilateral cleft lip and nose repair. *A,* Preoperative form. *B,* Nostril apex incisions extended down the columella to the bottom of the prolabial flap. *C,* Prolabial flap and nasal tip skin elevated away from the lower lateral cartilages in the manner of an open rhinoplasty. *D,* The nasal floors are closed and the domes are approximated in the midline under direct vision.

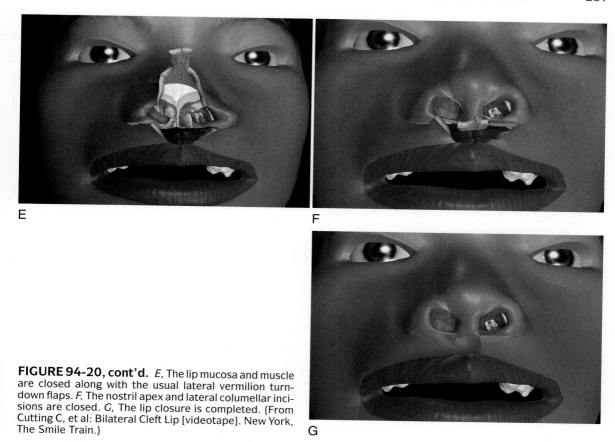

FIGURE 94-20, cont'd. *E,* The lip mucosa and muscle are closed along with the usual lateral vermilion turndown flaps. *F,* The nostril apex and lateral columellar incisions are closed. *G,* The lip closure is completed. (From Cutting C, et al: Bilateral Cleft Lip [videotape]. New York, The Smile Train.)

concepts from Mulliken's approach are incorporated into the cartilage paradigm. The nostril apex incisions elongate the columella and facilitate the placement of the horizontal mattress suture. In such patients, the scars at the nostril apices and the shortening of the skin distance from the nasal radix to the nostril apex are justified (Fig. 94-24).

It is useful to compare the relative strengths and weaknesses of the four cartilage paradigm repairs described. The McComb procedure does not require the application of presurgical molding. The lip adhesion at the time of the original nasal repair retracts the premaxilla such that alar base narrowing can be done at the time of the definitive lip repair. In complete bilateral clefts in infants, Mulliken and Cutting routinely employ presurgical retraction of the columella. The Trott repair would also benefit from columella retraction in infants. Older children with unrepaired bilateral clefts do not require as much premaxillary retraction as infants do. Presurgical molding in bilateral clefts is currently not widely available. The McComb procedure still has advantages in the infant with a severely projecting premaxilla when an ortho-

dontist trained in premaxillary retraction is not available. The McComb procedure also has the advantage that the skin from the nasal radix to the lip-columella junction is elongated surgically by a V-to-Y design. The Mulliken and Trott procedures elongate the columella by nostril apex incisions at the nasal tip. As a result, the skin distance between the nostril apex and the nasal radix is shortened. This tends to produce a "turned-up" nasal tip. Trott is aware of this problem and addresses it by dissecting over the nasal dorsum and drawing the skin down with a dermal suture to the septal angle. Mulliken reasons that if the lower lateral cartilages are in the correct position, any skin maldistribution will correct itself with growth.[127] However, a normal skin envelope over the repositioned lower lateral cartilage is preferable at the time of the initial operation, without the need for the bilateral Tajima "inverted U" incisions that sometimes do not scar well.[177,178] Normal skin envelope is most reliably achieved with presurgical nasoalveolar molding.

Malposition of the footplates of the medial crura should be corrected at the time of the primary lip repair. As described in the section on pathologic

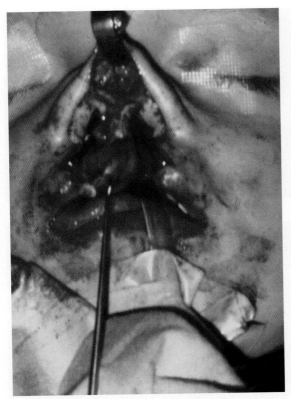

FIGURE 94-21. Intraoperative photograph of one of the author's Trott repairs after approximation of the domes in the midline. The Trott and McComb procedures offer the best view of the pathologic anatomy of the lower lateral cartilages.

anatomy, these footplates rest in a cul-de-sac between the quadrangular cartilage of the septum and the body of the premaxilla. These would normally project from the prominence of the anterior nasal spine. The anterior nasal spine is absent or diminutive in these patients, and a cul-de-sac deficient in bone replaces it (Fig. 94-25). The retrograde repair advances the footplates of the medial crura anteriorly and places them on top of the muscle pennants of the alar bases that have been brought together in the midline. This allows the alar bases to be brought more closely together than in the other repairs of this type and provides support for the footplates of the medial crura. This produces somewhat better tip projection.

Cleft surgeons are frequently asked to see an infant who has recently undergone one of the earlier skin paradigm repairs. If the lip repair has gone badly, it is possible to treat the initial repair as a lip adhesion. The surgeon in this situation can redo the entire lip-nose complex with any one of the cartilage paradigm repairs described. Often, however, the lip repair has gone well, but the nose is left in the usual unsatisfac-

tory configuration. In this instance, the Mulliken procedure to the nose is used with preservation of the initial lip repair.[179] The first stage of the McComb procedure on the nose could be applied in this situation as well. The Cutting and the Trott procedures have the disadvantage that they require reopening of the lip and are not recommended.

POSTOPERATIVE CARE

Local wound care with half saline and half peroxide to remove dried blood clot facilitates suture removal a week later. The vertical lip wounds are taped in compression for 5 weeks after suture removal. This will produce the narrowest possible scar. Elbow restraints, which keep the elbows straight, are applied for 3 weeks. This prevents the child from manipulating the wound with his or her hands. A syringe feeder is usually used for 3 weeks after surgery.

In rare cases in which the posterior palate is intact and the child has been able to breast-feed preoperatively, breast-feeding may be continued in the postoperative period. It is the author's observation that infants with cleft lip breast-feed by latching on with the alveolus and palate to suck, rather than using the orbicularis muscle as in the normal infant. Use of the orbicularis muscle by a child with a cleft lip is not effective for suction. As a result, the infant learns to breast-feed without using that muscle. This behavior persists for several weeks after surgery. In the experience of the author, breast-feeding does no harm with the upper lip draped passively over the nipple-areola complex.

After cleft lip repair, transient wound contraction is universal. This phenomenon reaches its peak at 6 to 8 weeks after surgery. Parents should be warned that they will not like the appearance of the lip at this stage. They should be reassured that the wound will improve spontaneously in the first 9 to 12 months, with the final appearance of the lip taking 2 to 5 years to be fully appreciated.

COMPLICATIONS

The most serious complication that follows bilateral cleft lip and nose repair is airway obstruction in the immediate postoperative period. In the older repairs in which primary nasal reconstruction was not attempted, this was seldom a problem. Hematoma and edema of a bilaterally dissected nose can produce a transient but complete nasal obstruction the night after the procedure. This problem is more common if the surgeon forgets to lateralize the vestibular web as described. Obligate nose breathing in the neonate is a characteristic that is usually lost in the first few months of life. Neonatal complete nasal obstruction, for example, in choanal atresia, can result in death

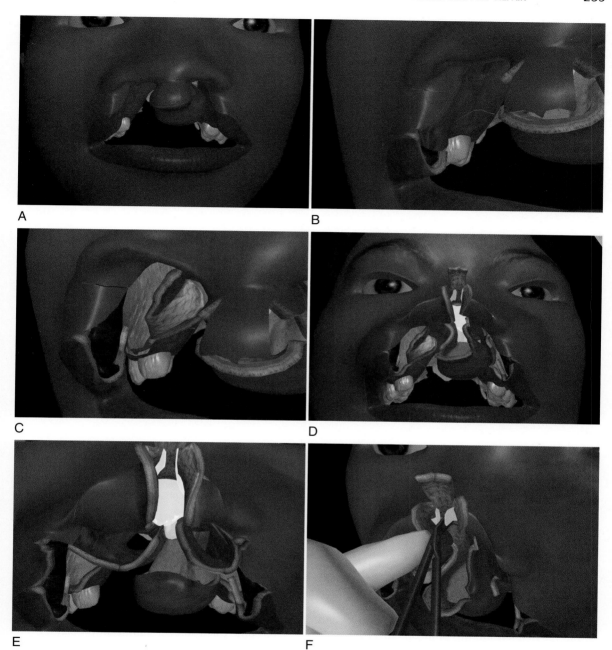

FIGURE 94-22. *A to J,* Cutting's technique. *B,* Millard's L flap cut, but note that it is pedicled on the lateral nasal wall and floor. *C,* L flap elevated, gingivobuccal sulcus and piriform aperture incisions made, and supraperiosteal undermining done as needed to allow the alar base to assume a normal position. *D,* Incision made up the membranous septum, elevating the composite chondrocutaneous columella and prolabial flap over the septal angle. *E,* The L flap is sutured into the piriform aperture defect. A septal flap is elevated and sutured to the inferior edge of the L flap to close the floor of the nose. *F,* Retrograde dissection is done to elevate the overlying skin and fat out from between the domes of the lower lateral cartilages.

Continued

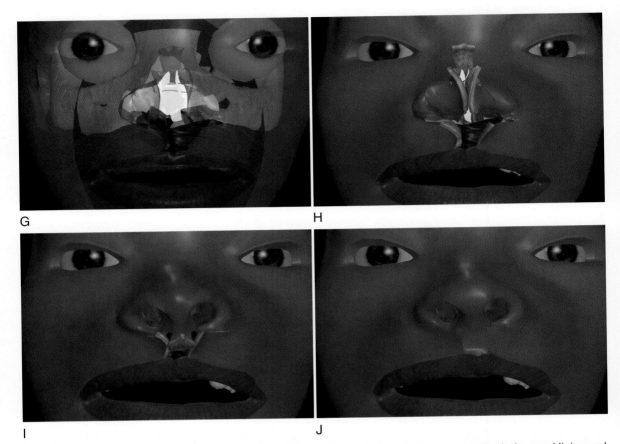

FIGURE 94-22, cont'd. *G,* A polydioxanone suture is placed as a horizontal mattress through the nasal lining and cartilages. Care must be taken not to include subcutaneous fat in the suture that will approximate the domes. *H,* The domes are approximated, the vestibular webs are lateralized, and the lip muscle is repaired in the midline. *I,* The nostril sills are closed. *J,* The lip is repaired in the usual manner. (From Cutting C, et al: Bilateral Cleft Lip [videotape]. New York, The Smile Train.)

if it is not treated promptly. Minor bouts of alternating nasal obstruction train the infant to open the mouth to breathe in the face of nasal obstruction within the first few months of life. Infants with clefts are less likely to learn mouth breathing because of the widely patent airway provided by the cleft. As a result, sudden lip closure and nasal obstruction can result in respiratory distress in the first postoperative evening. The child is observed to have nasal obstruction and simply does not open the mouth. This phenomenon has been observed after both unilateral and bilateral cleft lip and nose repairs. This situation is made worse by postoperative narcotics or lingering anesthetic agents. A pediatric nasal airway quickly resolves the problem. The nasal airway is sometimes anatomically patent but is obstructed by mucus and blood coagulation whose nidus is an intranasal stitch.

It is useful to have the mother apply saline nose drops several times a day to maintain patency of the nasal airway.

Bleeding can also be a significant problem. If the child is still in the hospital, a return trip to the operating room is sometimes required. The bleeding point is often buried deep under the repair, making surgical management difficult. On occasion, much of the repair will need to be reopened for access. It is much more difficult to handle late postoperative bleeding 5 to 10 days after surgery when the child has returned home. The child is usually taken to the local emergency department, where expertise in this type of surgery is not usually available. Blood transfusion and direct pressure may be required to stabilize the child before transfer to a more appropriate facility is possible. This problem is fortunately not common.

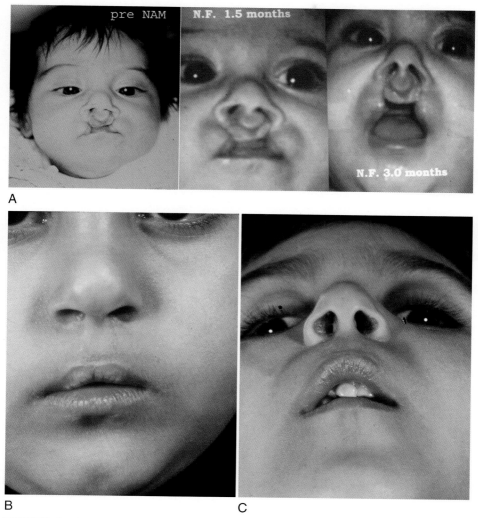

FIGURE 94-23. *A,* Nasoalveolar molding sequence (left to right) showing patient before molding with minimal columellar length, then after 1.5 and 3.0 months of molding. *B* and *C,* Frontal view and basal view 6 years after molding and the surgical procedure outlined in Figure 94-22. Note the maintenance of nasal shape with growth of the nose.

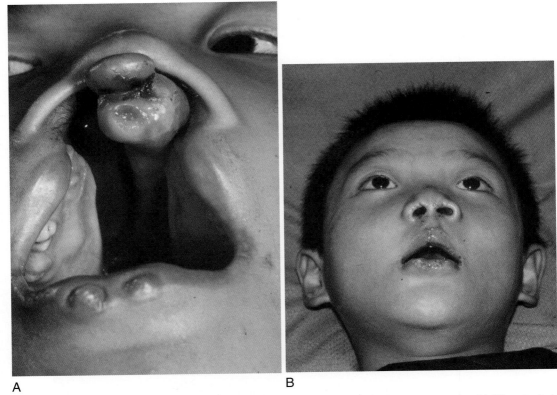

A   B

FIGURE 94-24. *A* and *B,* A 10-year-old child treated with a combination of the Cutting and Mulliken techniques without the benefit of presurgical molding. Note that a midline incision in the nasal tip is not used, as described recently by Mulliken.[173]

Infection after bilateral cleft lip repair is uncommon. If it occurs, it is usually an abscess around an absorbable suture. Although intravenous antibiotics are administered just before the procedure, the child is not sent home with a prescription for oral antibiotics. The inevitable oozing of serous fluid intraorally encourages bacterial growth. If the usual intraoral bacterial flora is suppressed by antibiotics, the fungi grow unopposed, resulting in a severe case of thrush.

Wound disruption will require either immediate or delayed return to the operating room. Disruption is common with lip adhesion procedures. Dehiscence is most common in an infant with a severely projecting premaxilla that has not been retracted presurgically. This complication is avoided with presurgical molding of the projecting premaxilla.

Ischemic loss of the prolabial flap is a distinct possibility in bilateral cleft lip repair. The possible production of ischemia to this essential piece of skin has been discussed in conjunction with a number of repairs mentioned earlier. Loss of the prolabial flap has been reported in conjunction with deep suturing of the prolabial dermis to the muscle repair in an attempt to produce a philtral dimple.[180] Full-thickness skin grafting provides the most immediate remedy.

Hypertrophic scarring and extremes of wound contraction can follow any surgical procedure in certain individuals. After cleft lip repair, patience is usually the best remedy. A lip repair wound will take 2 to 5 years to mature fully. Because the parents are usually the child's dominant social contact during this period, little psychosocial damage is done to the child if watchful waiting is employed. Depot steroid injection and scar revision are last resorts.

Abnormal premaxilla position is common after bilateral cleft lip repair. If the lip repair settles superior to the body of the premaxilla, the premaxilla may descend, prompting late orthognathic premaxillary repositioning (see Fig. 94-4). Similarly, the premaxilla may rotate severely to one side, requiring later repositioning. Midface growth deficiency is a common sequela of bilateral cleft palate. This deformity is the result of a combination of mesodermal deficiency inherent to the problem and growth restriction caused by the early surgical interventions to correct it. Should

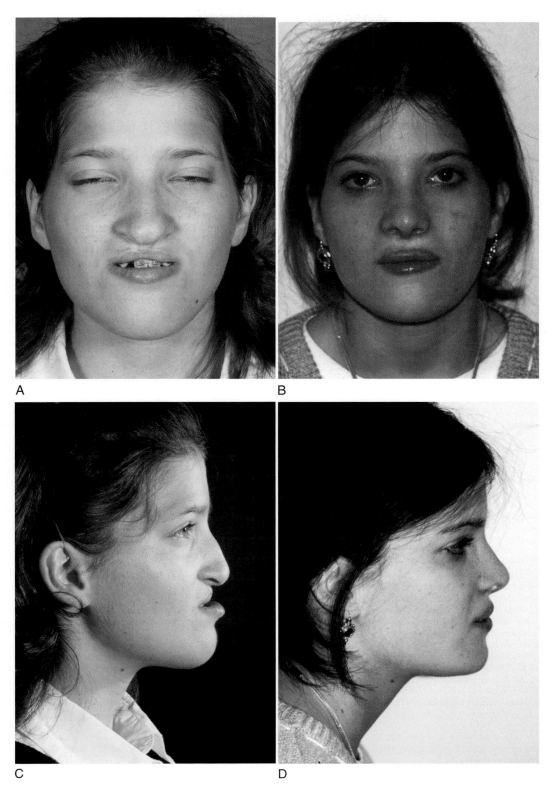

FIGURE 94-25. *A,* Preoperative frontal view of a teenage patient who had undergone a tight bilateral cleft lip repair in infancy. *B,* Postoperative frontal view after Le Fort I advancement, Abbe flap, and cleft nasal reconstruction. *C,* Preoperative lateral view showing midface retrusion and lack of nasal tip projection. *D,* Postoperative lateral view.

this occur, orthognathic surgery may be required to correct the problem in the late teen years.

REFERENCES

1. Murray JJ: Undescribed malformation of the lower lip occurring in four members of one family. Br Foreign Med Chir Rev 1860;26:502.
2. Van der Woude A: Fistula labii inferioris congenita and its association with cleft lip and palate. Am J Hum Genet 1954;6:244.
3. Stark R: The pathogenesis of harelip and cleft palate. Plast Reconstr Surg 1954;13:20.
4. Stark R, Ehrmann N: The development of the center of the face with particular reference to surgical correction of bilateral cleft lip. Plast Reconstr Surg 1958;21:177.
5. Baume L: The postnatal growth activity of the nasal cartilage septum. Helv Odontol Acta 1961;5:9.
6. Scott JH: Growth at facial sutures. Am J Orthod 1956;42:381.
7. Scott JH: Further studies on the growth of the human face. Proc R Soc Med 1959;52:263.
8. Scott JH: The growth of the nasal cavities. Acta Otolaryngol 1959;50:215.
9. King B, Workman C, Latham RA: An anatomical study of the columella and the protruding premaxillae in the bilateral cleft lip and palate infant. Cleft Palate J 1979;16:223.
10. Latham R, Workman C: Anatomy of the philtrum and columella: the soft tissue deformity in bilateral cleft lip and palate. In Georgiade N, Hagerty R, eds: Symposium on Management of Cleft Lip and Palate and Associated Deformities, vol 8. St. Louis, Mosby, 1974:10-12.
11. Latham RA: Facial Growth Mechanisms in the Human and Their Role in the Formation of the Cleft Lip and Palate Deformity. Liverpool, University of Liverpool, 1967.
12. Latham RA: The pathogenesis of the skeletal deformity associated with unilateral cleft lip and palate. Cleft Palate J 1969; 6:404.
13. Latham RA: Development and structure of the premaxillary deformity in bilateral cleft lip and palate. Br J Plast Surg 1973; 26:1.
14. Latham RA: A new concept of the early maxillary growth mechanism. Trans Eur Orthod Soc 1968;8:53.
15. Latham RA: Maxillary development and growth: the septopremaxillary ligament. J Anat 1970;107:471.
16. Latham RA, Scott JH: A newly postulated factor in the early growth of the human middle face and the theory of multiple assurance. Arch Oral Biol 1970;15:1097.
17. Huffman WC, Lierle DM: Studies on the pathologic anatomy of the unilateral hare-lip nose. Plast Reconstr Surg 1949;4:225.
18. McComb H: Primary correction of the unilateral cleft lip nasal deformity: a 10 year review. Plast Reconstr Surg 1985;75:791.
19. McComb H: Primary repair of the bilateral cleft lip nose: a 10-year review. Plast Reconstr Surg 1986;77:701.
20. Stenstrom SJ: The alar cartilage and the nasal deformity in unilateral cleft lip. Plast Reconstr Surg 1966;38:223.
21. Stenstrom SJ, Oberg TRH: The nasal deformity in unilateral cleft lip. Plast Reconstr Surg 1961;28:295.
22. Fara M: Anatomy and arteriography of cleft lips in stillborn children. Plast Reconstr Surg 1968;42:29.
23. Mulliken J, Pensler J, Kozakewich H: The anatomy of Cupid's bow in normal and cleft lip. Plast Reconstr Surg 1993;92:395.
24. Rees TD, Swinyard CA, Converse JM: The prolabium in the bilateral cleft lip: an electromyographic and biopsy study. Plast Reconstr Surg 1962;30:651.
25. Bardach J: Correction of the secondary bilateral nasal deformity: Bardach's technique. In Bardach J, Salyer K, eds: Surgical Techniques in Cleft Lip and Palate, 2nd ed. St. Louis, Mosby, 1991:201-211.
26. Bauer TB, Trusler HM, Tondra JM: Changing concepts in the management of bilateral cleft lip deformities. Plast Reconstr Surg 1959;24:321.
27. Bauer TB, Trusler HM, Tondra JM: Bauer, Trusler, and Tondra's method of cheilorrhaphy in bilateral lip. In Grabb WC, Rosenstein SW, Bzoch KR, eds: Cleft Lip and Palate: Surgical, Dental, and Speech Aspects. Boston, Little, Brown, 1971.
28. Cronin TD: Management of the bilateral cleft lip, palate, and nose. In Brent B, ed: The Artistry of Reconstruction Surgery. St. Louis, Mosby, 1987:242-252.
29. Manchester WM: The repair of double cleft lip as part of an integrated program. Plast Reconstr Surg 1970;45:207.
30. Salyer K: Primary bilateral cleft lip/nose repair: Salyer's technique. In Bardach J, ed: Atlas of Craniofacial and Cleft Surgery, vol II. Philadelphia, Lippincott-Raven, 1999:543-567.
31. Spina V, Kamakura L, Lapa F: Surgical management of bilateral cleft lip. Ann Plast Surg 1978;1:497.
32. Trusler HM, Bauer TB, Tondra JM: The cleft lip-cleft palate problem. Plast Reconstr Surg 1955;16:174.
33. Bardach J: The influence of cleft lip repair on facial growth. Cleft Palate J 1990;27:76.
34. Bardach J, Bakowska J, McDermott-Murray J, et al: Lip pressure changes following lip repair in infants with unilateral clefts. Plast Reconstr Surg 1984;74:476.
35. Bardach J, Eisbach K: The influence of primary unilateral cleft lip repair on facial growth. Cleft Palate J 1977;14:88.
36. Bardach J, Kelly K: The influence of lip repair with and without soft-tissue undermining on facial growth in beagles. Plast Reconstr Surg 1988;82:747.
37. Bardach J, Klausner E, Eisbach K: The relationship between lip pressure and facial growth after cleft lip repair: an experimental study. Cleft Palate J 1979;16:137.
38. Bardach J, Mooney M: The relationship between lip pressure following lip repair and craniofacial growth: an experimental study in beagles. Plast Reconstr Surg 1984;73:544-555.
39. Eisbach K, Bardach J: Effect of lip closure on facial growth in the surgically induced cleft rabbit. Otolaryngology 1978; 86:786.
40. Millard DR Jr: Adaptation of the rotation-advancement principle in bilateral cleft lip. In Wallace AB, ed: Transactions of the International Society of Plastic Surgeons, 2nd Congress. Edinburgh, E & S Livingstone, 1960:50.
41. Millard DR: Adaptation of the rotation-advancement principle in bilateral incomplete clefts. In Millard DR, ed: Cleft Craft, vol II. Boston, Little, Brown, 1977:189-213.
42. Noordhoff MS: Asymmetric bilateral cleft lip repair: Noordhoff's technique. In Bardach J, ed: Atlas of Craniofacial and Cleft Surgery, vol II. Philadelphia, Lippincott-Raven, 1999:568-593.
43. Berkowitz S: State of the art in cleft palate orofacial growth and dentistry. A historical perspective. Am J Orthod 1978; 74:564.
44. Berkowitz S: A comparison of treatment results in complete bilateral cleft lip and palate using a conservative approach versus Millard-Latham PSOT procedure. Semin Orthod 1996;2:169.
45. Berkowitz S: A multicenter retrospective 3D study of serial complete unilateral cleft lip and palate and complete bilateral cleft lip and palate casts to evaluate treatment: part 1—the participating institutions and research aims. Cleft Palate Craniofac J 1999;36:413.
46. Bardach J, Salyer K, Noordhoff MS: Bilateral cleft lip repair. In Bardach J, Salyer K, eds: Surgical Techniques in Cleft Lip and Palate, 2nd ed. Baltimore, Mosby–Year Book, 1991:113-172.
47. Spina V: The advantages of two stages in repair of bilateral cleft lip. Cleft Palate J 1966;3:56.

48. Motohashi N, Pruzansky S: Long-term effects of premaxillary excision in patients with complete bilateral cleft lips and palates. Cleft Palate J 1981;18:177.

49. Cronin TD: Surgery of the double cleft lip and protruding premaxilla. Plast Reconstr Surg 1957;19:389.

50. Padwa B, Sonis A, Bagheriz S, Mulliken J: Children with repaired bilateral cleft lip/palate: effect of age at premaxillary osteotomy on facial growth. Plast Reconstr Surg 1999;104:1261.

51. Hamilton R, Graham WP III, Randall P: Adhesion procedure on cleft lip repair. Cleft Palate J 1971;8:1.

52. Clodius L: Maxillary orthopedia by means of extraoral forces. In Hotz R, ed: Early Treatment of Cleft Lip and Palate. Bern, Hans Huber, 1964.

53. Desault P: Chorin: sur l'operation d'un bec-de-lievre double, avec fente; la voute du palais. J Chir Paris 1791;1:97.

54. Franco P: Traite des hernies. Lyon, Thiebaud Payen, 1561.

55. Griswold M, Sage W: Extra oral traction in cleft lip. Plast Reconstr Surg 1966;37:416.

56. Levret: Des nouvelles observations sur l'allaitement des enfants. J Med Chir Pharm Paris 1772;37:233.

57. Rutrick R, Black PW, Jurkiewicz MJ: Bilateral cleft lip and palate: presurgical treatment. Ann Plast Surg 1984;12:105.

58. Georgiade NG: The management of premaxillary and maxillary segments in the newborn cleft palate. Cleft Palate J 1970;7:411.

59. Georgiade NG: Improved technique for one-stage repair of bilateral cleft lip. Plast Reconstr Surg 1971;48:318.

60. Georgiade NG, Latham RA: Intraoral traction for positioning the premaxilla in the bilateral cleft lip. In Georgiade NG, Hagerty RF, eds: Symposium on Management of Cleft Lip and Palate and Associated Deformities. St. Louis, Mosby, 1974:123-127.

61. Georgiade NG, Latham RA: Maxillary arch alignment in the bilateral cleft lip and palate infant, using the pinned coaxial screw appliance. Plast Reconstr Surg 1975;56:52.

62. Latham RA: Orthopedic advancement of the cleft maxillary segment. A preliminary report. Cleft Palate J 1980;17:227.

63. Millard DR Jr, Latham RA: Improved primary surgical and dental treatment of clefts. Plast Reconstr Surg 1990;86:856.

64. Berkowitz S: The use of gingivoperiosteoplasty in CUCLP. Cleft Palate Craniofac J 1997;34:363.

65. Grayson B, Santiago P, Brecht L, Cutting C: Presurgical nasoalveolar molding in infants with cleft lip and palate. Cleft Palate Craniofac J 1999;36:486.

66. Burston WR: The early orthodontic treatment of cleft palate conditions. Dent Pract (Bristol) 1958;9:41.

67. Hotz M, Gnoinski W: Comprehensive care of the cleft lip and palate children at Zurich University: a preliminary report. Am J Orthod 1976;70:481.

68. McNeil C: Orthodontic procedures in the treatment of congenital cleft palate. Dent Rec 1950;70:26.

69. Prahl-Andersen B: State of the art—dental treatment of predental and infant patients with clefts and craniofacial anomalies. Cleft Palate Craniofac J 2000;37:528.

70. Ross R: Treatment variables affecting facial growth in complete unilateral cleft lip and palate. Part II. Presurgical orthopeadics. Cleft Palate Craniofac J 1987;24:24.

71. Ross RB, MacNamera M: Effect of presurgical infant orthopedics on facial esthetics in complete bilateral cleft lip and palate. Cleft Palate Craniofac J 1994;31:68.

72. Mishima K, Sugahara T, Mori Y, et al: Effects of presurgical orthopedic treatment in infants with complete bilateral cleft lip and palate. Cleft Palate Craniofac J 1998;35:227.

73. Brecht L, Grayson B, Cutting C: Nasoalveolar molding in early management of cleft lip and palate. In Taylor T, ed: Clinical Maxillofacial Prosthetics. Chicago, Quintessence Publishing, 2000:63-84.

74. Cutting C, Grayson B, Brecht L, et al: Presurgical columellar elongation and primary retrograde nasal reconstruction in one stage bilateral cleft lip and nose repair. Plast Reconstr Surg 1998;101:630.

75. Grayson B, Cutting C, Wood R: Preoperative columella lengthening in bilateral cleft lip and palate [brief communication]. Plast Reconstr Surg 1993;92:1422.

76. Grayson B, Santiago P: Presurgical orthopedics for cleft lip and palate. In Aston S, Beasley R, Thorne C, eds: Grabb and Smith's Plastic Surgery. Philadelphia, Lippincott-Raven, 1997:237-244.

77. Munoz Merino M, Rocabado Seaton M: New contributions to presurgical treatment of neonates with bilateral cleft lip with or without cleft palate [in Spanish]. Odontol Chil 1988;36:103.

78. Nakajima T: Early and one stage repair of bilateral cleft lip and nose. Keio J Med 1998;47:212.

79. Brown F, Colen L, Addante R, Graham J: Correction of congenital auricular deformities by splinting in the neonatal period. Pediatrics 1986;78:406.

80. Matsuo K, Hirose T: Preoperative nonsurgical overcorrection of cleft lip nasal deformity. Br J Plast Surg 1991;44:5.

81. Matsuo K, Hirose T, Otagiri T, Norose N: Repair of cleft lip with nonsurgical correction of nasal deformity in the early neonatal period. Plast Reconstr Surg 1989;83:25.

82. Matsuo K, Hirose T, Tomono T, et al: Nonsurgical correction of congenital auricular deformities in the early neonate: a preliminary report. Plast Reconstr Surg 1984;73:38.

83. Nakajima T, Yoshimura Y, Sakakibara A: Augmentation of the nostril splint for retaining the correct contour of the cleft lip nose. Plast Reconstr Surg 1990;85:182.

84. Maull D, Grayson B, Cutting C, et al: Long-term effects of nasoalveolar molding on three-dimensional nasal shape in unilateral clefts. Cleft Palate Craniofac J 1999;36:391.

85. Cutting C: Primary bilateral cleft lip and nose repair. In Aston S, Beasley R, Thorne C, eds: Grabb and Smith's Plastic Surgery. Philadelphia, Lippincott-Raven, 1997:255-262.

86. Lee C, Grayson B, Cutting C, Lin W: Presurgical nasal molding in bilateral cleft lip patients—the need for surgical revision before bone grafting age. Am Assoc Orthod 1999;6:22.

87. Lee C, Grayson B, Brecht L, et al: The need for surgical columella lengthening and nasal revision before the age of bone grafting in patients with bilateral cleft lip following presurgical nasal molding and columella lengthening. Am Cleft Palate Craniofac Assoc 1999;56:94.

88. Millard DR Jr: Cleft Craft, vol III. Boston, Little, Brown, 1980.

89. Millard DR Jr, Berkowitz S, Latham RA, Wolfe SA: A discussion of presurgical orthodontics in patients with clefts. Cleft Palate J 1988;25:403.

90. Skoog T: The use of periosteum and Surgicel for bone restoration in congenital clefts of the maxilla. Scand J Plast Reconstr Surg 1967;1:113.

91. Robertson NRE, Jolleys A: An 11-year followup of the effects of early bone grafting in infants born with complete clefts of the lip and palate. Br J Plast Surg 1983;36:438.

92. Brusati R, Mannucci N: The early gingivoalveoloplasty. Scand J Plast Reconstr Hand Surg 1992;26:65.

93. Pritchard J: Repair of fractures of the parietal bones in rats. J Anat 1946;80:55.

94. Millard DR, Latham R, Huifen X, et al: Cleft lip and palate treated by presurgical orthopedics, gingivoperiosteoplasty, and lip adhesion (POPLA) compared with previous lip adhesion method: a preliminary study of serial dental casts. Plast Reconstr Surg 1999;103:1630.

95. Santiago P, Grayson B, Cutting C, et al: Reduced need for alveolar bone grafting by presurgical orthopedics and primary gingivoperiosteoplasty. Cleft Palate Craniofac J 1998;35:77.

96. Santiago P, Grayson B, Gianoutsos M, et al: Elimination of alveolar bone grafting by presurgical orthopedics and primary gingivoperiosteoplasty. Proceedings of American Cleft Palate-Craniofacial Association, San Diego, Calif, 1996.

97. Lee C, Grayson B, Brecht L, et al: Long term study of midface growth in unilateral cleft lip and palate patients following gingivoperiosteoplasty. Am Cleft Palate Craniofac Assoc 1999; 56:95.

98. Wood R, Grayson B, Cutting C: Gingivoperiosteoplasty and growth of the midface. Plast Surg Forum 1993;16:229.

99. Wood R, Grayson B, Cutting C: Gingivoperiosteoplasty and midfacial growth. Cleft Palate Craniofac J 1997;34:17.

100. Abyholm F, Bergland O, Semb G: Secondary bone grafting of alveolar cleft. Scand J Plast Reconstr Surg 1981;15:127.

101. Axhausen G: Technik und Ergebnisse der Lippenplastik. Stuttgart, Georg Thieme Verlag, 1932.

102. Berkeley WT: The concepts of unilateral repair applied to bilateral clefts of the lip and nose. Plast Reconstr Surg 1961;27:505.

103. Brown JB: Elongation of the partially cleft palate. Am J Orthod 1938;24:878.

104. Davis WB: Methods preferred in cleft lip and cleft palate repair. J Int Coll Surg 1940;3:116.

105. Huffman WC, Lierle DM: The repair of the bilateral cleft lip. Plast Reconstr Surg 1949;4:489.

106. Manchester WM: A method of primary double cleft lip repair. In Huston JT, ed: Transactions of the 5th International Congress of Plastic and Reconstructive Surgery. Melbourne, Australia, Butterworths, 1971.

107. Millard DR Jr: Closure of bilateral cleft lip and elongation of columella by two operations in infancy. Plast Reconstr Surg 1971;47:324.

108. Millard DR Jr: Complete bilateral cleft lip; primary lip and nose correction. In Huston JT, ed: Transactions of the 5th International Congress of Plastic and Reconstructive Surgery. Melbourne, Australia, Butterworths, 1971:185.

109. Schultz LW: Bilateral cleft lips. Plast Reconstr Surg 1946;1:338.

110. Skoog T: The management of the bilateral cleft of the primary palate (lip and alveolus). Part 1. General considerations and soft tissue repair. Plast Reconstr Surg 1965;35:34.

111. Vaughn HS: Importance of premaxilla and philtrum in bilateral cleft lip. Plast Reconstr Surg 1946;1:240.

112. Adams WM, Adams LH: The misuse of the prolabium in the repair of bilateral cleft lip. Plast Reconstr Surg 1953;12:225.

113. Antia NH: Primary Abbe flap in bilateral cleft lip. Br J Plast Surg 1973;12:215.

114. Clarkson P: Use of the Abbe flap in the primary repair of double cleft lip. Br J Plast Surg 1954;7:175.

115. Honig CA: The operative treatment of bilateral complete clefts of the primary and secondary palate in the first year of life. In Hotz R, ed: Early Treatment of Cleft Lip and Palate. International Symposium. Zurich, University of Zurich Dental Institute, 1964.

116. Barsky A: Principles and Practice of Plastic Surgery. Baltimore, Williams & Wilkins, 1950.

117. Holdsworth W: Cleft Lip and Palate. New York, Grune & Stratton, 1951.

118. Smith F: Plastic and Reconstructive Surgery. Philadelphia, WB Saunders, 1950.

119. Veau V: Division palatine, anatomie, chirurgie, phonetique. Paris, Masson et Cie, 1931.

120. Mulliken JB: Principles and techniques of bilateral cleft lip repair. Plast Reconstr Surg 1985;75:477.

121. Manchester WM: The repair of bilateral cleft lip and palate. Br J Surg 1965;52:878.

122. Noordhoff MS, Cheng WS: Median facial dysgenesis in cleft lip and palate. Ann Plast Surg 1982;8:83.

123. Millard DR: Details of closing a complete bilateral cleft and banking the fork. In Millard DR, ed: Cleft Craft, vol II. Bilateral and Rare Deformities. Boston, Little, Brown, 1977:359.

124. Black PW: Bilateral cleft lip. Clin Plast Surg 1985;12:627.

125. Cutting C, Grayson B: The prolabial unwinding flap method for one-stage repair of bilateral cleft lip, nose, and alveolus. Plast Reconstr Surg 1993;91:37.

126. Mulliken JB: Correction of the bilateral cleft lip nasal deformity: evolution of a surgical concept. Cleft Palate Craniofac J 1992;29:540.

127. Mulliken JB: Bilateral complete cleft lip and nasal deformity: an anthropometric analysis of staged to synchronous repair. Plast Reconstr Surg 1995;96:9.

128. Trier WC: Repair of bilateral cleft lip: Millard's technique. Clin Plast Surg 1985;12:605.

129. Brauer RO, Foerster DW: Another method to lengthen the columella in the double cleft patient. Plast Reconstr Surg 1966; 38:27.

130. Converse JM: Corrective surgery of the nasal tip. Laryngoscope 1957;67:6.

131. Cronin TD: Lengthening the columella by use of skin from the nasal floor and alae. Plast Reconstr Surg 1958;21:417.

132. Duffy MM: Restoration of orbicularis oris muscle continuity in the repair of bilateral cleft lip. Br J Plast Surg 1971;24:48.

133. Marcks KM, Trevaskis AE, Payne MJ: Bilateral cleft lip repair. Plast Reconstr Surg 1957;19:401.

134. Marcks KM, Trevaskis AE, Payne MJ: Elongation of columella by flap. Plast Reconstr Surg 1957;20:466.

135. Millard DR Jr: Columella lengthening by a forked flap. Plast Reconstr Surg 1958;22:454.

136. Noordhoff MS: Bilateral cleft lip reconstruction. Plast Reconstr Surg 1986;78:45.

137. Peskova A, Fara M: Lengthening of the columella in bilateral cleft. Acta Chir Plast 1960;2:18.

138. Cronin T, Cronin E, Roper P, et al: Bilateral clefts. In McCarthy JG, ed: Reconstructive Plastic Surgery, vol 4. Philadelphia, WB Saunders, 1990:2653.

139. McComb H: Primary repair of the bilateral cleft lip nose: a 15 year review and a new treatment plan. Plast Reconstr Surg 1990;86:882.

140. Millard DR Jr: A primary compromise for bilateral cleft lip. Surg Gynecol Obstet 1960;111:557.

141. Millard DR Jr: Bilateral cleft lip and a primary forked flap: a preliminary report. Plast Reconstr Surg 1967;39:59.

142. Millard DR Jr: Results of surgical lengthening of the short nose in the bilateral cleft lip patient. Plast Reconstr Surg 1978;62:438.

143. Millard DR, Cassisi A, Wheeler J: Designs for correction and camouflage of bilateral clefts of the lip and palate. Plast Reconstr Surg 2000;105:1609.

144. Cutting C: Cleft lip nasal reconstruction. In Rees T, LaTrenta G, eds: Aesthetic Plastic Surgery. Philadelphia, WB Saunders, 1994:497.

145. Cutting C, Bardach J, Pang R: A comparative study of the skin envelope of the unilateral cleft lip nose subsequent to rotation-advancement and triangular flap lip repairs. Plast Reconstr Surg 1989;84:409.

146. McComb H: Primary repair of the bilateral cleft lip nose: a 4-year review. Plast Reconstr Surg 1994;94:37.

147. Anderl H: Simultaneous repair of cleft lip and nose in the unilateral cleft (a long term report). In Jackson I, Sommerlad B, eds: Recent Advances in Plastic Surgery, vol 3. London, Churchill Livingstone, 1985:1-11.

148. Berkeley WT: The cleft lip nose. Plast Reconstr Surg 1959;23:567.

149. Berkeley WT: Correction of the unilateral cleft lip nasal deformity. In Grabb WC, Rosenstein SW, Bzoch KR, eds: Cleft Lip and Palate: Surgical, Dental, and Speech Aspects. Boston, Little, Brown, 1971:227.

150. Boo-Chai K: Primary repair of the unilateral cleft lip nose in the Oriental: a 20 year followup. Plast Reconstr Surg 1987; 80:185.

151. Broadbent TR, Woolf R: Cleft lip nasal deformity. Ann Plast Surg 1984;12:216.

152. Brown JB, McDowell F: Simplified design for repair of single cleft lips. Surg Gynecol Obstet 1945;80:12.

153. Kernahan DA, Bauer BS, Harris GD: Experience with the Tajima procedure in primary and secondary repair in unilateral cleft lip nasal deformity. Plast Reconstr Surg 1980;66:46.

154. Lamont ES: Plastic surgery in reconstructing the primary cleft lip and nasal deformity. Am J Surg 1953;86:200.

155. McComb H: Primary repair of the bilateral cleft lip nose. Br J Plast Surg 1975;28:262.

156. McComb H: Treatment of the unilateral cleft lip nose. Plast Reconstr Surg 1975;55:596.

157. McComb H, Coghlan B: Primary repair of the unilateral cleft lip nose: completion of a longitudinal study. Cleft Palate Craniofac J 1996;33:23.

158. Ortiz-Monasterio F, Olmedo A: Corrective rhinoplasty before puberty: a long-term follow-up. Plast Reconstr Surg 1981; 68:381.

159. Pigott RW: "Alar leapfrog." A technique for repositioning the total alar cartilage at primary cleft lip repair. Clin Plast Surg 1985;12:643.

160. Salyer KE: Primary correction of the unilateral cleft lip nose: a 15-year experience. Plast Reconstr Surg 1986;77:558.

161. Sawhney CP: Nasal deformity in unilateral cleft lip. Cleft Palate J 1976;13:291.

162. Skoog T: Repair of unilateral cleft lip deformity: maxilla, nose and lip. Scand J Plast Reconstr Surg 1969;3:109.

163. Stenstrom SJ: Follow-up clinic: the alar cartilage and nasal deformity in unilateral cleft lip. Plast Reconstr Surg 1975;55:359.

164. Sugihara T, Yoshida T, Igawa H, Homma K: Primary correction of the unilateral cleft lip nose. Cleft Palate Craniofac J 1993;30:231.

165. Wynn SK: Primary nostril reconstruction in complete cleft lips. The round nostril technique. Plast Reconstr Surg 1972; 49:56.

166. Wellisz T, Cutting C, McCarthy J: The effects of unilamellar perichondrial dissection on the growth of rabbit ear cartilage. Plast Reconstr Surg 1987;79:935.

167. Morel-Fatio D, Lalardrie JP: External nasal approach in the correction of major morphologic sequelae of the cleft lip nose. Plast Reconstr Surg 1966;38:116.

168. Trott JA, Mohan N: A preliminary report on one stage open tip rhinoplasty at the time of lip repair in bilateral cleft lip and palate: the Alor Setar experience. Br J Plast Surg 1993;46: 215.

169. Cutting C: Coordinated presurgical columella elongation and one stage primary nasal correction of the bilateral cleft lip and nose. In Bardach J, ed: Atlas of Craniofacial and Cleft Surgery, vol II. Philadelphia, Lippincott-Raven, 1999:602.

170. Bardach J: Correction of secondary bilateral cleft lip and nasal deformities: Bardach's technique. In Bardach J, ed: Atlas of Craniofacial and Cleft Surgery, vol II. Philadelphia, Lippincott-Raven, 1999.

171. Bardach J, Salyer K: Correction of the nasal deformity associated with bilateral cleft lip. In Bardach J, Salyer K, eds: Surgical Techniques in Cleft Lip and Palate, 2nd ed. Baltimore, Mosby–Year Book, 1991:197-223.

172. Blair V, Brown J: Mirault operations for single harelip. Surg Gynecol Obstet 1930;51:81.

173. Mulliken J: Personal communication, 1997.

174. Trott J: Synchronous open rhinoplasty and primary bilateral cleft lip repair: Trott's technique. In Bardach J, ed: Atlas of Craniofacial and Cleft Surgery, vol II. Philadelphia, Lippincott-Raven, 1999:594-601.

175. Kohout M, Aljaro L, Farkas L, Mulliken J: Photogrammetric comparison of two methods for synchronous repair of bilateral cleft lip and nasal deformity. Plast Reconstr Surg 1998; 102:1339.

176. Monasterio L: Personal communication, 1997.

177. Cutting C, Grayson B, Brecht L: Columellar elongation in bilateral cleft lip [letter; comment]. Plast Reconstr Surg 1998; 102:1761.

178. Tajima S, Maruyama M: Reverse U incision for secondary repair of cleft lip nose. Plast Reconstr Surg 1977;60:256.

179. Uchida M, Kojima T, Hirase Y: Secondary correction of the bilateral cleft lip nose by excision of the columellar forked flap and nasal remodelling with reverse-U flaps: a preliminary report. Br J Plast Surg 1994;47:490.

180. Reinisch J, Sloan G: Complications of cleft lip repair. In Bardach J, Morris H, eds: Multidisciplinary Management of Cleft Lip and Palate. Philadelphia, WB Saunders, 1990:247.

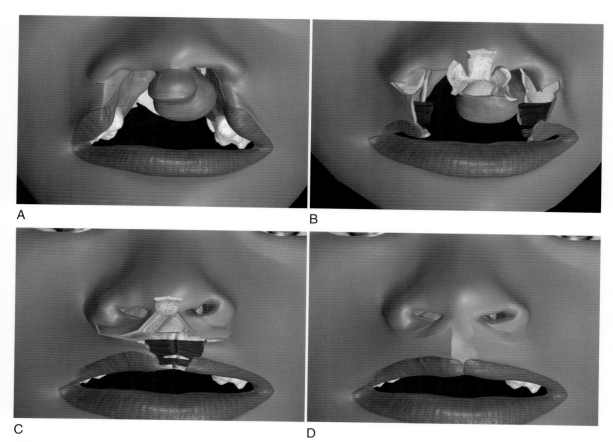

COLOR PLATE 94-1. First stage of the banked forked-flap procedure. *A,* Incisions marked. *B,* Lateral vermilion turndown flaps are developed, and the prolabium is divided into three vertical tines. The prolabial mucosa is folded back to set the height of the gingivobuccal sulcus. *C,* The muscle and the inner lip mucosa from the lateral elements are repaired. The lateral "forks" are inset into "whiskers" position. *D,* The lip is closed. (From Cutting C, et al: Bilateral Cleft Lip [videotape]. New York, The Smile Train.)

Cleft Palate Repair

WILLIAM Y. HOFFMAN, MD ✦ DELORA MOUNT, MD

HISTORY

The first recorded operative treatment of a cleft patient has been attributed to the period of the Chin (Tsin) Dynasty, circa AD 390.[1] The repair was of a cleft lip only, and no mention of cleft palate repair was made. Palatal clefts were confused with the more common fistulas resulting from tertiary syphilis and were not addressed surgically because of this association. The greater technical challenges of cleft palate repair no doubt presented a barrier to surgical treatment as well. Although the first known cleft palate repair was performed in the early 19th century, the introduction of anesthesia permitted a quantum leap in treatment as it did for many diseases.[2]

John Stephenson (1797-1842), a physician who was born with incomplete cleft palate, wrote the earliest recorded description of palatoplasty. As a medical student in Edinburgh, he traveled to Paris to observe the renowned surgeon Philibert Roux (1780-1854). While he was there, Roux noted his abnormal speech pattern; he performed the primary repair of his velum when Stephenson was 22 years old. In his thesis, Stephenson wrote in astute detail of his speech quality:

I always pronounced /th/ like /s/. As I grew up, the adjacent parts tended to close the defect, and by speaking slowly I articulated better. Thanks to the nasal quality of the language I used to speak French more clearly than English. Nature is kind and trying to correct her mistakes, did her best to improve my unpleasant voice by contracting as strongly as possible the muscles of the nasopharynx. . . . I believe that the nasal sound was due to faulty vibration of the air in its passage from lungs to nares, because the fissure prevented the soft palate from functioning.[3]

Following the description of his speech, Stephenson wrote in detail of the procedure, including the positioning (seated upright in front of Dr. Roux), anesthetic (none), difficulties (breathing and bleeding), and postoperative course (respiratory difficulty, nothing to eat or drink for 29 hours, and discomfort of suture removal). He also described the quality of the postoperative speech:

It must be confessed that some of the nasal quality is still present. Old habit and the above-mentioned muscular contraction were too much for me. The repaired instrument is not yet fulfilling its proper duties to giving the help it should to my vocal faculty. Who can deny the all-importance of habit?

The same problem often occurs today when cleft palate repair is delayed until later in life.

After the acceptance of his doctoral thesis, Stephenson returned to his home in Canada and eventually became principal founder of McGill Medical College, where he served as Professor of Anatomy, Physiology, and Surgery.[4] Roux later published his account of the procedure in 1825, describing the simple suture closure of the surgically freshened edges, which he termed staphyloraphie.[5]

The notoriety surrounding the publication of Stephenson's thesis angered Carl Ferdinand von Graefe (1787-1840), who proclaimed that he rather than Roux was the first surgeon to perform velar closure. Indeed, he had devised the surgery and performed it (unsuccessfully) before 1819. He had briefly mentioned the simple suture of the velum to the medical society of Berlin in 1816 but had failed to report it formally in the medical journals of the time. For von Graefe, "who appeared to have little interest in this procedure at the time, apparently deeming it of no importance, it now became the chief concern of his life."[6] Competition and national honor between surgical groups in Berlin and Paris split the European medical community on this topic. von Graefe eventually reported a successful repair in 1820.[7] The first successful closure of the soft palate in America was by John Collins Warren in 1820 in Boston.[2]

Johann Friedrich Dieffenbach (1792-1847) studied under von Graefe at the University of Berlin.[8] Dieffenbach expanded the technique of soft palate repair to include closure of the hard palate. Dieffenbach's palatoplasty method involved bringing together the cleft bony segments by a series of twisting silver or lead sutures passed through punch holes in the bony palate.[9] He eventually designed and advocated lateral mucosal relaxing incisions to aid successful soft tissue closure. Later, following von Graefe at Charité Hospital in Berlin in 1840, he not only improved the technique of palatoplasty but also advanced techniques of local flap closure and transplantation. Dieffenbach's possibly most important contribution to plastic surgery was the introduction of ether anesthesia to plastic surgical procedures.[9] Dieffenbach had been introduced to anesthetic technique during a demonstration at Massachusetts General Hospital in 1846 and began applying it to routine surgical procedures before his death in 1847. He was so revered in Germany that he received an official state burial.

After the death of Dieffenbach, Bernhard von Langenbeck (1810-1887) succeeded to the position at the University of Berlin. Incorporating his extensive work with bone and periosteum of the extremities during the Franco-Prussian war, he was the first to describe the mucoperiosteal plane of dissection and to use its advantage in mobility to cleft palate closure.[10] His technique, with various modifications, is still widely used today. The combination of Dieffenbach's introduction of general anesthesia and von Langenbeck's use of mucoperiosteal flaps ushered in the modern era of cleft palate surgery.

In the 180 years since the first cleft palate repair, the goals have remained the same: to attain normalization of speech and to minimize effects of surgery on midfacial growth. This chapter is designed to take the prin-

ciples learned from painstaking years of modifications of modern palatoplasty and to apply them to current care of patients.

CLEFT PALATE CLASSIFICATION

Careful anatomic evaluation of each patient is of paramount importance in considering palatoplasty. Anatomic variability within the broad diagnosis of cleft palate will influence the timing and sequence of surgical repair as well as the type of repair. Optimal functional results depend directly on accurate analysis of the available structures and understanding of their long-term significance to function and facial growth (Fig. 95-1).

Cleft Palate with Cleft Lip and Alveolus

Although the primary palate and the secondary palate form at different stages of embryonic development, cleft palate is most commonly seen in combination with cleft lip. The embryology of maxillary development is reviewed elsewhere; the failure of fusion of the frontonasal and maxillary processes gives rise to the cleft in the typical location between the premaxilla and the lateral maxilla, on either one or both sides.

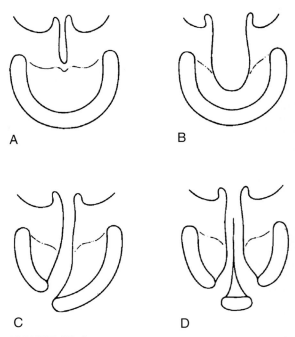

FIGURE 95-1. Cleft classification. *A,* Incomplete cleft of the secondary palate. *B,* Complete cleft of the secondary palate (extends forward to the incisive foramen). *C,* Complete unilateral cleft lip and palate. *D,* Bilateral complete cleft lip and palate. (After Veau V: Division Palatine. Paris, Masson et Cie, 1931.)

Displacement of the central premaxillary portion of the alveolus is commonly seen in complete cleft lip and palate, both unilateral and bilateral. The segment can be excessively protuberant, canted, rotated, or impacted. Preoperative molding of the alveolar gap before lip repair can better align the segment anatomically, thus reducing tension on the lip repair. Presurgical techniques vary from simple lip taping to pin-fixed alveolar appliances to mold the segments Controversy exists about which patients have indications for close-gap treatment, whether potential maxillary growth is disturbed, and also cost-effectiveness of presurgical orthodontic treatment.[11] Even without presurgical orthopedic management, the alveolar segments often come into close approximation after lip repair owing to the action of the repaired orbicularis oris muscle and its force on the premaxillary segment.

The alveolar portion of the cleft lies between the maxillary lateral incisor and canine tooth roots. This results in malposition of the maxillary lateral incisor and cuspid in both the deciduous and permanent dentition.[12,13] The maxillary lateral incisor on the cleft side is absent in 80% to 90% of cleft patients; when present, it may be smaller than the contralateral tooth or significantly dysmorphic.[13-15] Absence of other teeth is not uncommon,[16] but it may be related to the surgery itself because adults who have not been operated on do not show the same patterns of hypodontia.[17] Asymmetry is common, resulting in alterations in first maxillary molar position.[18-20] In comparison to noncleft individuals, patients with unilateral cleft lip and palate have overall reduction in crown size[21] and delay of eruption of permanent dentition.[22] These findings support the theory of global dental growth potential disturbance associated with clefting. Interestingly, eruption of deciduous dentition is not significantly delayed.[23]

Unilateral complete cleft palate is characterized by direct communication between the entire length of the nasal passage and oropharynx. The nasal septum is deviated and buckled toward the cleft side. The absence of a portion of the inferior piriform aperture and the hypoplasia of the lateral nasal bony platform at the maxillary wall contribute to the cleft nasal deformity; the nasal base is depressed, the ala collapses, and the floor widens. (See Chapter 98 for full description of the cleft nasal defect.) The unilateral complete cleft is thus a full-thickness palatal defect of nasal mucosa, bony palate, velar musculature, and oral mucosa; all of these deficiencies must be addressed during the cleft palate repair or later at the time of alveolar cleft bone grafting.

In the bilateral complete cleft lip and palate, the premaxillary segment containing the central and lateral incisor tooth roots is discontinuous from the alveolar arch. The lateral segments often collapse inward and lingually, resulting in "locking out" of the premaxilla

if appropriate preoperative management has not been used or is not successful. The anterior location of the premaxilla in this situation may result in anterior fistulas, which may in turn cause significant speech problems and nasal regurgitation of fluids. Later orthodontic treatment of the maxillary arch can align the segments before bone grafting.

The levator palatini muscle, in addition to being discontinuous across the cleft, runs more or less longitudinally along the cleft margin before it inserts aberrantly into the posterior border of the hard palate (Fig. 95-2).[24-26] This results in ineffective contraction and inability to close the palate against the posterior pharyngeal wall. Air escape through the nose during speech produces a characteristic hypernasal quality. In addition, aberrant levator positioning is thought to impair the function of the tensor palatini muscle, which normally assists eustachian tube function and is thought to be contributory to cleft otopathology.[27] A complete review of cleft otopathology is presented later in this chapter.

Clefts of the Secondary Palate

Also called incomplete cleft palate, a cleft of the secondary palate only may be variable, from an opening in the posterior soft palate to a cleft extending up to the incisive foramen. Most commonly, dentition is normal and symmetric. The levator palatini muscles are displaced as in the complete clefts.

Pierre Robin sequence is defined as micrognathia, glossoptosis, and respiratory distress.[28] Of the children diagnosed with Pierre Robin sequence, 60% to 90% have cleft palate[29,30]; the palatal cleft is usually isolated to the velum and can be V shaped or, more typically, U shaped.[31,32] In the past, this has been thought to be secondary to hyperflexion of the head in utero with secondary displacement of the tongue between the palatal shelves, preventing their fusion. More recently, extensive analysis of multiple syndromes associated with Pierre Robin sequence has delineated syndromic associations, indicating that the etiology may not be such a simple mechanical event.[33-35] Infants with Pierre Robin sequence also have increased incidence of associated anomalies, particularly cardiac and renal problems.[36]

Newborns with Pierre Robin sequence may have severe respiratory and feeding difficulty because of the posterior displacement of the tongue. Initial treatment consists of placing the child prone and use of gastric lavage feeding tubes or palatal obturators to push the tongue forward.[37] If these maneuvers fail, the child may need nasopharyngeal intubation to maintain a patent upper airway.[38] If these conservative measures fail, surgical management of the airway may be required. A tongue-lip adhesion has been used as an alternative to tracheostomy and is generally effective (Fig. 95-3).[39,40]

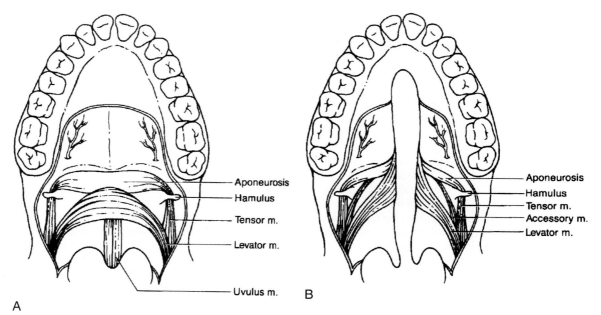

A

B

Aponeurosis
Hamulus
Tensor m.
Levator m.
Uvulus m.

Aponeurosis
Hamulus
Tensor m.
Accessory m.
Levator m.

FIGURE 95-2. *A,* Normal anatomy of the soft palate; the levator palatini muscle is seen as a sling across the posterior soft palate. *B,* Cleft palate anatomy. The levator palatini muscle is displaced longitudinally, almost parallel to the cleft. The tendon of the tensor palatini muscle can be seen coming around the hamulus to join the aponeurosis of the levator; division of this tendon is important to rotate the levator back into a posterior position. Note as well the position of the vascular pedicles, exiting through the palatine foramina. (After Millard DR Jr: Cleft Craft, vol III. Boston, Little, Brown, 1980:19, 30.)

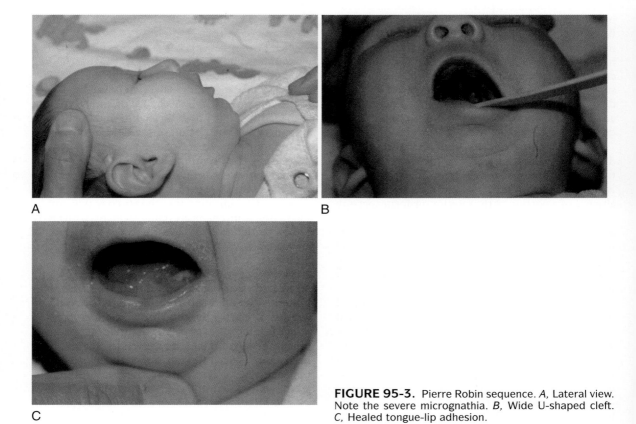

A

B

C

FIGURE 95-3. Pierre Robin sequence. *A,* Lateral view. Note the severe micrognathia. *B,* Wide U-shaped cleft. *C,* Healed tongue-lip adhesion.

Mandibular distraction osteogenesis has been used in neonates with success in averting tracheostomy, although long-term outcomes in regard to mandibular growth and dental development are not yet available.[41] In all cases, if management is focused on the upper airway, bronchoscopy should be performed to rule out any intrinsic subglottic problems (e.g., laryngomalacia) that might necessitate tracheostomy.

Palatoplasty in children with Pierre Robin sequence must be carefully timed with growth of the child, particularly the mandible. There is some controversy about "catch-up" growth of the mandible in children with Pierre Robin sequence; basically, there is good documentation of extra growth in the first year of life,[42,43] but growth is subsequently commensurate with that of normal children. Late cephalometric evaluation has consistently shown that the children with Pierre Robin sequence have smaller mandibles than normal.[44] If the mandible attains reasonable size in the first year of life, palate repair can still be performed safely before 1 year of age. Closure of the palate narrows the effective area for respiration and can lead to respiratory distress. In the rare patient who has previously undergone tracheostomy, the palate should be repaired before decannulation. The risk of airway compromise after palatoplasty reaches 25%, with an emergent tracheostomy or reintubation rate of 11% at one institution.[45]

Submucous Cleft Palate

Submucous cleft palate occurs when the palate has mucosal continuity but the underlying levator palatini muscle is discontinuous across the midline and longitudinally oriented, similar to the muscle anatomy in complete and secondary clefts. The classic triad of a midline clear zone, a bifid uvula, and a palpable notch in the posterior hard palate is diagnostic of this condition. With contraction of velar musculature, a distinct midline muscle diastasis may be seen.

The significance of a submucous cleft may be difficult to assess clinically; the child with submucous cleft palate is often undiagnosed in infancy. In a study screening a large population of schoolchildren in Denver, the overall incidence of submucous cleft palate in the population was found to be 1:1200.[46] Another similar cohort study reported that 45% to 55% of patients with isolated submucous cleft palate were symptomatic with regard to speech, serous otitis media, or hearing loss.[47,48] In a large series of children with submucous cleft palate in Mexico, examination with fiberoptic nasendoscopy showed about one third to have velopharyngeal insufficiency.[49] Other attempts to identify risk of speech problems with submucous cleft palate have been problematic because referrals to cleft palate clinics are usually based on the identification of speech issues rather than of the submucous cleft itself. Therefore, an infant identified with submucous cleft palate need not routinely undergo repair because a significant number of individuals with submucous cleft palate will not develop velopharyngeal insufficiency. Rather, these patients should be closely monitored with serial speech evaluations and audiometric surveillance.

Patients who present with velopharyngeal insufficiency and submucous cleft palate on examination require full evaluation, including speech evaluation and endoscopy.[50] Even in the absence of obvious findings on clinical examination, anatomic abnormalities are found in most patients (>90%) at the time of surgery[51,52]; thus, the so-called occult submucous cleft palate is simply one that is less obvious on clinical evaluation. There will still be rare patients, however, who have true palatopharyngeal disproportion and present with velopharyngeal insufficiency without any cleft, submucous or otherwise.[50]

Corrective surgical technique for submucous cleft palate is focused on anatomic correction of the velar muscle diastasis. Although pharyngeal flaps and sphincter pharyngoplasty have been proposed as primary means of treatment,[49] most surgeons focus on repair of the abnormal levator muscle position.[53] The Furlow double opposing Z-plasty (see later) is an ideal procedure for these patients because there is no width discrepancy to be overcome.[54] This avoids the potential for nasal obstruction and sleep apnea in these patients if a pharyngeal flap is used.

RATIONALE FOR REPAIR OF CLEFT PALATE

The normal palate serves several important functions, all related to functional separation of the oropharynx from the nasopharynx. Whereas the sine qua non for palate repair is normal speech, consideration of cleft palate surgery must balance developmental, dentofacial growth, and otologic issues as well.

Growth

At birth, the average weight is the same for cleft and unaffected newborns.[55,56] However, cleft infants have been shown to exhibit poor weight gain in early infancy. Studies observing infants with cleft lip and palate show initial growth retardation by the time they undergo surgical lip repair. When the same children reach the age for palatoplasty, they have significantly lagged on the growth curve. However, longitudinal studies show that after repair of the palate, average growth returns to normal compared with unaffected children by the age of 4 years. Stratification of risk within the longitudinal cohort shows pronounced growth retardation in associated syndromes and also in children with isolated clefts of the secondary palate.[57,58]

Cleft children stabilize and continue normal growth to at least 6 years of age, with no statistically significant differences in height and weight between cleft and unaffected children. In later childhood, however, average weight and height of children with cleft appear to diminish compared with those of control subjects. In a Danish study of skeletal maturity assessing both body height and radius length as an index of growth in male cleft patients, onset of puberty was found to be delayed on average 6 months, and the velocity of skeletal growth during puberty was blunted. However, duration of puberty and pubertal skeletal growth were prolonged an average of 1 year, resulting in final attained body height and radius length the same as those of control subjects.[59]

Numerous causes are thought to contribute to these differences in growth patterns. There are certainly feeding difficulties early in life before palate repair,[60] but it has also been suggested that intrinsic growth disturbances may be responsible for slow postnatal growth.[61] The increased frequency of ear and airway infections has been implicated in early growth retardation,[55] as have the multiple operative procedures that these children undergo.[60] Adding more confusion to the etiology is the fact that growth hormone levels may be diminished in cleft children. In summary, any growth disturbance is likely to be a multifactorial phenomenon throughout infancy, childhood, and puberty. Fortunately, families can be counseled that norms of height, weight, and development are attained by most children.

Feeding and Swallowing

The intact palate provides a barrier between the respiratory tract and the alimentary tract. To understand the difficulty cleft infants have with feeding, one must understand the normal role of the palate in sucking and swallowing. Oral intake is divided into two separate activities, generation of suction force (negative intraoral pressure) and swallowing. For negative intraoral pressure to be produced, the velum seals off the pharynx posteriorly; the lips close anteriorly, and negative pressure is produced by moving the tongue away from the palate and by opening the mandible. This effectively increases the intraoral volume within a closed system, resulting in generation of negative pressure. If the individual is unable to close the velopharynx or to generate a seal of the lips, or if the palate is not intact at the point of contact with the tongue, negative pressure cannot be produced. This failure of velopharyngeal closure is the basis of difficulty with breast-feeding or normal bottle-feeding in the patient with cleft palate.

Suction on the nipple in a breast-feeding infant is thought to stabilize the nipple position while motion of the tongue against the nipple pushes fluid into the mouth. Ingestion through an artificial nipple is different; infants learn to manipulate the nipple and flow rates by closing the alveolus against the artificial nipple. Tongue motion is primarily used to transfer the bolus to the pharynx for swallowing. In the cleft infant, the communication between the oropharynx and nasopharynx prevents a seal of the tongue against the palate, and negative pressure cannot be generated. Suckling is therefore not productive, and breast-feeding is ineffective.

Not all infants with clefts are unable to breast-feed. Infants with cleft limited to the velum can often use posterior tongue position to generate a partial negative seal. The exception to this is the child with Pierre Robin sequence and isolated velar cleft, who can develop respiratory distress or ineffective suction from glossoptosis. Obviously, patients with isolated cleft lip and an intact palate should and do have little difficulty with breast-feeding.[62]

Swallowing involves complex interaction of the tongue and pharynx. Coordinated swallowing is dependent on neuromuscular control and rhythmic coordinated contraction of the tongue and pharynx. Children with clefts generally do not have difficulty with swallowing and aspiration unless intrinsic neuromuscular abnormality of the tongue or pharynx is present. Children may cough or sputter with reflux of the ingested material into the nose, particularly if volume or rate of feeding is excessive. During normal deglutition, the tongue moves the food bolus to the pharynx by complex interaction of tongue against palate. When the palate is cleft, the food bolus may reflux into the nasal passage. Nasal reflux is irritating to the nasal mucosa and can predispose to sinusitis and ulceration. In the older child, a persistent communication through a fistula in the palate may result in incontinence of food through the nose, which is socially unacceptable. It is an error to ascribe aspiration simply to the presence of a cleft palate; indeed, aspiration with swallowing should stimulate an appropriate diagnostic evaluation, including thin barium swallow studies, bronchoscopy, and gastroscopy.

Infants who are unable to breast-feed because of cleft palate have a number of options for feeding. Regimens and devices have evolved to nourish the infant, including specialty nipples such as lamb's nipples, crosscutting of standard nipples, and long soft nipples that place the liquid at the posterior tongue.[62-65] Special flow bottles, such as gravity flow bottles, and squeeze bottles allow the caregiver to carefully control the flow rate. The strategy of each technique is low resistance to flow, with controllable flow rate for optimal volume and minimal effort by the infant. All of these techniques are effective, and selection is generally by personal preference and the baby's acceptance of the method. Other key considerations are elevated head positioning during feeding and careful observation of feeding time and volume ingested.

Weight gain and skeletal growth confirm success of the feeding regimen. Once the palate is successfully closed surgically, special feeding methods are generally unnecessary.

Speech

The primary goal of palatoplasty is normal speech. Patients can grow and even thrive despite feeding difficulties, but speech cannot be normalized if the palate is not closed. The ability to partition the oropharynx and nasopharynx is crucial for normal speech production. The palate elevates during production of any sounds requiring positive pressure in the oropharynx; the levator palatini is primarily responsible for this movement, creating the genu or "knee action" that can be seen on radiographs (Fig. 95-4).

Speech is a complex issue, and many factors may influence speech development in a child with a cleft palate. In addition to the importance of the palate itself, speech development may be influenced by motor or neurologic developmental delay (often seen in syndromes), by hearing (see later), and by environmental stimuli. It is important to distinguish between speech production, which is primarily dependent on normal anatomic function, and speech development, which is influenced more by global developmental issues. Speech production also requires normal articulation, which in turn depends on tongue placement, lip competence, and dental position, all of which may be abnormal in cleft patients.

If palate function is not corrected, velopharyngeal insufficiency results, with speech that is hypernasal, often with hoarse quality due to difficulty in directing airflow through the mouth. When complete closure cannot be anatomically or functionally obtained, compensatory mechanisms for sound production are learned. These are maladaptive patterns that interfere with global intelligibility and include glottal stops and pharyngeal fricatives. In addition, tongue placement for various phonemes is altered to achieve the most normal production of sounds. Eliminating these learned compensatory articulations is difficult, even with the best of speech and language therapy. Compensatory articulations may persist even in the face of a functioning palate repair, especially in later repairs or secondary correction of velopharyngeal insufficiency.

Eustachian Tube

Alt[66] was the first physician to note a correlation between ear disease and cleft palate in 1878. Numerous studies have linked the presence of a cleft palate to abnormalities in eustachian tube function. In multicenter studies, incidence of otitis media effusion has been found to be 96% to 100% in cleft patients, measured by both middle ear effusions on otoscopy and impedance testing and middle ear aspiration.[67,68] In the cleft palate, impairment of tubal dilation is thought to occur from complex misalignment of the paratubal musculature.[69,70] Both radiologic and manometric testing techniques have demonstrated abnormalities in active dilation of the eustachian tube.[71] In addition, intrinsic abnormalities of tubal cartilage framework rendering a eustachian tube more collapsible have been noted. Although anatomic studies show that the levator veli palatini muscle does not directly actively

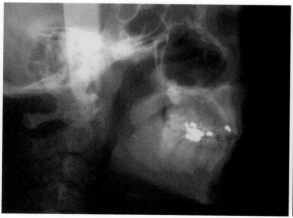
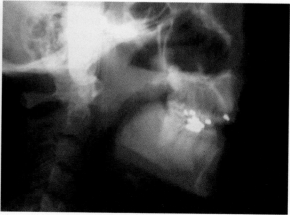

A   B

FIGURE 95-4. Elevation of the soft palate with speech. These are both lateral cephalograms obtained after cleft palate repair with a Furlow double opposing Z-plasty. *A,* Resting; the palate actually appears a little short, and there is a fairly large posterior airway. *B,* Radiograph obtained during sustained *s* sound; the posterior pharynx is completely closed by the elevation of the soft palate.

open the eustachian tube orifice, it is likely to have a secondary effect by influence on the tensor veli palatini and also with passive position of the orifice. The levator and tensor do share a common tendinous insertion near the hamulus and pulley position around the hamulus. In the cleft patient, the levator is connected solidly against the rigid posterior hard palate; the pulley effect around the hamulus cannot be activated and impairs opening of the tube. In addition, some theorize that constant bathing of the tube orifice with oropharyngeal refluxed material leads to inflammation and obstruction of drainage. Other studies have demonstrated adenoidal tissue at the level of the tubal dilator that could potentially contribute to mechanical obstruction.[72] Anatomic paratubal abnormalities and risk for serous otitis media and chronic audiologic sequelae are present regardless of cleft type, although Pierre Robin sequence has been postulated to be at even higher risk for hearing loss because of potential for concomitant ossicular malformation.[73]

Chronic obstruction of drainage leads to serous otitis media, and long-standing effusion can result in hearing loss. Estimates are 20% to 30% incidence of pure tone hearing loss in cleft patients by audiography[74]; decreased hearing has been found in as many as half of cleft palate patients by other authors.[75] Untreated children with clefts and severe effusions may have total deafness. Obviously, whereas hearing loss is significant in any child, it may be even more so in a cleft patient in whom speech development may be abnormal.

It has long been suggested that closure of the palate reduces risk of permanent hearing loss. In retrospective studies, children who had undergone palatoplasty had significantly lower incidence of permanent hearing loss than did children with unrepaired cleft palates.[76] Although still controversial, palatoplasty is thought by most surgeons to reduce risk of chronic serous otitis media and hearing loss, although not by universal agreement. Nevertheless, serous otitis persists in most cleft patients for several years after palate repair, and myringotomy with placement of ventilating tubes remains the mainstay of treatment for this difficult problem.

TIMING OF PALATOPLASTY
Speech Outcome

The driving force for palatoplasty is the development of normal speech. Two crucial aspects of palatoplasty are important in optimal speech outcome: (1) surgical technique, discussed in the next section, and (2) timing of palate repair. Victor Veau[24] first made the observation of a correlation between age at repair and speech outcome in 1931. He noted that children who

had undergone repair before 12 months of age were much more likely to have normal speech than those with repair between 2 and 4 years of age. Children who underwent repair after 9 years of age had the worst speech outcome. The optimal time of palatoplasty still remains scientifically unproven. Confounding variables of technique, surgeon's skill, lack of standardization of speech evaluations, and therapies preclude exact determination of optimal age at repair.[77]

Most would agree that the best speech results are correlated with closure of the palate near the time of the infant's beginning language acquisition, which for the normal-developing child is before 12 months of age.[78,79] Indeed, there is a body of evidence that phonologic development actually begins earlier, at 4 to 6 months of age.[80,81] Most studies of the timing of palatal repair have looked at secondary outcomes; increased compensatory articulations were shown in one study and increased need for pharyngeal flaps in another when the palate was repaired after 1 year of age. Although repairs before 1 year of age are now common, this is not a rigid chronologic milestone; rather, repair should be related to the child's phonologic development. Some studies have shown that if correction occurs even as late as 21 months, compensatory maladaptive patterns are infrequent. Despite the absence of hard evidence supporting earlier palate repairs, a growing body of opinion seems to support palate repair around 9 to 10 months of age for children with apparently normal development.[82,83] Very early repair of the palate has been proposed by some surgeons,[84-87] primarily as a means of improving feeding; however, long-term results are lacking for any large cohort of these patients. Prospective longitudinal assessment is currently in progress to attempt to better define the optimal timing of cleft repair.

Maxillary Growth

Palatoplasty has been shown to detrimentally affect maxillary growth. Cephalometric analysis of adults with unrepaired cleft palate has shown normal maxillary dimensions and growth.[88,89] There is experimental evidence that the lip repair may restrict sagittal growth of the maxilla,[90] but in most patients, it seems that the palate repair is more significant. Many children with repaired cleft palate display typical findings of transverse maxillary deficiency requiring orthodontic widening of the maxilla once permanent teeth have erupted (permanent first molars are necessary for the forces required).

Transverse growth of the maxillary arch is narrowed in comparison with that in noncleft patients, resulting in typical malocclusion traits of crowding, lateral crossbite, and open bite.[18,92-94] Whether the narrowed arch and maxillary growth inhibition result from cicatrix[95,96] or intrinsic maxillary underdevelopment remains a matter of debate; most likely it is a combination of the two. There may be a sagittal growth deficiency as well; whereas 35% to 40% of children will develop an anterior crossbite, 15% to 20% of children with cleft palate go on to require a Le Fort I maxillary advancement in some series. There is some evidence that the development of crossbite and maxillary hypoplasia may be related to the severity of the original cleft.[97,98]

Although it might seem preferable to wait until a more advanced age for palate repair given the growth effects on the maxilla, it is far more difficult to establish normal speech in older children after cleft repair than to correct occlusion with a combination of orthodontic treatment and orthognathic surgery.

Syndromic Child with Cleft Palate

Multiple malformations or syndromes have been found frequently in cleft patients.[99] Children with cleft palate associated with an identified syndrome must be evaluated thoroughly and have individualized planning and timing of therapy. Infants with profound developmental delay and severely shortened life span projection should have surgical intervention delayed or should undergo palatoplasty under special circumstances only. In addition, syndromic children may have increased incidence of cardiac anomalies, requiring specific anesthetic and postoperative considerations. Repair of cleft palate in the hope that this will stimulate or allow a severely disabled child to speak gives unreasonable expectations and hope to parents; as noted before, it is critical to explain that palate repair may aid speech production but not speech develop-ment. Palate repair in severely disabled children can lead to altered airway status and obstructed upper airway in those with neuromuscular delay.

TECHNIQUES OF PALATE REPAIR

A number of perioperative considerations must be addressed regardless of the type of repair used. The general health and the developmental status of the child play a role in the timing of the palate repair and are also important for anesthetic and surgical management. Audiologic evaluation is routinely obtained preoperatively so that the otolaryngologist can place ventilating tubes in the tympanic membranes if indicated, saving the child an additional anesthetic.

The use of a RAE endotracheal tube facilitates placement of the Dingman gag without kinking the tube. The airway must be assessed constantly for problems; if lower central teeth are present, this can be a source of tube compression against the retractor. The Dingman gag, the most commonly used instrument for exposure, compresses the tongue and causes ischemia; if it is used for longer than 2 hours, significant postoperative tongue swelling can occur (Fig. 95-5). Lidocaine 0.5% and epinephrine 1 : 200,000 are infiltrated into the palate 7 to 10 minutes before incision; use of a 3-mL syringe makes the injection into the hard palate somewhat easier than with a larger syringe. A maximum of 1 mL/kg is used.

Palate repair is performed with the surgeon at the child's head, with use of a fiberoptic headlight or retractor. A rolled towel under the shoulders will extend the neck; it is important to check that the child does not have any syndromes that predispose to cervical spine anomalies. The use of curved needle

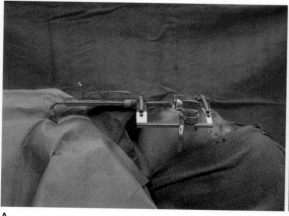

A

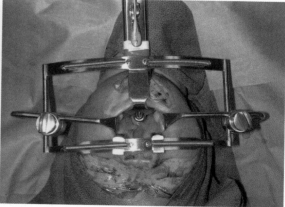

B

FIGURE 95-5. Operative preparation for cleft palate repair. *A,* The head is extended with the Dingman gag in place. *B,* Surgeon's view from above the head.

holders facilitates suture placement without obstruction of vision.

The most important aspect of surgical anatomy is the location of the greater palatine neurovascular bundle, which emerges through the greater palatine foramen through the lateral posterior hard palate. Incisions on each side are best made with the surgeon's contralateral hand to bevel the incision away from the vascular pedicle. Circumferential freeing of the palatal attachments around the pedicle and stretching of the pedicle out of the foramen are essential to obtain a tension-free closure of the oral flap.[100] In general, the goal is to obtain complete nasal and oral closure from front to back. In wide clefts, this may not be possible, particularly on the nasal surface, and the most difficult area for closure, around the junction of the hard and soft palate, is the most common location for fistulas.

It is easier to understand cleft palate surgery by separating techniques used for the hard palate from those used for the soft palate. In general, all techniques use some form of mucoperiosteal flap for the hard palate closure; the soft palate repair emphasizes correction of the abnormal position of the levator palatini muscles. The location of the incision along the cleft margin can be varied to include more or less mucosa to be turned over for nasal lining.

von Langenbeck

Langenbeck introduced the use of mucoperiosteal flaps to close clefts of the secondary palate. The initial description of the technique involved a simple approximation of the cleft margins with a relaxing incision that began posterior to the maxillary tuberosity and followed the posterior portion of the alveolar ridge (Fig. 95-6). The Langenbeck repair is still used commonly for clefts of the secondary palate. Intravelar veloplasty, or repair of the levator palatini muscle, is usually added today to reproduce the normal muscle sling.

Pushback (Veau-Wardill-Kilner)

George Dorrance (1877-1949) of Philadelphia realized that a distinct number of patients with cleft would develop velopharyngeal dysfunction caused by inability of the soft palate to touch the posterior pharyngeal wall.[101,102] In fact, he advocated muscle transposition but did so by fracturing the hamulus, which he believed would change the vector of muscle contraction and in combination with techniques of Langenbeck would lengthen the palate. He also advocated division of the major palatine neurovascular bundles to assist with the pushback. Thomas Kilner (1896-1964) was important in development of the V-Y palate repair

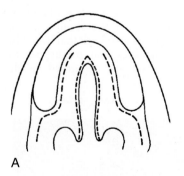

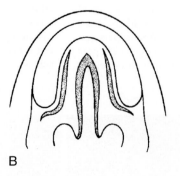

Lambeaux bipédiculés

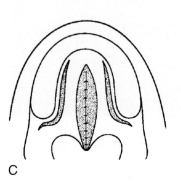

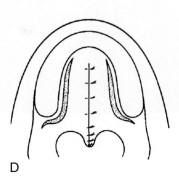

FIGURE 95-6. The von Langenbeck palate repair. *A,* Markings for incisions. *B,* Mucoperiosteal flaps elevated from lateral relaxing incisions to cleft margins. *C,* Closure of nasal mucosa. *D,* Final appearance after oral closure. Note: closure of levator palatini muscle across midline is not illustrated here. (From Randall P, LaRossa D: Cleft palate. In McCarthy JG, ed: Plastic Surgery. Philadelphia, WB Saunders, 1990: 2743.)

along with Victor Veau and William E. M. Wardill (1893-1960). In addition, he pushed for palate repair at an earlier age, 12 to 18 months.[103]

The essence of the pushback repair is the V to Y incision and closure on the hard palate. The initial description included osteotomy of the posterior hard palate at the greater palatine foramina to release the palatine vessels; circumferential dissection with release of the periosteum behind the vessels was subsequently advocated to stretch the vessels, which works as well with less risk of injury to this vital blood supply.[100,104] The nasal tissue is released and left open; some authors have proposed providing nasal lining either with septal flaps[105] or with buccal mucosa.[106] The soft palate is addressed with repair of the cleft margins and transverse closure of the levator muscle (Fig. 95-7).

The pushback technique has the advantage of providing increased length for the palate and placing the levator muscle in a more favorable position. Large open areas are left anteriorly; however, this may result in loss of maxillary width anteriorly, a situation more difficult to correct than posterior maxillary narrowing. The arch may also be flattened anteriorly, which is also a difficult problem for the orthodontist. The closure anteriorly in a complete cleft is a single layer of nasal mucosa only, which gives rise to a higher fistula rate in pushback repairs than in other techniques.[107]

Two-Flap Palatoplasty

Bardach[108] originally described a technique of freeing mucoperiosteal flaps from the cleft margins only, arguing that the arch of the cleft would provide the length needed for central closure. This is certainly not a universal finding, and it is probably most applicable in relatively narrow clefts. The more extensive two-flap palatoplasty is a modification of the Langenbeck technique, extending the relaxing incisions along the alveolar margins to the edge of the cleft. This designs flaps entirely dependent on the circulation from the palatine vessels but also much more versatile in terms of their placement. In a complete unilateral cleft, the flap from the greater (medial) segment can be shifted across the cleft and closed directly behind the alveolar margin. This virtually eliminates fistulas in the anterior hard palate (Fig. 95-8).[109]

The soft palate closure is accomplished again with a straight-line closure in the typical two-flap technique. Intravelar veloplasty is an essential part of this closure in the most successful reports.

Double Opposing Z-Plasty

Furlow[110] first described his technique for palate closure in the 1980s, adapting the Z-plasty principle

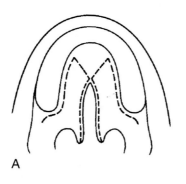

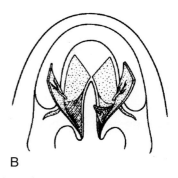

A

B

FIGURE 95-7. V-Y pushback repair (Veau-Wardill-Kilner). *A*, Markings for incisions. *B*, Mucoperiosteal flaps raised; note the greater palatine vessels preserved on both sides. *C*, Intravelar veloplasty; repair of the levator palatini muscle, after repair of nasal mucosa. *D*, Oral closure completed. Note raw areas. If a complete cleft is present through the alveolus, only nasal mucosa is closed anteriorly. (From Randall P, LaRossa D: Cleft palate. In McCarthy JG, ed: Plastic Surgery. Philadelphia, WB Saunders, 1990:2744.)

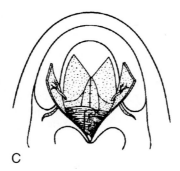

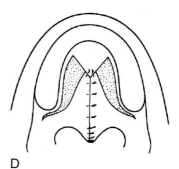

C

D

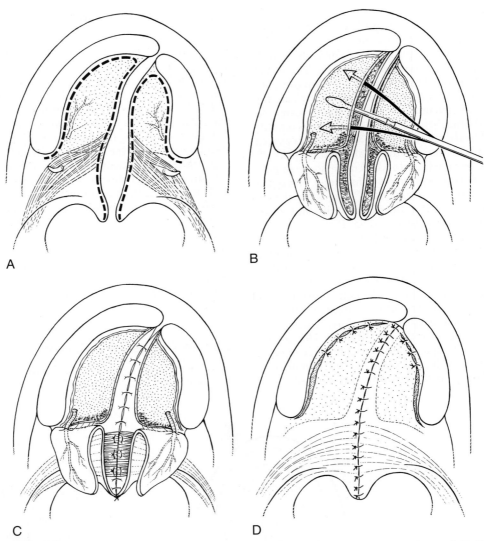

FIGURE 95-8. Two-flap palatoplasty. *A*, Markings for repair. *B*, Incisions made. *C*, Flaps elevated. *D*, Closure.

to palatal closure. By alternating reversing Z-plasties of the nasal and oral flaps and keeping the levator palatini within the most posterior flaps, he reported initial early success in both speech outcomes and skeletal growth.

A Z-plasty is developed on both the oral and nasal surfaces of the soft palate but in opposite directions. For both of the Z-plasties, the central limb is the cleft margin, and the posteriorly based flap is designed to include the levator muscle. Furlow recommended that the posteriorly based oral flap be on the left side for a right-handed surgeon because the elevation of the muscle from the nasal mucosa is the most difficult part of the dissection (Fig. 95-9).

This technique addresses closure of the soft palate in a manner that provides complete nasal and oral

closure as it re-establishes the levator sling. Because the nasal Z-plasty is placed more laterally, a higher and presumably more functional sling is formed. The theoretical disadvantage of this technique is that it is nonanatomic in that it completely ignores the small longitudinal uvular muscle, but overall speech results have been comparable to or better than those with other techniques.[111,112]

Furlow described the use of relaxing incisions when necessary. The authors' preference is to combine a double opposing Z-plasty of the soft palate with a two-flap technique for the hard palate, resulting in a low fistula rate with good speech results. The chief problem may arise in very wide clefts, in which the distance to be traversed by the Z-plasty may be excessive. The anteriorly based oral flap can be joined to the relaxing

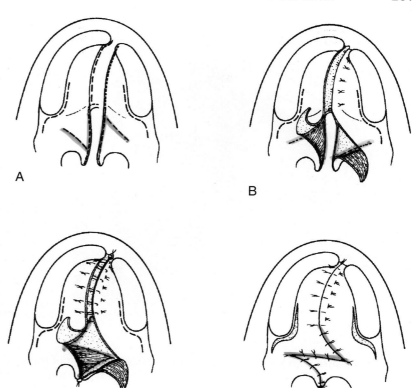

[handwritten notes at top left:]
FURLOW
• Allonge le palais mou
• Double la fermeture du palais mou (2 épaisseurs)

FIGURE 95-9. Furlow double opposing Z-plasty. *A,* Markings are made for the Z-plasty. In a wide cleft, the relaxing incisions can be carried anteriorly to the cleft margin for a two-flap repair. *B,* Elevation of the oral flaps; note that the muscle is elevated with the posteriorly based flap. The incisions are marked for the nasal flaps in a reverse fashion. The nasal lining anteriorly is closed with a vomer flap. *C,* The nasal flaps are transposed, and the oral closure is started anteriorly. *D,* Final closure of the oral mucosa. The relaxing incisions are left open. (From Randall P, LaRossa D: Cleft palate. In McCarthy JG, ed: Plastic Surgery. Philadelphia, WB Saunders, 1990:2740.)

A   B   C   D

incision to design an island flap based on the palatine vessels and giving considerably greater mobility, although this will shift the closure to the side of the posteriorly based flap. Alternatively, a straight-line closure may be employed in these wide cases, reserving the Z-plasty as a secondary procedure if needed.[113]

Intravelar Veloplasty

Although Victor Veau actually first advocated midline levator palatini reapproximation, Braithwaite[114] was the first to perform more extensive muscle dissection for posterior repositioning and tension-free approximation. He emphasized careful dissection and freeing of the levator palatini from the posterior edge of the hard palate before approximation in the midline.

Cutting[115] has described a technique of veloplasty that includes division of the tensor palatini tendon and repositioning of the muscle at the hamulus. This method requires an extensive dissection of the levator muscle, freeing it from both nasal and oral mucosa. Although there is a reasonable thickness of oral mucosa, the adherence of the nasal mucosa to the muscle makes the dissection difficult on this side and at times results in perforation of the mucosa. The tensor tendon is released just medial to the hamulus, and the levator muscle may be overlapped to provide

appropriate tension on the repair. This is presumably similar to the muscle overlap accomplished by Furlow's method. This technique has shown excellent speech outcomes in early evaluations. Both Cutting and Sommerlad[116] have proposed "re-repair" of the levator muscle when primary palatoplasty still results in velopharyngeal insufficiency (Fig. 95-10).

Vomer Flaps *[handwritten:] ⌐ incision sur ligne médiane*
[handwritten:] ∟ lambeaux basés supérieurement

There is confusion about the terminology applied to anterior closure of the nasal mucosa in complete cleft lip and palate. The original vomer flap is described as inferiorly based; an incision is made high on the septum, and the flap is reflected downward to provide a single-layer closure on the oral side. A number of European centers noted a high number of patients with maxillary retrusion, presumably from injury to the vomer-premaxillary suture, as well as a high fistula rate and changed to a two-layer anterior closure.[117-119]

Similar problems have not been found with superiorly based vomer flaps. This technique involves reflecting the mucosa from the septum near the cleft margin, dissecting only enough to close the nasal mucosa of the opposite side. In bilateral cleft palate, this requires a midline incision along the septum, and two flaps are reflected in each direction. This technique results in a

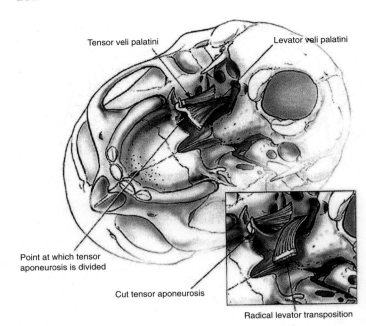

Tensor veli palatini

Levator veli palatini

Point at which tensor
aponeurosis is divided

Cut tensor aponeurosis

Radical levator transposition

FIGURE 95-10. Cutting's technique for release of the levator palatini muscle with division of the tendon of the tensor palatini. The main drawing shows detachment of the levator from the posterior border of the hard palate; *inset,* the release of the tensor tendon and posterior rotation of the levator. (From Cutting C, Rosenbaum J, Rovati L: The technique of muscle repair in the cleft soft palate. Operative Techniques Plast Surg 1995;2:215-222.)

two-layer closure, with low fistula rates and less effect on maxillary growth.[107,113]

Two-Stage Palatal Repair

Despite success in reliable palatal closure techniques, the late result of midface protrusion in the cleft population remained a problem. With publication of large series of patients with unrepaired clefts who had normal skeletal cephalometric relationships,[88,89] the association between closure technique and midface retrusion evolved. All cleft palate repairs at this time resulted in a midline sagittal scar band. This led to the conclusion that excessive scar tension in the anterior-posterior vector impeded normal growth of the midface.[120]

The problem with maxillary growth has led some surgeons to advocate a two-stage approach to palatoplasty, with earlier repair of the soft palate only and later repair of the hard palate. The general protocol, originally introduced by Schweckendiek,[121] entailed repair of the soft palate at the same time as the cleft lip repair, around 4 to 6 months. The hard palate was obturated and repaired at about 4 to 5 years of age. Earlier ages have subsequently been proposed for hard palate repair, usually around 18 to 24 months.[122]

The rationale for this approach has been that the hard palate cleft narrows during the time between procedures, requiring less dissection and thus resulting in less maxillary growth disturbance. Although it is intriguing on a theoretical basis, numerous studies have shown poorer speech results from these two-stage procedures, with marginal if any salutary effect on the

growth of the maxilla.[123-125] Optimal timing of palate repair must be balanced between optimal speech outcome and optimal maxillary growth. However, as noted before, good speech outcomes become more difficult to achieve with increasing age, whereas most maxillary growth problems can be addressed with orthodontic treatment and, if needed, maxillary osteotomies.

Primary Pharyngeal Flap

Repair of cleft palate with immediate placement of a posterior pharyngeal flap is another technique that has had support over the years.[126] The argument is that speech outcomes are improved; the problem is that most patients will receive a flap without needing it, as most busy centers are reporting good speech in at least 80% to 90% of patients after palatoplasty. Pharyngeal flaps have a significant incidence of sleep apnea, which is observed more frequently when they are performed in younger children. Thus, a large number of patients are unnecessarily placed at risk for respiratory embarrassment.

OUTCOMES OF CLEFT PALATE REPAIR

Complications after palate repair include bleeding, respiratory problems, dehiscence, and fistula formation. Although it has been suggested that palate repair may actually improve airway function,[127] in general the palate repair acutely reorganizes the child's airway and may partially obstruct the nasal airway.

A relatively small amount of bleeding combined with swelling of the soft palate can cause respiratory insufficiency. Because infants are obligate nose breathers, this may cause a varying degree of respiratory difficulty in the acute postoperative period. The pushback palatoplasty has been shown to cause greater degrees and duration of hypoxemia than the von Langenbeck technique[128]; although this has not been reported with the Furlow repair, presumably the results would be similar to the pushback results because of the posterior pharyngeal crowding.

Almost all patients will recover from the initial respiratory depression,[129] but this is an important issue in the early postoperative period. Use of a nasopharyngeal tube to evacuate the stomach of any air and monitoring of pulse oximetry are important considerations. A large silk suture is usually placed in the posterior tongue for traction, allowing the tongue to be brought forward without use of nasal or oral airways during emergence from anesthesia; the suture can be removed the following day. Intensive care monitoring may be necessary for a small number of infants who are struggling early after surgery.

Bleeding is not uncommon after palate repair. There are inevitably raw surfaces, which may ooze for 12 to 24 hours. Bleeding can be reduced by surgery that takes less than 90 to 120 minutes because the epinephrine will still have some effect during emergence from anesthesia. Light pressure on the hard palate repair at the conclusion of the procedure will often control bleeding as well. We have found that application of ice packs to the posterior neck is almost always effective in stopping postoperative bleeding in recovery or on the ward; this is a technique that has not been documented previously but has been used by experienced surgeons.[130]

Fistula formation is one complication that has been studied in some detail. Fistulas may be a source of persistent nasal air loss even in the face of a functioning soft palate; they are also a source of nasal regurgitation of fluids. In one particularly extensive review of fistulas at a single institution, use of the Furlow repair was shown to markedly reduce fistulas relative to the V-Y pushback or von Langenbeck technique. The width of the cleft was the other factor in this multivariate analysis.[107] Late closure of fistulas may be difficult, especially in the hard palate, and the use of large mucoperiosteal flaps on the oral side is recommended to give the best outcome (Fig. 95-11).[131] If there is reason for delay of repair, a palatal plate may aid in obturating a fistula for speech purposes until surgical correction can be achieved.

ALVEOLAR BONE GRAFTING

Children with complete cleft lip and palate have a cleft through the alveolus that must be addressed as part of the staged reconstruction of the cleft deformity. In most cases, there is a small fistula from the buccal vestibule into the nose. Complete rehabilitation of the cleft deformity mandates closure of this alveolar cleft, either with bone grafting or with periosteoplasty.

[handwritten: A faire avant l'éruption de la canine du côté de la fente]

Rationale for Bone Grafting

There are four primary reasons for alveolar cleft bone grafting: closure of the fistula; stabilization of the maxillary arch; support for the roots of teeth adjacent to the cleft on each side; and support for a prosthesis. Although the fistula through the alveolus can be closed without bone, the success rate is much lower than when bone is placed. The bone grafting is usually delayed until the maxillary arch width has been restored by expansion; the graft then prevents relapse. Long-term studies have shown that the teeth adjacent to the cleft, generally the central incisor and cuspid (when the lateral incisor is absent), are often lost in the third or fourth decade of life if bone grafting is not performed, although long-term follow-up is not yet available of patients who underwent bone grafting in the 1970s or 1980s, when the practice became more routine. Last, prosthetic restoration of the missing lateral incisor requires stability of the adjacent teeth for a fixed bridge or adequate bone stock for placement of an osseointegrated implant.

An additional rationale for bone grafting is related to the appearance of the nose. The typical cleft nasal deformity has multiple components, not the least of which is the hypoplasia of the maxilla at the piriform aperture on the affected side. At the time of bone grafting, additional bone is placed around the piriform aperture, adding support to the alar base on the cleft side.

Timing of Bone Grafting

Primary bone grafting refers to the placement of bone (usually rib) in the alveolar and hard palate cleft, usually at the time of palate repair. This has been proposed as a means of avoiding later operation. Although this procedure is used at a handful of institutions,[132,133] most investigators have found that there is a negative effect on maxillary growth from primary bone grafting.[134]

Latham[135,136] was one of the first to introduce the use of presurgical appliances for manipulation and alignment of the cleft segments. Presurgical orthopedic manipulation of the alveolar segments followed by primary gingivoperiosteoplasty at the time of lip repair (see Chapter 94) has provided a method for early closure of anterior fistula. Long-term reports, even of the same cohort of patients, have differed on the efficacy of this technique when later dentofacial characteristics are examined.[137,138] Early reports show that at least half of the children treated with this technique may not require secondary alveolar bone grafting,[11,139] although methods of restoring the absent lateral

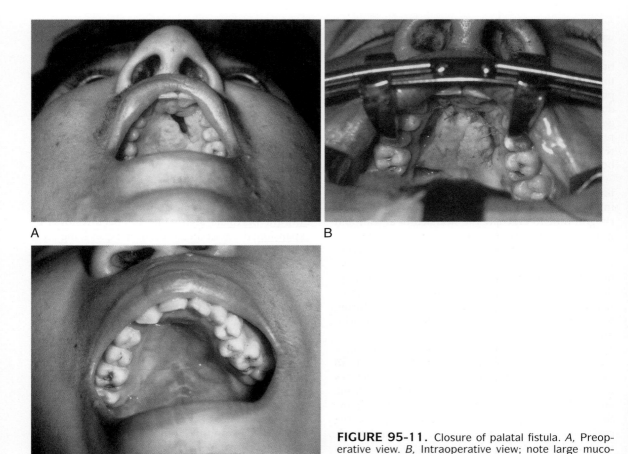

A

B

C

FIGURE 95-11. Closure of palatal fistula. *A,* Preoperative view. *B,* Intraoperative view; note large mucoperiosteal flap used for oral closure. *C,* Postoperative; complete healing of fistula closure.

incisor are not addressed. Today, long-term data are still lacking in regard to dental eruption patterns, maxillary growth, and orthodontic-surgical outcomes of a large cohort of children treated with gingivoperiosteoplasty.

Secondary bone grafting of the alveolar cleft gained popularity in the 1970s and 1980s. At present, this technique is still preferred for closure of the alveolar cleft at most centers. The ideal timing for secondary bone grafting is before eruption of the cuspid into the cleft[140]; if the grafting is done after eruption of the cuspid, there is a greater possibility (10% to 15%) of late root resorption.[141]

Timing of secondary bone grafting must be coordinated with orthodontic treatment. Ideally, the maxillary arch has been expanded and the existing permanent teeth are in reasonable position before the procedure. The ultimate goal of replacement of the missing lateral incisor must be kept in mind. The two best choices are a fixed bridge and an osseointegrated implant, and both require good bone stock in the cleft; for a fixed bridge, the bone prevents later root

resorption and loss of the teeth adjacent to the cleft, whereas the osseointegrated implant is placed in the grafted bone.[142,143]

Bone Graft Material

The usual sources of bone grafts exist for alveolar clefts; however, one must recognize that the intraoral and intranasal location of the graft is relatively inhospitable and that later placement of implants requires excellent retention of bone stock. Iliac crest cancellous bone is the "gold standard" with reported success rates above 95%.[144] The primary problem with this donor material is the associated pain; this may be mitigated by the use of marrow harvesting instruments or trephines.[145-147] Cranial bone, which offers the advantage of a nearly pain-free donor site, has been used by a number of surgeons with reasonable success, but because this is a mixture of cancellous and ground cortical bone, the need for nearly perfect flap healing is greater and the success rate somewhat lower.[148,149] Results may be somewhat better if only bone from the diploic space is harvested.[150] The tibia has also been reported as a source of cancellous bone with favorable outcomes.[151-153] The mandibular symphysis has also been used, mostly for augmentation of existing grafts.[154]

Technique

Secondary bone grafting of alveolar clefts is a technically demanding three-dimensional procedure. After the margins of the cleft along the alveolus on each side are incised, mucoperiosteal flaps are elevated on the anterior surface of the alveolus, particularly on the lateral segment, where the gingival attachments of the first two teeth (often the primary cuspid and the permanent first bicuspid) are elevated with the flap. The lateral incision is carried up into the vestibule

lateral to the first two teeth. The anterior maxilla and the piriform aperture are exposed. The lining of the cleft is then elevated, off the alveolus laterally and off the septum medially. These two flaps are followed posteriorly to the back of the fistula if there is one present or to the bony posterior margin of the cleft. They are then divided on each side near the hard palate, forming two flaps above to close the floor of the nose and two flaps below to close the palatal surface. A space is thus made with alveolar bone on each side and flaps above and below. Posteriorly, scar or bone ends the space.

The anterior opening is now used to pack cancellous bone into the cleft. Some bone is usually placed along the piriform aperture to elevate the alar base on the cleft side. The key to a tension-free closure is division of the periosteum on the lateral mucoperiosteal

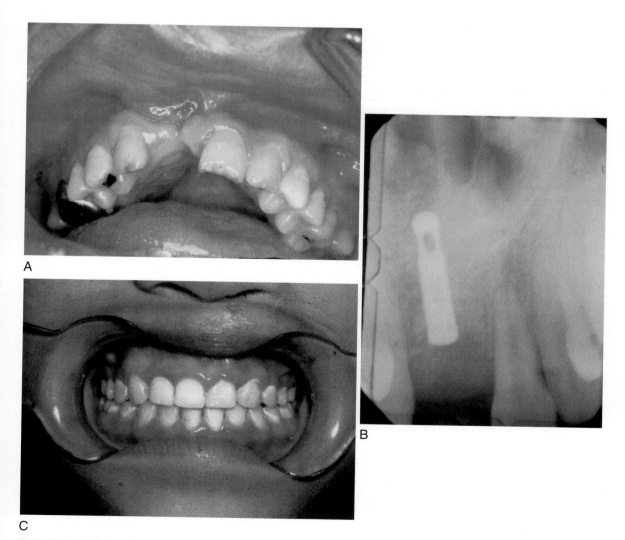

FIGURE 95-12. Alveolar cleft bone grafting. *A,* Alveolar defect. *B,* Radiograph showing implant in grafted alveolus. *C,* Final result with prosthetic tooth on implant.

flap from the maxilla, which permits advancement of this flap across the anterior defect.

Liquids are maintained postoperatively until early healing is adequate, followed by soft foods for a total of 6 weeks after grafting. Radiographic assessment of the graft is not done for several months. If an implant is to be placed in the graft, it is best done at about 4 to 6 months after bone grafting because there will be some resorption of the graft if it is not stressed.[143] Attempts to place implants at the same time as bone grafting have had higher complication rates and should be avoided (Fig. 95-12).[142]

CONCLUSION

Cleft palate repair has undergone major changes in the past quarter century. Overall, results have improved as far as speech outcomes; this is probably due to the growth of centers for cleft care as well as to refinement of techniques. The team approach has decreased the number of operations needed to obtain better outcomes as the surgeon has gained knowledge from the other specialists involved in cleft care. The increased application of methods that incorporate reconstruction of the levator palatini muscle has produced much more predictable speech results. Current trends of earlier surgical intervention for cleft palate and presurgical alignment of the dental arches should result in still more predictable outcomes.

REFERENCES

1. Boo-Chai K: An ancient Chinese text on a cleft lip. Plast Reconstr Surg 1966;38:89-91.
2. Rogers BO: History of cleft lip and cleft palate treatment. In Grabb WC, ed: Cleft Lip and Palate. Boston, Little, Brown, 1971.
3. Stephenson J: Repair of cleft palate by Philibert Roux in 1819. Plast Reconstr Surg 1971;47:277-283.
4. Entin MA: Dr. Roux's first operation of soft palate in 1819: a historical vignette. Cleft Palate Craniofac J 1999;36:27-29.
5. Roux PJ: Memoire sur la staphyloraphie, ou il suture a voile du palais. Arch Sci Med 1925;7:516-538.
6. McDowell F: The classic reprint: Graefe's first closure of a cleft palate. Plast Reconstr Surg 1971;47:375-376.
7. May H: The classic reprint. The palate suture. A newly discovered method to correct congenital speech defects. Dr. Carl Ferdinand von Graefe, Berlin. Plast Reconstr Surg 1971;47:488-492.
8. Mau A, Biemer E: Johann-Friedrich Dieffenbach: the pioneer of plastic surgery. Ann Plast Surg 1994;33:112-115.
9. Goldwyn RM: Johann Friedrich Dieffenbach (1794-1847). Plast Reconstr Surg 1968;42:19-28.
10. Goldwyn RM: Bernhard von Langenbeck. His life and legacy. Plast Reconstr Surg 1969;44:248-254.
11. Pfeifer TM, Grayson BH, Cutting CB: Nasoalveolar molding and gingivoperiosteoplasty versus alveolar bone graft: an outcome analysis of costs in the treatment of unilateral cleft alveolus. Cleft Palate Craniofac J 2002;39:26-29.
12. Suzuki A, Takahama Y: Maxillary lateral incisor of subjects with cleft lip and/or palate. Part 1. Cleft Palate Craniofac J 1992;29:376-379.
13. Vichi M, Franchi L: Eruption anomalies of the maxillary permanent cuspids in children with cleft lip and/or palate. J Clin Pediatr Dent 1996;20:149-153.
14. Jordan RE, Kraus BS, Neptune CM: Dental abnormalities associated with cleft lip and/or palate. Cleft Palate J 1966;3:22-55.
15. Werner SP, Harris EF: Odontometrics of the permanent teeth in cleft lip and palate: systemic size reduction and amplified asymmetry. Cleft Palate J 1989;26:36-41.
16. Shapira Y, Lubit E, Kuftinec MM: Hypodontia in children with various types of clefts. Angle Orthod 2000;70:16-21.
17. Lekkas C, Latief BS, ter Rahe SP, et al: The adult unoperated cleft patient: absence of maxillary teeth outside the cleft area. Cleft Palate Craniofac J 2000;37:17-20.
18. Sofaer JA: Human tooth-size asymmetry in cleft lip with or without cleft palate. Arch Oral Biol 1979;24:141-146.
19. Ranta R: A review of tooth formation in children with cleft lip/palate. Am J Orthod Dentofacial Orthop 1986;90:11-18.
20. Kipelainen PVJ, Laine-Alava MT: Palatal asymmetry in cleft palate subjects. Cleft Palate Craniofac J 1996;33:483-488.
21. Foster TD, Lavelle CL: The size of the dentition in complete cleft lip and palate. Cleft Palate J 1971;8:177-184.
22. Peterka M, Tvrdek M, Mullerova Z: Tooth eruption in patients with cleft lip and palate. Acta Chir Plast 1993;35:154-158.
23. Poyry M, Ranta R: Formation of anterior maxillary teeth in 0-3-year-old children with cleft lip and palate and prenatal risk factors for delayed development. J Craniofac Genet Dev Biol 1986;6:15-26.
24. Veau V: Division palatine. Anatomie, chirurgie, phonetique. En collaboration avec Mme. Borel. Paris, Masson et Cie, 1931.
25. Kriens OB: Anatomy of the velopharyngeal area in cleft palate. Clin Plast Surg 1975;2:261.
26. Fara M: The musculature of cleft lip and palate. In McCarthy JG, ed: Plastic Surgery. Philadelphia, WB Saunders, 1991:2598-2626.
27. Huang MH, Lee ST, Rajendran K: A fresh cadaveric study of the paratubal muscles: implications for eustachian tube function in cleft palate. Plast Reconstr Surg 1997;100:833-842.
28. Robin P: Glossoptosis due to atresia and hypotrophy of the mandible. Am J Dis Child 1934;48:541-547.
29. Dykes EH, Raine PA, Arthur DS, et al: Pierre Robin syndrome and pulmonary hypertension. J Pediatr Surg 1985;20:49-52.
30. Caouette-Laberge L, Bayet B, Larocque Y: The Pierre Robin sequence: review of 125 cases and evolution of treatment modalities. Plast Reconstr Surg 1994;93:934-942.
31. Cohen MM Jr: The Robin anomalad—its nonspecificity and associated syndromes. J Oral Surg 1976;34:587-593.
32. Shprintzen RJ: Pierre Robin, micrognathia, and airway obstruction: the dependency of treatment on accurate diagnosis. Int Anesthesiol Clin 1988;26:64-71.
33. Shprintzen RJ: The implications of the diagnosis of Robin sequence. Cleft Palate Craniofac J 1992;29:205-209.
34. Sadewitz VL: Robin sequence: changes in thinking leading to changes in patient care. Cleft Palate Craniofac J 1992;29:246-253.
35. Cohen MM Jr: Robin sequences and complexes: causal heterogeneity and pathogenetic/phenotypic variability. Am J Med Genet 1999;84:311-315.
36. Shprintzen RJ: Palatal and pharyngeal anomalies in craniofacial syndromes. Birth Defects 1982;18:53-78.
37. Singer L, Sidoti EJ: Pediatric management of Robin sequence. Cleft Palate Craniofac J 1992;29:220-223.
38. Sher AE: Mechanisms of airway obstruction in Robin sequence: implications for treatment. Cleft Palate Craniofac J 1992;29:224-231.
39. Smith JD: Treatment of airway obstruction in Pierre Robin syndrome. A modified lip-tongue adhesion. Arch Otolaryngol 1981;107:419-421.

40. Parsons RW, Smith DJ: Rule of thumb criteria for tongue-lip adhesion in Pierre Robin anomalad. Plast Reconstr Surg 1982;70:210-212.

41. Denny AD, Talisman R, Hanson PR, Recinos RF: Mandibular distraction osteogenesis in very young patients to correct airway obstruction. Plast Reconstr Surg 2001;108:302-311.

42. Figueroa AA, Glupker TJ, Fitz MG, BeGole EA: Mandible, tongue, and airway in Pierre Robin sequence: a longitudinal cephalometric study. Cleft Palate Craniofac J 1991;28:425-434.

43. Vegter F, Hage JJ, Mulder JW: Pierre Robin syndrome: mandibular growth during the first year of life. Ann Plast Surg 1999;42:154-157.

44. Laitinen SH, Ranta RE: Cephalometric measurements in patients with Pierre Robin syndrome and isolated cleft palate. Scand J Plast Reconstr Surg Hand Surg 1992;26:177-183.

45. Lehman JA, Fishman JR, Neiman GS: Treatment of cleft palate associated with Robin sequence: appraisal of risk factors. Cleft Palate Craniofac J 1995;32:25-29.

46. Weatherley-White RC, Sakura CY Jr, Brenner LD, et al: Submucous cleft palate. Its incidence, natural history, and indications for treatment. Plast Reconstr Surg 1972;49:297-304.

47. Stewart JM, Ott ME, Lagace R: Submucous cleft palate. Birth Defects 1971;7:64-66.

48. Stewart JM, Ott JE, Lagace R: Submucous cleft palate: prevalence in a school population. Cleft Palate J 1972;9:246-250.

49. Ysunza A, Pamplona MC, Mendoza M, et al: Surgical treatment of submucous cleft palate: a comparative trial of two modalities for palatal closure. Plast Reconstr Surg 2001;107:9-14.

50. Peterson-Falzone SJ: Velopharyngeal inadequacy in the absence of overt cleft palate. J Craniofac Genet Dev Biol Suppl 1985;1:97-124.

51. Trier WC: Velopharyngeal incompetency in the absence of overt cleft palate: anatomic and surgical considerations. Cleft Palate J 1983;20:209-217.

52. Kaplan EN: The occult submucous cleft palate. Cleft Palate J 1975;12:356-368.

53. Pensler JM, Bauer BS: Levator repositioning and palatal lengthening for submucous clefts [see comments]. Plast Reconstr Surg 1988;82:765-769.

54. Chen PK-T, Wu J, Hung KF, et al: Surgical correction of submucous cleft palate with Furlow palatoplasty. Plast Reconstr Surg 1996;97:1136-1146.

55. Seth AK, McWilliams BJ: Weight gain in children with cleft palate from birth to two years. Cleft Palate J 1988;25:146-150.

56. Becker M, Svensson H, Kallen B: Birth weight, body length, and cranial circumference in newborns with cleft lip or palate. Cleft Palate Craniofac J 1998;35:255-261.

57. Jones WB: Weight gain and feeding in the neonate with cleft: a three-center study. Cleft Palate J 1988;25:379-384.

58. Lee J, Nunn J, Wright C: Height and weight achievement in cleft lip and palate. Arch Dis Child 1997;76:70-72.

59. Jensen BL, Kreiborg S, Dahl E, Fogh-Andersen P: Cleft lip and palate in Denmark, 1976-1981: epidemiology, variability, and early somatic development. Cleft Palate J 1988;25:258-269.

60. Drillien CM, Thomson AJ, Burgoyne K: Low-birthweight children at early school-age: a longitudinal study. Dev Med Child Neurol 1980;22:26-47.

61. Bowers EJ, Mayro RF, Whitaker LA, et al: General body growth in children with clefts of the lip, palate, and craniofacial structure. Scand J Plast Reconstr Surg Hand Surg 1987;21:7-14.

62. Clarren SK, Anderson B, Wolf LS: Feeding infants with cleft lip, cleft palate, or cleft lip and palate. Cleft Palate J 1987;24:244-249.

63. Brine EA, Rickard KA, Brady MS, et al: Effectiveness of two feeding methods in improving energy intake and growth of infants with cleft palate: a randomized study. J Am Diet Assoc 1994;94:732-738.

64. Pashayan HM, Lewis MB: Clinical experience with the Robin sequence. Cleft Palate J 1984;21:270-276.

65. Paradise JL, McWilliams BJ: Simplified feeder for infants with cleft palate. Pediatrics 1974;53:566-568.

66. Alt A: Ein Fall von gespaltenem Gaumen mit acquirinter Taubstummheit Staphyloraphie. Heilung. Arch Angenheilk 1878;7:211-215.

67. Paradise JL: Middle ear problems associated with cleft palate. An internationally-oriented review. Cleft Palate J 1975;12:17-22.

68. Dhillon RS: The middle ear in cleft palate children pre and post palatal closure. J R Soc Med 1988;81:710-713.

69. Doyle WJ: Functional eustachian tube obstruction and otitis media in a primate model. A review. Acta Otolaryngol Suppl (Stockh) 1984;414:52-57.

70. Fara M, Hrivnakova J, Horak I: Middle ear complications in clefts. Results of stage I in longterm studies of hearing defects, considering type of cleft and age of patient. Acta Chir Plast 1973;15:7-10.

71. Fara M, Jelinek R, Peterka M, et al: Orofacial clefts. A theoretical basis for their prevention and treatment. Acta Univ Carol Med Monogr 1988;124:1-143.

72. Finkelstein Y, Zohar Y, Nachmani A, et al: The otolaryngologist and the patient with velocardiofacial syndrome. Arch Otolaryngol Head Neck Surg 1993;119:563-569.

73. Gould HJ: Audiologic findings in Pierre Robin sequence. Ear Hear 1989;10:211-213.

74. Gordon AS, Jean-Louis F, Morton RP: Late ear sequelae in cleft palate patients. Int J Pediatr Otorhinolaryngol 1988;15:149-156.

75. Yules RB: Hearing in cleft palate patients. Arch Otolaryngol 1970;91:319-323.

76. Yules RB: Current concepts of treatment of ear disease in cleft palate children and adults. Cleft Palate J 1975;12:315-322.

77. Peterson-Falzone SJ: The relationship between timing of cleft palate surgery and speech outcome: what have we learned, and where do we stand in the 1990s? Semin Orthod 1996;2:185-191.

78. Chapman KL, Hardin MA: Phonetic and phonologic skills of two-year-olds with cleft palate. Cleft Palate Craniofac J 1992;29:535-543.

79. Dorf DS, Curtin JW: Early cleft palate repair and speech outcome. Plast Reconstr Surg 1982;70:74-81.

80. Kemp-Fincham SI, Duehn DP, Trost-Cardamone JE: Speech development and the timing of primary palatoplasty. In Bardach J, Morris HL, ed: Multidisciplinary Management of Cleft Lip and Palate. Philadelphia, WB Saunders, 1990:736-745.

81. O'Gara MM, Logemann JA, Rademaker AW: Phonetic features in babies with unilateral cleft lip and palate. Cleft Palate Craniofac J 1994;31:446-451.

82. Evans D, Renfrew C: The timing of primary cleft palate repair. Scand J Plast Reconstr Surg 1974;8:153-155.

83. Dalston RM: Timing of cleft palate repair: a speech pathologist's viewpoint. Prob Plast Reconstr Surg 1992;2:30-38.

84. Kaplan EN: Cleft palate repair at 3 months? Ann Plast Surg 1981;7:179.

85. Desai SN: Early cleft palate repair completed before the age of 16 weeks: observations on a personal series of 100 children. Br J Plast Surg 1983;36:300-304.

86. Copeland M: The effects of very early palatal repair on speech. Br J Plast Surg 1990;43:676-682.

87. Nunn DR, Derkay CS, Darrow DH, et al: The effect of very early cleft palate closure on the need for ventilation tubes in the first years of life. Laryngoscope 1995;105(pt 1):905-908.

88. Ortiz-Monasterio F, Serrano A, Barrera G, et al: A study of untreated adult cleft palate patients. Plast Reconstr Surg 1966;38:36-41.

89. Boo-Chai K: The unoperated adult cleft of the lip and palate. Br J Plast Surg 1971;24:250.

90. Bardach J, Klausner EC, Eisbach KJ: The relationship between lip pressure and facial growth after cleft lip repair: an experimental study. Cleft Palate J 1979;16:137-146.

91. Bardach J: The influence of cleft lip repair on facial growth. Cleft Palate J 1990;27:76-78.

92. Wada T, Tachimura T, Satoh K, et al: Maxillary growth after two-stage palatal closure in complete (unilateral and bilateral) clefts of the lip and palate from infancy until 10 years of age. J Osaka Univ Dent Sch 1990;30:53-63.

93. Kipelainen PVJ, Laine-Alava MT, Lammi S: Palatal morphology and type of clefting. Cleft Palate Craniofac J 1996;33:477-482.

94. Hellquist R: Team work and clinical research in the treatment of cleft lip and palate. Sven Tandlak Tidskr 1973;66:145-155.

95. Rudolph W: Follow-up investigations on operated cleft palates. Int J Oral Surg 1978;7:281-285.

96. Kremenak CR, Huffman WC, Olin WH: Growth of maxillae in dogs after palatal surgery. Cleft Palate J 1967;4:6.

97. Hellquist R, Ponten B, Skoog T: The influence of cleft length and palatoplasty on the dental arch and the deciduous occlusion in cases of clefts of the secondary palate. Scand J Plast Reconstr Surg 1978;12:45-54.

98. Peltomaki T, Vendittelli BL, Grayson BH, et al: Associations between severity of clefting and maxillary growth in patients with unilateral cleft lip and palate treated with infant orthopedics. Cleft Palate Craniofac J 2001;38:582-586.

99. Jones MC: Etiology of facial clefts: prospective evaluation of 428 patients. Cleft Palate J 1988;25:16-20.

100. Edgerton MT: Surgical lengthening of the cleft palate by dissection of the neurovascular bundle. Plast Reconstr Surg 1962;29:551.

101. Dorrance GM: Lengthening the soft palate in cleft palate operations. Ann Surg 1925;82:208.

102. Dorrance GM, Bransfield JW: The pushback operation for repair of cleft palate. Plast Reconstr Surg 1946;1:145.

103. Wallace AF: A history of the repair of cleft lip and palate in Britain before World War II. Ann Plast Surg 1987;19:266-275.

104. Dellon AL, Edgerton MT: Correction of velopharyngeal incompetence by retrodisplacement of the levator veli palatini muscle insertion. Surg Forum 1969;20:510-511.

105. Cronin TD: Method of preventing raw areas on the nasal surface of soft palate in push-back surgery. Plast Reconstr Surg 1957;20:474.

106. Kaplan EN: Soft palate repair by levator muscle reconstruction and a buccal mucosal flap. Plast Reconstr Surg 1975;56:129.

107. Cohen SR, Kalinowski J, LaRossa D, Randall P: Cleft palate fistulas: a multivariate statistical analysis of prevalence, etiology, and surgical management. Plast Reconstr Surg 1991;87:1041-1047.

108. Bardach J, Salyer K: Surgical Techniques in Cleft Lip and Palate. Chicago, Year Book, 1987.

109. Bardach J: Two-flap palatoplasty: Bardach's technique. Operative Techniques Plast Surg 1995;2:211-214.

110. Furlow LT Jr: Cleft palate repair by double opposing Z-plasty. Plast Reconstr Surg 1986;78:724.

111. Randall P, LaRossa D, Solomon M, Cohen M: Experience with the Furlow double-reversing Z-plasty for cleft palate repair. Plast Reconstr Surg 1986;77:569-576.

112. Gunther E, Wisser JR, Cohen MA, Brown AS: Palatoplasty: Furlow's double reversing Z-plasty versus intravelar veloplasty. Cleft Palate Craniofac J 1998;35:546-549.

113. Furlow L: Cleft palate repair by double opposing Z-plasty. Operative Techniques Plast Surg 1995;2:223-232.

114. Braithwaite F, Maurice DG: The importance of the levator palatini muscle in cleft palate closure. Br J Plast Surg 1968;21:60-62.

115. Cutting C, Rosenbaum J, Rovati L: The technique of muscle repair in the soft palate. Operative Techniques Plast Surg 1995;2:215-222.

116. Sommerlad BC, Henley M, Birch M, et al: Cleft palate re-repair—a clinical and radiographic study of 32 consecutive cases. Br J Plast Surg 1994;47:406-410.

117. Friede H, Johanson B: A follow-up study of cleft children treated with vomer flap as part of a three-stage soft tissue surgical procedure. Facial morphology and dental occlusion. Scand J Plast Reconstr Surg 1977;11:45-57.

118. Delaire J, Precious D: Avoidance of the use of vomerine mucosa in primary surgical management of velopalatine clefts. Oral Surg Oral Med Oral Pathol 1985;60:589-597.

119. Molsted K, Palmberg A, Dahl E, Fogh-Andersen P: Malocclusion in complete unilateral and bilateral cleft lip and palate. The results of a change in the surgical procedure. Scand J Plast Reconstr Surg Hand Surg 1987;21:81-85.

120. Ross RB: Treatment variables affecting facial growth in complete unilateral cleft lip and palate. Cleft Palate J 1987;24:54-77.

121. Schweckendiek W, Doz P: Primary veloplasty: long-term results without maxillary deformity—a 25 year report. Cleft Palate J 1978;15:268.

122. Rohrich RJ, Byrd HS: Optimal timing of cleft palate closure. Speech, facial growth, and hearing considerations. Clin Plast Surg 1990;17:27-36.

123. Witzel MA, Salyer KE, Ross RB: Delayed hard palate closure: the philosophy revisited. Cleft Palate J 1984;21:263-269.

124. Bardach J, Morris HL, Olin WH: Late results of primary veloplasty: the Marburg Project. Plast Reconstr Surg 1984;73:207-218.

125. Cosman B, Falk AS: Delayed hard palate repair and speech deficiencies: a cautionary report. Cleft Palate J 1980;17:27-33.

126. Stark RB, Dehaan CR, Frileck SP, Burgess PD Jr: Primary pharyngeal flap. Cleft Palate J 1969;6:381-383.

127. Milerad J, Ideberg M, Larson O: The effect of palatoplasty on airway patency and growth in infants with clefts and failure to thrive. Scand J Plast Reconstr Surg Hand Surg 1989;23:109-114.

128. Xue FS, An G, Tong SY, et al: Influence of surgical technique on early postoperative hypoxaemia in children undergoing elective palatoplasty. Br J Anaesth 1998;80:447-451.

129. Iida S, Kogo M, Ishii S, et al: Changes of arterial oxygen saturation (SpO_2) following push-back operation. Int J Oral Maxillofac Surg 1998;27:425-427.

130. Ousterhout DK: Personal communication, 1986.

131. Emory RE Jr, Clay RP, Bite U, Jackson IT: Fistula formation and repair after palatal closure: an institutional perspective. Plast Reconstr Surg 1997;99:1535-1538.

132. Dado DV, Rosenstein SW, Alder ME, Kernahan DA: Long-term assessment of early alveolar bone grafts using three-dimensional computer-assisted tomography: a pilot study. Plast Reconstr Surg 1997;99:1840-1845.

133. Eppley BL: Alveolar cleft bone grafting. Part I. Primary bone grafting. J Oral Maxillofac Surg 1996;54:74-82.

134. Trotman CA, Long RE Jr, Rosenstein SW, et al: Comparison of facial form in primary alveolar bone-grafted and nongrafted unilateral cleft lip and palate patients: intercenter retrospective study. Cleft Palate Craniofac J 1996;33:91-95.

135. Latham RA, Kusy RP, Georgiade NG: An extraorally activated expansion appliance for cleft palate infants. Cleft Palate J 1976;13:253.

136. Latham RA: Orthopedic advancement of the cleft maxillary segment: a preliminary report. Cleft Palate J 1980;17:227.

137. Millard DR, Latham RA: Improved primary surgical and dental treatment of clefts. Plast Reconstr Surg 1990;86:856-871.

138. Berkowitz S: A comparison of treatment results in complete bilateral cleft lip and palate using a conservative approach versus Millard-Latham PSOT procedure. Semin Orthod 1996;2:169-184.

139. Santiago PE, Grayson BH, Cutting CB, et al: Reduced need for alveolar bone grafting by presurgical orthopedics and primary gingivoperiosteoplasty. Cleft Palate Craniofac J 1998;35:77-80.

140. Bergland O, Semb G, Abyholm FE: Elimination of the residual alveolar cleft by secondary bone grafting and subsequent orthodontic treatment. Cleft Palate J 1986;23:175-205.

141. Enemark H, Sindet-Pedersen S, Bundgaard M: Long-term results after secondary bone grafting of alveolar clefts. J Oral Maxillofac Surg 1987;45:913-919.

142. Jensen J, Sindet-Pedersen S, Enemark H: Reconstruction of residual alveolar cleft defects with one-stage mandibular bone grafts and osseointegrated implants. J Oral Maxillofac Surg 1998;56:460-466, discussion 467.

143. Kearns G, Perrott DH, Sharma A, et al: Placement of endosseous implants in grafted alveolar clefts. Cleft Palate Craniofac J 1997;34:520-525.

144. Canady JW, Zeitler DP, Thompson SA, Nicholas CD: Suitability of the iliac crest as a site for harvest of autogenous bone grafts. Cleft Palate Craniofac J 1993;30:579-581.

145. Caminiti MF, Sandor GK, Carmichael RP: Quantification of bone harvested from the iliac crest using a power-driven trephine. J Oral Maxillofac Surg 1999;57:801-805, discussion 805-806.

146. Burstein FD, Simms C, Cohen SR, et al: Iliac crest bone graft harvesting techniques: a comparison. Plast Reconstr Surg 2000;105:34-39.

147. McCanny CM, Roberts-Harry DP: A comparison of two different bone-harvesting techniques for secondary alveolar bone grafting in patients with cleft lip and palate. Cleft Palate Craniofac J 1998;35:442-446.

148. LaRossa D, Buchman S, Rothkopf DM, et al: A comparison of iliac and cranial bone in secondary grafting of alveolar clefts. Plast Reconstr Surg 1995;96:789-797, discussion 798-799.

149. Denny AD, Talisman R, Bonawitz SC: Secondary alveolar bone grafting using milled cranial bone graft: a retrospective study of a consecutive series of 100 patients. Cleft Palate Craniofac J 1999;36:144-153.

150. Wolfe SA, Berkowitz S: The use of cranial bone grafts in the closure of alveolar and anterior palatal clefts. Plast Reconstr Surg 1983;72:659-671.

151. Besly W, Ward Booth P: Technique for harvesting tibial cancellous bone modified for use in children. Br J Oral Maxillofac Surg 1999;37:129-133.

152. Kalaaji A, Lilja J, Elander A, Friede H: Tibia as donor site for alveolar bone grafting in patients with cleft lip and palate: long-term experience. Scand J Plast Reconstr Surg Hand Surg 2001;35:35-42.

153. Sivarajasingam V, Pell G, Morse M, Shepherd JP: Secondary bone grafting of alveolar clefts: a densitometric comparison of iliac crest and tibial bone grafts. Cleft Palate Craniofac J 2001;38:11-14.

154. Enemark H, Jensen J, Bosch C: Mandibular bone graft material for reconstruction of alveolar cleft defects: long-term results. Cleft Palate Craniofac J 2001;38:155-163.

Orthodontics in Cleft Lip and Palate Management

ALVARO A. FIGUEROA, DDS, MS ◆ JOHN W. POLLEY, MD

INFANCY
    Unilateral Cleft Lip
    Bilateral Cleft Lip
    Wide Palatal Clefts: Articulation Development
        Prosthesis
PRIMARY DENTITION
    Posterior Crossbite
    Anterior Crossbite

TRANSITIONAL DENTITION
    Surgical Management of Protrusive Premaxilla in
        Bilateral Clefts
PERMANENT DENTITION
    Orthognathic Surgery and Distraction Procedures

Optimal management of patients with orofacial clefts requires a multidisciplinary approach because various structures, traditionally treated by several specialists, are involved. In the oral cavity, the cleft affects not only the soft and hard palate but also the alveolus and dentition. The structural rehabilitation of these patients requires surgical correction of the soft and hard tissue defects as well as the secondary effects of the cleft on maxillary development and dental-occlusal alignment. The role of the orthodontist in cleft management is essential; the orthodontist can assist the surgeon during all stages of reconstructive care. The orthodontist's role may include presurgical nasal and maxillary orthopedics. During the transitional dentition stage, the orthodontist may assist with alignment of the maxillary segments and in preparation for secondary alveolar bone grafting. During the permanent dentition and late adolescent years, the orthodontist may assist by obtaining satisfactory dental and occlusal relationships and prepare the dentition for prosthetic rehabilitation and orthognathic surgery if required. In addition, it has been the role of the orthodontist to monitor the craniofacial growth and dental development as well as to monitor treatment effects through the use of roentgencephalometry.

With this approach, the management of the cleft patient has evolved dramatically in recent years. The reason for improved outcomes is based on refinements in primary surgery techniques as well as timing and incorporation of other procedures, such as presurgical orthopedics, orthodontics, and the new prosthetic

approaches with resin-bonded prostheses or osseointegrated implants.

Patients treated within the context of the multidisciplinary approach can obtain excellent outcomes related to speech, ideal occlusion, satisfactory lip aesthetics, and skeletal balance (Fig. 96-1). However, it is the secondary cleft nasal deformity that may still give the patient "cleft stigmata."

In recent years, new treatment modalities have become available that may further improve outcomes in patients with orofacial clefts. These include presurgical nasoalveolar molding techniques in infancy and, as early as childhood, distraction osteogenesis to improve the position of the maxilla in those patients with severe maxillary hypoplasia. In the past, these patients often had disappointing results after conventional surgery. Efforts toward improvement of these challenging problems are a welcome addition to the new treatment protocols for the cleft patient.

In this chapter, the orthodontic management of the cleft patient by use of a developmental approach from infancy through adulthood is presented. Only general guidelines can be given; the final treatment plan is highly individualized for the particular patient, especially because we know that "not all congenital cleft lips and palates are alike"[1] and that they present with a wide spectrum of anatomic variability and severity.

INFANCY

The surgeon is often presented with an infant who has a severe cleft with marked distortions not only of the

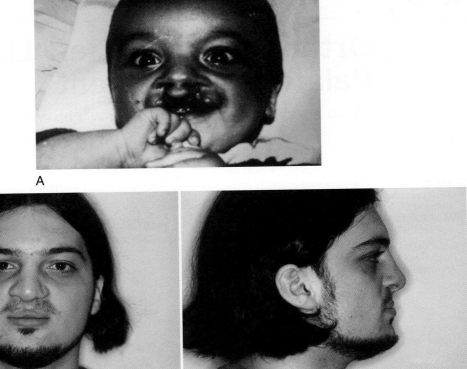

A

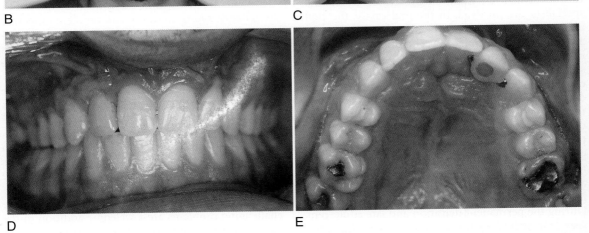

B   C

D   E

FIGURE 96-1. *A* to *C,* Facial photographs of a patient born with bilateral cleft lip and palate before and after rehabilitation. *D* and *E,* Frontal and occlusal (reverse mirror) images of the same patient demonstrate occlusion after orthodontic treatment and prosthetic rehabilitation with an osseointegrated implant.

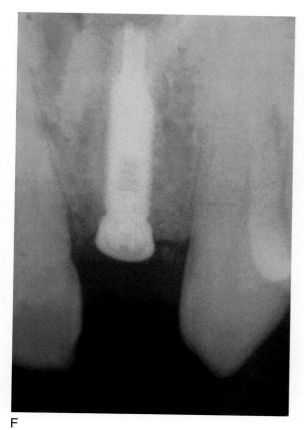

FIGURE 96-1 cont'd. *F,* Radiograph demonstrates a well-integrated implant. Note excellent facial balance, aesthetics, and occlusion.

maxillary segments but also of the cartilages of the nose. This situation can occur in the patient with unilateral and bilateral cleft lip and palate.

In the past, many surgeons chose not to perform any presurgical maxillary orthopedics because it was believed that the effect of lip repair was sufficient to rearrange the maxillary segments into favorable position for arch form and also to narrow the secondary palatal cleft (Fig. 96-2). Proponents of primary closure of the alveolus by bone grafting or gingival periosteoplasty must use maxillary orthopedics to narrow the alveolar segments so appropriate soft tissue closure of the alveolar defect can be accomplished. At this time, evidence available in the literature still supports the approach of delaying reconstruction of the alveolus until a later date to minimize the possible negative effects of surgery on future maxillary growth.[2-4] The authors currently adhere to this protocol but watch with interest the reports from those practicing early alveolar reconstruction with newer surgical techniques and maxillary orthopedics.[5]

For the past 10 years, the authors have followed the reports from Grayson et al,[6-9] who use premaxillary and maxillary orthopedics with the additional purposes of aligning the maxillary segments and repositioning the nasal cartilages before lip repair. This approach has now been included in our protocol of infant management before lip surgery in all patients with moderate to severe nasal deformities in unilateral cases and bilateral clefts with premaxillary protrusion and hypoplastic columella.

Unilateral Cleft Lip

Evaluation of the cleft nose demonstrates the presence of severely distorted nasal cartilage with deviation of the nasal tip toward the noncleft side and severe angulation of the columella also to the noncleft side. In addition, soft tissues caudal to the lateral nasal cartilage are often hyperplastic and prominent. Repair of the lip under these conditions, even with surgical repositioning of the nasal cartilages, results in a suboptimal outcome concerning nasal morphology even though the lip repair is satisfactory. For this reason, orthopedic repositioning of the nasal cartilages, columella, nasal tip, and lateral wall of the vestibule is preferable to provide patients with the best possible primary nasal reconstruction with minimally invasive surgical techniques. The procedure of presurgical infant nasal remodeling using a modified intraoral plate was first described in the literature by Bennun and his coworkers in Argentina.[9a,9b] Since then, it has been popularized in the United States as nasoalveolar molding by Grayson et al.[6-9] The authors have used this technique since 1995 and have made some modifications.

Once it has been determined that the severity of the nose is such that a surgical outcome would be suboptimal, the patient is referred for nasal molding. All patients who undergo this procedure have a preoperative impression of the maxillary arch as well as a facial moulage of the upper face from the upper lip to the forehead. In addition, intraoral and facial photographs are obtained so graphic and three-dimensional records of the deformity are kept in the registry. These records are also used to fabricate the maxillary plate that will be used to deliver the orthopedic forces to mold the nasal cartilages. The maxillary plate is made with a light-cured orthodontic resin. A wire may be incorporated as a clinical guide to assist with the direction required to reposition the nasal structures. Once the appropriate direction is obtained, this wire can be covered with light-cured acrylic, and the portion that will do the actual lifting and repositioning of the nose is lined with acrylic covered with a soft denture liner to avoid any irritation to the delicate tissues of the nasal mucosa. At this point, the maxillary aspect of the plate is relined with soft tissue liner to obtain an

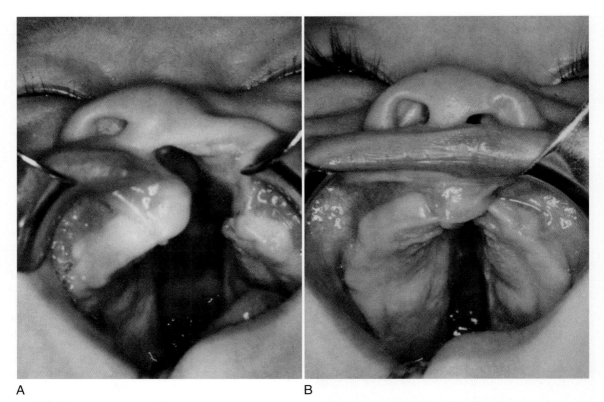

A   B

FIGURE 96-2. Intraoral views of a patient with complete unilateral cleft lip and palate before *(A)* and after *(B)* lip repair. Note changes on maxillary arch form and narrowing of the alveolar and palatal clefts after lip repair. Presurgical maxillary orthopedics were not used.

exact copy of the maxillary undercuts made by the cleft (Figs. 96-3 and 96-4). An exact fit of the plate is required for adequate retention, especially because we do not rely on external adhesive tape to maintain the plate in position. Denture adhesive cream should be used after drying the plate and the oral mucosa before insertion. The parents are instructed to clean and replace the denture adhesive one to three times per day. Patients return on a weekly basis for additional adjustments in the form of increases to the nasal prong until the surgeon is satisfied with the newly repositioned nasal structures. While the nasal molding is taking place, one can also elect to narrow the maxillary segments by selectively grinding acrylic medial to the palatal shelves and adding acrylic lateral to the alveolar processes. In addition, facial taping can apply transverse pressure to the cleft segments and help with the cleft narrowing process (Fig. 96-5).

The results expected from this technique include repositioning of the nasal tip toward the noncleft side with straightening of the columella and equalization of the height on the nasal domes as much as possible. In addition, the nasal prong is adjusted in such a way as to exert lateral pressure on the lateral nasal wall against the hyperplastic soft tissues caudal to the lateral

nasal cartilage. This treatment results in a straighter nose with convex nasal cartilages and flattened hyperplastic lateral wall vestibular tissues (see Fig. 96-5).

At the time of surgery, the lip repair is performed with a triangular flap or the rotation-advancement operation with medial repositioning of the base of the nose and narrowing of the nasal domes with tacking of the vestibular tissues to the lateral nasal wall. This combined effort will provide these patients with better noses that will require less extensive secondary revisions. The outcomes obtained with this technique are consistent and predictable, and these variations of the molding technique have been incorporated with favorable results (Fig. 96-6). This treatment protocol has been used for a few years, and there are not enough long-term data to demonstrate the effects of the technique on the fully developed nasal structures. Long-term follow-up and intercenter prospective studies are on the way to try to demonstrate the long-term effects and stability of this technique.[10]

In patients with severe nasal distortion, nasal molding by postsurgical nasal stenting with commercially available removable nasal stents is recommended.[11,12] However, custom acrylic stents have also

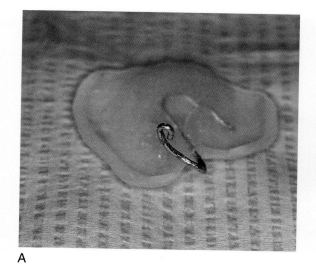

A

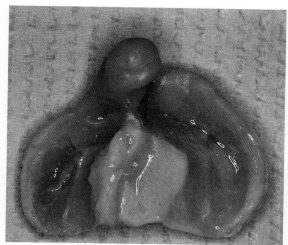

B

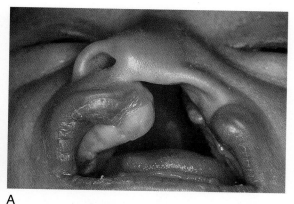

A

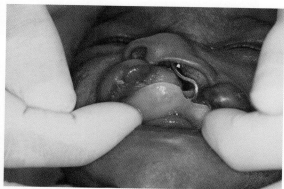

B

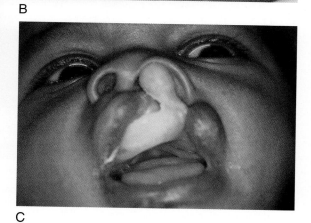

C

FIGURE 96-3. *A,* Frontal view of nasoalveolar molding plate demonstrating guide wire before relining. *B,* Superior view after covering of the guide wire with soft resin to be used as the nasal lifting prong and plate relining.

FIGURE 96-4. *A,* Patient with complete unilateral left cleft lip and palate and severe nasal distortion before treatment. *B,* At the time of initial fitting of the nasal molding plate with guide wire in place. *C,* Plate in position; note direction of the nasal prong elevating the depressed nasal dome and straightening of the columella.

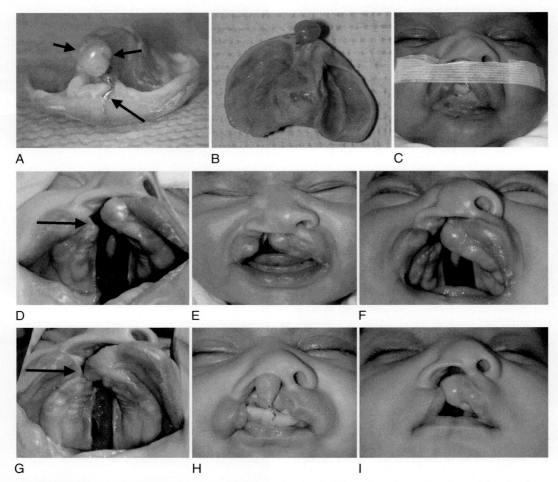

FIGURE 96-5. *A,* Frontal view and detail of nasoalveolar molding plate demonstrating guide wire *(long arrow)* used for accurate placement of the nasal molding bulb *(short arrows). B,* Occlusal view of the plate demonstrating the anatomic maxillary detail after relining. *C,* Child with complete right cleft lip and palate undergoing nasoalveolar molding supported with facial taping. *D,* Intraoral view of the same child demonstrating the alveolar *(arrow)* and palatal clefts as well as distortion of the greater maxillary segment. *E* and *F,* Frontal and inferior views of the nose before treatment. Note severely distorted ala cartilages and severe deviation of the nasal tip and columella to the cleft side. *G,* After nasoalveolar molding, note narrowing of the alveolar and palatal clefts *(arrow). H,* Patient undergoing nasoalveolar molding. Note direction of the nasal prong elevating the nasal tip and columella and reshaping of the ala cartilages. *I,* Before lip surgery and after nasoalveolar molding, note convexity of the nasal cartilages with elevation of the cleft-side nasal dome and straightening of the columella.

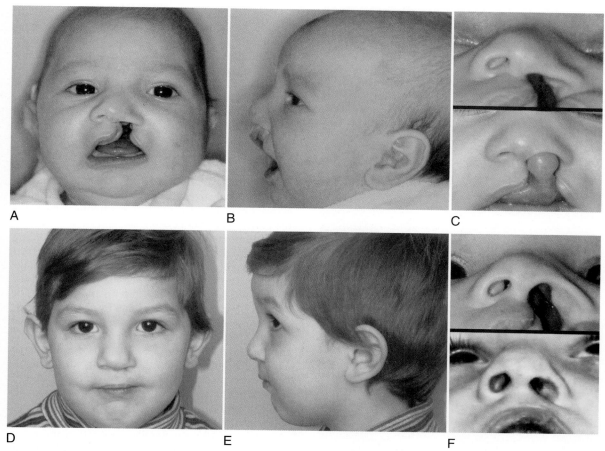

FIGURE 96-6. Frontal and profile photographs of a child with a complete left cleft lip and palate who underwent nasoalveolar molding, before molding (*A* and *B*) and 3 years after lip repair (*D* and *E*). Close-ups of the original nasal distortion and the molding process are shown (*C*), as well as the nasal improvement after molding (increased nasal cartilage convexity, columella elongation, and overall symmetry) and after lip repair (*F*).

been used.[13] The stent is usually kept in place with facial taping (Fig. 96-7) and is maintained for at least 2 to 3 months or for as long as the patient can deal with it comfortably. This protocol has been well tolerated by the patients and readily accepted by the parents.

Bilateral Cleft Lip

The patient with bilateral cleft lip and palate represents the most challenging condition for the reconstructive team. What makes these patients so difficult is that commonly, the premaxilla is extremely protrusive, the premaxilla and prolabium can be of variable size, the columella is deficient or almost nonexistent, the palatal clefts are wider than usual, and, occasionally, the maxillary palatal shelves are collapsed. In addition, the nasal domes are usually wide apart and the tip projection is decreased (Figs. 96-8 and 96-9). In patients with bilateral cleft lip and palate with

a protrusive premaxilla, it becomes imperative for the premaxilla to be repositioned into a more favorable relationship with the maxillary segments to achieve definitive lip closure with minimal tension. If this is not performed, a poor repair or failure with unfavorable consequences may occur (Fig. 96-10). For this purpose, one may choose to use premaxillary orthopedics with an intraoral appliance that is retained with denture adhesive and has an elastic strap for premaxillary retraction.[14,15] This approach allows the surgeon to close the lip satisfactorily.

In the patient with bilateral cleft lip and palate, the approach requires repositioning of the premaxilla before the nasal molding technique. In the past, these patients have been managed with various approaches, few of them leading to satisfactory results. This management included the use of lip adhesions followed by definitive lip repair, a two-stage repair in which one side is repaired first followed by

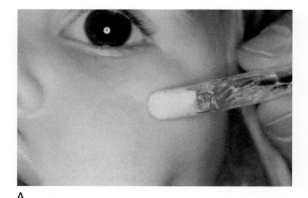

A

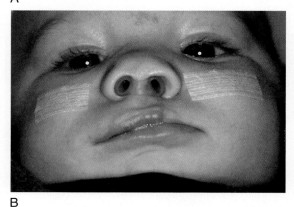

B

C

FIGURE 96-7. *A,* Application of liquid skin adhesive to the cheek. *B,* On the painted sections, a base section of tape is applied. Note nasal stent in position. *C,* Support of the nasal stent with perforated tape across the nose. Tape adheres to base tape glued over skin and not directly to skin to avoid irritation.

the contralateral side. In patients with extreme premaxillary protrusion, there have been reports of surgical excision of the premaxilla. The premaxilla has also been set back surgically in infancy, and various techniques for orthopedic repositioning of the protrusive premaxilla have been used, including extra-

oral and intraoral appliances. The extraoral appliances include facial taping and bonnets. The intraoral approaches include appliances that are retained with pins and those that are self-retained by undercuts of the clefts. For the last 15 years, the authors have used a self-retaining intraoral plate[15] that has been modified from the original design.[14] Initially, an elastic strap made of dental rubber dam was used. This approach had to be modified because the half-life of the strap was limited. The modification included placing orthodontic buttons on the plate to which an elastomeric chain was attached. The elastomeric chain was modified to have a lining of a soft material around the area of the chain over the prolabium. This modification allowed easy adjustments and less frequent visits for the patient (Fig. 96-11).

Grayson et al[6,7,9] have used nasoalveolar molding for bilateral clefts. The appliance was intended to retract the premaxilla as well as to mold the nasal cartilage and elongate the columella. Their plate design included retention through extraoral taping and elastics. The authors have modified the design by use of our principles of a self-retained appliance[14,15] to avoid facial taping. The appliance is constructed in the following manner. An intraoral impression of the maxillary arch and face is obtained. On the maxillary cast, a light-cured resin plate is constructed to which orthodontic buttons are attached for retraction of the premaxilla (see Fig. 96-11). In addition, the plate is relined with soft tissue conditioner for close adaptation to the maxillary tissues. After premaxillary retraction and repositioning are completed, the plate is modified by the addition of two wire prongs that go into each nasal vestibule. The ends of the wires are covered with a soft denture lining material. In addition, loops are bent about the level of the superior aspect of the prolabium for attachment of an elastomeric chain that has been covered with a soft tissue denture liner. The purpose of the elastomeric chain across the prolabium is to hold it down, while the nasal prongs at the end of the wires are gradually elevated, lifting and medially repositioning the nasal domes and at the same time elongating the hypoplastic columella. The plate is used for 24 hours, removed daily for cleaning, and held in position with the aid of a denture adhesive cream. In addition, the intraoral aspect of the plate can be modified by adding material on the lateral aspects of the plate and removing acrylic on the medial aspects. This will allow gentle and gradual repositioning of the maxillary segments, resulting in narrowing of the cleft if necessary. In patients in whom the maxillary palatal segments are collapsed, it is then necessary to expand them before premaxillary retraction by placing a midline expansion screw. After the expansion is completed, a new plate is fabricated for retention of the new arch form, continuation of premaxillary repositioning, columella lengthening, and nasal cartilage

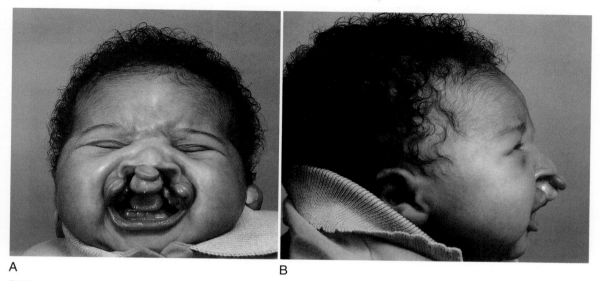

FIGURE 96-8. Frontal (A) and profile (B) views of an infant born with a complete bilateral cleft lip and palate. Note protrusive premaxilla, absent columella, broad nasal dimensions, and limited nasal tip projection.

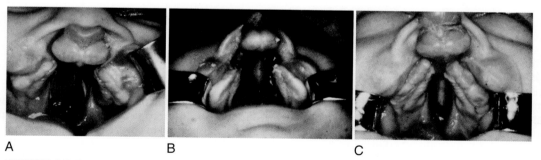

FIGURE 96-9. Variability observed in patients with complete bilateral cleft lip and palate. A, Symmetric position of the premaxilla and wide palatal cleft with a small prolabium. B, Severe premaxillary protrusion with small prolabium and wide palatal cleft. C, Protrusive premaxilla and collapsed palatal segments.

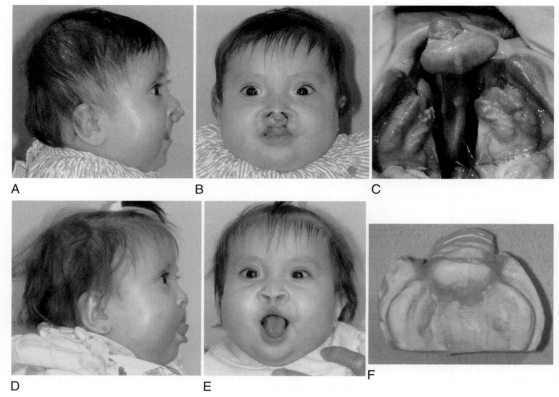

FIGURE 96-10. *A to C,* Profile, frontal, and intraoral views of an infant born with bilateral cleft lip and palate who underwent two unsuccessful attempts for bilateral cleft lip repair elsewhere. Note premaxillary protrusion and diminutive residual prolabium. *D to F,* Postoperative views after bilateral cleft lip repair with simultaneous surgical repositioning of the premaxilla, as demonstrated by the maxillary cast. Note acceptable lip repair, but retrusion of the upper lip is already evident.

molding. This technique not only has given the surgeon an improved situation for obtaining adequate lip repair but also has provided a better situation for primary nasal reconstruction with remodeling of the nasal domes and nasal tip and elongation of the hypoplastic columella (see Fig. 96-10). The main advantage of this procedure is that it eliminates the need for secondary procedures for columella elongation in the early childhood years. All of the patients in whom this technique has been used have adjusted extremely well to the use of the appliance, and the families have been extremely pleased with the results (see Fig. 96-11) as well as with the ease in which the orthopedic phase is carried out.

In those patients with incomplete bilateral clefts, especially those involving one side in which the premaxilla and the prolabium are asymmetric, it is preferable to surgically remove the soft tissue band to obtain symmetric repositioning of the premaxilla, prolabium, columella, and nasal domes.

Wide Palatal Clefts: Articulation Development Prosthesis

In patients with palatal clefts that are extremely wide, the surgeon is forced to delay palate surgery. A prosthesis may be used to cover the palatal defect until the time the palate surgery can be completed in either one stage or two stages, with closure of the soft palate preceding closure of the hard palate. The purpose of this plate is to provide the child with a more normal oral environment so the child can start to use the oral mechanism for speech production without the development of compensatory articulations that are difficult for the speech pathologist to treat later in life.[16] These plates are not used for feeding purposes because children with open clefts can feed adequately with appropriate feeding techniques. However, the use of the plate facilitates feeding according to parents and also nurses and speech pathologists who observe the children during these early months.

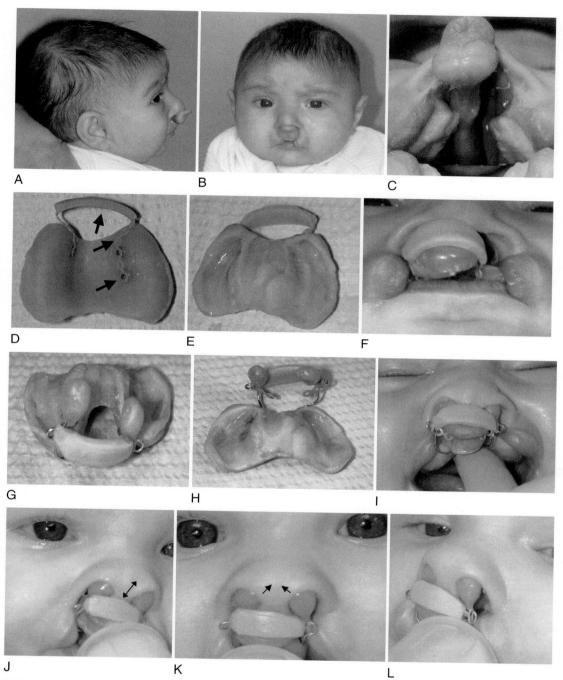

FIGURE 96-11. *A to C,* Profile, frontal, and intraoral photographs of an infant born with a complete bilateral cleft lip and palate. Note premaxillary protrusion and absent columella. *D and E,* Inferior and superior views of premaxillary repositioning appliance. Note the asymmetric position of the orthodontic buttons to exert force toward the left side to center and retract the deviated and protrusive premaxilla. Note the orthodontic elastomeric chain covered by soft denture lining material *(forward arrows). F,* The patient is shown wearing the intraoral plate to reposition and retract the premaxilla. *G to I,* After premaxillary repositioning, the plate was modified by the addition of intranasal wire extensions that ended in an acrylic nasal prong. The plate is in place; also note the transverse elastomeric chain covered with soft tissue conditioner exerting posterior and inferior pressure over the prolabium while the nasal extensions lift the nasal tip and narrow the displaced nasal domes. *J to L,* Oblique and frontal close-up views after wearing of the nasal orthopedic plate. Note elongation of the columella *(double arrow)* as well as approximation of the nasal domes toward the midline *(arrows).*   *Continued*

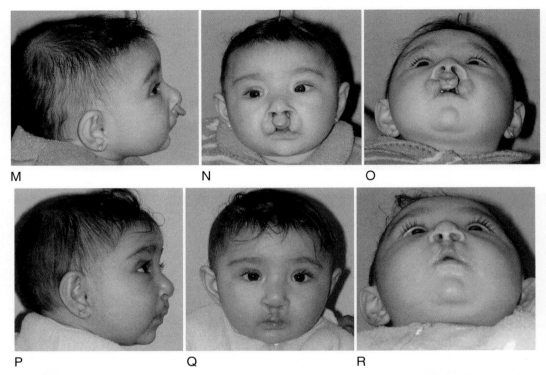

FIGURE 96-11, cont'd. *M to O,* Profile, frontal, and inferior views after orthopedic premaxillary repositioning with medial repositioning of the nasal domes and elongation of the columella. Note nasal definition and symmetry. *P to R,* Profile and frontal photographs after premaxillary repositioning, nasal and columellar molding, and one-stage bilateral cleft lip repair.

PRIMARY DENTITION

Orthodontic treatment at this stage is limited to the correction of certain posterior crossbites and anterior crossbites of mild to moderate degree.

Posterior Crossbite

In the cleft patient, posterior crossbites are of both skeletal and dental origin. They are skeletal because the maxillary segments are usually collapsed after cleft palate surgery, especially in the canine region (Fig. 96-12). In most instances, this change in arch form occurs before the eruption of the primary canines; therefore, at the time of eruption of these teeth, the maxillary cleft-side primary canine erupts medially to the lower one. In addition, this early relationship causes minor palatal displacement of the maxillary primary canine and labial displacement of the mandibular one. This is an important observation because this is the reason that cleft patients in the primary dentition rarely have occlusal or functional shifts. Patients in whom an occlusal shift is detected are the ones who are candidates for either selective tooth grinding or expansion procedures. Expansion

can readily be accomplished; but after it is completed, unless a bone graft is placed, it has to be retained until the time of alveolar reconstruction with a bone graft. For this reason, it is preferable to delay transverse expansion in the primary dentition until the patient is older and just before secondary alveolar bone grafting procedures usually undertaken in the transitional dentition.

Anterior Crossbite

Anterior crossbite of mild to moderate degree can be managed in the primary dentition by use of elastic protraction forces delivered through a facial mask.[17-19] However, if this crossbite is related to a moderate to severe skeletal maxillary hypoplasia, the patient is best managed with a surgical approach. If it is thought that the maxillary advancement is important at an early age because of the severity of the crossbite, it can be instituted by means of distraction osteogenesis (discussed later in the chapter).

When it is determined that protraction facemask therapy is indicated, it is performed by manufacturing an intraoral splint that is anchored to the second primary molars; it has protraction hooks just lateral

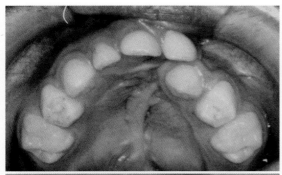

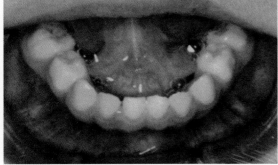

A

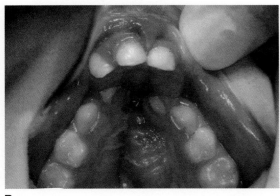

B

FIGURE 96-12. Occlusal views of a child with a repaired unilateral cleft lip and palate *(A)* and of a child with a repaired bilateral cleft lip and palate *(B)*. Note the medial collapse of the cleft segment in the unilateral patient and the collapse of both maxillary segments posterior to the premaxilla in the bilateral patient.

to the maxillary primary lateral incisors. Two 6- or 8-ounce elastics per side are used to deliver a force between 24 and 32 ounces. The device is worn for at least 10 to 12 hours per day. It is important to incorporate an expansion screw to improve arch form and also to activate and increase the response of the maxillofacial sutures to the maxillary protraction (Fig. 96-13). Results are observed within 3 months. If no response or a limited one is noted, the treatment is

discontinued and management of the anterior crossbite is delegated to a combined surgical and orthodontic approach at a later time.

Facemask protraction in the cleft patient usually yields advancement ranging from 2 to 4 mm.[19] The overall effects of facemask therapy include a modest maxillary advancement with some clockwise mandibular repositioning (Fig. 96-14). To date, the long-term stability of this approach has not been documented in a large series of cleft patients. With the advent of new surgical approaches, it is not justified to subject the patient to long-term therapy that may need to be repeated several times because of the unpredictable response of the procedure in the cleft patient. The reason that facemask therapy is not as effective in the cleft patient as in the noncleft patient is that the palatal tissues, including the transverse palatal suture and pterygomaxillary junctions, are commonly scarred from previous palatal surgery.[20]

TRANSITIONAL DENTITION

This is the developmental stage in which a patient who had a cleft lip and palate also involving the alveolus will be receiving the next or third surgical procedure after lip and secondary palate repair. In most instances, the dentition around the cleft presents with severe malpositions that limit surgical access to the alveolar site (Fig. 96-15). For this purpose, the dentition adjacent to the cleft has to be orthodontically repositioned to prepare the cleft site for the secondary alveolar bone graft. Reconstruction of the cleft alveolus and anterior aspect of the maxilla is deferred until this stage to minimize the risk of affecting growth as a result of surgical trauma and scarring.[3,20,21]

In those patients in whom the maxillary segments and dentition on either side of the cleft are well aligned, it is not necessary to do presurgical orthodontics. Orthodontic treatment is then postponed until after the bone graft, when most of the permanent dentition is complete. If it is determined that the patient requires orthodontic treatment for preparation of the surgical site, it should be based on the stage of dental development of the permanent teeth that will be orthodontically moved rather than on chronologic age.[22,23] It is known that cleft patients present a delay of dental development and eruption.[23,24] Orthodontic treatment should not be initiated until the development of the incisor roots, on which orthodontic brackets will be placed, is almost complete (Fig. 96-16). Adherence to this guideline will result in minimal resorptive changes on the roots of the maxillary incisors. If the necessary treatment for secondary bone grafting of the maxilla is based on dental development rather than on chronologic age, a safeguard for the adverse effects of surgery on growth is added. The author's studies[23] indicate that development and

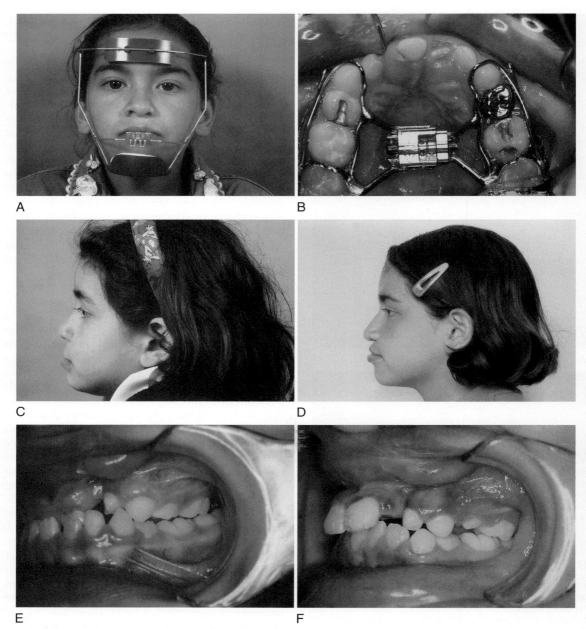

FIGURE 96-13. *A* and *B,* Patient with a repaired unilateral cleft with mild maxillary hypoplasia with anterior dental crossbite. The patient was in the early transitional dentition and underwent maxillary protraction with an intraoral expander and a facemask. *C* and *D,* Note the profile changes after treatment with increased facial convexity and position of the upper lip. *E* and *F,* The anterior crossbite present before treatment was corrected after maxillary protraction and minor orthodontic alignment of the maxillary incisors.

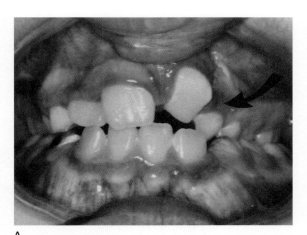

A

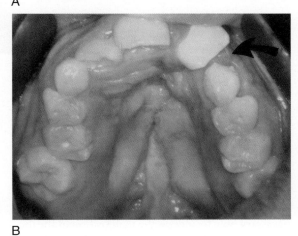

B

FIGURE 96-15. Frontal *(A)* and occlusal *(B)* views of a patient in the transitional dentition with a repaired right cleft lip and palate. Note abnormal position of the left central incisor into the area of the alveolar cleft *(arrows)*.

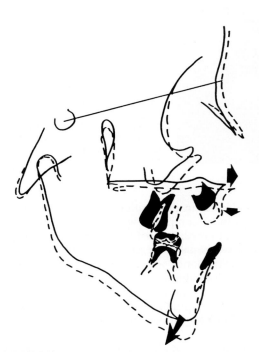

FIGURE 96-14. Cephalometric tracings of a patient after orthopedic facemask treatment. Note anterior maxillary movement with downward and backward rotation of the mandible.

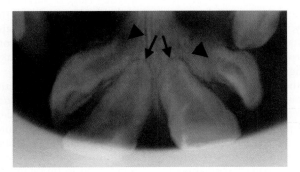

FIGURE 96-16. Occlusal radiograph of a patient with a bilateral cleft lip and palate before orthodontic treatment. Note closed apex in both central incisors *(arrows)* and wide-open apex in both maxillary lateral incisors *(arrowheads)*.

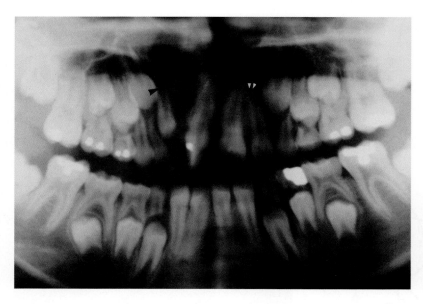

FIGURE 96-17. Panoramic radiograph of a patient with unilateral cleft lip and palate demonstrating delayed dental development of the cleft-side lateral incisor *(black arrowhead)* compared with the contralateral lateral incisor *(white arrowheads)*.

eruption of the cleft lateral incisor are markedly delayed compared with a contralateral one (Fig. 96-17). This observation allows placement of orthodontic appliances on the remaining incisors while the cleft lateral incisor has not yet erupted. When a viable cleft maxillary lateral incisor is present, this ensures its preservation and adequate bone support for eruption after the bone graft.

To prepare the maxillary arch for a bone graft, it is necessary only to address the malposition of the incisors and the anterior collapse of the maxillary arch. The first stage is usually obtained through the use of a bonded edgewise appliance (Fig. 96-18). The expansion of the arch can also be done with this appliance, but it occasionally has to be supported with a maxillary expander. The expander commonly used in our protocol is the quad helix expander (Fig. 96-19). A screw expander is rarely used unless the palatal tissues are severely scarred; fortunately, with the use of more delicate surgical techniques, this situation is uncommon. The expansion that is required for alveolar bone grafting should provide well-aligned maxillary segments with a minimal increase in the size of the alveolar gap. Wider alveolar gaps are difficult to close with local flaps. In patients in whom the required expansion of the maxilla or repositioning of the premaxilla will cause a wider gap between the maxillary segments, expansion and bone grafting procedures are deferred until adolescence. At this time, the maxillary segments can be surgically mobilized and approximated to each other for closure with local flaps at the time of final orthognathic surgery.

After the maxillary segments and dentition are placed in their ideal positions, the patient is referred for secondary alveolar bone grafting.[25] Presurgical orthodontics in preparation for this reconstructive stage can be completed within a period of 6 to 12 months. Immediately before the bone graft, all appliances over the palate are removed and the labial aspects of the orthodontic wire are segmentalized for surgical access. In addition, supernumerary or primary teeth in the surgical site are extracted 8 to 12 weeks before surgery. This will allow the surgeon to have intact gingival tissues for proper coverage of the alveolar bone graft.

The presence of alveolar bone is dependent on the presence of teeth. When the lateral incisor is present, with adequate crown and root anatomy and in favorable position, every attempt should be made to preserve it. If the lateral incisor erupts through the bone graft, suitable alveolar bone will be available in the alveolar ridge as well as for the erupting canine on the cleft side (Fig. 96-20). If the permanent lateral incisor on the cleft side is missing or needs to be extracted because of its poor anatomy or position, the actively erupting canine could take its place and preserve the reconstructed alveolus.

Orthodontic treatment can be continued 8 to 12 weeks after bone graft surgery. As soon as appropriate maxillary arch and dental relations are achieved, the orthodontic appliances are removed and the patient is placed in retention until the full permanent dentition. Teeth that were severely rotated before treatment need to be retained (Fig. 96-21). Absent teeth can be replaced with a removable prosthetic appliance to improve aesthetics and limit the effects on speech production (Fig. 96-22).

Patients treated with the protocol outlined complete the preparatory phase of orthodontic treatment in the preteen or early teen years. Patients are

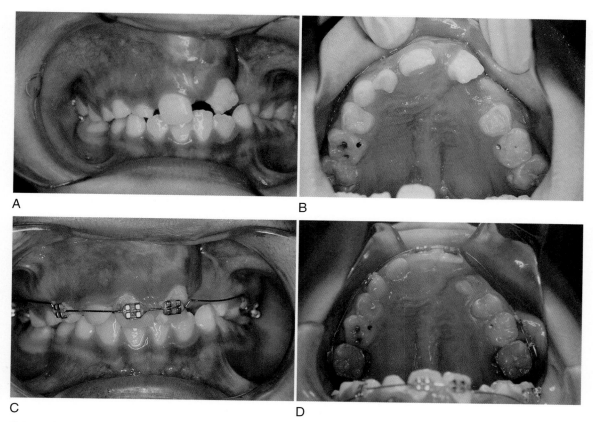

FIGURE 96-18. *A* and *B,* Frontal and occlusal photographs of a patient in the transitional dentition with a repaired left cleft lip and palate. Note position of the cleft-side central incisor into the residual alveolar cleft. *C* and *D,* After segmental orthodontic treatment in the maxillary arch only, the cleft-side incisor has been moved from the alveolar cleft, leaving the site ready for secondary alveolar bone grafting.

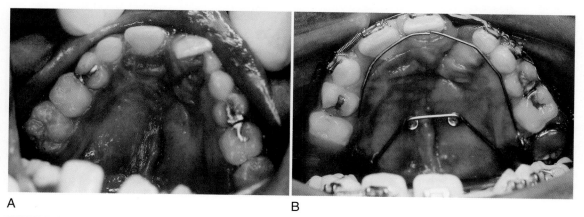

FIGURE 96-19. Occlusal views of a patient in the transitional dentition with a repaired left cleft lip and palate before *(A)* and after *(B)* orthodontic treatment in preparation for secondary alveolar bone grafting. Note collapsed cleft segment as well as the position of the cleft-side central incisor into the residual alveolar cleft. The arch form has been improved by use of a quad helix expander in conjunction with a segmental orthodontic appliance. The patient is clinically missing both the cleft-side and noncleft-side lateral incisors.

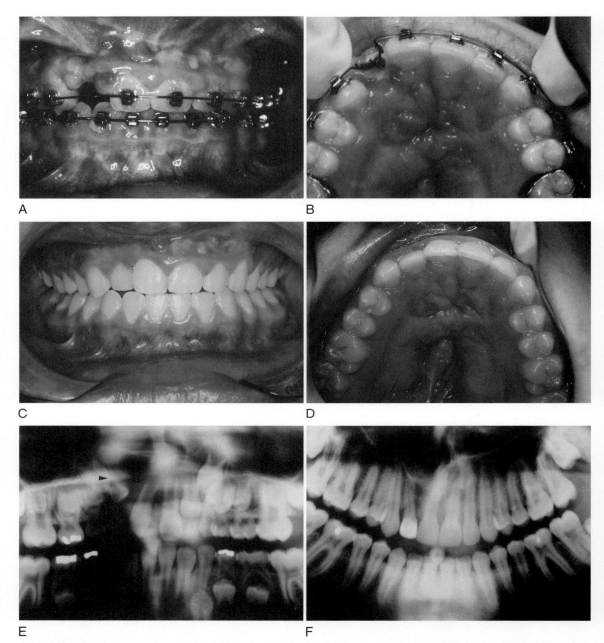

FIGURE 96-20. *A* and *B,* Frontal and occlusal views of a patient with a repaired right cleft lip and palate after secondary alveolar bone grafting. Note that the maxillary lateral incisor is erupting in the area of the alveolar cleft and the permanent cleft-side canine has been properly positioned with the orthodontic appliance. *C* and *D,* Post-orthodontic frontal and occlusal views demonstrating the intact alveolar cleft area and presence of a complete dentition. The crown of the cleft-side lateral incisor has been aesthetically enlarged with a resin restoration. *E,* Panoramic radiograph taken before bone grafting demonstrates the presence of the cleft-side lateral incisor *(arrowhead).* *F,* After treatment, note crown restoration on the cleft-side lateral incisor, good bone levels adjacent to the cleft-side maxillary canine, but decreased alveolar bone levels surrounding the cleft-side maxillary lateral incisor.

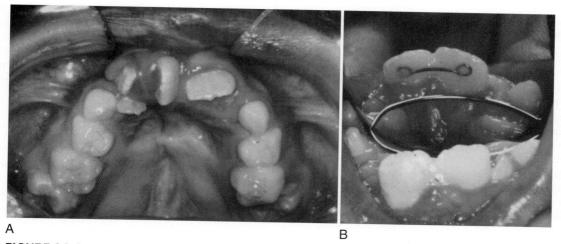

A   B

FIGURE 96-21. *A,* Pre-orthodontic occlusal view of a patient with a complete right cleft lip and palate. Note severe rotation of the cleft-side central incisor. *B,* After orthodontic treatment, the central incisor has been aligned and is being retained with a bonded lingual wire.

observed every 6 months to determine their craniofacial growth and dental development, especially eruption of the maxillary lateral incisor and canine on the cleft side. On occasion, the maxillary canine is impacted and requires surgical exposure and orthodontic incorporation into the arch. Impacted or severely malpositioned cleft-side maxillary lateral incisors are usually extracted.

Finally, if it is determined that there is anterior-posterior skeletal disharmony, the reconstructive team has to decide whether it is convenient to do the bone grafting in the transitional dentition or whether it should be performed in combination with future orthognathic surgical procedures. Patients in whom there is marked tissue deficiency, including maxillary

hypoplasia and congenitally missing teeth, are likely to be candidates for postponement of the traditional approach for secondary alveolar bone grafting and will be treated later in the permanent dentition in combination with orthognathic surgery. If it is deemed important to preserve the dentition adjacent to the alveolar cleft, orthodontics are therefore indicated even in the presence of a skeletal disharmony. The purpose of the orthodontic treatment is then to prepare the dentition for the alveolar bone graft and also to coordinate the maxillary arch to the mandibular arch for future orthognathic surgery that will be performed in the teen years. This approach minimizes the required orthodontic treatment before orthognathic surgery in the adolescent years.

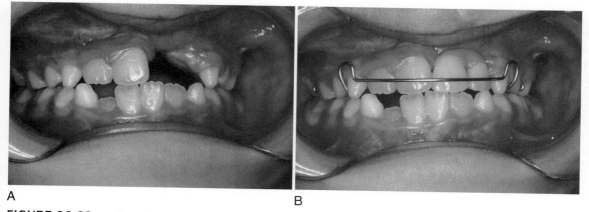

A   B

FIGURE 96-22. *A,* Frontal intraoral view of a patient with a left cleft lip and palate after orthodontic treatment. *B,* The patient was missing the cleft-side central and lateral incisors, which were temporarily replaced with a removable prosthesis.

Surgical Management of Protrusive Premaxilla in Bilateral Clefts

Even after initial successful premaxillary orthopedics in infancy, some patients with bilateral cleft lip and palate end up with a protrusive premaxilla that needs to be managed usually at the time of secondary bone grafting. The ideal approach for these patients is a combined surgical and orthodontic procedure that minimizes orthodontic treatment and maximizes the benefits of surgical intervention. These patients usually have a protrusive or retropositioned premaxilla with increased overjet and overbite as a result of horizontal and vertical displacement of the premaxilla. The buccal segments can be in either class I or class II molar relationships, and it is not uncommon to find a collapsed arch at the level of the maxillary canines. In addition, these patients may present with large alveolar fistulas and a palatal fistula posterior to the premaxilla (Fig. 96-23).

The patients should be treated with the following sequence of procedures. Orthodontic treatment is initiated with the necessary expansion, especially at the canine level with a quad helix-type expander; this is followed by continuous or segmental alignment of the buccal segments and the teeth in the premaxilla (see Fig. 96-23). The teeth in the premaxilla are usually severely rotated; therefore, it becomes necessary to place appliances for their alignment. In addition, the orthodontic appliances will be used for fixation at the time of premaxillary repositioning. Once the segments are individually aligned, a set of dental impressions is obtained and the working maxillary cast is sectioned to reposition the premaxilla in its ideal anatomic position. The clinician must keep in mind that the axial inclination of the teeth needs to be improved to an ideal position relative to the palatal plane and the lower incisors. As this is done, the clinician will note that the areas that need to be closed during the bone grafting procedure are tightly approximated, facilitating soft tissue closure of the alveolar bone graft and the residual fistula posterior to the premaxilla. With the premaxilla in its new position, the splint is made of self-curing orthodontic resin to assist the surgeon during the fixation period after the surgical repositioning and bone grafting (Fig. 96-24). With this approach, all patients with bilateral clefts and severely displaced premaxilla have complete closure of the oronasal and palatal fistulas with successful bone grafting of the alveolus and ideal position of the maxillary incisors (see Fig. 96-23).

The main advantage of this approach is that minimal orthodontic forces are required during the alignment of the incisors, which may have abnormally short roots in bilateral cleft patients. Obviously, the premaxilla can be repositioned through orthodontic means, but the time and force levels exerted on the incisors during repositioning can be high and result in severe root resorption, jeopardizing the long-term prognosis for these teeth. After premaxillary repositioning, the patient is placed in retention until the permanent dentition is complete to initiate the final stage of orthodontic treatment.

PERMANENT DENTITION

At the time of almost complete or complete permanent dentition, the orthodontist must perform definitive orthodontic treatment in the cleft patient. The goals are no different from those for noncleft patients, but certain conditions must be kept in mind during treatment planning. The specific goals include maintenance of the integrity of the dentition and supporting structures, especially for teeth adjacent to the alveolar cleft; correction of unusual dental positions; correction of impactions, dental transpositions, congenitally missing teeth, or severely abnormal teeth that may need to be extracted—these will need replacement either with a prosthesis or with orthodontic space closure, especially in the cleft region; correction of maxillary and mandibular dental midlines and their relation to the facial midline; and correction of anterior-posterior, transverse, and vertical relationships of the maxilla and mandible to each other and to the face.[22,26,27]

Every attempt should be made to give the patients class I cuspid and molar relationships with ideal overjet and overbite (see Figs. 96-1 and 96-20). If the cleft-side lateral incisor is missing, the clinician must decide whether this tooth needs to be replaced with a prosthesis or the space closed with orthodontics or a combined surgical-orthodontic approach. Prosthetic replacement is usually reserved for those cases in which ideal class I cuspid relationships and overjet and overbite are present. In these patients, if the anatomy of the teeth adjacent to the dental gap is sound, a bonded prosthesis or an osseointegrated fixture can be used (see Fig. 96-1).[22,26-28]

In those patients with a missing lateral incisor in whom the maxillary canine has migrated forward and is erupting into the grafted alveolar ridge (Fig. 96-25), one must consider replacement of the lateral incisor by the canine and movement of all the posterior teeth forward. The cleft side will be finished with class II relations (Fig. 96-26). In patients in whom the outcome of the alveolar bone graft is not ideal, the clinician may want to move the canine forward into it to improve bone morphology rather than replacing the lateral incisor with an osseointegrated fixture or a prosthesis that might need additional bone grafting. One may also have to decide how to manage the missing cleft-side maxillary incisor, including the shape,

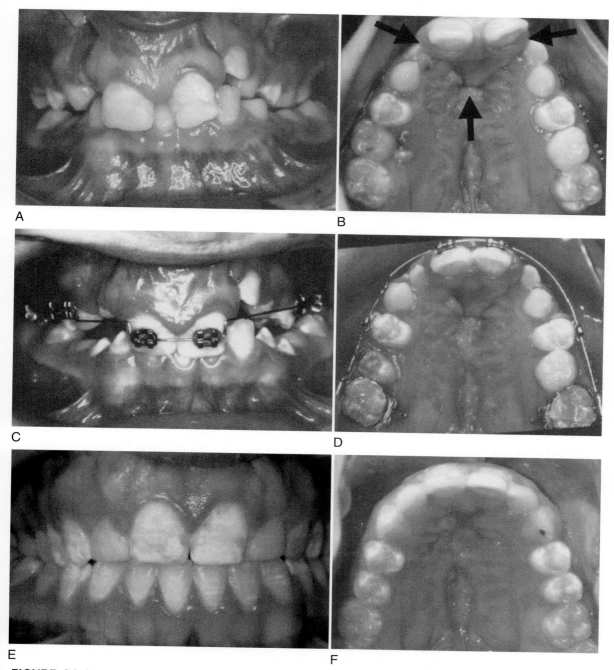

FIGURE 96-23. *A* and *B,* Patient with a bilateral cleft lip and palate with protrusive and downward displaced premaxilla and residual alveolar and anterior palatal fistulas *(arrows).* *C* and *D,* Fixed orthodontic appliance treatment was instituted in the maxillary arch with independent alignment of the teeth on each of the three segments. *E* and *F,* After successful premaxillary repositioning with simultaneous bone grafting and closure of alveolar and palatal fistulas, the patient's maxillary arch integrity has been restored.

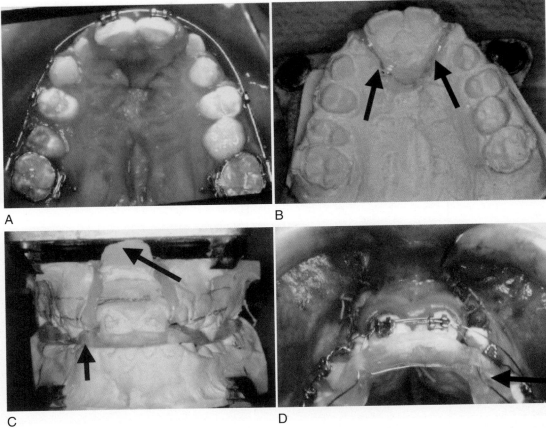

A

B

C

D

FIGURE 96-24. *A* and *B*, Intraoral occlusal view of the maxillary arch from the patient shown in Figure 96-23 after orthodontic alignment and dental cast with repositioning of the premaxilla. *Arrows* point to repositioned segment. *C*, Frontal view of the cast, illustrating superior repositioning of the premaxilla *(upper arrow)*. The surgical splint *(lower arrow)* is made with the premaxilla in its new position. *D*, Surgical splint wired in place to the orthodontic appliance, after surgical premaxillary superior repositioning with simultaneous bilateral alveolar cleft closure and bone grafting.

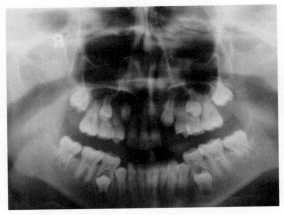

FIGURE 96-25. Panoramic radiograph of a patient with a left cleft lip and palate demonstrating absence of the cleft-side lateral incisor with eruption of the cleft-side permanent canine adjacent to the central incisor. This is a clear indication for replacement of the lateral incisor with the naturally erupting canine.

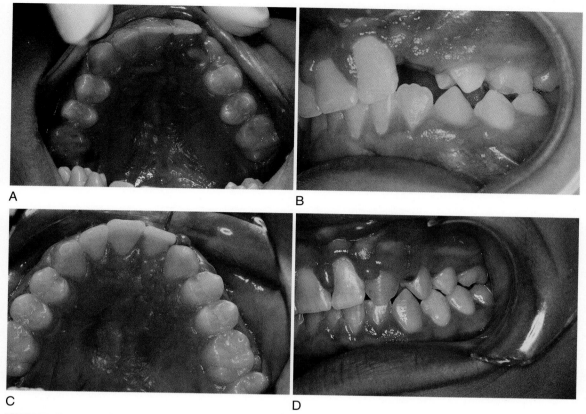

FIGURE 96-26. *A* and *B,* Occlusal and lateral views of a patient with a left cleft lip and palate in which the maxillary canine erupted adjacent to the central incisor after secondary alveolar bone grafting. *C* and *D,* After orthodontic treatment, the permanent canine was kept adjacent to the permanent central incisor with adequate buccal interdigitation (class II relations) on the cleft side.

size, and color of the canine as well as the gingival contour in the area of the cleft.[22] If they are properly planned, both the prosthetic and orthodontic options to manage the missing cleft-side lateral incisor can provide outstanding results (see Figs. 96-1 and 96-26).

In situations in which the alveolar cleft is too wide for conventional bone grafting, the clinician may elect to surgically shift the cleft-side posterior segment forward and place the canine in the position of the missing lateral incisor. This ensures not only closure of the alveolar defect but also closure of the dental gap made by the missing cleft-side maxillary lateral incisor (Fig. 96-27).[22,29]

After bone grafting, it is not uncommon to find that the cleft-side maxillary canine has an unusual eruption path and is impacted. These teeth need to be managed surgically by exposing them so the orthodontist can incorporate them into the dental arch (Fig. 96-28).

Orthodontic management following the developmental approach outlined previously allows the clinician to take advantage of developmental and growth changes and permits the patient and family to recognize the need for distinct phases of orthodontic treatment that also allows sufficient rest space between stages. This approach ensures the patient's and family's acceptance, compliance, and cooperation with the treatment protocol.

Orthognathic Surgery and Distraction Procedures

Skeletal and dental discrepancies between the maxilla and mandible are not uncommon in cleft patients. These discrepancies can be in the sagittal, transverse, and vertical planes. If the discrepancies are moderate to severe, they are best managed with a combined surgical and orthodontic approach. This approach results in substantial functional and aesthetic improvements in the cleft patient.

It is generally accepted that patients with orofacial clefts have mandibles that are of normal size or slightly smaller.[30] For this reason, in most of the patients in

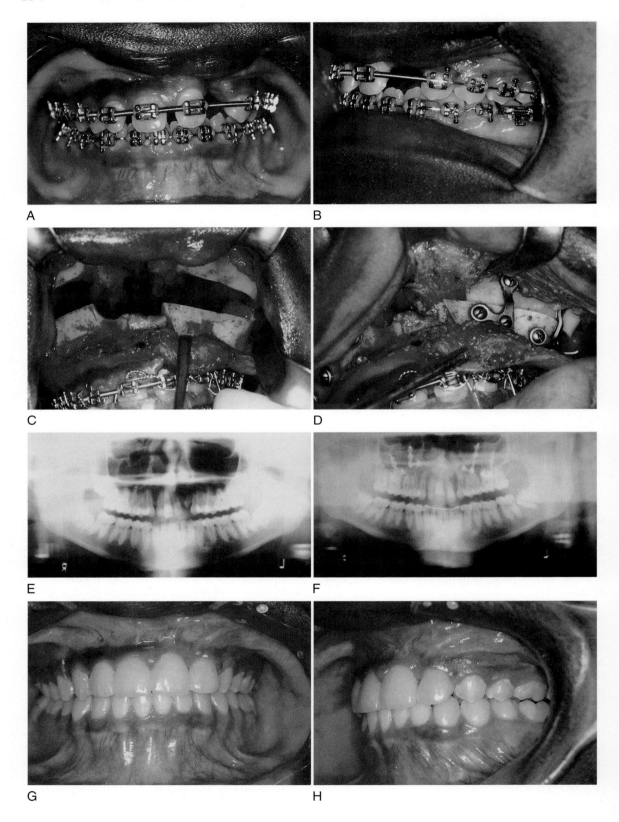

A

B

C

D

E

F

G

H

FIGURE 96-27. *A* and *B,* Intraoral frontal and lateral views of a patient with a large residual left alveolar cleft and dental gap as a result of loss of the cleft-side lateral incisor. *C* and *D,* The alveolar cleft and dental gap were closed by surgical shifting of the cleft-side posterior segment forward through a two-piece Le Fort I osteotomy with rigid fixation and bone grafting. *E* and *F,* The preoperative and postoperative panoramic radiographs demonstrate the extent of the original alveolar cleft and its closure by advancement of the cleft segment. Note approximation of the cleft-side canine and central incisor as well as rigid fixation plates. *G* and *H,* Post-treatment frontal and lateral occlusal views demonstrating resolution of the alveolar defect and dental gap. The maxillary incisors had cosmetic resin-bonded procedures, and the cleft-side canine was reshaped to resemble a lateral incisor.

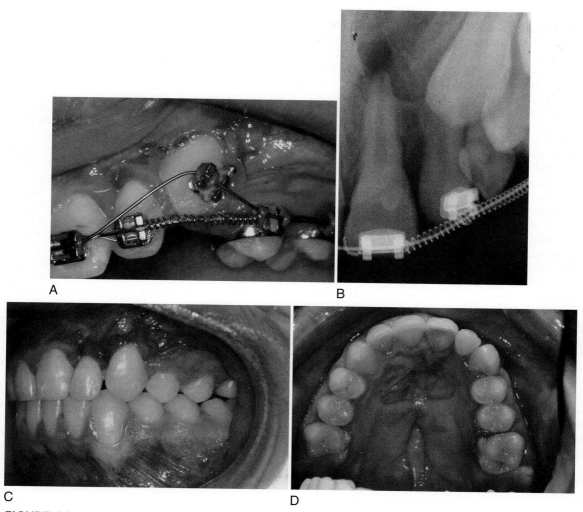

A

B

C

D

FIGURE 96-28. *A* and *B,* Intraoral view of a patient with a left cleft lip and palate who had an impacted cleft-side maxillary canine with corresponding radiograph. The patient underwent surgical exposure and orthodontic treatment to incorporate the tooth into the arch. *C* and *D,* Lateral and occlusal views of the patient at the completion of orthodontic treatment. Note the presence of all teeth on the maxillary arch with good occlusion. The gingival contour around the cleft-side lateral incisor is irregular as a result of the cleft, and the one around the maxillary canine is slightly high as a result of the impaction with subsequent exposure and orthodontic movement.

whom the maxilla is extremely hypoplastic, the surgeon may want to do most of the sagittal correction with surgery just in the maxillary bone. In patients in whom there is skeletal open bite and marked mandibular deficiency or asymmetry, a two-jaw approach must be undertaken. The advantage of this surgical-orthodontic approach is that with one operation, the reconstructive team can provide the patient with close to ideal occlusal relations as well as markedly improved function and aesthetics.

At the time of orthognathic surgery, the surgeon has the added advantage of access to the nasal cavity, including deviated septum, large turbinates, and residual nasal floor defects. In addition, the segments can be approximated in such a way to facilitate closure with locally elevated flaps.

To ensure success, close cooperation between the orthodontist and surgeon is required. It is the responsibility of the orthodontist to support the surgeon so that at the time of operation, adequate occlusal relationships can be obtained that, in turn, add stability to the orthognathic surgical procedure.

The planning of orthognathic surgery for the cleft patient is no different from that for the patient with a noncleft dentofacial deformity (see Chapter 58). This includes a detailed clinical examination and collection of pertinent records before orthodontic treatment and again before surgery. In the cleft patient, particular attention is given to the nose and upper lip, which are usually asymmetric. This asymmetry is evident not only at rest but also during function. All patients with palatal clefts who undergo maxillary advancement surgery are at risk for velopharyngeal insufficiency; therefore, preoperative evaluation by the team speech and language pathologist is required before and after surgery to discuss potential risks and postoperative correction if necessary. After all the necessary records are obtained, the orthodontist will perform a cephalometric analysis and prediction surgical tracing to determine the required surgical movements (see Chapter 41). This can be done by hand tracing the x-rays or by use of computerized video imaging and cephalometric analysis (Fig. 96-29). All these preoperative evaluations give the clinician a close approximation of outcome, but he or she must be aware of the limited knowledge on soft tissue responses relative to skeletal movement, especially in cleft patients.

Dental study models are obtained and also used to determine the changes required in dental arch form to provide a stable occlusion. In cases in which a double-jaw approach is used, a face-bow transfer must be done and the casts are mounted in a semiadjustable articulator (Fig. 96-30). After the maxilla has been moved and fixed to its new position in the articulator, an interocclusal space is made between the maxilla and mandible. This space represents the new relation

between the repositioned maxilla and the unoperated mandible. This space is then filled with self-curing orthodontic resin to make the intermediate splint (see Fig. 96-30). The use of this splint is critical because it is the guideline to reposition the maxilla when anatomic spatial relations are difficult to establish during surgery. In instances in which only the maxilla will be mobilized, it can be mounted in a hinge articulator (see Fig. 96-30). Cleft patients usually require expansion at the time of surgery as well as segmentalization for movement of posterior segments forward to close the cleft site. These movements are done in the dental model and incorporated into the final splint that is given to the surgeon during execution of the surgical procedure. The splint will guide the surgeon in repositioning the segments as well as assist in postsurgical stabilization.

Before surgery, the orthodontist must position all teeth within their supporting basal bones with the maxillary incisors in ideal position relative to the palatal plane and the mandibular incisors in ideal axial inclination relative to the mandibular plane. Both arches need to be properly coordinated to allow ideal occlusal interdigitation at the time of surgery. In addition, the orthodontist must make interdental spaces to facilitate instrumentation if interdental osteotomies are anticipated. The orthodontic appliance is used during the period of intermaxillary fixation and immediately after surgery for postsurgical elastic therapy and detailing of the occlusion. Close cooperation between the orthodontist and surgeon during the planning and initial orthodontic treatment stages should yield favorable occlusal, functional, and aesthetic outcomes (Figs. 96-31 to 96-35).

In patients in whom the maxillary deficiency is severe and there is substantial scarring or existing pharyngeal flaps, conventional orthognathic procedures are not reliable because of the inherent lack of stability and high relapse tendencies.[31,32] In addition, in young patients with severe maxillary hypoplasia, one must wait until adolescence for surgical correction because these techniques rely on rigid fixation, which requires substantial bone for placement of the hardware. Further, unerupted tooth buds might be injured during application of rigid fixation plates. For these patients, distraction osteogenesis with a rigid external distraction device may be used. This technique may be applied to children as young as 5 years and also to adults. Distraction osteogenesis in the craniofacial skeleton is a technique that was initially introduced in 1992 by McCarthy et al,[33] who applied it to elongate the hypoplastic mandible. Since that time, the technique has been applied to other parts of the craniofacial skeleton.[34-40]

The technique of maxillary distraction with a rigid external distraction device consists of five steps:

Text continued on p. 303

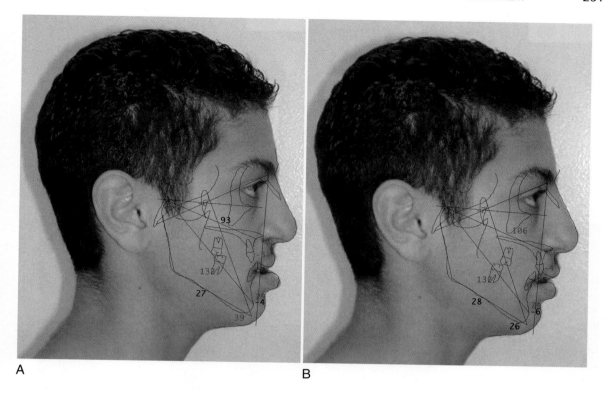

A   B

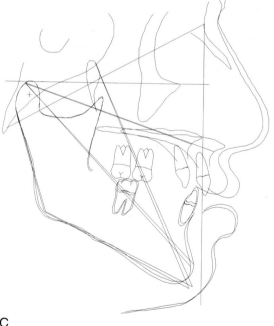

FIGURE 96-29. *A,* Preoperative cephalometric tracing superimposed through video imaging on the profile photograph of a patient with maxillary hypoplasia and cleft lip and palate. *B,* Prediction cephalometric tracing with soft tissue profile facial morphing done through video imaging techniques. Note predicted improvement of skeletal and dental relations as well as position of the upper lip. *C,* Computer-generated cephalometric tracings demonstrating the intended maxillary advancement with the projected changes in the lip and nose.   C

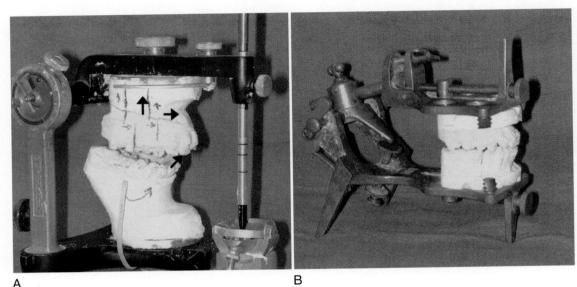

A   B

FIGURE 96-30. Photographs illustrating articulators used during orthognathic surgery. *A,* Semiadjustable articulator used in double-jaw cases. In this example, the maxillary cast has been raised and advanced as shown by
the horizontal and vertical arrows. The oblique arrow represents the interocclusal space made after the maxillary
impaction and advancement. The intermediate splint will fill this space. The surgeon uses the splint as a guide
during maxillary repositioning. *B,* Hinge articulator used to mount casts and fabricate a final interocclusal splint.

FIGURE 96-31. Profile and frontal preoperative (*A* to *C*) and postoperative (*D* to *F*) photographs of a patient with
left cleft lip and palate, maxillary deficiency, and mandibular asymmetry. Note improvement in facial harmony after
maxillary and mandibular orthognathic surgery and corrective rhinoplasty.

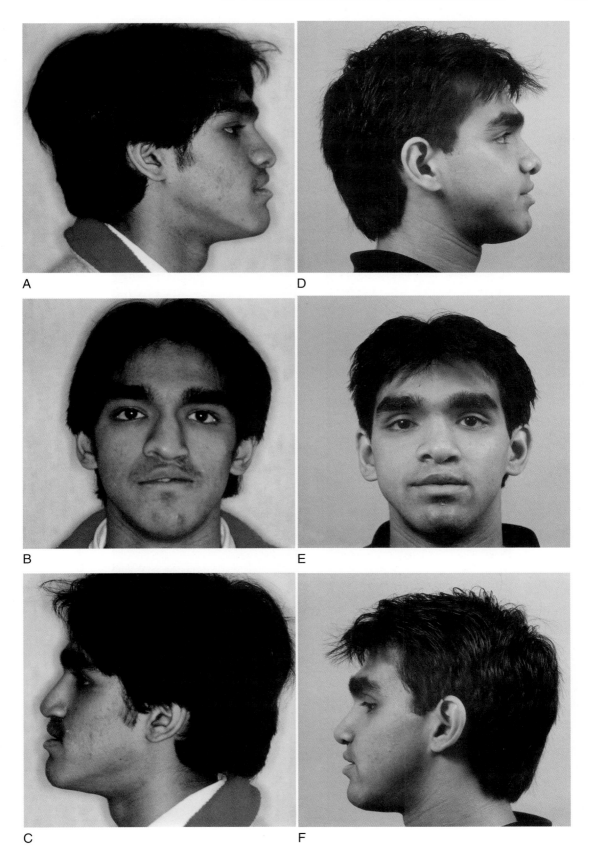

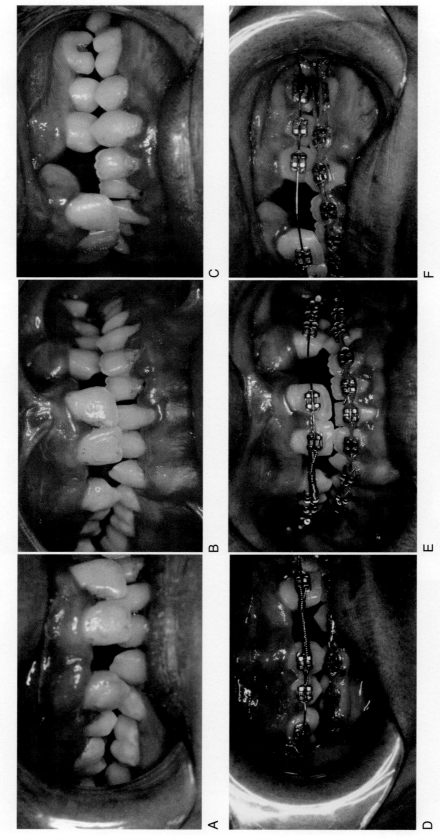

FIGURE 96-32. *A* to *F*, Frontal and lateral views of patient shown in Figure 96-31 before and after orthodontic preparation.

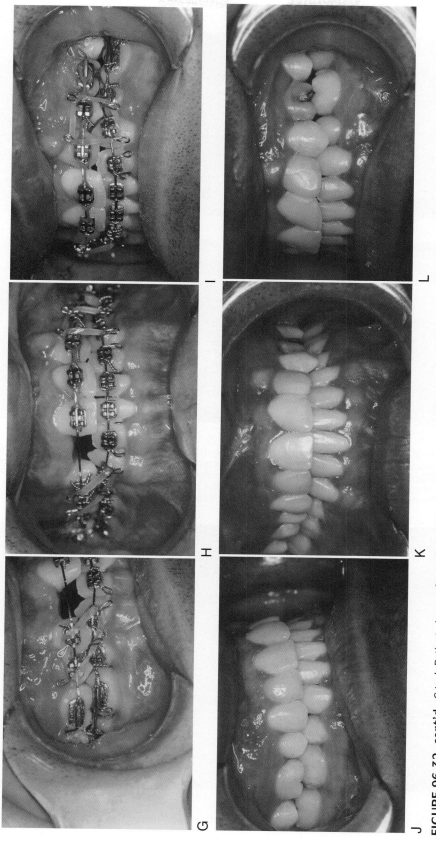

FIGURE 96-32, cont'd. *G* to *I*, Patient shown after orthognathic surgery undergoing elastic therapy. *J* to *L*, Patient shown at the completion of treatment with replacement of the noncleft-side lateral incisor with an osseointegrated fixture. Note that the patient was initially missing both maxillary lateral incisors and had a large left alveolar cleft and dental gap. At surgery, the cleft-side posterior segment was shifted forward so the cleft-side canine was in contact with the central incisor, effectively closing the preoperative dental gap.

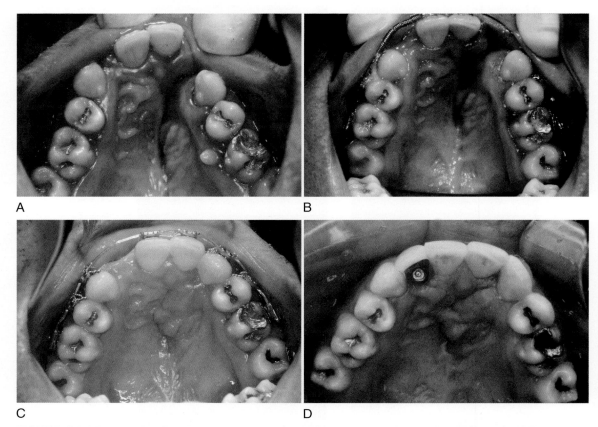

FIGURE 96-33. Occlusal view of patient in Figure 96-31. *A,* Before treatment demonstrating absence of both maxillary lateral incisors as well as right first bicuspid and impacted left second bicuspid. *B,* After orthodontic alignment and space redistribution. Note the large palatal fistula, alveolar cleft, and large interdental gap. *C,* Postsurgical view after surgical consolidation of the arch with simultaneous bone grafting. *D,* After surgical, orthodontic, and dental treatment with replacement of the missing noncleft-side lateral incisor with an osseointegrated fixture.

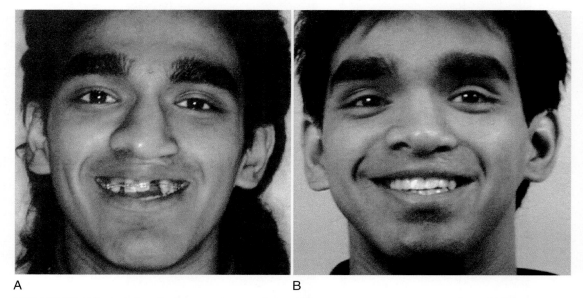

FIGURE 96-34. *A,* Preoperative smile view of patient in Figure 96-31 demonstrating an unattractive smile and cleft-side dental gap and nasal asymmetry. *B,* Post-treatment smile photograph demonstrating marked improvement after orthognathic surgery, orthodontics, prosthetic rehabilitation, and corrective rhinoplasty.

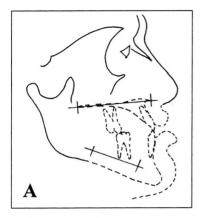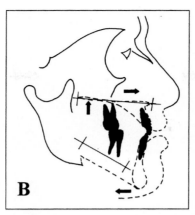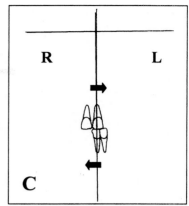

FIGURE 96-35. Cephalometric tracings demonstrating the surgical plan for the patient illustrated in Figures 96-31 to 96-34. *A,* The preoperative cephalometric tracing. *B,* The surgical plan with maxillary advancement and posterior impaction and mandibular setback. *C,* Because of midline asymmetry, the patient required movement of the maxillary midline to the left and the mandibular one to the right.

(1) fabrication of an intraoral splint that is used to deliver the distraction forces to the maxilla through the teeth; (2) complete high Le Fort I osteotomy with septal and pterygomaxillary disjunction; (3) placement of a cranial halo with an external adjustable distraction screw system; (4) distraction; and (5) rigid and removable retention.[41-45]

The intraoral splint (Fig. 96-36) is fabricated by soldering an orthodontic cervical headgear to either maxillary bands fitted in the second primary molars or first permanent molars. In addition, a palatal bar is placed for added rigidity. The outer bows of the cervical headgear are bent outward to clear the lip and bent at the level of the palatal plane into an eyelet that will be used with surgical wire to connect the intraoral splint to the distraction screws mounted on the halo, or the intraoral splint can be manufactured with removable traction hooks. The splint is cemented in place and further secured with circumdental wires at the time of surgery. After completion of the Le Fort I osteotomy performed at the desired vertical level, depending on the degree of vertical midfacial hypoplasia, the halo is secured with two or three scalp pins per side about 2 to 3 cm above the ear helix (Figs. 96-37 and 96-38).

Three to 5 days later, the distraction screws are connected to the external eyelets of the intraoral splint with surgical wire; distraction is initiated at the rate of 1 mm per day, which is achieved with two turns of the screws per day. After the desired amount of advancement is obtained, activation is stopped and the system is left in place for at least 3 to 4 weeks to allow consolidation of the newly repositioned maxilla. In this period, the clinician must be aware that the external traction hooks will bend and tension is accumulated.

After the desired advancement is achieved, the clinician may need to turn the screws backward to decrease tension and avoid excessive maxillary advancement. After this period, the halo is removed and the external distraction hooks of the intraoral appliance are either cut with a rotating disk or just removed if they were made with a removable system. Subsequently, elastic traction by means of a removable facemask (see Fig. 96-13) is applied for another 6 to 8 weeks with a force of 12 to 16 ounces for 8 to 10 hours per day.

This technique has been applied to young children as well as to adolescents and adults with excellent functional and aesthetic results (Figs. 96-39 and 96-40). The stability of the procedure has been remarkable and superior to that reported for conventional orthognathic surgical approaches.[41,43] The soft tissue changes have also been superior to those reported when conventional orthognathic surgical techniques are used in cleft patients.[46] The velopharyngeal mechanism of these patients is minimally affected, especially for those patients having pharyngeal flaps, who report improved articulation and resonance. Patients without pharyngeal flaps who require major advancements can have velopharyngeal incompetence that needs to be managed after distraction with a pharyngeal flap or another type of pharyngoplasty.[47] To date, negative effects on dental development have not been observed, although when surgery is done in children younger than 6 years, rotation of a permanent second molar tooth bud as a result of posterior arch length increases or surgical trauma has been observed (Fig. 96-41).

Maxillary distraction now offers a solution for the difficult cleft maxillary hypoplasia deformity. In addition, the technique has been expanded to other patients

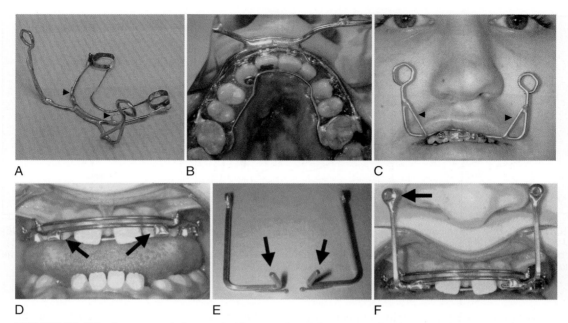

A   B   C

D   E   F

FIGURE 96-36. Custom-made intraoral splints used to deliver distraction forces to the maxilla with a rigid external distraction system. *A,* Note the long external traction hooks with round eyelets and the short hooks *(arrowheads)* soldered to the labial wire to be used during the retention phase for elastic traction with a face-mask. *B,* Intraoral splint cemented in place. At the time of surgery, circumdental wiring will further secure the splint for improved anchorage. *C,* Heavy support wires *(arrowheads)* soldered to strengthen the external traction hook. *D,* Intraoral view of newly designed splint with rectangular tubes *(arrows)* to receive removable rectangular traction hooks *(E). F,* Removable traction hooks connected to intraoral splint. Note traction eyelet *(arrow)* to connect with twisted surgical wire to the distraction screws mounted on the halo system.

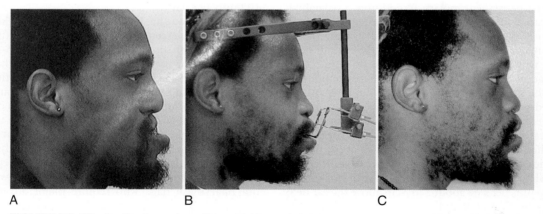

A   B   C

FIGURE 96-37. Profile views of a patient with bilateral cleft lip and palate and severe maxillary hypoplasia before treatment with rigid external distraction *(A),* during distraction *(B),* and after treatment *(C).* Note significant improvement in facial balance and aesthetics.

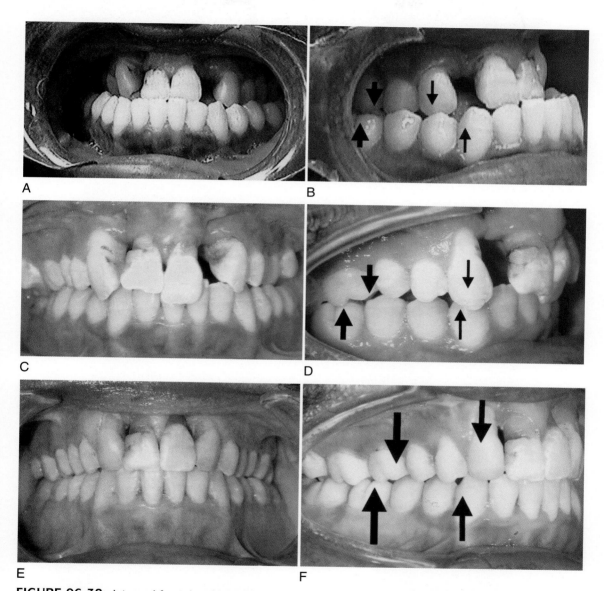

FIGURE 96-38. Intraoral frontal and lateral views of patient shown in Figure 96-37 before distraction (*A* and *B*), after distraction (*C* and *D*), and after completion of orthodontic treatment (*E* and *F*). Note correction of anterior and right buccal crossbite with substantial advancement of the maxillary buccal segment (arrows delineate the changes at the molar and canine levels).

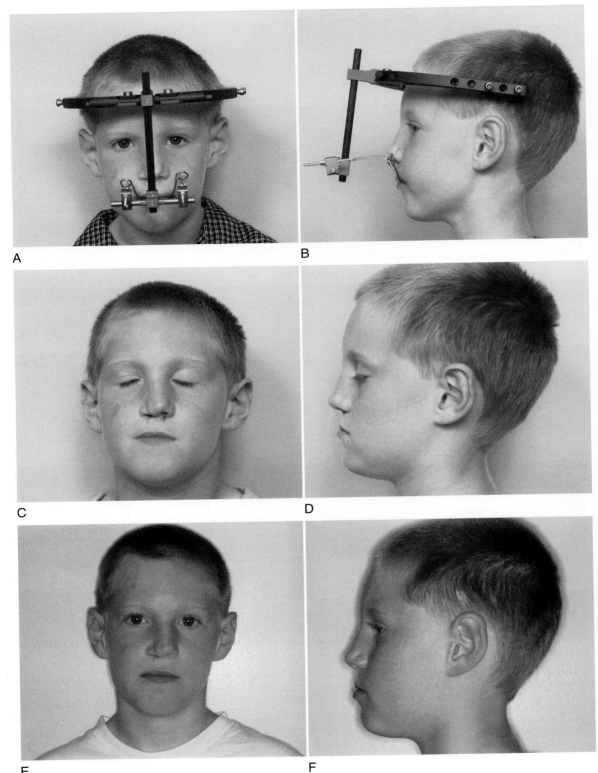

FIGURE 96-39. Frontal and profile views of an 8-year-old boy with left cleft lip and palate and maxillary hypoplasia wearing a rigid external distraction system (*A* and *B*), before treatment (*C* and *D*), and after maxillary advancement with rigid external distraction (*E* and *F*). Note symmetric position of the halo and placement of the fixation skull screws. Also note the positive changes in the position of the paranasal region as well as in upper lip and nose position.

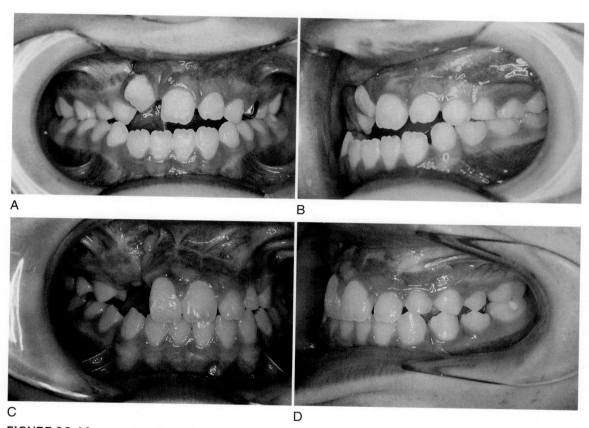

FIGURE 96-40. Frontal and lateral occlusal views of the patient shown in Figure 96-39 before (*A* and *B*) and after (*C* and *D*) maxillary advancement with a rigid external distraction system. Note correction of the anterior crossbite and open bite.

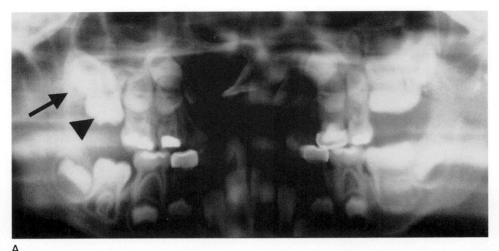

A

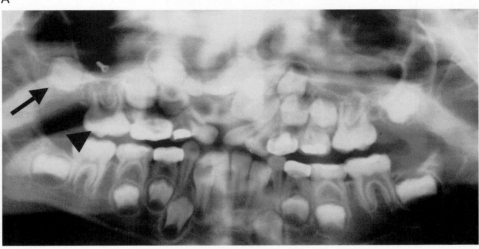

B

FIGURE 96-41. Panoramic radiograph of a 5-year-old patient before *(A)* and after *(B)* distraction. In the postoperative view, note the rotation of the developing second molar tooth bud *(arrow)*. The first permanent molars have erupted uneventfully *(arrowhead)*.

with syndromic conditions such as Apert and Crouzon syndromes and traumatic deformities.

SUMMARY

The important contribution of the orthodontist to the comprehensive surgical-orthodontic management of the cleft patient is well documented. The role of the orthodontist is to support the surgeon with all aspects of dental development, occlusion, and treatment planning so ideal outcomes can be obtained. With the addition of nasoalveolar molding as well as maxillary distraction osteogenesis, the traditional protocols for cleft management have been expanded. It is hoped that these modifications will provide clinicians with new strategies for the difficult management of the cleft patient and provide the patient with an outstanding outcome. The treatment plan should be developed around the patient's anatomic, functional, and developmental needs. Close cooperation between the surgeon and orthodontist is imperative for a successful outcome.

REFERENCES

1. Pruzansky S: Description, classification, and analysis of unoperated clefts of the lip and palate. Am J Orthod 1953;39:590-611.
2. Bergland O, Semb G, Abyholm F, et al: Secondary bone grafting and orthodontic treatment in patients with bilateral complete clefts of the lip and palate. Ann Plast Surg 1986;17:460-474.

3. Semb G: Effect of alveolar bone grafting on maxillary growth in unilateral cleft lip and palate patients. Cleft Palate J 1988;25:288-295.

4. Shaw WC, Asher-McDade C, Brattstrom V, et al: A six center international study of treatment outcome in patients with clefts of the lip and palate. Part 1. Principles and study design. Cleft Palate Craniofac J 1992;29:393-397.

5. Santiago PE, Grayson BH, Gianoutsos MP, et al: Reduced need for alveolar bone grafting by presurgical orthopedics and primary gingivoperiosteoplasty. Cleft Palate Craniofac J 1998;35:77-80.

6. Grayson BH, Cutting CB, Wood R: Preoperative columella lengthening in bilateral cleft lip and palate. Plast Reconstr Surg 1993;92:1422-1423.

7. Grayson BH, Santiago PE: Presurgical orthopedics for cleft lip and palate. In Aston SJ, Beasley RW, Thorne CHM, eds: Grabb and Smith's Plastic Surgery, 5th ed. Philadelphia, Lippincott-Raven, 1997:237-244.

8. Maull DJ, Grayson BH, Brecht LE, Cutting CB: Long-term effects of nasoalveolar molding on three-dimensional nasal shape. Cleft Palate Craniofac J 1999;36:391-397.

9. Grayson BH, Santiago PE, Brecht LE, Cutting CB: Presurgical nasoalveolar molding in infants with cleft lip and palate. Cleft Palate Craniofac J 1999;36:486-498.

9a. Dogliotti P, Bennun R, Losoviz E, Ganiewich E: Tratamiento no quirúrgico de la deformidad nasal en el paciente fisurado. Rev Ateneo Arg de Odontol 1991;27:31-35.

9b. Bennun RD, Perandones C, Sepliarsky VA, et al: Nonsurgical correction of nasal deformity in unilateral complete cleft lip: a 6-year follow-up. Plast Reconstr Surg 1999;104:616-630.

10. Lin WY, Grayson BH, Figueroa AA, et al: The effect of presurgical molding of nasal form in patients with unilateral cleft lip and palate: an intercenter report. American Cleft Palate-Craniofacial Association, 56th Annual Meeting, Scottsdale, Arizona, 1999.

11. Matsuo K, Hirose T, Otagiri T, Norose N: Repair of cleft lip with nonsurgical correction of nasal deformity in the early neonatal period. Plast Reconstr Surg 1989;83:25-31.

12. Yeow VK, Chen PK, Chen YR, Noordhoff SM: The use of nasal splints in the primary management of unilateral cleft nasal deformity. Plast Reconstr Surg 1999;103:1347-1354.

13. Friede H, Lilja J, Johanson B: Lip-nose morphology and symmetry in unilateral cleft lip and palate patients following a two-stage lip closure. Scand J Plast Reconstr Surg 1980;14:55-64.

14. Reisberg DJ, Figueroa AA, Gold HO: An intraoral appliance for management of the protrusive premaxilla in bilateral cleft lip. Cleft Palate J 1988;25:53-57.

15. Figueroa AA, Reisberg DJ, Polley JW, Cohen M: Intraoral-appliance modification to retract the premaxilla in patients with bilateral cleft lip. Cleft Palate Craniofac J 1996;33:497-500.

16. Dorf DS, Reisberg DJ, Gold HO: Early prosthetic management of cleft palate. Articulation development prosthesis: a preliminary report. J Prosthet Dent 1985;53:222-226.

17. Subtelny JD: Oral respiration: facial maldevelopment and corrective dentofacial orthopedics. Angle Orthod 1980;50:147-164.

18. Friede H, Lennartsson B: Forward traction of the maxilla in cleft lip and palate patients. Eur J Orthod 1984;3:21-40.

19. Tindlund RS, Rygh P: Maxillary protraction: different effects on facial morphology in unilateral and bilateral cleft lip and palate patients. Cleft Palate Craniofac J 1993;30:208-221.

20. Friede H: The vomero-premaxillary suture—a neglected growth site in mid-facial development of unilateral cleft lip and palate patients. Cleft Palate J 1978;15:398-404.

21. Ross RB: Treatment variables affecting facial growth in complete unilateral cleft lip and palate. Part 3. Alveolus repair and bone grafting. Cleft Palate J 1987;24:33-44.

22. Figueroa AA, Polley JW, Cohen M: Orthodontic management of the cleft lip and palate patient. Clin Plast Surg 1993;20:733-753.

23. Solis A, Figueroa AA, Cohen M, et al: Maxillary dental development in complete unilateral alveolar clefts. Cleft Palate Craniofac J 1998;35:320-328.

24. Ranta R: A review of tooth formation in children with cleft lip and palate. Am J Orthod 1986;90:11-18.

25. Abyholm FE, Bergland O, Semb G: Secondary bone grafting of alveolar clefts. Scand J Plast Reconstr Surg 1981;15:127-140.

26. Aduss H, Figueroa AA: Stages of orthodontic treatment in complete unilateral cleft lip and palate. In Bardach J, Morris HL, eds: Multidisciplinary Management of Cleft Lip and Palate. Philadelphia, WB Saunders, 1990:607-615.

27. Figueroa AA, Aduss H: Orthodontic management for patients with cleft lip and palate. In Cohen M, ed: Mastery of Plastic and Reconstructive Surgery, vol 1. Boston, Little, Brown, 1994:648-668.

28. Verdi FJ Jr, Lanzi GL, Cohen S, Powell R: Use of the Branemark implant in the cleft palate patient. Cleft Palate Craniofac J 1991;28:301-303.

29. Posnick, JC, Witzel MA, Dagys AP: Management of jaw deformities in the cleft patient. In Bardach J, Morris HL, eds: Multidisciplinary Management of Cleft Lip and Palate. Philadelphia, WB Saunders, 1999:530-543.

30. da Silva Filho OJ, Normando AD, Capelozza Filho L: Mandibular growth in patients with cleft lip and/or cleft palate: the influence of cleft type. Am J Orthod Dentofacial Orthop 1993;104:269-275.

31. Hochban W, Gans C, Austermann KH: Long-term results after maxillary advancement in patients with cleft. Cleft Palate Craniofac J 1993;30:237-243.

32. Posnick JC, Dagys AP: Skeletal stability and relapse patterns after LeFort I maxillary osteotomy fixed with miniplates: the unilateral cleft lip and palate deformity. Plast Reconstr Surg 1994;94:924-932.

33. McCarthy JG, Schreiber J, Karp N, et al: Lengthening the human mandible by gradual distraction. Plast Reconstr Surg 1992;89:1-8.

34. Molina F, Ortiz Monasterio F, de la Paz Aguilar M, Barrera J: Maxillary distraction: aesthetic and functional benefits in cleft lip palate and prognathic patients during mixed dentition. Plast Reconstr Surg 1998;101:951-963.

35. Polley JW, Figueroa AA, Charbel FB, et al: Monobloc craniomaxillofacial distraction osteogenesis in a newborn with severe craniofacial synostosis: a preliminary report. J Craniofac Surg 1995;6:421-423.

36. Polley JW, Figueroa AA: Management of severe maxillary deficiency in childhood and adolescence through distraction osteogenesis with an external adjustable rigid distraction device. J Craniofac Surg 1997;8:181-185.

37. Cohen SR, Rutrick RE, Burstein FD: Distraction osteogenesis of the human craniofacial skeleton: initial experience with a new distraction system. J Craniofac Surg 1995;6:368-374.

38. Guerrero CA, Bell WH, Contasti GI, Rodriguez AM: Intraoral mandibular distraction osteogenesis. Semin Orthod 1999;5:35-40.

39. Rachmiel A, Pottaric Z, Jackson IT, et al: Midface advancement by gradual distraction. Br J Plast Surg 1993;46:201-207.

40. Liou EJW, Chen PKT, Huang CS, Chen YR: Interdental distraction osteogenesis and rapid orthodontic tooth movement: a novel approach to approximate a wide alveolar cleft or bony defect. Plast Reconstr Surg 2000;105:1262-1272.

41. Figueroa AA, Polley JW: Management of severe cleft maxillary deficiency with distraction osteogenesis: procedure and results. Am J Orthod Dentofacial Orthop 1999;115:1-12.

42. Figueroa AA, Polley JW, Ko EW: Maxillary distraction for the management of cleft maxillary hypoplasia with a rigid external distraction system. Semin Orthod 1999;5:46-51.

43. Polley JW, Figueroa AA: Rigid external distraction (RED): its application in cleft maxillary deformities. Plast Reconstr Surg 1998;102:1360-1372.

44. Polley JW, Figueroa AA: Rigid external maxillary distraction. In McCarthy JG, ed: Distraction of the Craniofacial Skeleton. New York, Springer-Verlag, 1999:321-336.

45. Polley JW, Figueroa AA: Maxillary distraction osteogenesis with rigid external distraction. Atlas Oral Maxillofac Surg Clin North Am 1999;7:15-28.

46. Ko EW, Figueroa AA, Polley JW: Soft tissue profile changes after maxillary advancement with distraction osteogenesis by use of a rigid external distraction device: a 1-year follow-up. J Oral Maxillofac Surg 2000;58:959-969.

47. Ko EW, Figueroa AA, Guyette TW, et al: Velopharyngeal changes after maxillary advancement in cleft patients with distraction osteogenesis using a rigid external distraction device: a 1-year cephalometric follow-up. J Craniofac Surg 1999;10:312-320.

Velopharyngeal Dysfunction

GERALD M. SLOAN, MD, FACS ✦ DAVID J. ZAJAC, PhD, CCC-SLP

Velopharyngeal insufficiency is a generic term for inability to achieve complete closure of the velopharyngeal apparatus during speech. The velopharyngeal apparatus is the combination of soft palate and pharyngeal structures that regulate airflow from the lungs and larynx through the mouth for oral sounds and through the nose for nasal sounds (Figs. 97-1 and 97-2).

Loney and Bloem[1] have subdivided velopharyngeal insufficiency by etiology. Velopharyngeal incompetence is used to describe imperfect closure of the velopharyngeal apparatus that is caused by a neuromuscular dysfunction. On the other hand, velopharyngeal inadequacy is used to refer to imperfect closure of the velopharyngeal apparatus caused by a tissue deficit. Their nomenclature, however, has not been universally accepted. Trost-Cardamone[2] has recommended a different classification that uses velopharyngeal inadequacy as the generic term for any type of abnormal velopharyngeal function and divides that into three categories by etiology: velopharyngeal insufficiency, velopharyngeal incompetence, and velopharyngeal mislearning. Velopharyngeal insufficiency is used by Trost-Cardamone to refer to "any structural defect of the velum or pharyngeal wall at the level of the nasopharynx; there is not enough tissue to accomplish closure, or there is some kind of mechanical interference to closure. Most often these problems are congenital." Velopharyngeal incompetence, as used by Trost-Cardamone, "includes neurogenic etiologies that result in impaired motor control or impaired motor programming of the velopharynx." Velopha-

ryngeal mislearning is used to describe a third category that "includes etiologies that are not caused by structural defect or neuromotor pathologies of the velopharyngeal complex." Because of the disagreement and potential confusion in nomenclature, velopharyngeal dysfunction is used as the generic term for any type of abnormal velopharyngeal function regardless of etiology, as has been proposed by D'Antonio.[3]

For the plastic surgeon evaluating and treating velopharyngeal dysfunction, the etiology is an important factor in clinical decision-making and planning of therapeutic interventions. The most common cause of velopharyngeal dysfunction seen by most plastic surgeons is clefting of the secondary palate. In such cases, there is often lack of sufficient soft palate tissue to allow closure of the velopharyngeal apparatus, and scar tissue may interfere with such closure. Velopharyngeal dysfunction can be caused by a fistula in the hard or soft palate, which allows nasal air escape with speech. Another possible cause is enlarged tonsils,* which can actually prevent velopharyngeal closure by physically blocking closure. In such a situation, tonsillectomy, usually without adenoidectomy, can be the appropriate treatment.[4,5] Neuromotor impairment involving the muscles of the velopharyngeal apparatus, as seen in congenital abnormalities, neurologic diseases, or head injury, can cause velopharyngeal dysfunction. Finally, another cause can be mislearning, as in so-called phoneme-specific nasal emission, a term that refers to nasal air emission isolated to specific pressure consonants such as /s/ and /z/.[6,7] Phoneme-specific nasal emission is an articulation error that requires

* can poids trop élevé des amygdales oubien leur pôle sup. obstrue.

311

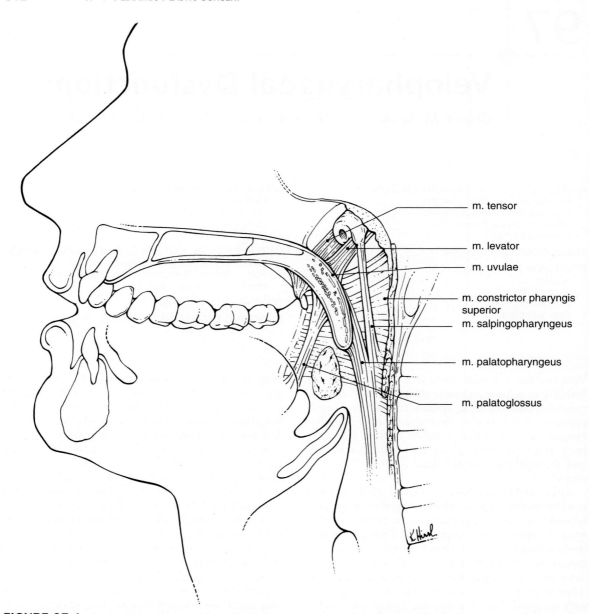

m. tensor

m. levator

m. uvulae

m. constrictor pharyngis superior

m. salpingopharyngeus

m. palatopharyngeus

m. palatoglossus

FIGURE 97-1. Sagittal view of the normal adult palate showing the relationships of the levator palatini, the uvula, and the palatoglossus and palatopharyngeus muscles within and beyond the palate. The adjacent superior pharyngeal constrictor muscle is also shown.

Mauvais candidats chx:
- ex. Steinert → risque d'apnée
    ⇒ prothèses, obturateurs
        (tolérance difficile re N°)

- déplacement des carotides sur la ligne médiane

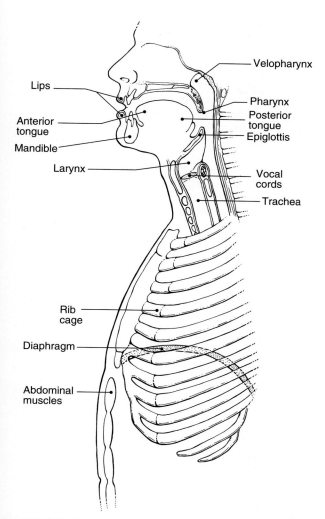

FIGURE 97-2. Cross-sectional diagram of the vocal tract showing the structures that are important for phonation, articulation, and vocal resonance.

behavioral therapy for effective treatment, not surgical intervention.

ASSESSMENT OF VELOPHARYNGEAL FUNCTION

The complexity of the terminology and potential causes of velopharyngeal dysfunction should make obvious the need for a thorough multispecialty evaluation and assessment before any therapeutic intervention is undertaken.

Perceptual Speech Evaluation

Evaluation by a well-trained speech pathologist, preferably one with extensive cleft experience, is the cornerstone of any diagnostic work-up. To communicate properly with the speech pathologist, the plastic surgeon must understand some of the terms used to describe resonance, articulation, and phonation disorders that can be seen in the context of velopharyngeal dysfunction. Therefore, a brief glossary of terms is listed:

Hypernasality: the perception of inordinate nasal resonance during the production of *vowels*.

Nasal emission: the escape of nasal air associated with the production of *consonants* that require high oral pressure (examples of such high oral pressure consonants are *s*, *p*, and *k*).

Hyponasality: a decrease in normal nasal resonance that is usually caused by blockage of the nasal airway. Causes of such blockage can include upper respiratory infection, enlarged turbinates, and postsurgical changes such as an obstructing posterior pharyngeal flap.

Mixed hypernasality and hyponasality: presence of hypernasality and hyponasality in the same individual. This is often the result of velopharyngeal dysfunction in the presence of significant but not complete blockage of the nasal airway.

Nasal substitutions: the articulators (such as the tongue and lips) are positioned appropriately for an intended oral consonant, such as *b*, but velopharyngeal dysfunction causes the sound that is produced to be a nasal consonant, in this case *m*. Similarly, *d* can become *n*.

Compensatory articulations (also called compensatory substitutions): inappropriate use of articulators to form plosive (e.g., *p*) or fricative (e.g., *s*) sounds despite velopharyngeal dysfunction. Because the patient cannot build up oral pressure at the level of the velopharyngeal apparatus, compensatory articulations substitute closure at the glottal or pharyngeal level.

Sibilant distortion: incorrect tongue placement—often due to malocclusion—for the sounds /s/ and /z/.

In addition to listening for hypernasality, nasal emission, nasal substitutions, compensatory articulations, and sibilant distortions (all of which can be particularly confusing in a setting with a component of hyponasality or mixed hypernasality and hyponasality, which is not unusual with the septal deviation and nostril stenosis that can be seen with a repaired cleft lip), the speech pathologist will assess overall speech intelligibility. After all, appropriate speech intelligibility is the ultimate goal of any surgical or nonsurgical intervention. Furthermore, the speech pathologist will be trying to distinguish phoneme-specific nasal emission, which is isolated to specific pressure consonants such as /s/ and /z/, from the consistent nasal emission that is heard when the velopharyngeal apparatus is not capable of any proper closure.[6,7]

Pressure-Flow Measurements

The pressure-flow technique[8-10] allows quantitative measurement of pressure, airflow, and timing variables associated with velopharyngeal closure (Fig. 97-3). This technique does require the subject to have the intellectual capacity and neuromuscular integrity necessary to perform the tasks required for the testing. Where the proper equipment is available, the technique can consistently be applied in most intellectually normal 4-year-olds and even in some particularly cooperative 3-year-olds.

To perform pressure-flow testing, one catheter is placed within the mouth and another in one nostril, where it is secured by a cork that blocks that nostril. Both of those catheters are connected to pressure transducers to allow measurement of static air pressure. Pressure drops across the velopharyngeal orifice can thus be measured. Nasal airflow is measured by a heated pneumotachograph (flowmeter) connected by plastic tubing to the subject's other nostril. A formula allows calculation of the cross-sectional area of the velopharyngeal orifice. Warren[11] suggests that the word *hamper* be used during pressure-flow testing because the /mp/ sequence requires dynamic closure of the velopharyngeal portal. At an orifice opening of more than 20 mm^2 during production of the nonnasal /p/ sound, oral air pressure is generally reduced and overlaps with nasal airflow associated with the /m/ segment (Figs. 97-4 and 97-5). Vocal resonance is generally perceived as hypernasal.[11] Velopharyngeal orifice size between 10 and 20 mm^2 generally results in airflow patterns that are not normal and are similar to those associated with velopharyngeal dysfunction. Although vocal resonance may be variable, it is usually perceived as mildly to moderately hypernasal. At orifice size less than 10 mm^2, pressure and airflow patterns are usually normal, but in some

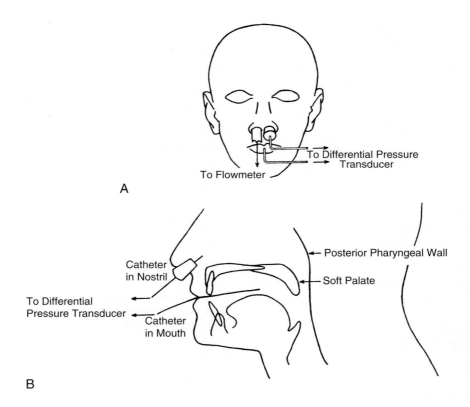

A

B

NORMAL SUBJECT

FIGURE 97-3. *A,* Frontal view of the pressure-flow technique showing placement of the oral and nasal air pressure catheters and the nasal airflow tube. *B,* Lateral view showing placement of the oral air pressure catheter below the velopharyngeal portal and the nasal air pressure catheter above the portal. Differential oral-nasal air pressure and nasal airflow are used to calculate the size of the velopharyngeal portal during speech.

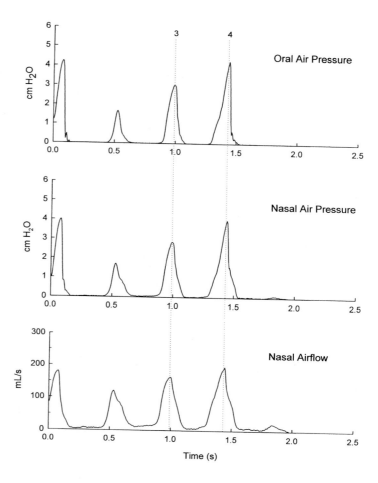

FIGURE 97-4. Pressure-flow recordings of four productions of the syllable /pi/ by an 8-year-old boy with velopharyngeal inadequacy due to tonsillectomy-adenoidectomy. Nasal air pressure *(middle graph)* is almost the same magnitude as oral air pressure *(top graph)*. This indicates a severe inability to separate the oral and nasal cavities during speech. Nasal airflow *(bottom graph)* is consistently above 100 mL/s. Calculated velopharyngeal areas during the third and fourth productions of /p/ were approximately 43 mm² (not shown).

instances a trained listener will perceive speech as mildly hypernasal, even at orifice sizes between 5 and 10 mm².

Studies have provided descriptive pressure-flow measurements for a large sample of normally speaking noncleft children and adults.[12,13] These studies indicate that velopharyngeal closure is essentially airtight during production of nonnasal syllables such as /pi/. Airtight closure is defined as nasal airflow of 20 mL/s or less. This criterion is used because the normal occurrence of "velar bounce" may cause the displacement of small magnitudes of nasal airflow during nonnasal syllables. During production of the word *hamper*, normal nasal airflow is typically less than 30 mL/s at the point of the stop-plosive /p/.[12]

The advantage of pressure-flow testing is that it provides relatively instantaneous, quantitative data that are easy to interpret and highly reliable. Indeed, pressure-flow information provides an index of the structural integrity of the palate that is not influenced by behavioral factors. Conversely, the perception of

hypernasality is a complex phenomenon that is influenced by factors such as respiratory effort and tongue placement. Another advantage is that pressure-flow instrumentation can potentially be used for biofeedback therapy. Disadvantages are that the equipment is relatively expensive and is not available at all cleft centers, testing cannot consistently be performed in children younger than 4 years, and even some older children have difficulty cooperating.

Nasopharyngeal Endoscopy

Another method that allows objective although not quantitative determination of velopharyngeal function is videonasopharyngeal endoscopy. This permits direct observation of the velopharyngeal apparatus during speech. Movement of the soft palate, posterior pharynx, and lateral pharyngeal walls is directly observed.[14,15] For these studies, the endoscopist visualizes the velopharyngeal apparatus by use of a small nasopharyngolaryngoscope inserted through an anesthetized

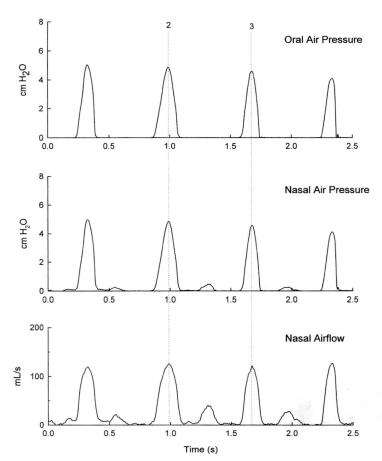

FIGURE 97-5. Pressure-flow recordings of four productions of the word *hamper* by the same 8-year-old boy as in Figure 97-4. Calculated velopharyngeal areas during the second and third productions of /p/ were approximately 60 to 70 mm². Nasal air pressure and nasal airflow also completely overlap with oral air pressure during the /mp/ sequence. These findings are characteristic of severe velopharyngeal inadequacy.

nostril (Fig. 97-6). A high-resolution video camera is used to display the image on a video screen and to record the evaluation on a videocassette recorder. Simultaneous audio recording is obtained on the audio channel of the video recorder. A speech pathologist prompts the subject to repeat words and phrases that are part of a speech protocol. The videotape can then be reviewed and evaluated for velopharyngeal closure and closure pattern and motion of the soft palate, the two lateral walls of the pharynx, and the posterior wall of the pharynx (Fig. 97-7).

Nasopharyngeal endoscopic evaluations can be reliably performed in most cooperative and intellectually normal 5-year-olds and in some younger children. The advantage of endoscopic assessment is that it provides instantaneous data on the function of the velopharyngeal apparatus with continuous speech. Like pressure-flow technology, it can also be used for biofeedback therapy. A disadvantage of the technique is that it requires a fair amount of skill and experience on the part of the endoscopist, particularly with younger children. Furthermore, the equipment is relatively

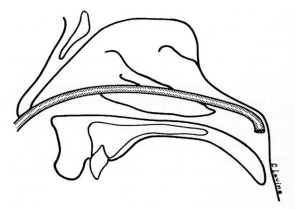

FIGURE 97-6. Ideal pathway of insertion of endoscope through the middle nasal meatus to view the nasopharynx during speech production. (From Kummer AW: Cleft Palate and Craniofacial Anomalies, Therapy Tech "Kit." © 2001. Reprinted with permission of Nelson, a division of Thomson Learning: *www.thomsonrights.com*. Fax 800-730-2215.)

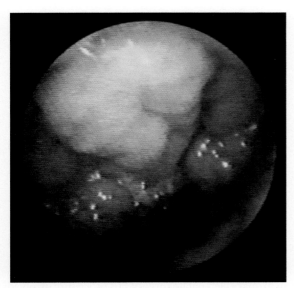

FIGURE 97-7. Endoscopic image of a preschool-aged girl with severe velopharyngeal inadequacy secondary to repaired cleft palate. The girl produced the sentence "Buy Bobbie a puppy." In addition to a large velopharyngeal gap, a small Passavant pad is formed at the posterior pharyngeal wall.

expensive and is not generally available at all cleft centers. Whereas a good endoscopic study will determine whether there is velopharyngeal closure with speech, the study is not truly quantitative. The size of the velopharyngeal orifice can be estimated but cannot be accurately measured. One advantage over pressure-flow technology is that endoscopy does give direct visualization of the dynamic velopharyngeal apparatus. Such anatomic information is considered helpful by some surgeons.

Cinefluoroscopy

Cinefluoroscopy of the velopharynx, like endoscopy, can provide dynamic visualization of the velopharyngeal apparatus. It is generally easier for a young child to tolerate cinefluoroscopy, but the technique does involve radiation exposure. As a compromise, resting and phonating lateral cephalometric radiographs involve much less radiation exposure than with cinefluoroscopy. Lateral cephalometric radiographs do not provide the dynamic visualization of the velopharynx that can be obtained with nasopharyngeal endoscopy or cinefluoroscopy, but even a static picture can be useful in combination with other available information (Fig. 97-8).

Advantages of cinefluoroscopy and lateral still radiography are that they are generally available at most medical centers and are relatively easy to perform. Data are somewhat limited, being two-dimensional, but are

somewhat quantitative; the films are easy to interpret, and reliability is fair to good.

For the interested reader, Dalston and Warren[16] have reviewed and summarized the relative advantages and disadvantages of various techniques for assessment of velopharyngeal function.

SUBMUCOUS CLEFT PALATE

The earliest description of what we now call submucous cleft palate was by Roux[17] of a young girl with severe hypernasality and unintelligible speech who had a split of the posterior soft palate and separation of the two sides of the bony hard palate beneath an intact mucosa. Calnan[18] described three findings that, present simultaneously, defined an entity he called submucous cleft palate. Those three findings were (1) bifid uvula, (2) separation of the soft palate musculature in the midline but with intact mucosa, and (3) midline notching at the posterior edge of the hard palate. The combination of those three findings is still the most widely accepted definition of submucous cleft palate.

The best data on the incidence of submucous cleft palate are from a study by Weatherley-White et al.[19] They examined 10,836 schoolchildren in the Denver, Colorado, area. Nine of those children were found to have physical findings of a submucous cleft palate, an incidence of about 1 in 1200 or 0.08%. Only one of the nine children with submucous cleft palate had

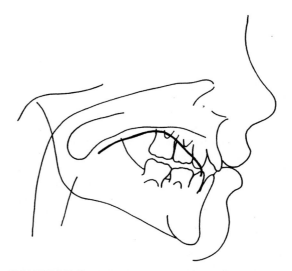

FIGURE 97-8. Tracing of a lateral cephalometric radiograph that facilitated diagnosis of phoneme-specific nasal emission in a 4-year-old boy without cleft palate. The illustration shows incomplete velopharyngeal closure in conjunction with tongue-palate contact during production of a sustained /s/ sound. Note tongue-palate contact that occludes the oral cavity. This child exhibited normal velopharyngeal closure, however, during production of other nonnasal speech sounds.

abnormal speech, which was able to be corrected with speech therapy without requiring surgery.

Whereas many questions are still unanswered, the following guidelines are recommended:

1. The term *submucous cleft palate* should be used only when the triad of findings described by Calnan[18] is present, specifically, a bifid uvula, midline separation of the soft palate musculature beneath an intact mucosa, and a notch in the bony posterior hard palate. A bifid uvula alone is not sufficient for the diagnosis of submucous cleft palate.

2. It is not clear that the presence of a bifid uvula, or even the full triad of findings that constitute a submucous cleft palate, absolutely contraindicates adenoidectomy, and it is almost certainly not a contraindication to tonsillectomy. However, one should have particularly strong indications before proceeding with adenoidectomy in that setting, and a conservative adenoidectomy, with preservation of the upper portion of the adenoid pad at the level of Passavant ridge, is advisable.

3. The occurrence of velopharyngeal insufficiency after tonsillectomy or adenoidectomy does not a priori mean that there was a previously unrecognized submucous cleft palate, unless the classic triad of findings is present.

4. Velopharyngeal dysfunction after tonsillectomy-adenoidectomy, in most cases, merits conservative treatment and speech therapy for several months before surgical intervention is seriously considered for treatment of the velopharyngeal dysfunction.

The traditional surgical treatment of velopharyngeal dysfunction related to presence of submucous cleft palate has been attachment of a posterior pharyngeal flap.[17,20-22] More recent reports have emphasized the efficacy of other approaches. Pensler and Bauer[23] used levator muscle repositioning with palatal lengthening in 15 patients with submucous cleft palate. Their best results were in patients who had surgery before the age of 2 years. However, even five of the seven patients who had later surgery had improved speech, a success rate of 71%. Chen[24] performed surgery in 35 patients with submucous cleft palate who had velopharyngeal dysfunction between 1988 and 1993. A Furlow palatoplasty was used in 30 of those patients. Twenty-nine patients (97%) achieved competent velopharyngeal function after the Furlow palatoplasty, including three patients who were older than 20 years. Seagle[25] treated 29 patients with submucous cleft palate between 1986 and 1996. The largest group, 18 patients, were treated with Furlow palatoplasty. A successful speech outcome was obtained in 15 of those 18 patients (83%). The Furlow palatoplasty was found to have the highest

success for patients with a velopharyngeal gap of 8 mm or less by preoperative videofluoroscopy; it was less likely to be successful when the preoperative gap exceeded 8 mm.

POSTERIOR PHARYNGEAL FLAP
History

The predecessor of the modern posterior pharyngeal flap was reported by Passavant,[26] who performed surgical adhesion of the posterior border of the soft palate to the posterior pharyngeal wall. The first true attachment of a posterior pharyngeal flap to the palate was described by Schoenborn[27] and was an inferiorly based flap. Schoenborn had performed 20 such procedures by 1886, and his surgical technique had evolved to a superiorly based flap.[28] Rosenthal[29] was the first to report use of the posterior pharyngeal flap in primary cleft palate surgery. His procedure involved a modified von Langenbeck palatoplasty in combination with attachment of an inferiorly based posterior pharyngeal flap. The posterior pharyngeal flap was popularized in the United States by Padgett,[30] who used a superiorly based flap as a salvage procedure in patients whose primary repair of cleft palate had failed. His preference for the superiorly based flap was based on his belief that it was difficult to achieve adequate length with an inferiorly based flap.

The question of the width of the posterior pharyngeal flap, and the size of the lateral port on either side, was addressed by Hogan,[31] who introduced the concept of lateral port control in pharyngeal flap design. His flap was a wide superiorly based posterior pharyngeal flap, which he lined with nasal mucosal flaps from the posterior soft palate. The operation was performed with a 4-mm-diameter catheter positioned through the lateral port on either side of the flap, as a guide to calibration of the size of the lateral ports. Using lateral port control, Hogan reported restoration of velopharyngeal competence in 91 of 93 patients (98%). On the other hand, only 3 of the 93 patients (3%) ended up with hyponasality that lasted more than 6 months after posterior pharyngeal flap surgery. Hogan's choice of port diameter was based on the pressure-flow studies of Warren et al.[8-10] The concept of calibrating the width of the posterior pharyngeal flap was taken a step further by Shprintzen et al,[32] who introduced the concept of the "tailor-made" pharyngeal flap. They proposed that the width of the flap should be determined by the amount of lateral pharyngeal wall motion seen by endoscopy or by videofluoroscopy before surgery. In their report, 60 patients were studied retrospectively, and another 60 were assigned prospectively to three different types of pharyngeal flap surgery (narrow, moderately wide, or very wide flaps). All flaps were superiorly based. In the prospective portion of the study, patients were given a narrow flap when the preoperative lateral pharyngeal wall motion had been rated excellent, a moderately wide flap when the preoperative lateral wall motion had been rated moderate, or a very wide pharyngeal flap when the preoperative lateral wall motion had been rated poor. Of the 60 prospectively treated patients, vocal resonance after surgery was normal in 47 (78%), hyponasal in 11 (18%), and still hypernasal in 2 (3%).

In addition to the superiorly based and inferiorly based designs that have already been discussed, Kapetansky[33] has advocated transversely based flaps. He thought that the transverse design would preserve nerve supply and therefore maintain more bulk as well as the potential for contractile function. To this end, he made an S-shaped incision in the posterior pharyngeal wall and elevated two laterally based flaps, each 30 to 35 mm in length and 15 to 20 mm in width. One was sutured in place to provide nasal lining, and the other was sutured below it to provide oral lining. Despite the theoretical advantages of nerve preservation, neither Kapetansky nor any subsequent investigator has demonstrated a functional speech advantage to this design, and it has never been as popular as the traditional superiorly based flap.

Surgical Technique

In the preferred surgical technique (Fig. 97-9), the patient is intubated orally with a midline oral RAE endotracheal tube. This tube is secured, and the mouth is held open by a Dingman retractor. The posterior pharyngeal wall and midline of the soft palate are injected with 1.0% lidocaine with epinephrine 1:100,000. After a wait of 7 minutes, parallel incisions are made in the posterior pharyngeal wall, approximately 2.5 cm apart. Dissection is carried down to the prevertebral fascia. The flap is undermined and elevated with its superior as well as inferior attachments still intact, and the inferior attachment is then divided. The soft palate is split in the midline, and lining flaps are incised and elevated from the nasal surface of the soft palate, based on the posterior edge of the soft palate. The tip of the superiorly based posterior pharyngeal flap is then sutured into the defect on the nasal surface of the soft palate with absorbable horizontal mattress sutures. These are left untied until all have been placed, and they are then sequentially tied. It can be helpful to pass a 10 or 12 French nasal catheter through the planned lateral port on each side to define the ports and to prevent their obliteration. The lateral edge of the posterior pharyngeal flap on each side can then be sutured to the lateral edge of the soft palate to better define the lateral ports. The oral lining of the soft palate and the nasal lining flaps of the soft palate are then repaired in the midline. The flap donor defect

in the posterior pharyngeal wall is repaired in the midline if it can be easily closed. Otherwise, in most cases, it is left open and will rapidly heal by secondary intention.

If the patient shows any significant upper airway obstruction at the end of surgery, the oral RAE tube is changed to a cuffed endotracheal tube, and the patient is mechanically ventilated for the next 24 to 72 hours until the edema has decreased. Even if the patient can be extubated in the operating room, all patients who have undergone pharyngeal flap attachment are observed in the intensive care unit for the first night after surgery because of the risk of early postoperative airway complications.

Outcomes

There is no agreement as to the relative advantages and disadvantages of the superiorly based versus the inferiorly based design for posterior pharyngeal flaps. Skoog[34] believed that the position of the base of the flap made no difference in long-term outcome on the basis of his review of 82 flaps, 45 of which were superiorly based and 33 inferiorly based. Similarly, Hamlen[35] reviewed the cases of 95 patients, aged 4 to 19 years, who had undergone attachment of a posterior pharyngeal flap with follow-up as long as 13 years. There were 64 patients who had undergone attachment of a superiorly based flap and 27 who had undergone attachment of an inferiorly based flap. No differences in short-term or long-term speech results were seen between the two groups. In a prospectively randomized study, Whitaker[36] compared 17 patients who received a superiorly based posterior pharyngeal flap for treatment of velopharyngeal insufficiency with 18 patients who underwent attachment of an inferiorly based flap. No differences were found in length of hospital stay, complications, speech outcome, or hearing results.

Karling et al[37] compared attachment of posterior pharyngeal flaps into either a transverse split of the soft palate or a longitudinal midline split. Their hypothesis was that the transversely split soft palate would result in a wider, more caudally based flap. On examination of the flaps by videoradiography and nasopharyngoscopy, however, they found that there were no differences in flap position or flap width at rest between 22 patients with a transversely split soft palate attachment and 20 patients with a midline split. The flaps that had been inserted into a transversely split soft palate did show significantly more widening of the flap base during phonation, but no differences were noted in speech outcome. Karling et al[38] also studied lateral pharyngeal wall adduction as a function of flap width. Nasopharyngoscopy was used to determine flap width in 53 patients who had undergone posterior pharyngeal flap attachment, and

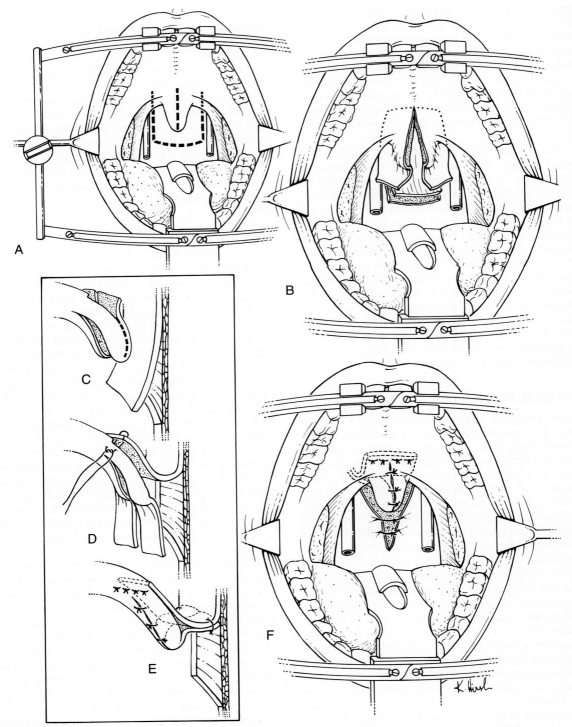

FIGURE 97-9. *A* to *H,* The authors' preferred technique for attachment of posterior pharyngeal flap.

Soulèvement de la paroi post. du pharynx vers le nez
La constriction des parois latérales ferme les espaces
qu'on laisse en latéral

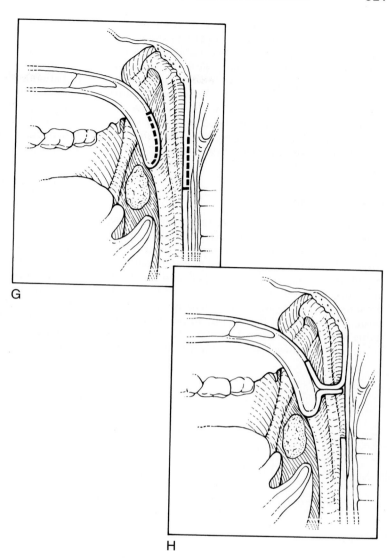

G

H

FIGURE 97-9, cont'd.

videoradiography was used to determine lateral pharyngeal wall adduction. They found that patients who started with limited preoperative adduction showed a greater increase in lateral pharyngeal wall adduction with a narrow flap than with a wide flap. On the other hand, patients who started with better preoperative adduction showed a decrease in postoperative adduction, and that also correlated with flap width. Pressure-flow recordings of a typical patient after flap attachment are shown in Figures 97-10 and 97-11, and endoscopy in Figure 97-12.

Complications

Several authors have documented acute postoperative airway obstruction, chronic obstructive sleep apnea, and even death after posterior pharyngeal flap surgery.[39-44] Orr et al[45] performed polysomnographic monitoring 1 to 2 days before surgery and 2 to 3 days after surgery as well as 3 months postoperatively in 10 patients undergoing attachment of a superiorly based posterior pharyngeal flap and in 10 patients undergoing von Langenbeck palatoplasty. No patients in either group showed any significant abnormalities

preoperatively. Of the patients who had palatoplasty, one had a significant change in the early postoperative period, which had completely resolved by 3 months postoperatively. On the other hand, 9 of the 10 patients who had attachment of a posterior pharyngeal flap showed a significant increase in the number of obstructive episodes per hour in the early postoperative period. By 3 months, seven of those patients had returned to normal, but two continued to show increased frequency of obstructive episodes. There were no differences in central apneas, in either group of patients, during the entire study.

A large series of patients undergoing attachment of a superiorly based posterior pharyngeal flap was reviewed by Valnicek et al.[46] They described 219 children at the Hospital for Sick Children in Toronto who underwent such surgery between 1985 and 1992. There was one death, with autopsy showing cerebral edema of unknown cause. Other complications included airway obstruction in 20 patients (9.1%); bleeding in 18 (8.2%), 5 of whom required blood transfusion; and documented obstructive sleep apnea after discharge from the hospital in 9 children (4.1%). Reintubation in the early postoperative period was necessary in

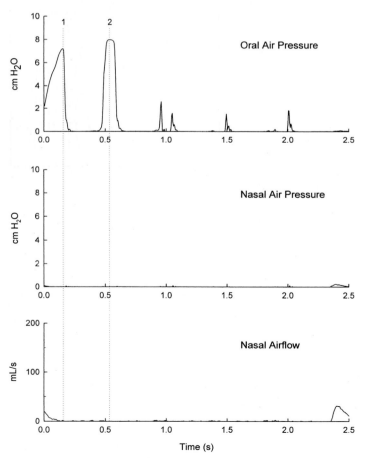

FIGURE 97-10. Pressure-flow recordings of five productions of the syllable /pi/ by the same 8-year-old boy as in Figure 97-4 after pharyngeal flap surgery. Inappropriate nasal air pressure and nasal airflow are essentially eliminated. Oral air pressures during the third to fifth syllables were reduced because of faulty placement of the oral catheter.

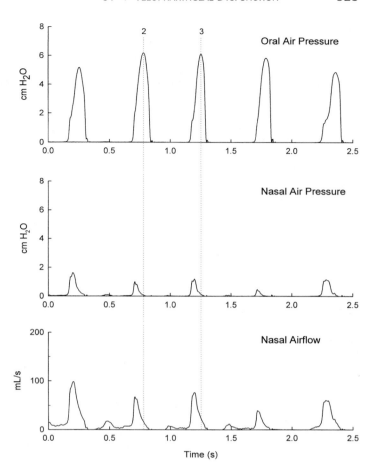

FIGURE 97-11. Pressure-flow recordings of five productions of the word *hamper* by the same 8-year-old boy as in Figure 97-4 after pharyngeal flap surgery. Calculated velopharyngeal areas during the second and third productions of /p/ were below 1 mm². Nasal air pressure and nasal airflow are separated from the oral air pressure peak, typical of the normal production of the /mp/ sequence.

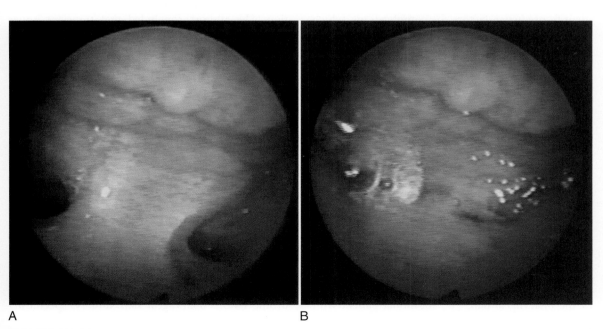

A   B

FIGURE 97-12. Endoscopic views of a boy with cleft palate after pharyngeal flap surgery. *A,* Open lateral velopharyngeal ports during production of /mama/. *B,* Closed velopharyngeal ports during production of /sasa/.

3 patients, and 11 eventually needed surgical revision, including complete division of the flap in 4. Fraulin et al,[47] from the same institution, compared 164 patients who underwent attachment of a superiorly based posterior pharyngeal flap between July 1985 and December 1990 with 222 patients who underwent the same surgery between January 1991 and June 1996. They questioned whether changes in their patient care protocol, instituted after a patient's death in the recovery room in 1990, had led to any change in the number of acute complications (in the first 24 hours after surgery). Changes that were instituted after the 1990 death included closer observation and monitoring in the intensive care unit by use of apnea, oxygen saturation, and cardiac monitors. Also, there were fewer operating surgeons—four surgeons performed 222 operations in the later period versus the seven who performed 164 operations in the earlier period. There was also more frequent use of nasopharyngeal airways in the later patients. Furthermore, the later patients had fewer simultaneous major procedures, such as fistula repair, alveolar bone grafting, or maxillary osteotomies, and the later patients were also more likely to have direct closure of the posterior pharyngeal wall flap donor site. There were no differences between the two groups in age, gender, or associated medical conditions. Airway complications decreased from 11% in the earlier group to 3.2% in the later group ($P = .0012$). Bleeding complications decreased from 7.3% to 1.4% ($P = .0027$). Total complications decreased from 19.5% to 6.3% ($P = .0001$). Furthermore, the mean hospital stay decreased from 5.8 to 3.8 days ($P = .0001$). Perhaps of most significance, the authors were able to identify predictive factors for complications, which included other associated medical problems, simultaneous performance of another major surgical procedure, not closing the posterior pharyngeal flap donor site, and specific operating surgeon. They did not compare speech outcome for the two groups, nor did they evaluate late complications such as obstructive sleep apnea.

Ysunza et al[48] described 585 patients who had undergone surgical management of velopharyngeal dysfunction. Of those patients, 571 had attachment of a superiorly based pharyngeal flap, and 14 underwent a Jackson-type sphincter pharyngoplasty. Of the 585 patients, 15 had findings on polysomnographic evaluation that were diagnostic of obstructive sleep apnea, for which they eventually underwent further surgery. Fourteen of those 15 patients had previously undergone attachment of a posterior pharyngeal flap. All 14 were successfully treated with uvulopalatopharyngoplasty, although one also required complete division of the pharyngeal flap. The additional patient with obstructive sleep apnea had previously undergone Jackson-type pharyngoplasty and was found to have a prominent uvula that was obstructing the pharyn-

goplasty port. That patient was successfully treated with partial resection of the uvula.

Sirois et al[49] further investigated the question of sleep apnea after pharyngeal flap attachment by performing preoperative and postoperative polysomnographic recordings for 40 children undergoing pharyngeal flap attachment. Postoperatively, 26 patients (65%) had normal sleep studies. Of the 14 with abnormal studies, 6 showed obstructive apneas, 6 central apneas, and 2 both central and obstructive apneas. Ten of those 14 patients underwent repeated sleep studies in the following months. Eight had normal recordings and two showed continued central apneas. Of the two children with persistent abnormal recordings, one remained free of clinical symptoms. The other patient had snoring, restless sleeping, sweating, and daytime lethargy, and division of the pharyngeal flap was recommended. These authors concluded that significant sleep apnea after posterior pharyngeal flap surgery might not be as frequent or permanent as had previously been suggested.

Posterior pharyngeal flap surgery is a delicate balance between hypernasal resonance and airway obstruction, and this concept is underscored by Lesavoy et al.[50] They described 29 patients who underwent superiorly based posterior pharyngeal flap attachment. Of those patients, 11 (38%) had signs or symptoms of sleep apnea or upper airway obstruction during sleep in the early period after surgery. This resolved in all but two patients within 5 months. Interestingly, the patients who showed postoperative upper airway obstruction were only half as likely to have residual postoperative velopharyngeal dysfunction. The authors concluded that transient upper airway obstruction may be a necessary price to pay for successful treatment of velopharyngeal dysfunction. Despite data suggesting spontaneous resolution of obstructive symptoms, it would be better still to successfully treat velopharyngeal dysfunction without postoperative airway problems, transient or otherwise.

Finally, an important anatomic consideration is highlighted by Mitnick et al,[51] who studied 20 consecutive patients with velocardiofacial syndrome by magnetic resonance angiography. All 20 patients showed anomalies of the vertebral arteries, the carotid arteries, or both, and two patients had internal carotid arteries close to the pharyngeal midline, at the level of the first cervical vertebra, where they could easily be encountered during elevation of a posterior pharyngeal flap. On the basis of their results, the authors recommended that magnetic resonance angiography be used in all patients with velocardiofacial syndrome before pharyngeal flap surgery, specifically looking for such carotid or vertebral artery anomalies. This diagnostic study allows identification of high-risk patients.

SPHINCTER PHARYNGOPLASTY

History

The origin of the sphincter pharyngoplasty dates to Wilfred Hynes of Sheffield, England, who used the salpingopharyngeus muscles and their overlying mucosa, which he dissected, based superiorly, and transplanted into a transverse surgical defect in the mucosa of the posterior wall of the nasopharynx. He reported this operation for repair of "failed cleft palate."[52] His initial attempts were performed as two-staged procedures. In the first stage, the soft palate was divided and the salpingopharyngeus muscles were attached to the posterior pharyngeal wall, and to each other, in a side-to-side design (Fig. 97-13). At a separate operation, the soft palate was repaired, and in some of his early cases, palatal pushback was performed as well. His first report described 12 patients, 8 of whom had completed both stages of surgery. All eight were reported as showing improvement in speech, which was described as "dramatic" in three.

In his 1953 Hunterian Lecture, Hynes[53] described 55 sphincter pharyngoplasties. As the technique evolved, he advocated bulkier flaps, which now included salpingopharyngeus, palatopharyngeus, and part of the superior constrictor muscle as well. The flaps were now sutured together in an end-to-end fashion, but with some overlap of the tips of the flaps to achieve sufficient tightening of the sphincter. By 1953, Hynes was performing the procedure as a single operation, simply by retracting rather than dividing the soft palate, in most cases (see Fig. 97-13). When Hynes found it necessary to divide the soft palate for access to the nasopharynx, he still recommended that it be repaired at a separate time, with the possibility of palatal pushback at that same time. By 1953, 36 patients had completed one- or two-staged sphincter pharyngoplasty and had been observed for at least 1 year after the last operation. Of those patients, 19 (53%) were rated as having "perfect, or almost perfect" speech. Another 13 patients (36%) had improvement but still were found to have some nasal air escape. Only four patients (11%) were thought to have had no speech improvement.

A different sphincter pharyngoplasty design was proposed by Miguel Orticochea[54] of Bogotá, Colombia. Orticochea inset the pharyngoplasty flaps at a much lower level than Hynes did, significantly below the level of usual velopharyngeal closure. Orticochea also raised a separate, inferiorly based flap from the posterior pharyngeal wall and sutured the tips of his pharyngoplasty flaps to the raw surface of that flap (Fig. 97-14). Orticochea used his pharyngoplasty design in all of his patients with cleft palate and did not reserve it for those whose initial palatoplasty had failed. All patients underwent sphincter pharyngoplasty 6 months after their initial palate repair.

Jackson and Silverton[55] introduced a third technique for sphincter pharyngoplasty. In their technique, bilateral superiorly based flaps from the posterior tonsillar pillars, including the palatopharyngeus muscles, were elevated. These flaps were then sutured together in the midline and also to the undersurface of a superiorly based posterior pharyngeal flap (Fig. 97-15). The Jackson and Silverton technique should produce a higher positioning of the pharyngoplasty flaps than in the original Orticochea operation, thus bringing the level of the sphincter pharyngoplasty closer to the normal level of velopharyngeal closure. Jackson and Silverton described 74 patients who underwent their pharyngoplasty. They found speech improvement in 67 patients (91%).

Surgical Technique

A sphincter pharyngoplasty technique that is similar to Hynes' 1953 modification[53] (Fig. 97-16) is currently recommended. The patient is intubated with an oral RAE endotracheal tube. The Dingman mouth retractor is used to stabilize the endotracheal tube and to provide exposure for the procedure. Incisions for elevation of superiorly based flaps from the posterior tonsillar pillars, bilaterally, and the posterior pharyngeal wall transverse incision, above the resting position of the soft palate, are marked. An adenoid retractor is used to elevate the soft palate for the markings as well as for the surgical dissection and suturing in that area.

The area of planned incisions is injected with 1% lidocaine with epinephrine 1 : 100,000. After a wait of 7 minutes, the posterior tonsillar pillar flaps are incised and elevated, including the bulk of the palatopharyngeus muscle on both sides. The transverse incision is made in the posterior pharyngeal wall; this incision is continuous with the superior medial extent of the posterior tonsillar pillar dissection. The muscle flaps are sutured together in an end-to-end fashion and then into the defect in the posterior pharyngeal wall with absorbable sutures. At the completion of the procedure, the velopharyngeal port is markedly reduced in transverse as well as in anterior to posterior dimension. In some cases, a decision can be made to suture the palatopharyngeus muscle flaps together in a partially overlapping manner to produce a tighter sphincter. In all cases, a great effort is made to suture the flaps into the posterior pharyngeal wall at the highest level that is technically feasible.

Outcomes

Hynes[56] reviewed his experience with sphincter pharyngoplasty in a paper entitled "Observations on Pharyngoplasty." On the basis of his 20 years of experience, he emphasized the importance of elevating as

Text continued on p. 330

Lambeau du muscle salpingopharyngien

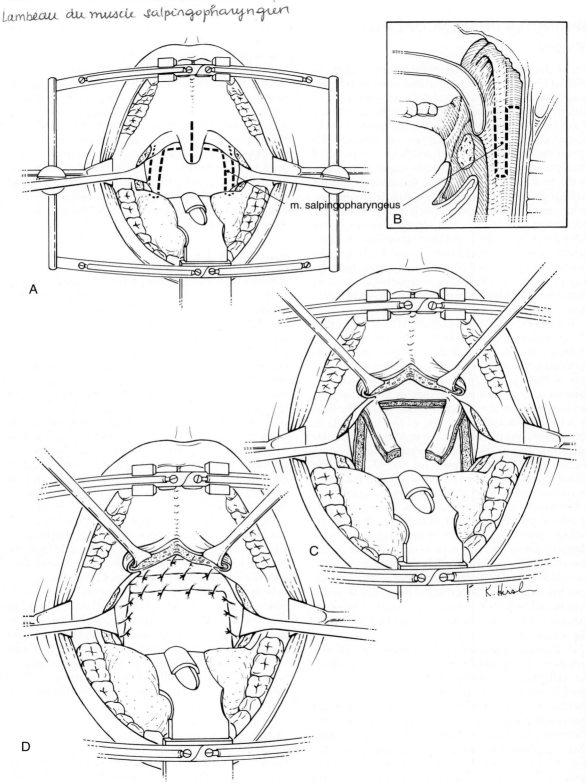

m. salpingopharyngeus

B

A

C

D

K. Hirsh

FIGURE 97-13. *A* to *D*, The original Hynes pharyngoplasty.

Paroi pharyngée latérale rabattue ds l'ouverture vélopharyngée
c'est le palais (sa mobilité) qui ferme l'orifice central qu'on laisse.
• Evaluer 1) la mobilité du palais
2) la hauteur de la pharyngoplastie] en pré-op

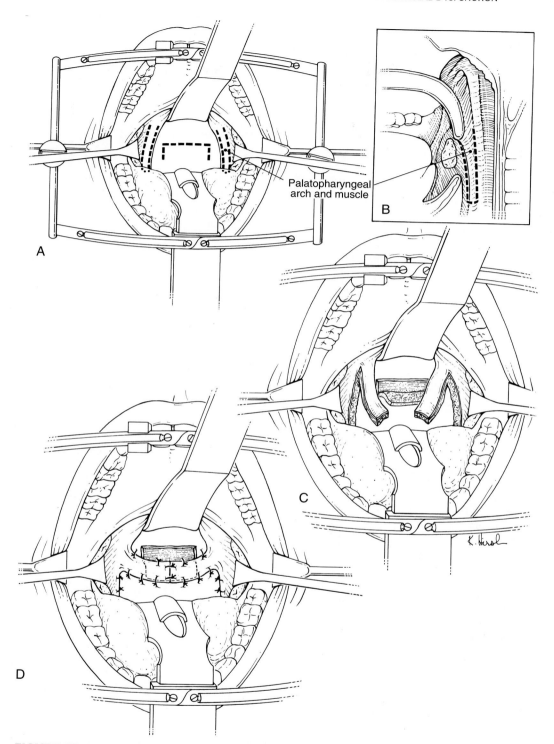

Palatopharyngeal arch and muscle

FIGURE 97-14. *A to D,* Orticochea's pharyngoplasty technique.

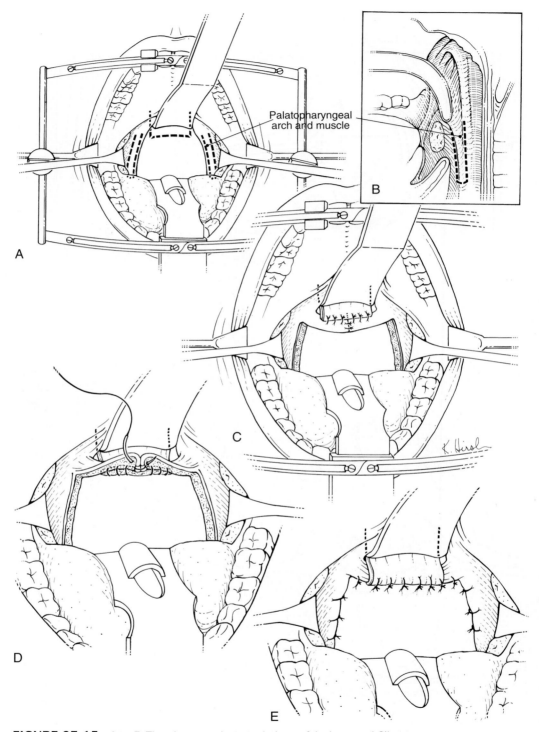

Palatopharyngeal arch and muscle

FIGURE 97-15. *A to E,* The pharyngoplasty technique of Jackson and Silverton.

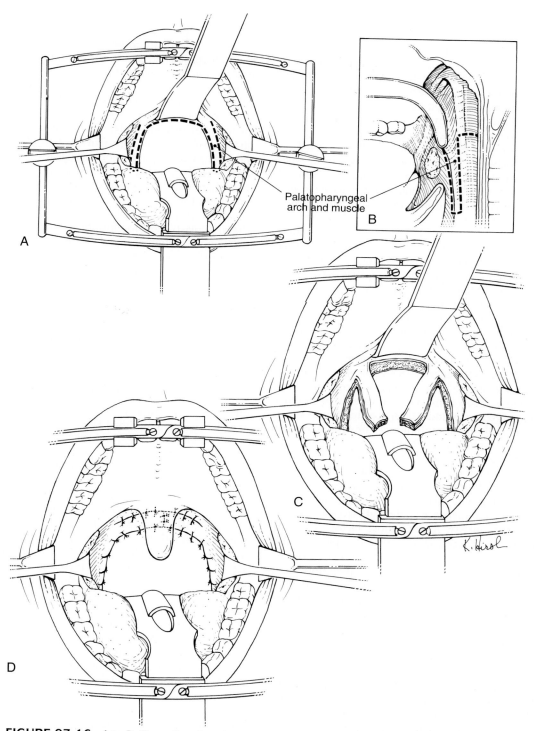

Palatopharyngeal arch and muscle

FIGURE 97-16. *A to D,* The authors' preferred technique for modified Hynes pharyngoplasty.

much muscle bulk as possible with the pharyngoplasty flaps. He still thought that it was advisable, in some cases, to split an intact soft palate to allow better exposure for inset of the pharyngoplasty flaps in the posterior pharyngeal wall. He did, however, after 20 years believe that it was possible to repair the soft palate at the same surgical procedure. He thought that 20% of pharyngoplasty patients would require even further surgical treatment, such as a palatal lengthening procedure, after the pharyngoplasty had fully healed.

Orticochea[57,58] has reviewed his longer term experience with his sphincter pharyngoplasty. In the 1983 report, he stated that all patients with cleft palate treated by him since 1958 had undergone construction of a sphincter pharyngoplasty. He divided these patients into four groups. Group 1 (104 patients) had undergone palatoplasty at the age of 2 years and sphincter pharyngoplasty 6 months later. Group 2 (94 patients) had undergone sphincter pharyngoplasty between the ages of 3 and 11 years. Sixteen of those patients who had tonsillar hypertrophy also underwent tonsillectomy at the same time. Group 3 (27 patients) underwent sphincter pharyngoplasty surgery between the ages of 11 and 18 years. Group 4 (11 patients) underwent sphincter pharyngoplasty construction in two stages between the ages of 18 and 32 years. Contractile capacity of the pharyngoplasty flaps and speech outcome were best in the younger patients. In the older patients (groups 3 and 4), Orticochea found many patients with poor mobility of the sphincter and residual velopharyngeal dysfunction in speech, and more of the older patients required further surgery.

In his 1999 review, Orticochea made personal observations based on 40 years of experience with the sphincter pharyngoplasty. He believed that several factors could influence the potential success of sphincter pharyngoplasty. Among those factors were the amount of air that escapes through the sphincter and the mobility of the sphincter. He thought that the patient's age at the time of surgery was an important factor, with better results in younger children than in older children or adults. He also thought that the ability of the patient to modify learned speech habits, the language spoken by the patient, and the size of the pharynx were other factors that influenced outcome. His protocol is strict and not commonly followed by most clinics. Specifically, he does not allow any speech therapy before surgery. He also has patients refrain from speaking for 17 days after surgery and confines them to a completely liquid diet for that entire time. However, the major criticism of Orticochea's pharyngoplasty is the low level of inset of the pharyngoplasty flaps, which does not make as much anatomic and physiologic sense as the higher level of inset advocated by virtually all others. The specific issue of the level of flap inset was addressed by Riski et al.[59] They reviewed their experience with the original Orticochea

pharyngoplasty as well as a modification of it. They identified 26 patients whose pharyngoplasty flaps were below the level of attempted velopharyngeal closure. Only 16 (62%) had successful resolution of hypernasality. On the other hand, 27 of 29 patients (93%) whose flaps were inserted at the level of attempted velopharyngeal closure showed resolution of hypernasal resonance. They therefore recommended that Orticochea's original design be modified to place the pharyngoplasty flaps higher in the nasopharynx, at the level of attempted velopharyngeal closure. The same group[60] revisited this issue 8 years later. By this time, there were 139 patients to assess. As with their first study, they found that the major cause of failure of sphincter pharyngoplasty was insertion of the pharyngoplasty flaps too low, that is, below the level of attempted velopharyngeal closure.

Pigott[61] reviewed the 1953 modification of the Hynes pharyngoplasty. He theorized that the operation might work in any of three ways: (1) augmenting the posterior pharyngeal wall, (2) statically reducing the lateral pharyngeal recess, and (3) truly producing a dynamic sphincter. Similar to the findings of Riski et al, Pigott emphasized that the transverse incision for inset of the palatopharyngeus flaps should be made at the highest level the surgeon can technically achieve. In fact, he stated that "it cannot be placed too high."

Several others have reviewed results of sphincter pharyngoplasty surgery. Moss et al[62] reviewed their experience with a modified Hynes pharyngoplasty in 40 patients between 1980 and 1984. Ages ranged from 4 to 52 years. Speech was assessed before surgery and at least 6 months after pharyngoplasty. Additional radiologic and nasendoscopic evaluations were also performed. The authors found that postoperatively, 38 patients (95%) had no nasal air escape or only intermittent nasal air escape, and 33 patients (82%) had normal or slightly hyponasal resonance. They had only one complication, which was a "bucket-handle" flap separation from the posterior pharyngeal wall. That patient had normal speech. Another 13 patients had minor side effects, which included catarrh, snoring, swallowing problems, nasal obstruction, and difficulty in blowing the nose. None of these required further surgical treatment. Their conclusion was that patients suitable for the modified Hynes sphincter pharyngoplasty are those with slight or moderate nasal escape, good palate mobility, and anterior-posterior gap of 5 mm or less.

Witt et al[63] evaluated 20 patients who had undergone sphincter pharyngoplasty. Their procedure is reported as a Jackson-type pharyngoplasty, but their description and illustrations appear to be virtually identical to the modified Hynes design. Patients underwent perceptual speech evaluations as well as endoscopic study. Of the 19 patients who had good preoperative and postoperative speech samples, 15 (79%) showed improvement in hypernasality. Nasal emission decreased in 14 of the 19 patients (74%). However, only 7 of 20 patients (35%) demonstrated complete velopharyngeal closure postoperatively, and 13 patients (65%) were still thought to be candidates for additional surgical management.

James et al[64] retrospectively studied 54 patients who had been treated by the Orticochea pharyngoplasty, by a single surgeon, between 1984 and 1994. Interestingly, the procedure used was the original Orticochea procedure, not the modification that had been suggested by Riski et al.[59,60] Of the 54 patients, 49 (91%) showed improvement in nasal escape, and 5 (9%) remained unchanged. No patient was made worse by surgery. A detailed analysis showed that 40 patients (75%) had complete resolution of nasal escape. Nasal resonance was assessed as normal in 46 patients (85%). The authors therefore question the need for positioning the pharyngoplasty flaps at the high level recommended by Moss et al[62] and Riski et al.[59,60]

In an interesting report, Georgantopoulou et al[65] studied 24 pharyngoplasty patients with preoperative and postoperative videotape speech recordings and lateral videofluoroscopy; 11 of the patients had undergone Jackson pharyngoplasty, 10 Orticochea pharyngoplasty, and 3 modified Hynes pharyngoplasty. After pharyngoplasty, 9 patients (38%) were thought to have an excellent result with completely normal speech, 12 (50%) had a good speech result, 1 (4%) had little improvement, and only 2 (8%) showed no speech improvement. Videofluoroscopy demonstrated a highly significant increase in the range of palatal movement postoperatively. However, there was no correlation between the degree of the increase of palatal movement and the postoperative speech improvement.

Kasten et al[66] retrospectively investigated the revision rate for sphincter pharyngoplasty. They described 30 patients who underwent sphincter pharyngoplasty between 1988 and 1994 by seven different surgeons. Surgical techniques varied. Of the 30 patients, 7 (23%) had residual moderate to severe hypernasality that required further surgery, and 1 patient (3%) had hyponasality severe enough to require reoperation. Seven of the eight patients who underwent revision of pharyngoplasty had acceptable speech after revision. The original surgery was considered to have failed in four of the eight patients requiring revision because of dehiscence of the palatopharyngeal flaps. The original operation was thought to have failed in an additional patient requiring revision because of inferior positioning of the flaps. The authors believed that there was a "learning curve," with fewer failures occurring after the individual surgeon had 9 months of experience with the procedure.

Potential abnormal location of the carotid and vertebral arteries in patients with velocardiofacial syndrome has already been mentioned as a danger with posterior pharyngeal flap attachment.[51] Witt et al[67] have reported encouraging results with use of sphincter pharyngoplasty as an alternative to pharyngeal flap in the management of velopharyngeal dysfunction in patients with velocardiofacial syndrome. Between 1984 and 1996, 19 patients with velocardiofacial syndrome underwent sphincter pharyngoplasty. Successful surgical outcome was defined as elimination of hypernasality, nasal emission, and turbulence by perceptual speech assessment and 100% velopharyngeal orifice closure by nasendoscopy or fluoroscopy. By such a definition, 18 of their 19 patients (95%) had successful management of velopharyngeal dysfunction with sphincter pharyngoplasty.

The question has often been raised as to how truly dynamic the so-called dynamic sphincter pharyngoplasty is. Several reports have addressed this issue. Witt et al[68] reviewed speech videofluoroscopy evaluations before and after surgery in 20 patients who underwent sphincter pharyngoplasty. They found a quantifiable and statistically significant difference in maximum to minimum excursion of the velopharyngeal apparatus after sphincter pharyngoplasty compared with preoperatively. In a related study, Witt et al[69] demonstrated that the sphincteric-type movement was not caused by preexisting posterior pharyngeal wall motion.

Ysunza et al[70] may have resolved the issue of active sphincteric motion. They evaluated 25 patients who had undergone sphincter pharyngoplasty between 1985 and 1996. All patients were examined by simultaneous electromyography and videonasopharyngoscopy. All of the pharyngoplasties were performed by the Jackson and Silverton technique, and efforts had been made to insert the flaps at the level of attempted velopharyngeal contact as determined preoperatively by videonasopharyngoscopy and videofluoroscopy. For the postoperative studies, wire electrodes were inserted orally, under direct vision, on the bellies of the levator veli palatini muscle, the superior constrictor pharyngeus muscle, and the palatopharyngeus muscle. None of the patients showed electromyographic activity of the palatopharyngeus muscle in the superiorly based flap. However, all patients showed normal electromyographic activity at the superior constrictor pharyngeus and the levator veli palatini muscles. Although 23 of the 25 patients demonstrated complete velopharyngeal closure on videonasopharyngoscopy, active sphinctering was not demonstrated by electromyography. It was concluded that the observed sphinctering was passive and caused by contraction of the superior constrictor pharyngeus.

Complications

Moss et al[62] reported one surgical complication (2.5%) in a series of 40 patients who underwent modified

Hynes pharyngoplasty. The complication was a bucket-handle flap separation of the pharyngoplasty flaps from the posterior pharyngeal wall. An additional 13 patients (32%) had what were described as side effects. These included catarrh, snoring, swallowing problems, nasal obstruction, and difficulty in blowing the nose. None of these required surgical management. In the series of 54 Orticochea pharyngoplasties reported by James et al,[64] there were five complications (9%). These included one each of postoperative hemorrhage, streptococcal infection, respiratory obstruction requiring admission to the intensive care unit, complete pharyngoplasty dehiscence, and persistent snoring.

Kasten et al[66] did not specifically look at complications that followed the original pharyngoplasty but rather concentrated on the need for subsequent revision. Still, one striking statistic from their study is that of 30 patients undergoing pharyngoplasty between 1988 and 1994, 4 (13%) were found to have had dehiscence of the original palatopharyngeal myomucosal flaps at the time of reoperation or re-evaluation.

There has been only one report of perioperative and postoperative airway compromise after sphincter pharyngoplasty. Witt et al[71] retrospectively assessed 58 patients who had undergone sphincter pharyngoplasty, after previous palatoplasty, for velopharyngeal dysfunction. Eight patients (14%) had perioperative or postoperative upper airway problems. Five of the eight patients had Pierre Robin sequence and micrognathia; the other three had histories of perinatal respiratory and feeding difficulties without micrognathia or an identified genetic disorder. All but two of the eight patients had complete resolution of airway problems within 3 days postoperatively. The two whose airway problems did not resolve were discharged home with apnea monitors, and both required readmission for recurrent airway dysfunction. Continuous positive airway pressure was successfully used, and neither required takedown of the sphincter pharyngoplasty.

OTHER SURGICAL AND NONSURGICAL APPROACHES
Palatal Lengthening Procedures

Any of several so-called palatal lengthening procedures can be applied to the management of velopharyngeal dysfunction. Such procedures have generally been described for primary management of cleft palate and include the techniques of Dorrance,[72] Wardill,[73] Kilner,[74] and Furlow.[75] The efficacy of any of these procedures for secondary surgical management of velopharyngeal dysfunction has never been established. The concept of palatal lengthening is theoretically appealing and may have appropriate clinical applications. These procedures should be limited, however, to situations in which the gap in the velopharyngeal

orifice is relatively small. The Furlow palatoplasty has been used for secondary management of velopharyngeal dysfunction in eight patients. Results have been best in patients who started with small gaps.

Augmentation of Posterior Pharyngeal Wall

For more than a century, there has been interest in treatment of velopharyngeal dysfunction by augmentation of the posterior pharyngeal wall. Passavant[76] unsuccessfully attempted to surgically augment the posterior pharyngeal wall in 1879. Gersuny[77] injected paraffin to augment the posterior pharyngeal wall. Several major complications, including at least one death, resulted in the abandonment of this technique.[78] Hollweg and Perthes[79] suggested insertion of autogenous cartilage into the posterior pharyngeal space by an external cervical approach. Bentley[80] reported poor long-term results with autogenous cartilage augmentation of the posterior pharynx, although a report by Denny et al[81] shows that there may still be interest in such a technique. Halle[82] used autogenous fascia and von Gaza[83] used fat and fascia from the abdominal and gluteal regions of adults and fascia lata in children inserted into the retropharyngeal space. Hagerty[84] advocated the use of cartilage allograft for augmentation of the posterior pharyngeal wall, recognizing that there would be gradual absorption of this material. However, he believed the increased palatal mobility that would develop after the implantation would compensate for the eventual loss of the pharyngeal wall projection.

Several different alloplastic materials have been used for posterior pharyngeal wall augmentation. These include silicone,[85,86] Teflon,[75,87-89] and Proplast.[90] As has been the case in so many other surgical applications of alloplastic materials, posterior pharyngeal wall augmentation with synthetic materials has been complicated by exposure, infection, extrusion, and migration. In a series of 23 patients treated with liquid, solid, shredded, or sponge implants of Silastic with less than 1 year of follow-up,[85] three implants (13%) needed to be totally or partially removed because of infection or exposure. Similarly, in a series of 26 patients treated with Proplast pharyngeal wall implants,[90] four patients (15%) lost their implants 4 weeks to 5 months after surgery.

Prosthetic Management

Modern prosthetic management of velopharyngeal dysfunction dates back more than 100 years.[91] There are two types of appliances that can be used, the palatal lift and the pharyngeal bulb. In general, a lift-type appliance is used when there is a long but adynamic palate. The palate is physically lifted by the appliance to assist velopharyngeal closure. The pharyngeal bulb is generally selected when there is a short palate to partially obturate the velopharyngeal port. Bulbs can also be helpful when lateral pharyngeal wall motion is minimal or absent. In general, because of their passive nature, bulb-type appliances are more easily tolerated by patients. The two types of appliances can also be combined as a bulb-lift appliance.

Prosthetic management requires a tremendous investment of time by the dental specialist who will be making the appliance and by the patient and family. McGrath and Anderson[92] have listed criteria for the selection of patients, which include the following:

1. The patient has the mental capacity and is compliant with requests to imitate speech.
2. The patient or the parents prefer nonsurgical management.
3. The patient has good oral hygiene.
4. The patient and family are committed to this course of therapy.
5. The patient and family are willing to take responsibility to maintain good oral hygiene and to keep the appliance clean.
6. The patient must be able to cooperate for treatment.

In addition, it almost goes without saying that the patient should have well-documented velopharyngeal dysfunction that the patient and family perceive as a problem and that is not phoneme specific.

COMPARING OUTCOMES

There have been few publications comparing the outcome of different treatment approaches for velopharyngeal dysfunction. A retrospective study compared 30 patients who underwent attachment of a posterior pharyngeal flap with another 30 patients who were treated with modified Hynes pharyngoplasty.[93] There was a tendency toward hyponasality in the pharyngeal flap patients, with 13 patients (43%) having mild, moderate, or severe hyponasality after surgery. On the other hand, there was a tendency toward residual hypernasality in the pharyngoplasty patients, with 13 (43%) being rated as mildly, moderately, or severely hypernasal even after surgery. Further surgery was necessary in three (10%) of the pharyngoplasty patients, two because of persistent hypernasality and one because of nasal obstruction. On the other hand, eight (27%) of the pharyngeal flap patients required further surgery, three for persistent hypernasality and five for obstructive symptoms. All five of the obstructed patients required division of the pharyngeal flap, and three were subsequently successfully converted to pharyngoplasty. There were three complications (10%) in the pharyngoplasty group and 11 (37%) in the pharyngeal flap group. The

complications for the pharyngoplasty patients were one partial flap separation, one patient with sinusitis, and one with obstructive symptoms. In the pharyngeal flap group, two patients had flap dehiscence, six had significant obstructive symptoms, two had postoperative bleeding (including one who required reoperation), and one had aspiration pneumonia. On the basis of this retrospective experience, the modified Hynes pharyngoplasty had fewer complications and could more easily be surgically revised but may not be as effective in correcting velopharyngeal dysfunction, particularly when the patient has a large gap preoperatively.

To further explore these issues, an international multicenter prospective randomized trial was organized to compare superiorly based posterior pharyngeal flap and modified Hynes pharyngoplasty. During an 8-year-period, the trial has enrolled patients at centers in the United States as well as in the United Kingdom, Norway, and Brazil. Data are being collected and analyzed under the direction of Professor William C. Shaw of Manchester, England.

Pensler and Reich[94] have retrospectively compared sphincter pharyngoplasty and pharyngeal flap. They studied 85 patients who underwent surgical treatment of velopharyngeal dysfunction during a 30-year-period. Of those patients, 75 underwent attachment of posterior pharyngeal flap and 10 had sphincter pharyngoplasty. They found that the majority of patients in each group experienced speech improvement, 56 of 75 (75%) of the pharyngeal flap patients and 7 of 10 (70%) of the sphincter pharyngoplasty patients. Three patients developed postoperative obstructive sleep apnea. All three of these patients had undergone attachment of a posterior pharyngeal flap.

Several authors have questioned whether the operation can be specifically tailored to the individual patient with velopharyngeal dysfunction on the basis of preoperative characteristics. Argamaso et al[95] hypothesized that preoperative lateral pharyngeal wall motion is necessary for the success of a posterior pharyngeal flap. Therefore, it was proposed that sphincter pharyngoplasty would be a better choice of operation in patients who do not have good preoperative lateral wall motion. Peat et al[96] tested this hypothesis by retrospectively studying 132 patients who had undergone surgical treatment of velopharyngeal dysfunction, with selection of the surgical procedure based on preoperative endoscopic findings, as follows:

1. Patients with poor palatal movement and little or no lateral wall adduction underwent combined attachment of superiorly based posterior pharyngeal flap and V-Y palatal pushback, or Honig operation.[97]

2. Patients with good palatal movement (anterior-posterior gap less than 0.5 cm) and little or no lateral wall adduction underwent modified Hynes pharyngoplasty.
3. Patients with poor palatal movement and good lateral wall adduction underwent attachment of a superiorly based posterior pharyngeal flap, the width of which was tailored to obturate the defect.
4. Patients with a small central defect were treated with a "fish flap."[98]

All patients had undergone speech and endoscopic or radiologic assessment preoperatively, and all patients also underwent such studies 6 months postoperatively. No statistical difference was found between the Honig, modified Hynes, and superiorly based pharyngeal flap groups in postoperative nasal resonance or nasal escape. More patients in the group that underwent the Honig operation had been severely hypernasal before surgery. No statistically significant difference was found between the modified Hynes and Honig operations in complications. Overall, 67 patients (51%) from the entire group reported catarrh or snoring postoperatively. The Honig operation achieved what was considered acceptable nasal resonance in 81% of patients, the modified Hynes operation also in 81% of patients, and the superiorly based pharyngeal flap in 63% of patients. The fish flap operation was successful in only 50% of patients, and the authors do not recommend it. The authors concluded that their selection criteria were valid, but this is not clear from their data, particularly because the speech results were virtually identical for their two largest groups and were similar to results that have been published in other series in which patients have not been subjected to similar selection criteria.

Another issue important in choosing a surgical procedure for management of velopharyngeal dysfunction is surgical salvage for patients whose first surgical attempt fails. Ease of revision has been emphasized by those who advocate the sphincter pharyngoplasty.[62] Kasten et al[66] studied their experience with surgical revision in a group of 30 children who underwent sphincter pharyngoplasty. They found that eight (27%) required revision of pharyngoplasty. Seven (23%) required revision because of persistent hypernasality and one (3%) because of postoperative hyponasality. Of the patients requiring revision for hypernasality, four were found to have had dehiscence of the pharyngoplasty flaps. All four had originally had end-to-end placement of the flaps. Revision consisted of re-elevation and repositioning of the flaps in a side-to-side configuration. In another patient with persistent hypernasality, the failure was thought to be due to low positioning of an end-to-end closure. The flaps were repositioned at a higher level at the time of revision. The one patient who was hyponasal after pharyngoplasty was treated by re-elevation of the flaps and widening of the port. Of the patients who were hypernasal before revision, four were still mildly hypernasal postoperatively, one was mildly hyponasal, one had mixed nasality, and one was lost to follow-up. The one patient who had revision because of hyponasality ended up still mildly hyponasal.

Revision of posterior pharyngeal flaps and sphincter pharyngoplasties was compared by Witt et al.[99] They evaluated 65 patients who underwent posterior pharyngeal flap attachment and 123 who underwent sphincter pharyngoplasty in a 7-year-period at a single center. They found that 13 (20%) of the posterior pharyngeal flap patients and 20 (16%) of the sphincter pharyngoplasty patients required further surgery. Seventeen of the 20 patients whose sphincter pharyngoplasty failed were salvaged with a single additional operation, and one patient was salvaged with two additional operations. Eight of the 13 patients whose pharyngeal flap failed were able to be corrected with one additional operation; the other five were successfully corrected with a second additional operation, one of whom was converted to a sphincter pharyngoplasty. All of the patients with secondarily corrected posterior pharyngeal flap were reported as being hyponasal after salvage, but with no other airway problems noted. These authors found that the most common cause of failure of either posterior pharyngeal flap or sphincter pharyngoplasty surgery was partial or complete flap dehiscence. Other causes of failure were excessively large ports and hypodynamic velopharynx. The conclusions from this review were that failed posterior pharyngeal flap attachment or sphincter pharyngoplasty can usually be salvaged with further surgery, although such additional surgery can often result in hyponasal speech.

CHOOSING TREATMENT IN SPECIFIC SITUATIONS

There is a role for various types of surgical as well as nonsurgical management of velopharyngeal dysfunction, depending on the specific clinical situation. Prosthetic management is reserved for patients who are not considered to be appropriate candidates for surgery and are good candidates for prosthetic management. Such patients include those with major associated medical problems that would increase their risk for surgery. Another situation in which we have found prosthetic management to be helpful is to obturate a large fistula in a child younger than 3½ years. Such obturation serves two functions. First, it can be a helpful test as to whether hypernasal speech is due to the fistula alone. A "quick test" with chewing gum or wax has not been as accurate for diagnosis. Obturating the fistula prosthetically gives the patient an opportunity to experiment and learn how to use the velopharyngeal apparatus, particularly in combination with speech therapy. This allows the surgeon to opt for fistula closure alone when age is appropriate. On the other hand, if satisfactory speech cannot be obtained with good obturation of the fistula and speech therapy, attachment of a posterior pharyngeal flap or sphincter pharyngoplasty can be combined with fistula closure. The second advantage of obturating the fistula is that when it is successful, it allows learning of proper articulation patterns, leading to the possibility of a better speech result once the problem is surgically corrected.

For patients who are candidates for surgical management, the choice of operation has been based on the size or magnitude of the velopharyngeal gap by pressure-flow testing, endoscopy, fluoroscopy, and other assessment modalities. When there is a large gap, which translates to more than 0.20 cm^2 on pressure-flow testing, attachment of a posterior pharyngeal flap has been used. When the gap is smaller, a modified Hynes pharyngoplasty can be considered. With very small but consistent gaps, palatal lengthening with muscle rearrangement by conversion to a Furlow repair (when the original repair was by a different technique) is thought to be a physiologic approach.

For patients who have had attachment of a posterior pharyngeal flap and who developed documented obstructive sleep apnea, initial management has been to institute nasal continuous positive airway pressure with sleep. Only when such conservative management is unsuccessful is the flap surgically divided. Interestingly, in our experience with seven such cases, the speech benefit of the flap is largely preserved, even after the flap is divided.[100] This is thought to be due to a combination of the bulk from the flap that remains on the posterior pharyngeal wall and surgical scarring, which tends to shrink the velopharyngeal orifice circumferentially.

REFERENCES

1. Loney RW, Bloem TJ: Velopharyngeal dysfunction: recommendations for use of nomenclature. Cleft Palate J 1987;24:334-335.
2. Trost-Cardamone JE: Coming to terms with VPI: a response to Loney and Bloem. Cleft Plate J 1989;26:68-70.
3. D'Antonio LL: Evaluation and management of velopharyngeal dysfunction: a speech pathologist's viewpoint. Probl Plast Reconstr Surg 1992;2:86-111.
4. Shprintzen RJ, Sher AE, Croft CB: Hypernasal speech caused by tonsillar hypertrophy. Int J Pediatr Otorhinolaryngol 1987;14:45-56.
5. Kummer AW, Billmire DA, Myer CM: Hypertrophic tonsils: the effect on resonance and velopharyngeal closure. Plast Reconstr Surg 1993;91:608-611.
6. Trost JE: Articulatory additions to the classical description of the speech of persons with cleft palate. Cleft Palate J 1981;18:193-203.
7. Peterson-Falzone SJ, Graham MS: Phoneme-specific nasal emission in children with withdrawal physical anomalies of the velopharyngeal mechanism. J Speech Hear Disord 1990;55:132-139.
8. Warren DW, DuBois AB: A pressure-flow technique for measuring velopharyngeal orifice area during continuous speech. Cleft Palate J 1964;1:52-71.
9. Warren DW, Devereux UL: An analog study of cleft palate speech. Cleft Palate J 1966;3:103-114.
10. Warren DW, Dalston RM, Trier WC, Holder MB: A pressure-flow technique for quantifying temporal patterns of palatopharyngeal closure. Cleft Palate J 1985;22:11-19.
11. Warren DE: Perci: a method for rating palatal efficiency. Cleft Palate J 1979;16:279-285.
12. Zajac D: Pressure-flow characteristics of /m/ and /p/ production in speakers without cleft palate: developmental findings. Cleft Palate Craniofac J 2000;37:468-477.
13. Zajac D, Hackett A: Temporal characteristics of aerodynamic segments in the speech of children and adults. Cleft Palate Craniofac J 2002;39:432-438.
14. D'Antonio LL, Marsh JL, Province MA, et al: Reliability of flexible fiberoptic nasopharyngoscopy for elevation of velopharyngeal function in a clinical population. Cleft Palate J 1989;26:217-225.
15. Shprintzen RJ: Evaluation of velopharyngeal insufficiency. Otolaryngol Clin North Am 1989;22:519-536.
16. Dalston RM, Warren DW: The diagnosis of velopharyngeal inadequacy. Clin Plast Surg 1985;12:685-695.
17. Gosain AK, Conley SF, Marks S, Larson D: Submucous cleft palate: diagnostic methods and outcomes of surgical treatment. Plast Reconstr Surg 1996;97:1497-1509.
18. Calnan JS: Submucous cleft palate. Br J Plast Surg 1954;6:264-282.
19. Weatherley-White RCA, Sakura CY Jr, Brenner LD, et al: Submucous cleft palate: its incidence, natural history, and indications for treatment. Plast Reconstr Surg 1972;49:297-304.
20. Crikelair GF, Striker P, Cosman B: The surgical treatment of submucous cleft palate. Plast Reconstr Surg 1970;45:58-65.
21. Abyholm FF: Submucous cleft palate. Scand J Plast Reconstr Surg 1976;10:209-212.
22. Porterfield HW, Mohler LR, Sandel A: Submucous cleft palate. Plast Reconstr Surg 1976;58:60-65.
23. Pensler JM, Bauer BS: Levator repositioning and palatal lengthening for submucous clefts. Plast Reconstr Surg 1988;82:765-769.
24. Chen PK-T, Wu J, Hung K-F, et al: Surgical correction of submucous cleft palate with Furlow palatoplasty. Plast Reconstr Surg 1996;97:1136-1146.
25. Seagle MB, Patti CS, Williams WN, Wood VD: Submucous cleft palate: a 10-year series. Ann Plast Surg 1999;42:142-148.
26. Passavant G: Über die Beseitigung der naselnden Sprache bei angeborenen Spalten des Harten und weichen Gaumens (Gaumensegel-Schlundnaht und Rucklagerung des Gaumensegels). Arch Klin Chir 1865;6:333-349.
27. Schoenborn K: Über eine neue Methode der Staphylorrhaphie. Verh Dtsch Ges Chir 1875;4:235-239.
28. Schoenborn K: Vorstellung eines Falle von Staphyloplastik. Verh Dtsch Ges Chir 1886;15:57-62.
29. Rosenthal W: Pathologie und Therapie der Gaumendefekte. Fortschr Zahnheilk 1928;4:55-56.
30. Padgett EC: The repair of cleft palates after unsuccessful operations, with special reference to cases with an extensive loss of palatal tissue. Arch Surg 1930;20:453-472.
31. Hogan VM: A clarification of the goals in cleft palate speech and the introduction of the lateral port control (L.P.C.) pharyngeal flap. Cleft Palate J 1973;10:331-345.
32. Shprintzen RJ, Lewin ML, Croft ML, et al: A comprehensive study of pharyngeal flap surgery: tailor made flaps. Cleft Palate J 1979;16:46-55.

33. Kapetansky DI: Bilateral transverse pharyngeal flaps for repair of cleft palate. Plast Reconstr Surg 1973;52:52-54.

34. Skoog T: The pharyngeal flap operation in cleft palate. Br J Plast Surg 1965;18:265-282.

35. Hamlen M: Speech changes after pharyngeal flap surgery. Plast Reconstr Surg 1970;46:437-444.

36. Whitaker LA, Randall P, Graham WP III, et al: A prospective and randomized series comparing superiorly and inferiorly based posterior pharyngeal flaps. Cleft Palate J 1972;9:304-311.

37. Karling J, Henningsson G, Larson O, Isberg A: Comparison between two types of pharyngeal flap with regard to configuration at rest and function and speech outcome. Cleft Palate Craniofac J 1999;36:154-165.

38. Karling J, Henningsson G, Larson O, Isberg A: Adaptation of pharyngeal wall adduction after pharyngeal flap surgery. Cleft Palate Craniofac J 1999;36:166-172.

39. Jackson P, Whitaker LA, Randall P: Airway hazard associated with pharyngeal flaps in patients who have the Pierre Robin syndrome. Plast Reconstr Surg 1976;58:184-186.

40. Robson MC, Stankiewicz JA, Mendelsohn JS: Cor pulmonale secondary to cleft palate repair. Plast Reconstr Surg 1977;59:754-757.

41. Wray C, Dann J, Holtmann B: A comparison of three techniques of palatorrhaphy: in-hospital morbidity. Cleft Palate J 1979;16:42-45.

42. Kravath RE, Pollak CP, Borowiecki B, Weitzman ED: Obstructive sleep apnea and death associated with surgical correction of velopharyngeal incompetence. J Pediatr 1980;96:645-648.

43. Thurston JB, Larson DL, Shanks JC, et al: Nasal obstruction as a complication of pharyngeal flap surgery Cleft Palate J 1980;17:148-154.

44. Schettler D: Intra- and postoperative complications in surgical repair of clefts in infancy. J Maxillofac Surg 1973;1:40-44.

45. Orr WC, Levine NS, Buchanan RT: Effects of cleft palate repair and pharyngeal flap surgery on upper airway obstruction during sleep. Plast Reconstr Surg 1987;80:226-230.

46. Valnicek SM, Zuker RM, Halpern LM, Roy WL: Perioperative complications of superior pharyngeal flap surgery in children. Plast Reconstr Surg 1994;93:954-958.

47. Fraulin FOG, Valnicek SM, Zuker RM: Decreasing the perioperative complications associated with the superior pharyngeal flap operation. Plast Reconstr Surg 1998;102:10-18.

48. Ysunza A, Garcia-Velasco M, Garcia-Garcia M, et al: Obstructive sleep apnea secondary to surgery for velopharyngeal insufficiency. Cleft Palate Craniofac J 1993;30:387-390.

49. Sirois M, Caouette-Laberge L, Spier S, et al: Sleep apnea following a pharyngeal flap: a feared complication. Plast Reconstr Surg 1994;93:943-947.

50. Lesavoy MA, Borud LJ, Thorson T, et al: Upper airway obstruction after pharyngeal flap surgery. Ann Plast Surg 1996;36:26-32.

51. Mitnick RJ, Bello JA, Golding-Kushner KJ, et al: The use of magnetic resonance angiography prior to pharyngeal flap surgery in patients with velocardiofacial syndrome. Plast Reconstr Surg 1996;97:908-919.

52. Hynes W: Pharyngoplasty by muscle transplantation. Br J Plast Surg 1950;3:128-135.

53. Hynes W: The results of pharyngoplasty by muscle transplantation in "failed cleft palate" cases, with special reference to the influence of the pharynx on voice production. Ann R Coll Surg Engl 1953;13:17-35.

54. Orticochea M: Construction of a dynamic muscle sphincter in cleft palates. Plast Reconstr Surg 1968;41:323-327.

55. Jackson IT, Silverton JS: The sphincter pharyngoplasty as a secondary procedure in cleft palates. Plast Reconstr Surg 1977;59:518-524.

56. Hynes W: Observations on pharyngoplasty. Br J Plast Surg 1967;20:244-256.

57. Orticochea M: A review of 236 cleft palate patients treated with dynamic muscle sphincter. Plast Reconstr Surg 1983;71:180-186.

58. Orticochea M: The timing and management of dynamic muscular pharyngeal sphincter construction in velopharyngeal insufficiency. Br J Plast Surg 1999;52:85-87.

59. Riski JE, Serafin D, Riefkohl R, et al: A rationale for modifying the site of insertion of the Orticochea pharyngoplasty. Plast Reconstr Surg 1984;73:882-890.

60. Riski JE, Ruff GL, Georgiade GS, et al: Evaluation of the sphincter pharyngoplasty. Cleft Palate Craniofac J 1992;29:254-261.

61. Pigott RW: The results of pharyngoplasty by muscle transplantation by Wilfred Hynes. Br J Plast Surg 1993;46:440-442.

62. Moss ALH, Pigott RW, Albery EH: Hynes pharyngoplasty revisited. Plast Reconstr Surg 1987;79:346-353.

63. Witt PD, D'Antonio LL, Zimmerman GJ, Marsh JL: Sphincter pharyngoplasty: a preoperative and postoperative analysis of perceptual speech characteristics and endoscopic studies of velopharyngeal function. Plast Reconstr Surg 1994;93:1154-1168.

64. James NK, Twist M, Turner MM, Milward TM: An audit of velopharyngeal incompetence treated by the Orticochea pharyngoplasty. Br J Plast Surg 1996;49:197-201.

65. Georgantopoulou AA, Thatte MR, Razzelle RE, Watson ACH: The effect of sphincter pharyngoplasty on the range of velar movement. Br J Plast Surg 1996;49:358-362.

66. Kasten SJ, Buchman SR, Stevenson C, Berger M: A retrospective analysis of revision of sphincter pharyngoplasty. Ann Plast Surg 1997;39:583-589.

67. Witt P, Cohen D, Grames LM, Marsh J: Sphincter pharyngoplasty for the surgical management of speech dysfunction associated with velocardiofacial syndrome. Br J Plast Surg 1999;52:613-618.

68. Witt PD, Marsh JL, Arlis H, et al: Quantification of dynamic velopharyngeal port excursion following sphincter pharyngoplasty. Plast Reconstr Surg 1998;101:1205-1211.

69. Witt PD, Myckatyn T, Marsh JL, et al: Does preexisting posterior pharyngeal wall motion drive the dynamism of sphincter pharyngoplasty? Plast Reconstr Surg 1998;101:1457-1462.

70. Ysunza A, Pamplona MC, Molina F, et al: Velopharyngeal motion after sphincter pharyngoplasty: a videonasopharyngoscopic and electromyographic study. Plast Reconstr Surg 1999;104:905-910.

71. Witt PD, Marsh JL, Muntz HR, et al: Acute and obstructive sleep apnea as a complication of sphincter pharyngoplasty. Cleft Palate Craniofac J 1996;33:183-189.

72. Dorrance GM: Congenital insufficiency of the palate. Arch Surg 1930;21:185.

73. Wardill WEM: Technique of operation for cleft palate. Br J Surg 1937;25:117.

74. Kilner TP: Cleft lip and palate repair technique. St Thomas Hosp Rep 1937;2:127.

75. Furlow LT: Cleft palate repair by double opposing Z-plasty. Plast Reconstr Surg 1986;78:724-736.

76. Passavant G: Über die Verbesserung der Sprache nach der Uranoplastik. Arch Klin Chir 1879;23:771.

77. Gersuny R: Über eine subcutane Prosthese. Z Heilk 1900;21:199-204.

78. Eckstein H: Demonstration of a paraffin prosthesis in defects of the face and palate. Dermatologica 1904;11:772-778.

79. Perthes H, as reported by Hollweg E: Beitrag zur Behandlung von Gaumenspalten [dissertation]. Tübingen, 1912.

80. Bentley FH, Watkins II: Speech after repair of cleft palate. Lancet 1947;2:862-865.

81. Denny AD, Marks SM, Oliff-Carneol S: Correction of velopharyngeal insufficiency by pharyngeal augmentation using autogenous cartilage: a preliminary report. Cleft Palate J 1993;30:46-54.

82. Halle H: Gaumennaht und gaumenplastik. Arch Ohr Nas Kehlkopfheilk 1925;12:377.

83. von Gaza WV: Transplantation of the face fatty tissue in the retropharyngeal area in cases of cleft palate. Lecture, German Surgical Society, April 9, 1926.

84. Hagerty RF, Hill MJ: Cartilage pharyngoplasty in cleft palate patients. Surg Gynecol Obstet 1961;112:350.

85. Blocksma R: Correction of velopharyngeal insufficiency by Silastic pharyngeal implants. Plast Reconstr Surg 1963;31:268.

86. Brauer RO: Retropharyngeal implantation of silicone gel pillows for velopharyngeal incompetence. Plast Reconstr Surg 1973;51:254.

87. Bluestone CD, Musgrave RH, McWilliams BJ: Teflon injection pharyngoplasty: status 1968. Laryngoscope 1968;78:558.

88. Sturim HS, Jacob CT: Teflon pharyngoplasty. Plast Reconstr Surg 1972;49:180.

89. Kuehn DP, Van Demark DR: Assessment of velopharyngeal competency following Teflon pharyngoplasty. Cleft Palate J 1978;15:145.

90. Wolford LM, Oelschlaeger M, Deal R: Proplast as a pharyngeal wall implant to correct velopharyngeal insufficiency. Cleft Palate J 1989;26:119.

91. Suersen W Sr: A new system of artificial palates. Am J Dent Sci 1867;1:373-379.

92. McGrath CO, Anderson MW: Prosthetic treatment of velopharyngeal incompetence. In Bardach J, Morris HL, eds: Multidisciplinary Management of Cleft Lip and Palate. Philadelphia, WB Saunders, 1990:809-815.

93. Sloan GM, Reinisch JR, Nichter LS, Downey SE: Surgical management of velopharyngeal insufficiency: pharyngoplasty vs. pharyngeal flap. Plast Surg Forum 1990;13:128-130.

94. Pensler JM, Reich DS: A comparison of speech results after the pharyngeal flap and the dynamic sphincteroplasty procedures. Ann Plast Surg 1991;26:441-443.

95. Argamaso RV, Shprintzen RJ, Strauch B, et al: The role of lateral pharyngeal wall movement in pharyngeal flap surgery. Plast Reconstr Surg 1980;66:214-219.

96. Peat BG, Albery EH, Jones K, Pigott RW: Tailoring velopharyngeal surgery: the influence of etiology and type of operation. Plast Reconstr Surg 1994;93:948-953.

97. Honig CA: The treatment of velopharyngeal insufficiency after palatal repair. Arch Chir Neerl 1967;19:71-81.

98. Pigott RW: Objectives for cleft palate repair. Ann Plast Surg 1987;19:247.

99. Witt PD, Myckatyn T, Marsh JL: Salvaging the failed pharyngoplasty: intervention outcome. Cleft Palate Craniofac J 1998;35:447-453.

100. Agarwal T, Sloan GM, Zajac D, et al: Speech benefits of posterior pharyngeal flap are preserved after surgical flap division for obstructive sleep apnea: experience with division of 12 flaps. J Craniofac Surg 2003;14:630-636.

Secondary Deformities of the Cleft Lip, Nose, and Palate

SAMUEL STAL, MD ✦ LARRY H. HOLLIER, JR., MD

Secondary deformities after cleft lip, cleft nose, and palatal repair are the rule, not the exception. Because essentially all patients are operated on within the first year of life, the long period of dramatic growth and the resultant scar after the repair of the cleft structures both profoundly affect the end result. Delaying the definitive repair until a child has reached adolescence or adulthood might minimize problems; however, early functional repair of the cleft deformity is mandatory for normal development. Unrestrained growth of the cleft margins may result in even more severe secondary deformities. It is ideal to allow the facial structures to develop in a normal relation to one another in the intended "functional matrix."[1]

Consequently, the correction of secondary deformities of the cleft lip, nose, and palate should be seen as an integral part of the care of these patients. In fact, these secondary procedures are in many ways more difficult than the primary repair. Unlike the relatively uniform nature of the initial deformity, secondary problems are widely varied in both their appearance and their etiology.[2] In addition, there are added psychosocial issues that must be dealt with in this population of older patients. Although many factors may contribute to a poor result in significant secondary deformities, the most prominent is poor preoperative analysis and design. The correct procedure must be appropriately matched with the correct deformity. This takes a great deal of experience and flexibility on the part of the surgeon. The cleft is the result of an embryologic insult, and in most severe cases, there is a significant primary tissue deficiency in the deformity. Even in the best of hands, the initial insult to the tissue will forever contribute to secondary deformities.

EVALUATION

Before any surgical procedure is undertaken for the correction of a secondary deformity, the specific nature of that deformity must be identified and documented. A careful evaluation must be performed of all of the involved structures. With respect to the lip, this includes examination of the lip scar, the orbicularis muscle, the vermilion and white roll, the shape and symmetry of Cupid's bow, and the mucosa. Elements of the nasal deformity that must be evaluated include the columella and the position of the alar bases, nostril shape and size, nasal tip anatomy, and deficiencies in nasal lining. The palate must be carefully evaluated for the presence of a fistula, the degree of scarring, and the anatomic length. All of these elements must be related in three dimensions to the underlying skeletal base on which they have developed. That is, maxillary hypoplasia, malposition and outward rotation of the cleft maxillary segments, and instability of the premaxilla may all contribute to the observed secondary deformity. This skeletal imbalance then has a significant impact on the quality of results obtained from the initial cleft repair. This is particularly true for the cleft lip rhinoplasty, as the platform on which the nasal repair rests is not only hypoplastic but also in a different plane, contributing to persistent problems with asymmetry of the nasal pyramid and the resultant stigmata of a columellar displacement or alar and nostril asymmetry.[2]

With this in mind, it must be appreciated that rarely do secondary deformities exist in isolation. For example, a widened lip scar may be secondary to failure to unite the orbicularis oris muscle at the time of initial evaluation or tension secondary to a paucity of tissue leading to a tight lip. In either case, simple revision of the scar is doomed to failure unless the underlying problem is addressed concomitantly. By careful, systematic evaluation of all the components of the cleft deformity, the secondary intervention can be designed to address the true problem, maximizing the chance for success and minimizing the number of secondary procedures necessary. Although there are classification schemes that attempt to simplify this evaluation, they tend to be cumbersome and serve as little more than checklists for evaluation.[3,4]

TIMING

The timing of intervention for secondary deformities in the cleft patient is highly variable. Despite Millard's belief that surgery from the ages of 8 to 18 years is followed by an exaggerated reaction involving long periods of exuberant scar formation, there are no absolute rules regarding the timing of surgery.[5] This having been said, all patients should be evaluated for secondary surgery before the start of kindergarten. At this time, peer interactions increase substantially and

may be a source of great distress for the cleft patient and the family. All other decisions in regard to timing are predicated on the severity of the problem relative to function and appearance balanced with the emotional and physical maturity of the patient (Fig. 98-1).

In early life, decisions relative to timing are the responsibility of the parents and the surgeon. The decision to perform a secondary intervention must be based on the surgeon's expectation that the deformity can be substantially improved by surgery and on a strong desire of the parents to facilitate a solution to the problem. In adolescence, the child becomes more capable of expressing opinions about his or her appearance and must be a significant contributor to surgical decisions and timing. The adolescent patient's input is critical, and no procedure should be undertaken unless some degree of desire for correction is expressed by the patient.

A critical factor that must be considered in this decision is the physical maturity of the patient. This is particularly pertinent with respect to cleft lip rhinoplasty. Whereas minor nasal revisions are perfectly acceptable in the very young patient, full osseocartilaginous vault surgery and septal modification are usually delayed until after nasal growth is complete. Nasal growth ceases in girls at approximately 11 to 12 years of age and in boys at approximately 14 years of age.[6] Once nasal growth is complete and the patient is thought to be mature enough to participate in the decision, there is no prohibition to a complete rhinoplasty in the cleft patient.

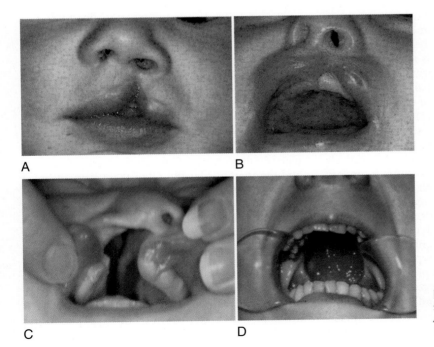

A

B

C

D

FIGURE 98-1. The spectrum of secondary cleft lip deformities. *A,* Mild. *B,* Moderate. *C* and *D,* Severe.

CLEFT LIP

Normal Lip Anatomy

The normal upper lip has as its central landmark the philtrum and Cupid's bow. The philtrum is composed of two columns on either side of the central dimple. The columns end at the level of the Cupid's bow peaks, at which point they are approximately 8 to 12 mm wide in the normal adult.[7] The philtrum columns gradually narrow as one approaches the columella, where they are approximately 6 to 9 mm apart. The normal philtrum is 17 mm or less in length.[7] These measurements are different in the young child. The most critical measurements at the time of primary lip repair (approximately 3 months) are the width of the philtrum at the level of the Cupid's bow peaks (6 mm) and the vertical height of the cleft prolabium (6 to 7.5 mm). Because the surgically reconstructed philtrum has a tendency to widen with time, it is critical that it not be designed any wider than this at the initial operation.

Another important anatomic structure in the normal lip is the white roll. This is the margin of tissue between the vermilion mucosa and the lip skin. This creates a smooth transition between these two structures. Incisions within this layer should be avoided because they cause distortion and pigment changes. There is no acceptable surgical technique to reconstruct this critical structure once this has occurred.

Appropriate anatomic repair of the lip musculature is an essential part of a successful cleft repair.[8] Orbicularis muscle fibers become atrophic and disorganized near the cleft margins.[8] Restoration of the normal muscle anatomy is essential to balanced facial growth, and failure to do so will lead to typical secondary deformities. It has been stated that the alar incision should be limited in the area of the cleft alar base to avoid denervation of the underlying nasolabial musculature. However, in patients with severe deformities, this is difficult because it is important to be able to move the lip and nose complex independently to achieve a better relationship. A superior plane can be designed by suturing the deep superior part of the lateral orbicularis muscle to the fibrous tissue at the base of the septum in front of the nasal spine, with the remainder of the muscle then joined by suturing to the orbicularis of the contralateral side. This suture junction should be just lateral to the midline to simulate a philtral ridge. These muscles can sometimes be overlapped to improve anteroposterior height.[8]

Also important with respect to lip anatomy is the relationship of the upper lip to the lower lip and dentition. At rest, the upper lip normally projects 2 to 3 mm anterior to the lower lip. There should be no lip incompetence. That is, the upper and lower lips should rest together when the patient is in the relaxed state. Incompetence of the lips is frequently disguised by overactivity of the mentalis muscle. The upper lip should rest so that approximately 2 to 4 mm of the mucosal edge of the maxillary incisors is exposed (incisor show). With maximal smile, no more than approximately 1 to 2 mm of gingiva should be exposed.

Common Secondary Deformities

In discussing secondary cleft deformities, one must emphasize prevention. In the majority of cases, it is easier to avoid a secondary deformity than it is to correct it. Consequently, before any surgery is undertaken, it is our strong belief that the patient needs to be evaluated for presurgical orthopedics. That is, the cleft segments can be manipulated either passively or actively by intraoral appliances or pin-retained devices to bring them into a more normal anatomic relationship.[9,10] Most recently, the technique of nasoalveolar molding has been used to improve the lip and nasal repair.[11] This technique places an intraoral appliance within the cleft margins that includes an extension anteriorly and applies pressure within the nasal vestibule (Fig. 98-2). The lip is then taped across the appliance. Weekly, the intraoral component is reduced in size to passively guide the cleft maxillary segments into a more normal relationship. By doing so, the gap at the level of the lip, alveolus, and palate is diminished, facilitating repair of these structures. The nasal component gradually reshapes the collapsed ala of the nose on the cleft side, greatly facilitating cleft lip rhinoplasty.[12] In patients in whom the alveolar segments have been well approximated, primary gingivoperiosteoplasty is possible. This reapproximates the gingiva and periosteum of the alveolar segments and decreases the need for secondary procedures to bone graft the alveolar cleft in some patients.[13]

In the operating room, accurate measurements are made when the patient is asleep, before local anesthesia is injected so there is no distortion. It is important to use precision instruments for both measurement and marking, that is, a caliper and a fine surgical marker. These markings should be made indelible with use of methylene blue and a 25-gauge needle or a No. 67 Beaver blade to ensure that they are not washed off during surgical preparation of the patient. After the cleft is released, the tissue is handled very carefully with hooks to avoid pressure necrosis.

The technique of lip repair has a significant influence on the overall result. In the triangular flap technique of Tennison and Randall, the tension is mostly placed in the lower third of the lip. In the Millard rotation-advancement repair, this tension is placed in the upper third. Whereas it is thought that the lower third has an excess of tissue relative to the upper third, it is preferable to place tension on the repair at the apex of the triangle of the philtrum. The Millard rotation-advancement technique also allows the

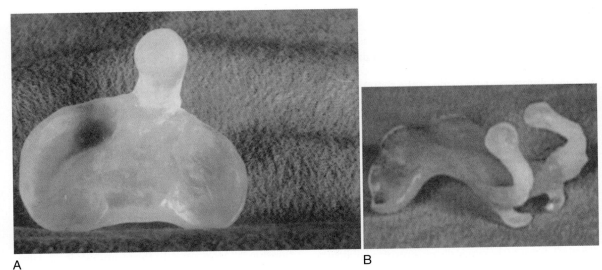

FIGURE 98-2. Nasoalveolar molding appliances. *A,* Unilateral appliance. *B,* Bilateral appliance.

development of a C flap to lengthen the columella and to give a greater fullness and width to the base. Consequently, with the additional tissue, the nasal sill and nose repair is optimized with the Millard technique (Fig. 98-3).

Every effort should be made at the time of the initial procedure to adequately release the soft tissue and to reconstruct the floor of the nose. This eliminates the anterior fistula so frequently seen in older patients. After the initial lip repair, this area is never as well visualized unless the entire lip repair is taken down. Consequently, the secondary correction of this problem is more difficult and not as successful.

Once secondary deformities have become established and the decision has been made to perform the surgical correction, this should be accomplished with as many procedures as necessary in one operation to minimize the number of interventions. The remainder of the chapter describes individual deformities and the surgical techniques that have been used successfully.

VERMILION ABNORMALITIES

Malalignment

Vermilion malalignment presents as a step-off in the vermilion border (Fig. 98-4). Step-offs in the alignment of the vermilion as small as 2 mm are

FIGURE 98-3. Untreated cleft nose with deformity of nostril sill and deviation after Tennison repair.

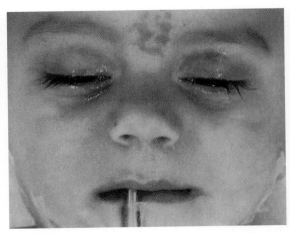

FIGURE 98-4. Lip repair demonstrating malalignment of the vermilion border.

noticeable because of the lack of color continuity; they are caused by inaccurate approximation of the vermilion border at the time of initial lip repair. Malalignment can be minimized by tattooing the lip at the level of the vermilion border with methylene blue and a 25-gauge needle or a No. 15 blade just lateral to the line of planned lip incision. This allows accurate reapproximation of the vermilion after rotation and advancement. Once a malalignment has been established, a Z-plasty rearrangement of the region of the step-off is usually successful in realignment and in minimizing scar formation (Fig. 98-5). Angles of 45 degrees are ideal, but a 30- to 60-degree Z-plasty can be done with local tissue rearrangement. This allows the re-establishment of the smooth vermilion-white roll line with minimal morbidity. It also observes the principle that only vermilion should be used to reconstruct vermilion. The use of mucosa in this area is contraindicated because it is different in color and texture and tends to dry and crust easily.

In the case of elevation of the vermilion border at the site of repair, the intervention depends on the severity of the deformity and the time course of its appearance. Early after the classic Millard rotation-advancement, this is often seen to a minor degree.[14] However, it most frequently resolves after scar maturation. Active massage with an emollient (Mederma, vitamin E, or aloe vera) can facilitate scar contracture. If significant elevation persists beyond the 12-month postoperative period, correction should be considered. For minor problems, diamond-shaped excision of the lip scar with pants-over-vest closure usually suffices (Fig. 98-6).[15] This increases the length of the scar and brings the vermilion down. This may also be achieved by use of a Z-plasty. In patients with moderate to severe deformities, the problem is more frequently the result of an inadequate rotation at the time of initial lip repair. The only recourse in such a situation is to take down the repair and to rerotate the lip. Care must be taken to reapproximate the orbicularis appropriately in these situations; failure to do so will lead to shortening of the scar.

Vermilion Deficiency: Unilateral Clefts

In considering deficiencies of the vermilion, one must approach unilateral and bilateral cleft lips differently. With respect to unilateral cleft lip deformities, deficiency of vermilion is a common problem. This is frequently referred to as a "whistle" deformity or a notch (Fig. 98-7). There is usually less vermilion on the medial portion of the lip than on the lateral lip segment. This builds in an asymmetry, which can lead to the secondary deformity even in the best designed skin alignment. This asymmetry can be prevented or minimized at the time of initial lip repair by back-cutting the mucosa in the gingivobuccal sulcus after advancement of the vermilion bulk of the lip. The resultant defect can usually be closed primarily or special attention paid to avoid a straight-line closure, which tends to contract and lend to notching. Closing these mucosal defects obliquely by half Z-plasties and filling in any residual defect with the M flap are helpful maneuvers.

Once the deformity has become established, most deficiencies can be addressed by local tissue rearrangement. In the majority of patients, there exists a relative paucity of tissue adjacent to a relative excess. The goal is to redistribute this tissue properly to achieve a natural-appearing vermilion. Direct excision of a notch only increases tension in the area of paucity. Resection of thick scar followed by incremental rearrangement of the relative excess to the area of tension with use of back-cuts and distal release will often address mild to moderate notches.

In attempting to bring the relative excess of tissue to the area of deficiency, the planned flaps must be designed carefully. One should minimize the amount of local infiltration used to avoid misjudging the available mucosa. By back-cutting the mucosa adjacent to

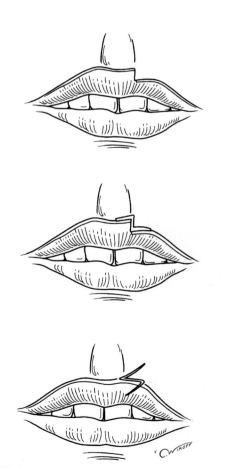

FIGURE 98-5. Z-plasty for realignment of white roll.

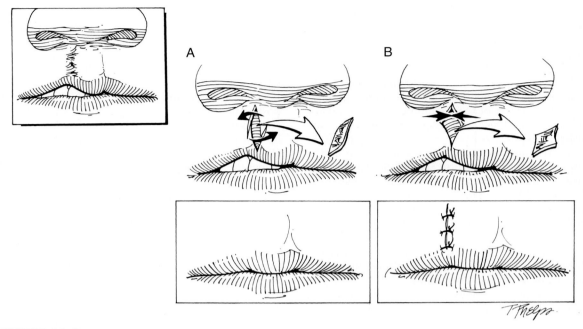

FIGURE 98-6. *A* and *B*, Diamond-shaped excision of the scar with linear closure lengthens the scar; the vest-over-pants closure adds bulk and prevents scar depression.

the region of deficiency, the tissue may be advanced and the primary defect closed.

Additional tissue may also be recruited by use of a V-Y advancement or a Z-plasty (Fig. 98-8). The location of these advancement flaps must be carefully planned with respect to the areas of tissue excess. The

leading edge of the flap must also be designed wide enough to adequately fill the vermilion deficiency. Kapetansky[16] described a double V-Y advancement that was horizontally based. However, in our opinion, although the lip looks good at rest, this frequently results in a significant amount of scarring that can

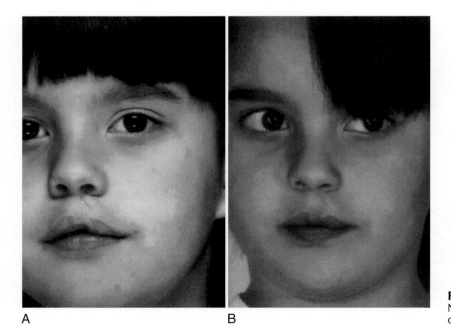

A   B

FIGURE 98-7. *A* and *B*, Notching or a "whistle" deformity of the vermilion.

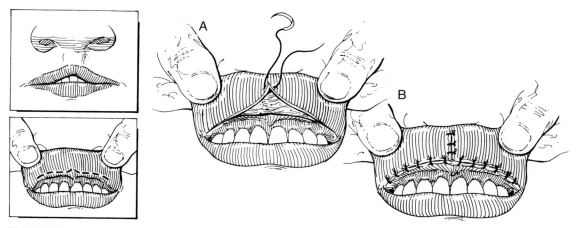

FIGURE 98-8. *A* and *B*, V-Y advancement may be used to recruit tissue into the area of vermilion deficiency.

give the lip an unnatural feel and appearance with animation.

It may also be helpful in these situations to perform an elliptical excision of tissue on the underside of the lip to help minimize areas of residual fullness. This may help in minimizing the residual vermilion asymmetry. Proper muscle closure is important to fill the dead space after these procedures, and meticulous hemostasis must be achieved; if not, the dead space formed may ultimately fill with blood and lead to a scar that compromises the final result.

For many years, dermal fat grafting has been used with limited success. In some patients in whom there is available mucosa but a paucity of underlying tissue, dermal fat grafts have occasionally been useful.

However, predictability of these grafts has been mixed. In the authors' experience, in approximately half of these patients, although the appearance is significantly improved, the resulting firmness of the lip is unacceptable.

With the increased popularity of fat injections,[17] they have been used for the correction of mild to moderate vermilion deficiencies with mixed success. It would seem that this technique is best used in minor deformities in lips with minimal scarring. In older patients with severely scarred lips, there may be difficulty in exerting sufficient force with the fat injections to fill out the area of deficiency and overcome the contracting forces of the vermilion scar (Fig. 98-9).

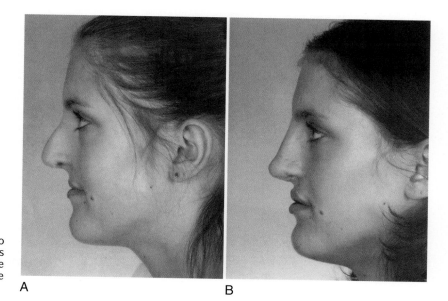

FIGURE 98-9. Fat injection to correct upper lip deficiencies after repair. *A*, Preoperative appearance. *B*, Postoperative appearance.   A   B

Vermilion Deficiency: Bilateral Clefts

Perhaps more common than unilateral vermilion deficiencies are deficiencies after bilateral cleft lip repair (Fig. 98-10). Although local tissue rearrangement as described before may suffice for minor deformities, the deficiency in the case of bilateral cleft lips is usually more severe and often requires an Abbe flap transfer for correction (Fig. 98-11). In addition to replacing vermilion bulk, the Abbe flap helps correct the discrepancy in projection between the upper and lower lip, which frequently exists in these patients. That is, the relative excess and pout of the lower lip is removed and transferred to the upper lip (Fig. 98-12).

With the improvement of techniques in repair of unilateral and bilateral cleft lips, Abbe flaps are used less frequently than they once were. Although this flap has historically been used primarily in the bilateral cleft lip, in unilateral clefts with malpositioned scars and extreme deficiencies in length or height, this flap may prove invaluable. However, in lips with reasonable dimensions, all local measures of tissue rearrangement and scar revision should be attempted first.

The procedure may be performed in children as young as 10 months of age as long as an airway such as a nasal trumpet is secured in the postoperative period. In performing this flap, it is critical to tattoo all markings with use of methylene blue and a Beaver blade to ensure appropriate alignment of the vermilion border. The labial artery should be carefully dissected with its location on the cut margin of the flap used as a guide. During formation of the recipient site, the surgeon should take the opportunity to fully release the floor of the nose and the columella, using tissue from the discarded philtrum if necessary. Once inset, the flap may be protected by 28-gauge wire used as an Ivy loop for intermaxillary fixation. This loop can be loosely tied so that the patient can open the mouth to insert a straw but not wide enough to disrupt the flap. The loop can be removed at the first postoperative visit.

CUPID'S BOW ABNORMALITIES

Significant abnormalities of Cupid's bow in unilateral cleft lip deformity are usually the result of malalignment or notching and can be corrected by the techniques described in the preceding section. In severe deformities, it is necessary to take down the previous lip repair and to repeat rotation-advancement. Although skin excision and vermilion advancement have been described in the correction of this deformity,[18] this procedure is not recommended because of the degree of scarring and artificial appearance that it induces.

In the bilateral cleft lip patient with significant Cupid's bow abnormalities, an Abbe flap as described in the preceding section is most frequently the best option because the lower lip has a Cupid's bow and philtral dimple. In the bilateral cleft lip repair with a degree of deformity not thought to warrant an Abbe flap, a direct skin excision and vermilion advancement could be performed with the Abbe flap reserved as a salvage procedure. However, if the deformity is severe enough to require surgery, it is preferable to proceed directly to the flap transfer.

SULCUS ABNORMALITIES

Deficiencies of the labial sulcus are most common after bilateral cleft lip repair and often reflect the underlying anatomy of the deformity rather than a deficiency

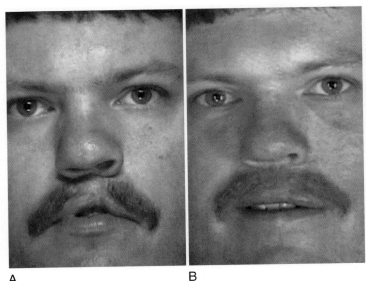

A   B

FIGURE 98-10. *A,* Vermilion deficiency after bilateral cleft lip repair. *B,* After repair with local tissue.

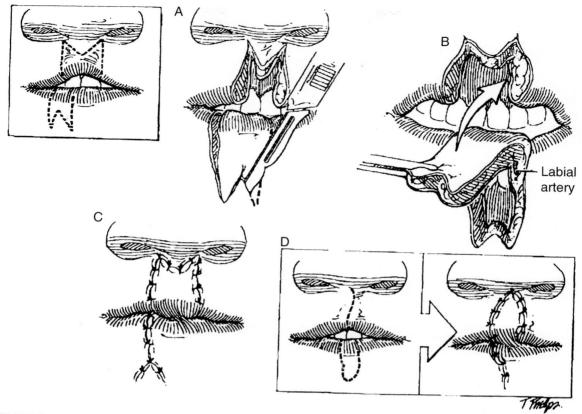

FIGURE 98-11. *A to D,* Abbe flap transfer uses lower lip tissue to augment the central upper lip with a pedicle based on the inferior labial artery.

in the initial technique used in the repair. Although the labial vermilion is most frequently turned down and used as the sulcus with vermilion flaps developed from tissue laterally, this is often not sufficient to construct an adequate sulcus. These patients most frequently present around the time of initiation of orthodontia before bone grafting. Although minor deficiencies may be corrected by local tissue rearrangements such as the V-Y advancement, the best solution is most frequently a release of the sulcus with a recreation of the defect and grafting. Buccal mucosa should be used as the graft material, and a dental amalgam should be used as a stent to maximize graft take. Although there are some advocates of prolonged stenting to minimize contraction,[2] this is usually unrealistic in children.

ORBICULARIS MUSCLE DEFORMITIES

The continuity of the orbicularis muscle is an important component in the appearance and function of the normal lip. Unilateral and bilateral clefts result in discontinuity of both the superficial and deep portions of the orbicularis (Fig. 98-13). Rather than forming a continuous sphincter, the muscles insert aberrantly in the region of the alar base.[19] In this area, the underlying maxilla as well as these muscles are hypoplastic, making a depression.

Failure to reposition and unite the orbicularis results in several problems. Most prominently, the patients may present with bulging on either side of the lip repair with attempted animation. It may also result in a widened and short lip scar that distorts the repair. The continuity of this sphincter is also important in shaping the underlying palatal shelves and premaxillary segment. After successful repair of the lip and orbicularis, the continuous action of the muscle helps bring the palatal shelves together and the premaxillary segment posteriorly. By doing so, it provides a more anatomic platform for the cleft nasal deformity and enables more efficient correction of this at subsequent procedures. As mentioned previously, appropriate tightening and cephalic suspension of the muscle in the upper lip help correct the depression commonly seen caudal to the nostril sill and alar base.

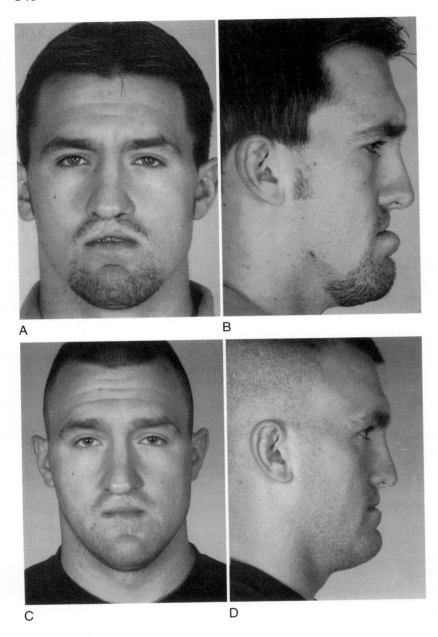

A

B

C

D

FIGURE 98-12. Abbe flap correction of a bilateral notch deformity. *A* and *B*, Preoperative appearance. *C* and *D*, Postoperative appearance.

If the evaluation of the secondary cleft lip deformity reveals discontinuity of the orbicularis, its repair should be incorporated into the secondary operation. This generally involves reopening the repair and dissecting the orbicularis for several millimeters from the skin in the subdermal plane. This provides a cuff for reapproximation to the contralateral orbicularis or to the prolabial segment. The muscle pedicle should be rotated down from its more vertical position to the appropriate horizontal orientation. In the unilateral deformity, care should be taken not to dissect the orbicularis beyond the midportion of the philtrum, or the normal philtral dimple may be distorted. In the bilateral deformity, it is unnecessary to attempt to reapproximate the muscle beneath the prolabial skin. It is sufficient to reattach it to the lateral aspects of the prolabium.

SCARS

The scar associated with a cleft lip often looks its best at the first office visit after the primary repair while it is approximated by sutures and anatomically aligned. The patient's family and the physician are often very

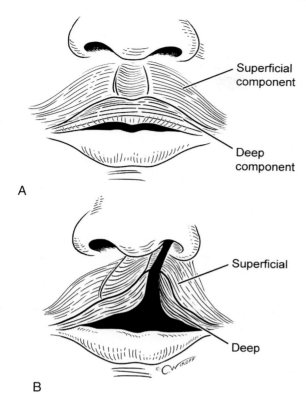

A

B

FIGURE 98-13. Orbicularis oris anatomy. *A,* Normal lip. Both the superficial and deep components of the orbicularis form a continuous sphincter. *B,* Cleft lip. The deep component to the orbicularis is interrupted by the cleft; the superficial component fans out at the cleft margins, becoming disorganized and inserting aberrantly into the region of the alar base.

happy. However, with time, the process of normal scar maturation may result in problems such as scar hypertrophy. There may also be scar contracture resulting in secondary deformities such as notching of the vermilion or shortening of the lip. Parents should be advised to massage the scar to soften it with vitamin E cream and Mederma. It allows the family to participate in the care of the child.

If the scar continues to be a problem after a minimum of 12 to 18 months have been given for scar maturation, consideration should be given to revision. The severity of the problem dictates the timing and method of correction. Generally speaking, scars are easiest to revise on the preschool-aged child. A skin-only excision with a vest-over-pants closure to add bulk will often suffice. The excision may be designed as an ellipse or a diamond and closed linearly to lengthen the scar if minor degrees of notching are a problem. If lack of muscle approximation is also a problem, a full-thickness excision should be used for access to accomplish correction of this. Scars that remain raised may simply be injected with steroids at the time of other

secondary procedures in young children or within the office in older patients. Dermabrasion is also an option if the scar is thought to require excision not for increased width but for its elevated appearance.

SHORT LIP

The short lip is defined as a cleft lip that is shorter than the normal length by approximately 3 to 4 mm and is usually accompanied by asymmetry of Cupid's bow. Scar contracture appears to be the most common cause of this secondary deformity, although inadequate initial rotation and advancement may be the problem. This can be prevented by taking careful measurements of the contralateral normal lip height and ensuring that the design of the rotation and advancement is adequate to duplicate these measurements.

Consideration should be given to correction of this secondary deformity only after the lip scar has completely matured. Operating during the active phase of scar hypertrophy may lead to further problems with contracture and shortening of the lip repair.

When the skin and vermilion are involved in the short lip, the difference in height of the lip between the normal and repaired sides is precisely measured to determine the amount of lengthening necessary. Unless the scar lines are totally outside of the philtral column, the initial scar may be used as the incision. In patients with minor deformities, the shortness may be treated by a diamond-shaped excision of the scar and closure to lengthen it as described before. However, for any significant degree of shortening, the entire repair should be taken down and repeated. One must also carefully reapproximate the orbicularis to reconstitute the oral sphincter mechanism. Failure to do so will result in postoperative shortening of the lip. In the case of the triangular flap repair, the lip may be readvanced, but it becomes increasingly difficult to maintain appropriate soft tissue for the triangle in the inferior third. This is one of the major shortcomings of the technique. A Z-plasty placed at the columella base or the nostril floor may be indicated to maintain the lip in a better position and to prevent recurrent contracture and shortening.

LONG LIP

With the popularity of the rotation-advancement repair, this is an exceedingly uncommon deformity. It most frequently presents after triangular flap repairs such as the Tennison. Most cleft palate centers no longer perform the Tennison technique, partly because of the difficulty this method presents for adequate cleft lip-nasal reconstruction.[20]

It is tempting in addressing this deformity to simply excise lip tissue from beneath the alar base in an effort to "hitch up" the elongated cleft side. Experience has demonstrated that this simply does not work because of the underlying muscle action and gravity. Even suspension with permanent sutures to bone is not always predictable. It is preferable to take down the entire repair and excise tissue in all dimensions to correct the deformity (Fig. 98-14). The long lip is only seen after a unilateral cleft lip repair. This deformity essentially does not exist in the bilateral cleft lip patient.

TIGHT LIP

This refers to a deficiency of tissue in the horizontal dimension. It is a secondary deformity most commonly seen in the bilateral cleft lip patient. The occurrence of this deformity is a reflection more of the initial severity of the cleft deformity than of inadequate technique. Bilateral cleft lip patients with a protruding premaxilla or a very wide cleft are susceptible to this problem. It is hoped that with increasing application of presurgical nasoalveolar molding, the secondary tight lip deformity will be seen with decreasing frequency.

However, when it is encountered, this deformity is best treated by the Abbe flap, transferring tissue from the central portion of the lower lip to reconstruct the philtrum of the upper lip. This helps not only by

increasing the available tissue for the upper lip but also by decreasing the relative excess in the lower lip. No other technique is worthwhile for addressing significant upper lip tissue deficiencies.

WIDE LIP

This refers to an excess of tissue in the horizontal dimension of the upper lip. Again, this is most frequently seen in the bilateral cleft lip patient in whom the prolabial philtral segment was designed too wide at the time of initial operation or the persistent presence of tension leads to a horizontal distention of the prolabial soft tissue (Fig. 98-15). Generally speaking, at the time of initial lip repair in a 3-month-old, the philtrum should be designed no greater than 6 mm in width at the level of the vermilion border. The philtrum will invariably stretch significantly with time owing to the action of the orbicularis. Initial design of philtral segments wider than this invariably results in an unnatural-appearing upper lip.

The solution to the problem is excision of the excess philtral tissue and reapproximation of the orbicularis to the newly designed philtrum. Regardless of the age

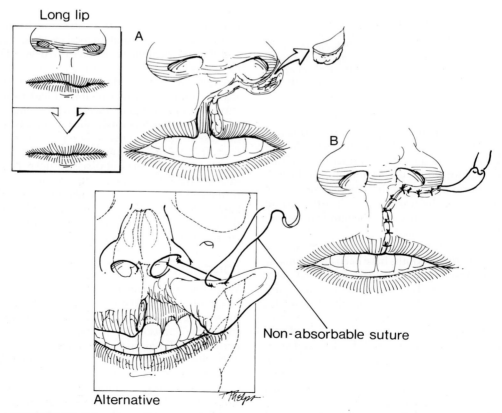

FIGURE 98-14. *A* and *B*, In the long lip deformity, the most successful procedure is to take down the entire repair and reduce the lip in all dimensions.

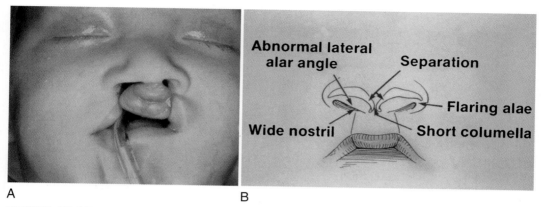

A   B

FIGURE 98-15. *A* and *B*, Problems with bilateral cleft lip after repair.

of the patient at the time of the secondary procedures, the philtrum should be cut smaller than the final desired size in anticipation of this subsequent stretching (Fig. 98-16).

CLEFT PALATE

Normal Palate Anatomy

The palate may be divided embryologically into primary and secondary segments. The primary palate is that anterior to the incisive foramen. The majority of the palate is considered the secondary palate and is posterior to this foramen. Posteriorly, the bony palate ends and at this point is considered the soft palate or velum. This section of the palate contains the levator veli palatini muscle. Although there are other muscles in the velum and oropharynx, the levator muscle complex is the most critical to the formation of a normal speech pattern. In the cleft palate deformity, the levator muscle is split in the midline where it normally unites with the contralateral levator to form a sling (Fig. 98-17). This acts to elevate and support the palate and close off the communication between the mouth and the nose during normal speech. In the cleft patient, the levator on each side of the cleft inserts aberrantly

FIGURE 98-16. The philtrum should be constructed from a prolabial segment no larger than 4 to 6 mm at the time of primary lip repair. *A*, Design at time of primary lip repair. *B*, Postoperative result at 3 years of age.

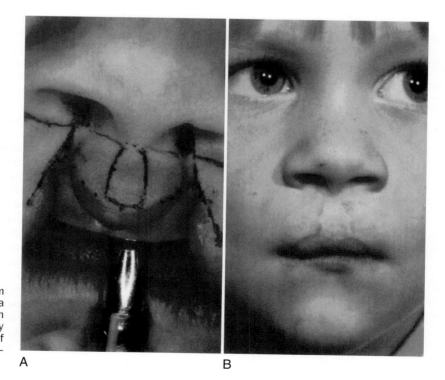

A   B

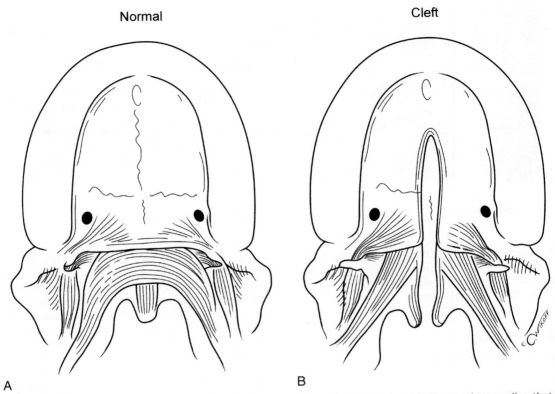

Normal   Cleft

A   B

FIGURE 98-17. Levator veli palatini muscle anatomy. *A,* Normally, the levator forms a continuous sling that acts to elevate the palate. *B,* In the cleft deformity, the levator inserts on the posterior aspect of the bony palate and cannot function properly.

on the posterior edge of the bony palate. This prevents efficient elevation of the soft palate. Misdirection of these fibers must be corrected at the time of primary palatoplasty to ensure an adequate speech pattern. Lateral release of the levator aponeurosis helps minimize tension on the muscle closure.

Another important aspect of the normal palatal anatomy is the greater palatine foramen. This is adjacent to the child's deciduous molars and carries the greater palatine vessels. It is the primary blood supply to the hard palate and should be preserved in elevating flaps to close the cleft. Just posterior to the greater palatine foramen is the lesser palatine foramen, which acts as the primary blood supply to the soft palate. Its preservation is important but not crucial in ensuring the vascularity of the region. Precise release of the vessels can be accomplished by skeletonizing the vessels along the mucomuscular pedicle or, in more difficult procedures, osteotomizing the foramen.

Palatal Fistula

The formation of fistulas after primary palatoplasty has a wide-ranging incidence in the literature and depends on several factors.[21-23] Wide clefts are obvi-

ously more susceptible to the formation of fistulas after palatoplasty because of placement of excessive tension on the flaps used for closure. This may lead to microischemia of the margins of the struggling closure with subsequent necrosis and breakdown. Hematoma and infection are also possible contributing causes of wound breakdown, as are postoperative issues such as coughing secondary to recent anesthesia and the very real issue of the child's putting the fingers or other objects into the mouth.

For the sake of discussion, the fistulas can be broken down into three groups: nasoalveolar fistulas, fistulas at the junction of the hard and soft palate, and soft palate fistulas. Nasoalveolar fistulas present in the region of the maxillary alveolus and most frequently represent not a fistula but a residual cleft not closed at the time of primary palatoplasty. More posterior fistulas represent failure of flap closure.

One consideration in the treatment of palatal fistulas is the presence or absence of symptoms. The most commonly reported symptoms are nasal regurgitation of food and difficulty with speech due to nasal escape of air. This may contribute to velopharyngeal incompetence (see Chapter 97). Food in the nasopharynx or lodged in the fistula presents a hygiene problem as well as a potential source of infection. Liquids or semisolid foods (ice cream, sodas) tend to cause more problems than solids do. There is no definite correlation between the size of the fistula and the severity of symptoms. Even relatively small defects may result in these problems. Small asymptomatic palatal fistulas do not necessarily need treatment.

Another consideration in the decision to treat these patients is the current state of their orthodontic treatment. For most nasoalveolar fistulas, bone grafting will be necessary to allow proper eruption of the adult dentition. Although primary gingivoperiosteoplasty, that is, reapproximation of the cleft and the alveolar gingiva and periosteum at the time of lip repair, holds some promise to eliminate or minimize the need for grafting, most patients will undergo this procedure at approximately 9 to 10 years of age or when the canine begins to position itself for eruption. Closure of the nasoalveolar fistulas before this point is not mandatory unless symptoms warrant closure for normal health, hygiene, or speech reasons. One must also consider the potential need for palatal expansion in cleft patients. Palatal expansion is an active dynamic process that stretches a contracted palate rapidly. Asymptomatic fistulas present at the time of palatal expansion may enlarge secondary to rapid expansion and need to be addressed surgically before or at the time of bone grafting. Even intact palates may experience

spontaneous tears with expansion that need to be closed at the time of bone grafting. Closure before this time may result in dehiscence of that closure and as such should be avoided.

It is obviously better to prevent the fistula than to treat it secondarily. As a general rule, the palate should be closed in two layers, and the flaps used should approximate in the midline without tension. Meticulous hemostasis should be achieved before closure, and the flaps should be approximated with horizontal mattress sutures.

OPTIONS FOR CLOSURE

Most established symptomatic palatal fistulas may be closed with local tissue flaps. However, certain principles must be observed in performing these procedures. Most important, as with the primary palatoplasty, fistula closure should be performed in a two-layer fashion. That is, there should be a separate nasal and oral layer (Fig. 98-18). Most frequently, the nasal layer may be formed by turnover flaps of the mucosa around the fistula, or flaps of mucosa elevated from the vomer may be used when this is not possible. The oral layer is then constructed from large flaps of palatal mucosa. It is critical to design these flaps much larger than the defect because the scarred palatal mucosa is inelastic and often covers less of an area than it appears to when the flap is designed. These flaps may

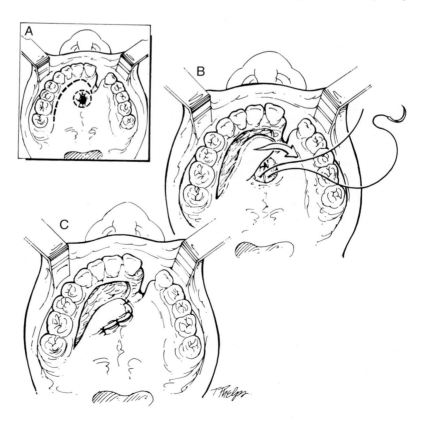

FIGURE 98-18. *A to C,* Palatal fistulas should always be closed in two layers, minimizing the chance for recurrent fistulization.

be designed unilaterally or bilaterally and may be elevated in either unipedicle or bipedicle fashion, much as the initial repair was performed. If at all possible, one should avoid overlapping the suture lines of the nasal and oral layers to decrease the chance for recurrent fistula formation if one of the layers breaks down. Obviously, there should be minimal tension on these flaps at the time of closure. It may be helpful to release the neurovascular bundle if it is tethering the flap, mobilizing the pedicle by osteotomizing the bone around the greater palatine foramen (Fig. 98-19).

If tissue adjacent to the fistula is not sufficient for closure, consideration should be given to other sources. The buccal mucosa is one such option, particularly for the nasal layer.[24] Large flaps of palatally based buccal mucosa may be tunneled into the defect and used for one layer of closure. The donor site can most often be closed primarily, but if not, it can be left open to heal secondarily without complications.

For very posterior fistulas, pharyngeal flaps may be used in the closure of the defect by adding fresh vascular tissue to the nasal layer. This is particularly attractive in patients with severe velopharyngeal incompetence. The pharyngeal flap not only closes the defect but also allows elevation of the palate and easier closure of the nasopharyngeal aperture during speech.

For particularly recalcitrant defects, the tongue flap may be a consideration. This has been described by Guerrerosantos and others.[25,26] It provides a large source of tissue for closure of the problematic palatal fistula. Basing these flaps anteriorly provides a greater degree of mobility for flap positioning. Because this is a pedicled flap, a second stage is necessary to divide the base of the flap approximately 3 weeks after the initial procedure. However, the texture, color, and consistency of the tongue are less than ideal for palatal repair. Intermaxillary fixation may be considered to decrease the likelihood that the patient will disrupt the flap inset, but this is most frequently not necessary.

One final option for fistula closure is microvascular tissue transfer. The radial forearm flap has been used to achieve closure of particularly large palatal defects resistant to other methods.[27,28] However, this should be reserved for a last option. Consideration must also be given in these cases to simple prosthetic obturation of these defects. Although the fit of the obturator and the ongoing care it requires may be a problem, these prostheses can also incorporate teeth to disguise residual clefts within the alveolus that have failed prior closure attempts.

CLEFT NASAL DEFORMITY

Anatomy

The anatomy of the cleft nasal deformity is important in understanding the rationale for the different techniques used in reconstructive procedures. In the unilateral cleft lip-nose, the cleft-side ala is laterally displaced, resulting in an obtuse alar-facial angle, deviation of the nasal tip to the cleft side, and deviation of the base of the septum to the noncleft side (Fig. 98-20). The development of this deformity also results in a significant loss of tip definition. These findings have been summarized in what has been termed the tripod concept.[29,30] Simply stated, nasal support is dependent on the septum centrally and the nasal sidewalls laterally. When support is removed by displacement of the cleft-side ala and the septum, the nose collapses, resulting in these findings.

The concept is the same for the bilateral cleft lip-nose (see Fig. 98-15). The support of the ala is diminished bilaterally, resulting in retropositioning of the entire nasal tip complex. This is manifested as a broad flat nose with minimal tip definition and projection. The severity of the nasal deformity is frequently made to appear worse by the position of the premaxilla. That is, the premaxillary segment may be anteriorly positioned, causing distortion of the columella.

Consequently, the distortion seen in the cleft lip-nose is the result of distortion of the lower lateral cartilages. Nasal tip definition depends on formation of an acute angle at the genu of the lower lateral cartilages or the middle crus. This can be maintained only when there is adequate support for the medial and lateral crura. With loss of this support in the cleft lip-nasal deformity, the angle formed at the genu of the lower lateral cartilage becomes obtuse and the tip broad and flat.

Timing of Repair

Primary repair of the cleft lip-nose is a widely practiced procedure in most centers.[31,32] This has been influenced greatly by the popularity of the Millard rotation-advancement procedure. The incisions used for this facilitate exposure and dissection of the nose. Other techniques, such as the Tennison triangular flap repair, do not allow the same access to the nose and consequently require other incisions for the nasal deformity to be addressed at the time of initial lip repair.

The timing of secondary surgery on the cleft lip-nose is predicated not only on the age of the patient but also on the severity of the deformity. In most situations, there is an attempt to address significant residual deformities in the preschool years, often at the time of secondary lip surgery. At this age, however, these procedures involve essentially no significant modification of the osseocartilaginous vault. Attention is mainly directed toward repositioning the lower lateral cartilage. Complete rhinoplasty with osteotomies and septal modification is usually deferred until the completion of nasal growth. Although classically this has been thought to be in the late teen years,

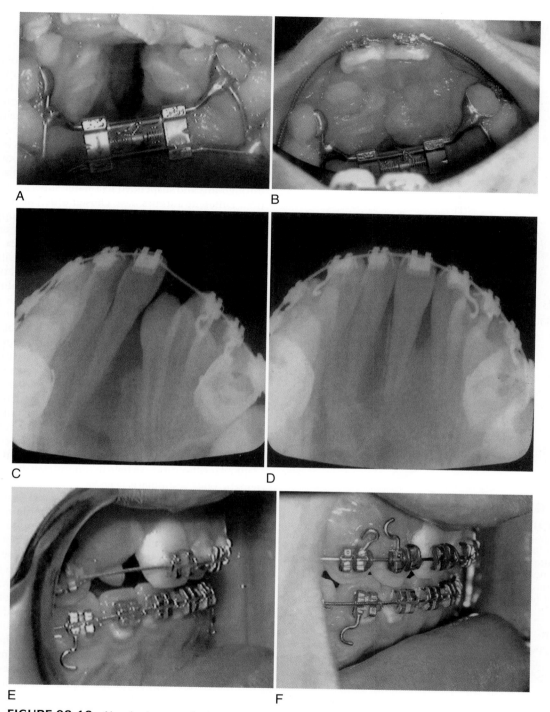

FIGURE 98-19. Alveolar bone graft. *A* and *B,* Significance of good closure of palate before bone graft. *C* and *D,* Radiographic views before and after bone graft. *E* and *F,* Preoperative and postoperative lateral views of bone graft.

Normal

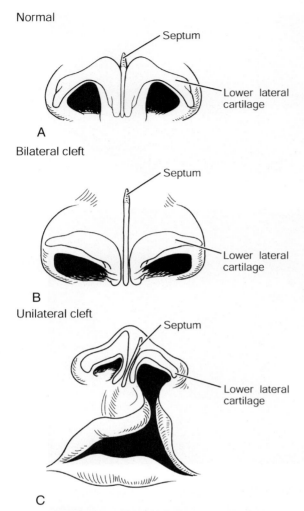

FIGURE 98-20. Cleft nasal anatomy. *A,* Normal. *B,* Bilateral cleft lip-nose. A broad flat nasal tip results from the lateral displacement of the lower lateral cartilages bilaterally, and the columella is short. *C,* Unilateral cleft lip-nose. The cleft-side ala is laterally displaced, resulting in a broad flat middle crus, loss of tip definition, obtuse alar-facial angle, and septal deviation.

firm anthropometric and cephalometric evidence supports the cessation of nasal growth at approximately the age of 11 to 12 years in girls and 13 to 14 years in boys.[6] One may perform a complete rhinoplasty at this time without fear of significantly influencing the growth pattern of the nose. However, the chief concern at this age is the emotional maturity of the patient. Complete rhinoplasty should be deferred until the patient is thought to be emotionally mature and capable of participating in the decision-making process preoperatively and assisting in the postoperative care. In the emotionally stable patient in his or her early teen years with a significant residual deformity, there should be no contraindication to complete rhinoplasty.

Techniques

The technique most frequently used to repair the unilateral cleft lip-nose is some sort of suspension of the lower lateral cartilage on the cleft side. To accomplish this, the lower lateral cartilage must first be freed from the overlying soft tissue. This may be performed through an infracartilaginous incision supplemented if necessary by medial dissection through the apex of existing lip incisions. Once the cleft-side ala has been completely freed, the desired position of the apex of the dome on the cleft side is chosen; suture is placed through this and suspended to a stable superior position. Different authors have chosen different points for this suspension, including to the contralateral upper lateral cartilage and tied over an external bolster or to the contralateral lower lateral cartilage dome apex.[33-36] It is preferable to stabilize the cleft-side apex with a taper needle on a polydioxanone suture to the dermis of the overlying skin envelope by taking the stabilizing suture out through the skin and re-entering it through the same point (Fig. 98-21). This may be facilitated by a small skin incision with a No. 11 blade. Although this sometimes causes a small dimple of the overlying skin, this always resolves during the course of several weeks. It also obviates the need for an external bolster that may cause scars on the nasal skin and that must be removed, eliminating the support that was established. The technique described maintains support for the repositioned ala as long as the suture maintains its integrity. These sutures are also an effective means of positioning the skin envelope in the defined position and can help in minimizing the problematic plica vestibularis (Fig. 98-22).

Much of the undercorrection associated with the unilateral cleft lip-nasal deformity can be minimized at the time of the initial lip and nasal repair by attention to certain details. Among these, it is important to mobilize the ala base thoroughly and to mobilize this medially, securing it to the contralateral ala base through the existing lip incisions. There is always a deficiency in nasal lining that is manifested at the time of this medial translocation of the ala. This defect should be filled by the L flap developed by the Millard rotation-advancement. The deviated septum should be dissected along the base and repositioned as much as possible in the midline with a suture. This helps establish the central support of the tripod and facilitates repositioning of the cleft-side ala.

For the bilateral cleft-nasal deformity, the techniques used for repair are somewhat different in practice from those for the unilateral cleft-nasal deformity but identical in principle. As in any surgical procedure, the three most important considerations are access, dissection, and fixation. Access can be achieved through an infracartilaginous incision supplemented as necessary with a medial dissection through the apex

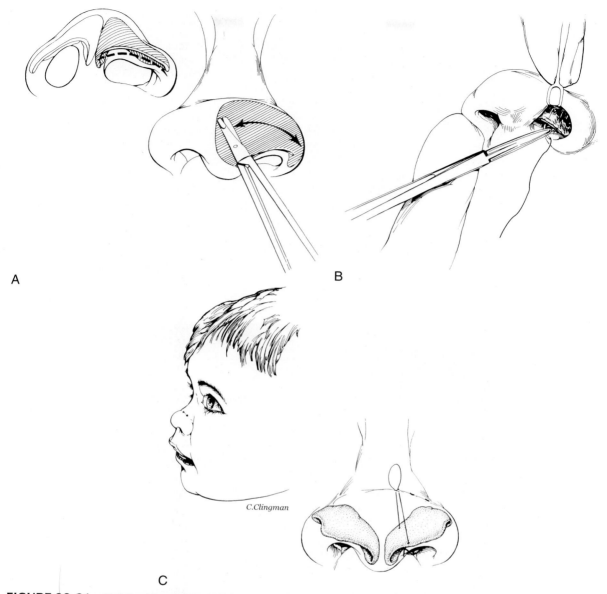

C.Clingman

FIGURE 98-21. Cleft lip rhinoplasty. *A,* Dissection of the lower lateral cartilage on the cleft side through an infracartilaginous incision. *B,* Exposure of the lower lateral cartilage and suture placement. *C,* Sutures are taken out through the skin and brought back in through the same site and tied in the nasal vestibule.

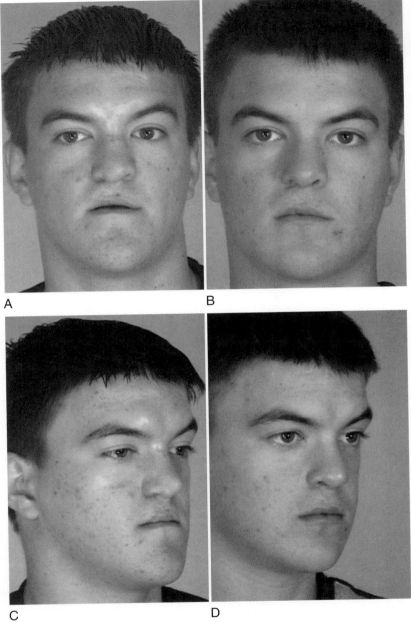

FIGURE 98-22. Preoperative and postoperative views of midface and cleft nose. *A* and *B*, Anteroposterior views. *C* and *D*, Oblique views.

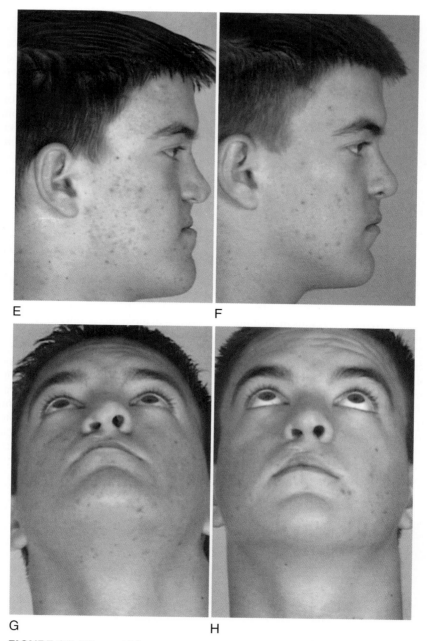

E

F

G

H

FIGURE 98-22, cont'd. *E* and *F,* Lateral views. *G* and *H,* Basal views.

of the existing lip incision. In most revisions, however, an infracartilaginous incision is safe and allows a good exposure medially and laterally; it also allows the occasional trimming of the skin or rolling of the alar rim as needed. Positioning the lower lateral cartilage is important after it is totally freed from its overlying attachments and redraped in lining. The cartilage and the underlying lining can then be repositioned to a more superior medial position and fixed with sutures to the contralateral alar cartilage or suspended transdermally.

In the past, procedures to correct the bilateral cleft-nasal deformity have been focused on the skin, not the underlying structural support.[37] In these procedures, nasal tip projection has been accomplished by advancing skin medially into the columella to support the new nasal tip position. Cronin[38] was among the first to describe this delayed columellar lengthening with

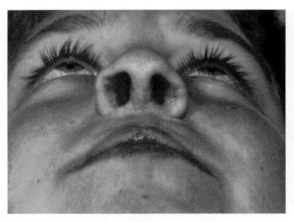

FIGURE 98-23. Long columella in the bilateral cleft lip-nasal deformity due to overaugmentation.

use of tissue from the nasal floor; others have used tissue from the broad prolabium.[39] However, columellar lengthening, when it is performed without addressing the deformed cartilage, frequently results in an abnormally long columella and significant secondary deformities (Fig. 98-23).

All techniques of repair of the cleft lip-nose, both unilateral and bilateral, are hampered by the lack of a stable platform on which to base the repair. That is, there is underlying skeletal deficiency that contributes to the lack of tip projection. Despite the best of efforts, suture modification of the tip as described in the preceding paragraph may be inadequate to correct the deformity completely. Although definitive treatment of this skeletal problem is Le Fort I osteotomy and advancement, this is not considered until the late teen years in most patients when maxillary and mandibular growth is complete. Therefore, when suture modification is thought to be inadequate, one must consider augmentation of nasal support with cartilage or grafts. Columellar struts or septal extension grafts with septal, ear, or rib cartilage fixed to the medial crura by sutures can achieve 2 to 3 mm of additional tip projection when performed properly. If this is still inadequate to address the tip position, one may consider the use of onlay cartilage grafts. Conchal cartilage is ideal for this purpose and can augment the projection of the cleft-side ala.

NASOALVEOLAR MOLDING

Cartilage in the neonate has a remarkable ability to be remodeled by external forces; this may be due to the high level of circulating estrogens in the immediate postnatal period.[40] Although there have been numerous reports in the past of the reshaping of the constricted ear deformity in the neonate through the process of molding,[40-42] only recently has this same technique been applied to the cleft lip-nasal deformity. Cutting and colleagues have used an extension of the palatal appliance placed during the period of presurgical orthopedics to shape the nose in the first several months of life.[43,44] The appliance is gradually reshaped on a weekly basis to guide the nose and palatal shelves into a more normal position. The anterior extensions of the device stretch the nasal lining and give a more acute angle to the middle crus by direct pressure under it. This greatly facilitates nasal repair (Figs. 98-24 and 98-25).

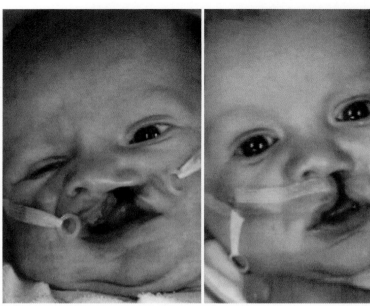

A   B

FIGURE 98-24. Nasoalveolar molding results. *A,* Appearance before molding. *B,* Appearance after molding before lip repair.

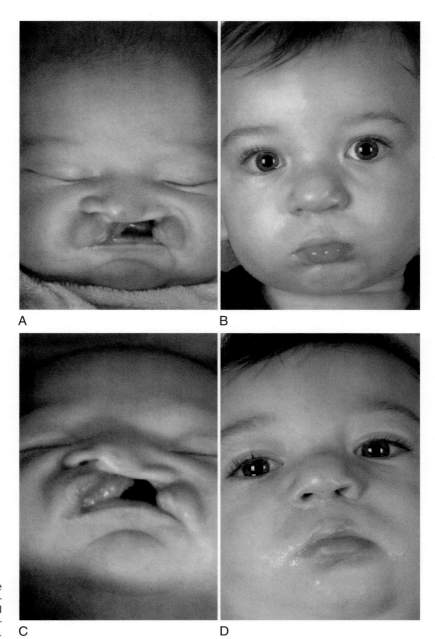

A   B

C   D

FIGURE 98-25. Preoperative and postoperative views. Unilateral complete cleft lip with nasal conformer. *A* and *B*, Anteroposterior views. *C* and *D*, Basal views.

Unfortunately, this technique is labor-intensive and requires a great deal of cooperation and effort on the part of the parents. The patients must be seen on a weekly basis and their appliance adjusted according to the changing shape of the nose and palatal shelves. In addition, the parents must remove the appliance daily for cleaning. Although the initial results of nasoalveolar molding have been very good, it is being practiced only at a few centers because of these difficulties.

OPEN VERSUS CLOSED APPROACH

There have been many arguments advocating both the open and the closed approach. Proponents of the open approach point out that the improved access afforded facilitates diagnosis and correction of the underlying anatomic problem. Surgeons using the closed or endonasal approach argue that all procedures in rhinoplasty can be accomplished through these incisions without causing the prolonged swelling that results from the open technique. Most frequently, the decision as to which technique to use depends on the surgeon's preference.

With respect to cleft lip rhinoplasty, the majority of procedures can be accomplished by the closed technique, particularly in the unilateral deformity. Because the primary goal is re-establishment of the position of the lower lateral cartilage on the cleft side, an open approach seems excessive in the majority of cases. The existing lip incisions and an infracartilaginous incision are usually sufficient to accomplish the necessary maneuvers. Because of the different nature of the lip incisions in the bilateral cleft lip-nasal deformity, the open technique is more common. Open dissection of the nose with the incisions for the flaps used to augment the skin of the columella is the most frequent approach. Partly because of this, in approaching a bilateral cleft lip-nasal deformity that has undergone multiple previous operations, one should take great care in designing the approach incisions so as not to devascularize the columella or limit subsequent secondary lip procedures.

In the older patient undergoing a definitive septorhinoplasty, the approach should be based on the degree of tip modification necessary. In those patients requiring minimal work on the tip, the closed approach is preferred. It is easier to address significant residual tip asymmetry in the secondary cleft lip-nose through the open approach.

WHEN "ENOUGH IS ENOUGH"

The array of secondary deformities possible in patients with cleft lip and palate is formidable. When deciding on which deformities to treat operatively, one must determine their impact on the patient and the likelihood that a surgical procedure will substantially improve the problem. At some point in the operative sequence, further surgical intervention is unlikely to improve the patient's appearance significantly. Consequently, it is important to know when "enough is enough,"[45] that is, when the patient is unlikely to be helped by any further intervention. Given the vast array of procedures to which these patients are subjected—lip and palatal repair, alveolar bone grafting, pharyngeal surgery, and orthognathic surgery—surgery for secondary deformities should be minimized by operating only on those problems that are bothersome to the patient and that are likely to be improved by the surgery. As Marsh[45] stated, the surgeon is at times more critical of the result than the patient is. Just as not every nasal dorsal hump needs to be removed, not every cleft lip-nasal deformity needs to be revised. The enemy of good is better, particularly when better is unlikely.

REFERENCES

1. Moss ML: A theoretical analysis of the functional matrix. Acta Biotheor 1995;18:195-202.
2. Bardach J, Salyer KE: Correction of secondary unilateral cleft lip deformities. In Bardach J, Salyer KE, eds: Surgical Techniques in Cleft Lip and Palate. Chicago, Year Book, 1987:225-246.
3. Williams H: A method of assessing cleft lip repairs: comparison of Le Mesurier and Millard techniques. Plast Reconstr Surg 1968;41:103-107.
4. Assuncao G: The VLS classification for secondary deformities in the unilateral cleft lip: clinical application. Br J Plast Surg 1992;45:288-296.
5. Millard DR Jr: Cleft Craft, vol 1: The Unilateral Deformity. Boston, Little, Brown, 1976.
6. Akguner M, Barutcu A, Karaca C: Adolescent growth patterns of the bony and cartilaginous framework of the nose: a cephalometric study. Ann Plast Surg 1998;41:66-69.
7. McCarthy J, Cutting C: Secondary deformities of cleft lip and palate. In Georgiade NG, Riefkohl R, Barwick W, eds: Textbook of Plastic, Maxillofacial and Craniofacial Surgery. Baltimore, Williams & Wilkins, 1992:307-319.
8. Schendel SA: Unilateral cleft lip repair—state of the art. Cleft Palate Craniofac J 2000;37:335-341.
9. Latham R, Qusy R, Georgiade N: An extraorally activated expansion appliance for cleft palate infants. Cleft Palate J 1976;13:253-261.
10. Georgiade N, Latham R: Maxillary arch alignment in the bilateral cleft lip and palate infant, using pinned coaxial screw appliance. Plast Reconstr Surg 1975;56:52-60.
11. Grayson BH, Santiago PE, Brecht LE, et al: Presurgical nasoalveolar molding in infants with cleft lip and palate. Cleft Palate Craniofac J 1999;36:486-498.
12. Maull DJ, Grayson BH, Cutting CB, et al: Long term effects of nasoalveolar molding on three dimensional nasal shape in unilateral clefts. Cleft Palate Craniofac J 1999;36:391-397.
13. Santiago PE, Grayson BH, Cutting CB, et al: Reduced need for alveolar bone grafting by presurgical orthopedics in primary gingivoperiosteoplasty. Cleft Palate Craniofac J 1998;35:77-80.
14. Millard DR Jr: Extensions of the rotation-advancement principle for wide unilateral cleft lips. Plast Reconstr Surg 1998;42:535-544.
15. Stal S, Spira M: Secondary reconstructive procedures for patients with clefts. In Sursin D, Georgiade NG, eds: Pediatric Plastic Surgery. St. Louis, CV Mosby, 1984:352-378.
16. Kapetansky DI: Double pendulum flaps for whistling deformities in bilateral cleft lips. Plast Reconstr Surg 1971;47:321-323.
17. Coleman SR: Facial recontouring with lipostructure. Clin Plast Surg 1997;24:347-367.
18. Gillies H, Kilner TP: Harelip operations for the correction of secondary deformities. Lancet 1932;2:1369.
19. Fara M: Anatomy and arteriography of cleft lips in stillborn children. Plast Reconstr Surg 1968;42:29-36.
20. Stal S, Klebuc M, Taylor TD, et al: Algorithms for the treatment of cleft lip and palate. Clin Plast Surg 1998;25:493-507.
21. Lin KY, Goldberg D, Williams C, et al: Long-term outcome analysis of two treatment methods for cleft palate: combined levator retropositioning and pharyngeal flap versus double-opposing Z-plasty. Cleft Palate Craniofac J 1999;36:73-78.
22. Folk SN, D'Antonio LL, Hardesty RA: Secondary cleft deformities. Clin Plast Surg 1999;24:599-611.
23. Emory RE Jr, Clay RP, Bite U, et al: Fistula formation and repair after palatal closure: an institutional perspective. Plast Reconstr Surg 1997;99:1535-1538.
24. Freedlander E, Jackson IT: The fate of buccal mucosal flaps in primary palatal repair. Cleft Palate J 1989;26:110-112.
25. Guerrerosantos J, Altamirano JT: The use of lingual flaps in repair of fistulas of the hard palate. Plast Reconstr Surg 1966;38:123-128.
26. Barrone CM, Argamaso RV: Refinements of a tongue flap for closure of difficult palatal fistulas. J Craniofac Surg 1993;4:109-111.

27. Chen HC, Ganos DL, Coessens BC, et al: Free forearm flap for closure of difficult oronasal fistulas in cleft palate patients. Plast Reconstr Surg 1992;90:757-762.

28. MacLaod AN, Morrison WA, McCann JJ, et al: Free radial forearm flap with and without bone for closure of large palatal fistulae. Br J Plast Surg 1987;40:391-395.

29. Hogan V: The tilted tripod: a theory of cleft lip nasal deformities. In Huston J, ed: Transactions of the 5th International Congress of Plastic and Reconstructive Surgery. Melbourne, Australia, Butterworths, 1971.

30. McCollough E, Mangap D: Systematic approach to correction of the nasal tip in rhinoplasty. Arch Otolaryngol 1981;107:12-16.

31. Millard D, Morovic C: Primary unilateral cleft nose correction: a ten-year follow-up. Plast Reconstr Surg 1998;102:1331-1338.

32. McComb H: Primary repair of the bilateral cleft lip nose: a four-year review. Plast Reconstr Surg 1994;94:37-47.

33. Tajima S, Maruyama M: Reverse-U incision for secondary repair of cleft lip nose. Plast Reconstr Surg 1977;60:256-261.

34. Reynolds J, Horton C: An alar lift in cleft lip rhinoplasty. Plast Reconstr Surg 1965;35:277.

35. Stenstrom S, Oberg T: The nasal deformity in unilateral cleft lip. Plast Reconstr Surg 1961;28:295.

36. Dibbell DG: Cleft lip nasal reconstruction: correcting the classic unilateral defect. Plast Reconstr Surg 1982;59:264-271.

37. Cutting CB: Primary bilateral cleft lip and nose repair. In Aston S, Beasley R, Thorne CHM, eds: Plastic Surgery. Philadelphia, Lippincott-Raven, 1997:257.

38. Cronin TD: Lengthening the columella by use of skin from the nasal floor and ala. Plast Reconstr Surg 1958;21:417-426.

39. Millard D: Closure of bilateral cleft lip and elongation of columella by two operations in infancy. Plast Reconstr Surg 1971;47:324-331.

40. Tan S, Abramson D, MacDonald D, et al: Molding therapy for infants with deformational auricular anomalies. Ann Plast Surg 1997;3:263-268.

41. Brown F, Colen L, Addante R, et al: Correction of congenital auricular deformities by splinting in the neonatal period. Pediatrics 1986;78:406-411.

42. Matsuo K, Hayashi R, Kiyono M, et al: Nonsurgical correction of congenital auricular deformities. Clin Plast Surg 1993;17:333-395.

43. Cutting C, Grayson B, Brecht L: Presurgical columella elongation with one-stage repair of the bilateral cleft lip and nose. Proceedings, American Cleft Palate-Craniofacial Association, 1995;52:58.

44. Maull D, Grayson B, Cutting C, et al: Long-term effects of nasoalveolar molding on three-dimensional nasal shapes in unilateral clefts. Cleft Palate Craniofac J 1999;36:391-397.

45. Marsh JL: When is enough enough? Secondary surgery for cleft lip and palate patients. Clin Plast Surg 1990;17:37-47.

Reconstruction: Orbital Hypertelorism

JOSEPH G. MCCARTHY, MD

HISTORY

The successful development of surgical techniques to correct orbital hypertelorism represents one of the most exciting achievements in the history of surgery. Surgeons had long identified the problem that the orbits (and the contained globes) were widely displaced. Not only did this condition prevent the development of binocular vision, but there was also an associated aesthetic deformity.

Radiographic studies had confirmed that the orbits were displaced laterally and that the intervening interorbital space, consisting of the nasal cavity and ethmoid sinuses, was overexpanded; the crista galli and cribriform plates were usually displaced inferiorly (see Fig. 99-1). Converse et al[1] had noted, though, that the optic foramina were not pathologically involved and were not malpositioned. Consequently, it would be possible to move the orbits (and globes) toward the midline if the orbits could be osteotomized and if some of the interorbital space could be reduced. One of the first attempts was by Converse and Smith[2] in 1962. They removed a central segment of bone containing nasal bone and ethmoid sinus and osteotomized and mobilized the medial wall, floor, and lateral wall of the orbit into the defect made by removal of the central segment. Alloplastic material was placed in the residual lateral defect, but the technique found little acceptance because it did not effectively mobilize the orbits (and globes) toward the midline.

Tessier et al[3] should be credited with the observation that the 360-degree orbit, including the roof (and floor of the anterior cranial fossa), had to be mobilized to ensure adequate medial translocation of the orbit. Tessier also reasoned that the "functional orbit" had to be mobilized, that is, that portion of the orbit posterior to the equator of the globe. Tessier[4-6] also made the observation that a combined craniofacial approach is essential to protect the frontal lobe of the brain while the osteotomy is being performed through the orbital roof (or floor of the anterior cranial fossa) as part of the 360-degree or circumferential osteotomy. The cribriform plate was resected to make a midline defect into which the orbits could be moved. This maneuver obviously had a negative impact on olfaction.

Schmid[7] probably performed the first successful orbital hypertelorism correction. In a line of thinking similar to that of Tessier, he postulated that the circumferential (360-degree) orbit had to be mobilized. He did not use a combined craniofacial approach but serendipitously performed the orbital roof osteotomy in a patient with an overexpanded frontal sinus, thus avoiding intracranial injury.

Converse et al[1] popularized a combined craniofacial route with preservation of the cribriform plate (unlike the two-stage technique of Tessier) and removal of paramedian segments, thus preserving the nasofrontal junction to serve as a base for bone grafting in the reconstruction of the nasal deformity. Long-term studies by McCarthy[8] demonstrated little change in olfactory or gustatory function after this technique.

van der Meulen[9] described the bipartition technique, and it was popularized by Ortiz Monasterio[10,11] and his group in Mexico City. It has the advantage of mobilizing the circumferential orbit and moving it to the midline, in association with the attached maxillary segments. It is especially indicated in the patient with an orbitofacial midline (zero) cleft[12] and an upward cant of the lateral segments of the maxilla. Working in conjunction with the orthodontist, the surgeon is able to correct the orbital hypertelorism, to close the midline maxillary cleft, and to restore the plane of the maxillary occlusion. Tessier also demonstrated its special utility in the patient with Apert syndrome.

PATHOLOGY

Orbital hypertelorism is not a syndrome but a physical finding usually associated with orbitofacial clefts[12] (see Chapter 100). With the unilateral clefts, the orbital hypertelorism tends to be asymmetric, and the more affected orbit tends to be inferiorly and laterally displaced. Such patients also have deformities of the nose, medial canthus, and cheek soft tissues. A meningoencephalocele or herniation of brain and overlying meninges exiting through a skeletal defect is often an associated component of the pathologic process. Frontoethmoidal meningoencephaloceles share a common bone defect in the anterior cranial fossa and are commonly associated with orbital hypertelorism.[13] They are also seen with dermoid cysts, glial tumors, and syndromic craniosynostosis, especially Apert syndrome. It is preferable to correct all deformities in the same surgical stage (see Chapter 101).

The skeletal pathologic process (Fig. 99-1) is characterized by an increased distance between the medial orbital walls or dacryons. The intervening ethmoid sinuses (interorbital space) are overexpanded, and in the more severe examples of orbital hypertelorism, there is an inferior displacement of the cribriform plate (Fig. 99-2). In such cases, there is also "lateralization" (temporal displacement) of the orbits, and the anteroposterior dimension of the lateral orbital wall is severely reduced. Associated abnormalities of the nasolacrimal apparatus are not uncommon. The optic foramina are usually spared. With extensive orbitofacial clefting, the maxillary dentoalveolus is interrupted, and there are a variety of malocclusions.

PREOPERATIVE PLANNING AND CONSIDERATIONS

In the preoperative planning, the patient should have an ophthalmologic evaluation to document the visual status and the absence or presence of associated amblyopia and extraocular dysfunction.[14]

Radiographic studies are essential in documenting the pathologic process and in planning the surgical reconstruction. Posteroanterior cephalograms (Fig. 99-3) are used to document the interorbital distance, as recorded between the dacryons. Hansman[15] documented the normal interorbital distances from birth to 25 years. Interorbital distance averages 16 mm at birth and increases to 25 mm by the age of 12 years. At approximately 13 years, the female curves begin to level off,

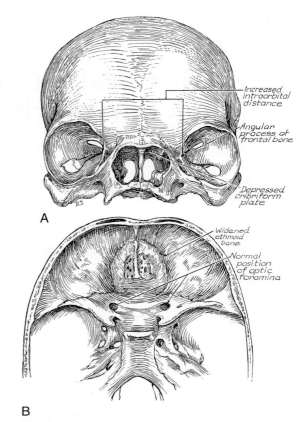

A

B

FIGURE 99-1. Infant skull demonstrating orbital hypertelorism. *A,* Frontal view. Note the increased interorbital distance and inferiorly displaced cribriform plate. *B,* Cranial view. There is widening of the roofs of the ethmoid labyrinth, but the optic foramina remain in normal position. (From McCarthy JG, Thorne CHM, Wood-Smith D: Principles of craniofacial surgery: orbital hypertelorism. In McCarthy JG, ed: Plastic Surgery. Philadelphia, WB Saunders, 1990:2974.)

but males show a continued increase in interorbital distance until approximately 21 years. The average adult interorbital distance is 25 mm in women and 28 mm in men. Tessier[4] classified orbital hypertelorism as follows: grade 1, 30 to 34 mm of interorbital distance; grade 2, 34 to 40 mm; and grade 3, greater than 40 mm (with lateral divergence of the orbits).

Computed tomographic scanning is absolutely essential. Axial and coronal cuts can be used to define the interorbital space (size of the ethmoid sinuses and configuration of the medial orbital walls) as well as the dimensions of the bony orbit (Fig. 99-4). In grade 3 hypertelorism, the anteroposterior dimension of the *lateral* orbital wall is generally reduced, a finding that affects the efficacy of the mobilization and translocation of the orbits. Munro[16] emphasized the variation in the shape of the *medial* orbital walls on computed tomographic study. This finding can also greatly affect the success of the orbital translocation.

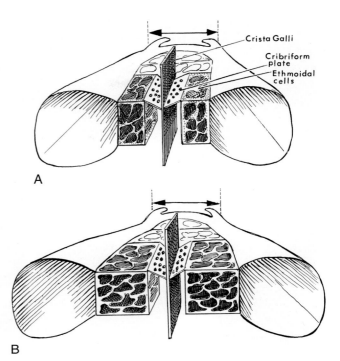

FIGURE 99-2. Diagrammatic representation of the interorbital space. *A,* Normal relationship between the orbit, the cribriform plate, and the ethmoid sinuses. *B,* In orbital hypertelorism, there is temporal divergence (lateralization) of the orbital cavities with overexpansion of the anterior ethmoidal cells. The posterior ethmoidal cells and the sphenoid sinus are not enlarged, and the distance between the optic foramina is usually not increased. The cribriform plate, although not illustrated, is usually inferiorly displaced. (From Converse JM, Ransohoff J, Mathews ES, et al: Ocular hypertelorism and pseudohypertelorism. Advances in surgical treatment. Plast Reconstr Surg 1970;45:1. Copyright © 1970, The Williams & Wilkins Company, Baltimore.)

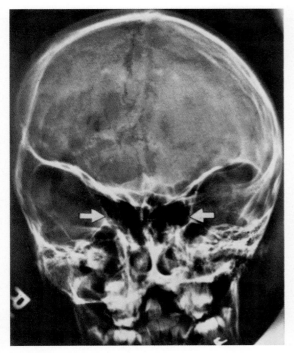

FIGURE 99-3. Posteroanterior cephalogram of a patient with orbital hypertelorism. Interorbital distance is measured between the two arrows. Note the lateral divergence of the orbits, the inferior displacement of the cribriform plate, and the increase of the horizontal dimension of the ethmoid sinuses. (From McCarthy JG, Thorne CHM, Wood-Smith D: Principles of craniofacial surgery: orbital hypertelorism. In McCarthy JG, ed: Plastic Surgery. Philadelphia, WB Saunders, 1990:2974.)

In planning surgical reconstruction, the postoperative interorbital distance should be reduced to the range of 16 to 18 mm. In a computed tomographic study, Hoffman et al[17] documented the arc of rotation that the orbits undergo during surgical translocation, a finding accounting for the observed postoperative undercorrection of the interorbital distance.

Ortiz Monasterio et al[18] have demonstrated that in the planning of a bipartition procedure, there is a clockwise-counterclockwise rotation of the orbits as the occlusal plane of the maxillary segments is leveled (Fig. 99-5). Such planning should be done jointly between the surgeon and orthodontist.

SURGICAL TECHNIQUES
Combined Craniofacial Osteotomy

In this technique,[5] the orbits are sectioned in a 360-degree fashion, with the osteotomies made posterior to the equator of the globes ("functional orbital volume"). The orbits and contained globes are mobilized toward the midline as individual cubes ("box osteotomies").

A bicoronal incision is made (Fig. 99-6*A*) and the dissection carried in a subperiosteal plane over the supraorbital rims, and the temporalis is reflected from the fossa bilaterally. The orbital contents are mobilized in a subperiosteal plane, with care being taken to preserve the optic nerve pedicle as well as the nasolacrimal apparatus. An anterior craniotomy is performed, and this maneuver allows retraction and

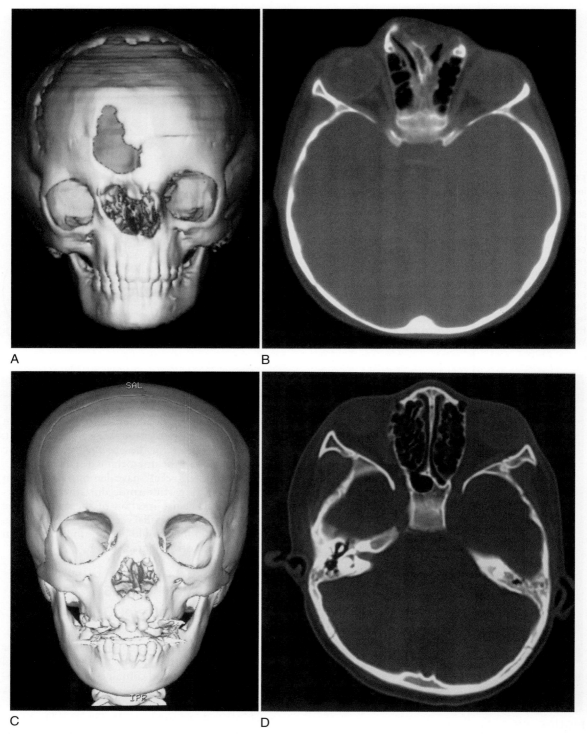

FIGURE 99-4. Three-dimensional computed tomographic scans detailing the skeletal configuration of the orbits. *A,* Frontal view showing increased interorbital distance and frontoethmoid defect. *B,* Axial cut demonstrating laterally displaced orbits, nasal defect, and parallel but slightly divergent *medial* orbital walls. *C,* Frontal view showing increased interorbital distance and bilateral dentoalveolar maxillary clefts. *D,* Axial cut demonstrating convex *medial* orbital walls and overexpanded interorbital space (ethmoid sinus). Note the lateralization of the lateral orbital walls.

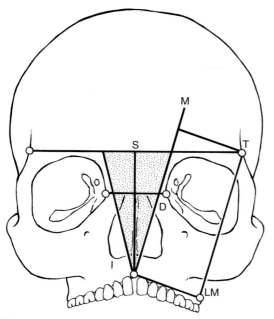

FIGURE 99-5. Geometric preoperative planning for the bipartition procedure. On a posteroanterior cephalogram, a line is drawn from sella (S) to interincisal point (I). The occlusal plane is outlined by line I-LM (lateral molar). A horizontal line is drawn between the temporal crests (T), 1 cm above the orbital rim and bisecting S. A line is drawn between LM and T. A line is drawn between I and M parallel to and equal in length to line LM-T (but slightly medial to D or dacryon). Line I-M represents the future midline and indicates the elongation that will be achieved at the midline.

protection of the frontal lobes in performing an osteotomy through the orbital roofs (floor of the anterior cranial fossa). It also gives exposure to the cribriform plate and crista galli (Fig. 99-6B). Exposure is often complemented by bilateral transcutaneous (Fig. 99-6C) or transconjunctival (Fig. 99-6D) eyelid incisions. The orbits, except for the optic nerve pedicle and nasolacrimal apparatus, are exposed in a subperiosteal plane (Fig. 99-6E).

The central defect (Fig. 99-7) can be made either by a single midline resection of nasal bone and ethmoid sinus (with or without the nasal septum) or, as popularized by Converse et al,[19,20] by two paramedian segments. The latter procedure, usually reserved for milder cases, preserves the nasofrontal junction as a recipient site for onlay bone grafting as part of the nasal reconstruction.

The lateral wall osteotomies are made in a full-thickness fashion at the junction of the lateral orbital wall and the cranium (see Fig. 99-7). The osteotomy is extended across the roof of the orbit (Fig. 99-8) posterior to the equator of the globe. The osteotomy is directed inferiorly along the medial orbital wall and carried through the floor of the orbit (Fig. 99-9) with or without the need for transconjunctival incisions. The zygomatic complex is completely sectioned. At this point in the procedure, the skeletal orbits are mobilized. The orbits can be translocated into the central defect (Fig. 99-10), and the residual lateral defects are filled with autogenous bone grafts (cranium, ilium, or rib). Rigid skeletal fixation is achieved with plates and

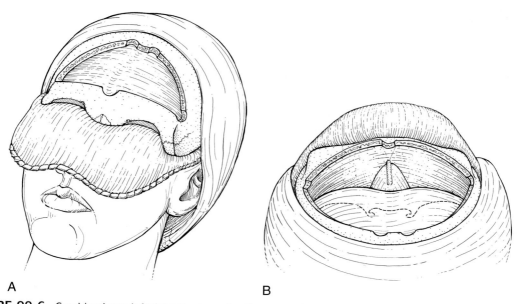

A   B

FIGURE 99-6. Combined craniofacial osteotomy for the correction of orbital hypertelorism. *A,* The bicoronal flap has been elevated, exposing the cranium, orbits, and root of the nose in a subperiosteal plane. The anterior craniotomy is completed. *B,* The craniotomy provides exposure of the anterior cranial fossa and cribriform plate.   *Continued*

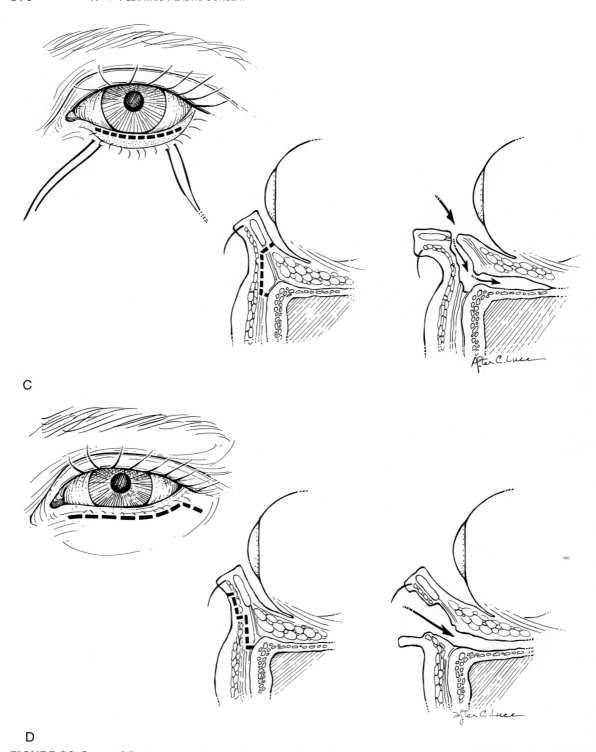

FIGURE 99-6, cont'd. *C,* Transconjunctival lower eyelid incision (anterior to the septum orbitale) to approach the inferior orbital rim. *D,* Transcutaneous lower eyelid incisions with a step-like approach (orbicularis muscle divided 8 mm below eyelid margin to expose the septum orbitale) to the inferior orbital rim.

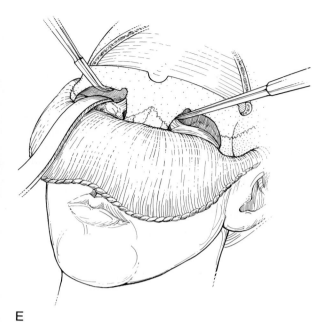

E

FIGURE 99-6, cont'd. *E,* Liberation of the supra-orbital nerves and exposure of the orbital roof.

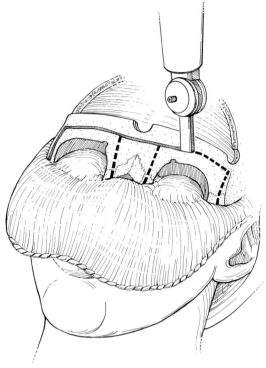

FIGURE 99-7. Outline of the central segment to be resected, the supraorbital osteotomy, and the lateral orbital wall osteotomies. Note the "frontal bandeau" that serves as a skeletal reference point.

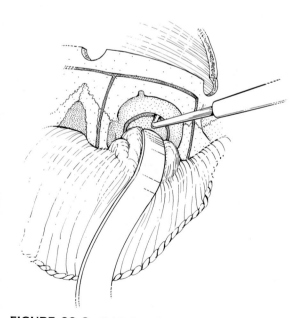

FIGURE 99-8. Orbital roof osteotomy with an oscillating saw.

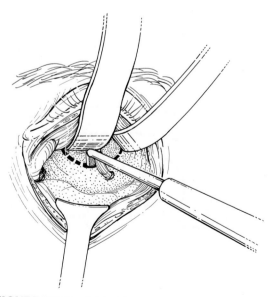

FIGURE 99-9. Orbital floor osteotomy with an oscillating saw. An osteotome can also be used.

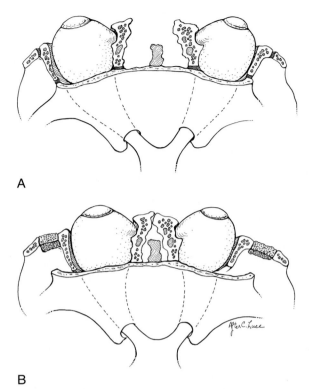

A

B

FIGURE 99-10. Transverse view of the medial translocation of the osteotomized orbits into the central defect. *A,* Lines of osteotomy and central defect. Note that the osteotomies are posterior to the equator of the globes. *B,* After medial mobilization of the orbits and bone grafting of the lateral defects.

screws (Fig. 99-11). Alternatively, paramedian defects can be made in lesser deformities, and this variation facilitates nasal bone grafting (Fig. 99-12).

A medial canthopexy (Fig. 99-13) is usually performed with transnasal wiring. It is essential to fixate the medial canthal mechanism or tendon in a posterosuperior position in the orbit.[21]

The transconjunctival incision is closed with plain catgut resorbable sutures, and the scalp incision is closed over a drain in a two-layer fashion. Nasal reconstruction with or without bone grafting usually complements the procedure (Figs. 99-14 and 99-15).

Bipartition Procedure

The bipartition procedure[9] is also done through a combined craniofacial route to mobilize the circumferential orbit and avoid injury to the frontal lobe of the brain (Fig. 99-16). It is especially indicated when there is an associated maxillary cleft and an inverted V deformity of the maxillary occlusion.

As in the combined craniofacial procedure, the osteotomies are made through the medial wall of the orbit, the roof, and the lateral walls of the orbit. However, the integrity of the floor is not disturbed so that it remains in continuity with the underlying maxillary segments.[22]

A midline defect is made as previously described. The lateral wall osteotomy is extended along the lateral aspect of the maxilla and through the pterygomaxillary junction. After the maxilla is liberated, the orbital-maxillary segments can be moved toward the midline.

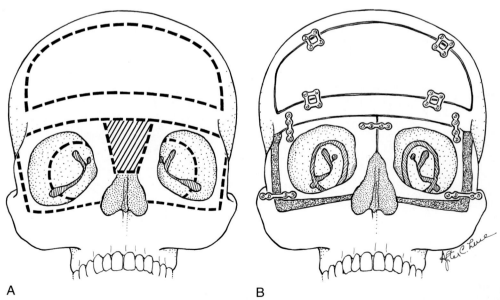

A   **B**

FIGURE 99-11. Central segment technique. *A,* Lines of osteotomy and central defect. *B,* After mobilization of the orbits and bone grafting of the lateral orbital walls (inlay) and anterior maxilla (onlay). Note the strategically placed plates and screws.

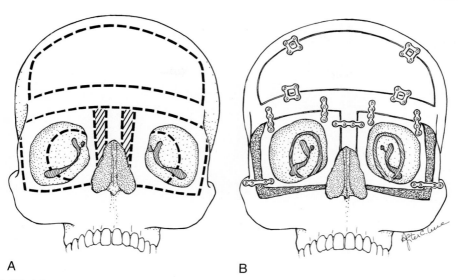

FIGURE 99-12. Paramedian segments technique. *A,* Lines of osteotomy and paramedian defects. *B,* After mobilization of the orbits and bone grafting of the lateral orbital walls (inlay) and anterior maxilla (onlay). Note the strategically placed plates and screws.

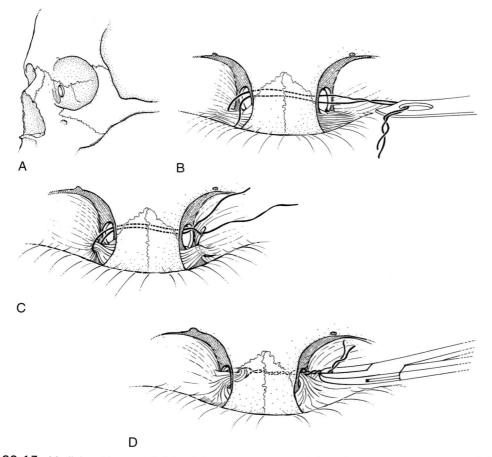

FIGURE 99-13. Medial canthopexy. *A,* Bone fenestrations have been made in a position high and posterior on the medial orbital wall. *B,* Passage of the transnasal wire (or wires) with a trocar and insertion into the contralateral canthal mechanism. *C* and *D,* The medial canthal mechanisms have been identified and transnasal No. 28 stainless steel wires passed through them. The wires are tightened with advancement of the medial canthal mechanisms into the bone fenestrations.

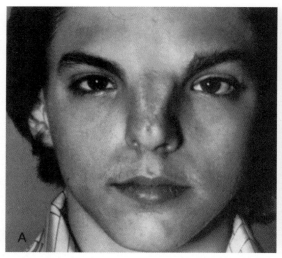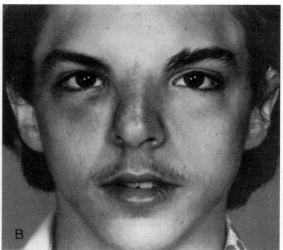

FIGURE 99-14. An adolescent boy with orbital hypertelorism, midline or zero cleft, and widow's peak. *A,* Preoperative view. *B,* Appearance after surgical correction, as illustrated in Figure 99-12. (From McCarthy JG, Thorne CHM, Wood-Smith D: Principles of craniofacial surgery: orbital hypertelorism. In McCarthy JG, ed: Plastic Surgery. Philadelphia, WB Saunders, 1990:2974.)

An occlusal splint that has been fashioned preoperatively ensures the position of the maxillary occlusion after mobilization of the segments. Autogenous bone grafts are placed in the defects of the lateral orbital wall and zygoma. Rigid skeletal fixation is achieved with plates and screws, and the closure is as previously described for the combined craniofacial correction of orbital hypertelorism. Medial canthopexy is also performed, and any nasal reconstruction is undertaken at the same surgical stage.

Subcranial or U-Shaped Osteotomy

The subcranial approach has few indications. First of all, it can be considered only if there is a superiorly positioned cribriform plate that would allow mobi-

lization of the medial orbital walls below that structure. There are few such patients.

A U-shaped osteotomy (Fig. 99-17) is performed after orbital exposure in the subperiosteal plane is obtained by a bicoronal incision. The osteotomy is made at the level of the frontozygomatic suture and carried through the full-thickness lateral orbital wall at its cranial attachment and extended through the zygomatic complex.[5] The floor of the orbit is sectioned with an osteotome after the lateral orbital wall osteotomy is completed. With the bicoronal flap reflected, the osteotomy is extended through the medial orbital wall, following which a central segment of nasal bone and ethmoid sinus is resected. The U-shaped orbital segments can then be moved toward the midline and autogenous bone grafts placed in the residual lateral defects. Rigid skeletal fixation is achieved with

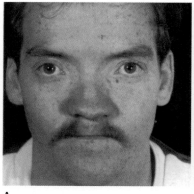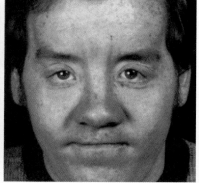

A   B

FIGURE 99-15. Orbital hypertelorism in an adult man. *A,* Preoperative appearance. *B,* After correction by the technique illustrated in Figure 99-11. (From McCarthy JG, Thorne CHM, Wood-Smith D: Principles of craniofacial surgery: orbital hypertelorism. In McCarthy JG, ed: Plastic Surgery. Philadelphia, WB Saunders, 1990: 2974.)

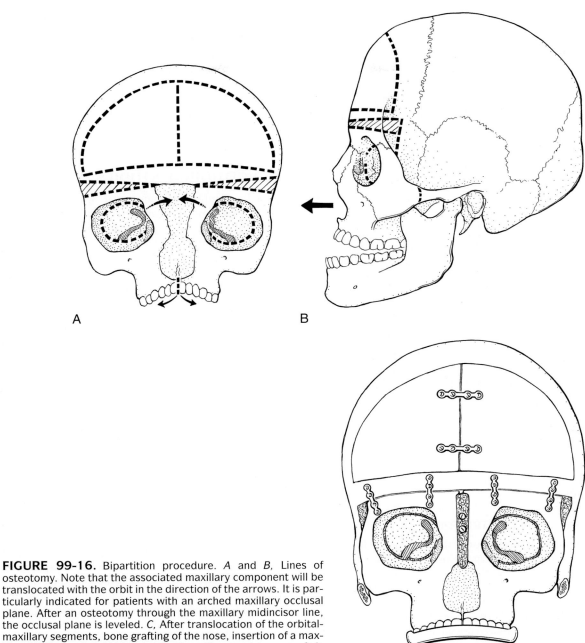

A

B

C

FIGURE 99-16. Bipartition procedure. *A* and *B,* Lines of osteotomy. Note that the associated maxillary component will be translocated with the orbit in the direction of the arrows. It is particularly indicated for patients with an arched maxillary occlusal plane. After an osteotomy through the maxillary midincisor line, the occlusal plane is leveled. *C,* After translocation of the orbital-maxillary segments, bone grafting of the nose, insertion of a maxillary splint, and rigid skeletal fixation. The nasal bone graft is secured with either wires or screws.

microplates and screws. Nasal reconstruction is performed at the same time.

Associated Procedures

MEDIAL CANTHOPEXY

Because the medial canthal mechanism is usually detached in the execution of the surgical procedure

for the correction of orbital hypertelorism, it should be reattached (medial canthopexy). As emphasized by Zide and McCarthy,[21] the medial canthal mechanism is best attached or fixated at a position superior and posterior on the medial orbital wall (see Fig. 99-13). The canthal mechanism is grasped and sutured with fine stainless steel wires passed transnasally through the septum and tightened

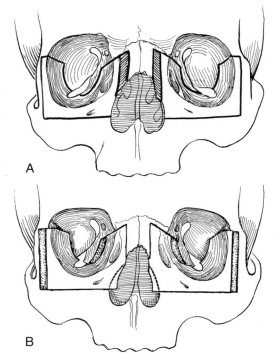

FIGURE 99-17. The subcranial approach. *A,* Lines of osteotomy (U shaped) and the paramedian bone resection. *B,* Mobilized orbits with bone grafts placed in the lateral defects. (From McCarthy JG, Thorne CHM, Wood-Smith D: Principles of craniofacial surgery: orbital hypertelorism. In McCarthy JG, ed: Plastic Surgery. Philadelphia, WB Saunders, 1990:2974.)

to re-establish the contours of the naso-orbital valley.

NASAL RECONSTRUCTION

In the execution of orbital translocation for the correction of orbital hypertelorism, nasal reconstruction is usually done at the same time because so many of the patients have associated nasal deformities characterized by naso-orbital clefts, nasal duplications, and bifidity. In the more severe types, it is necessary to make a midline nasal dorsal incision and, under direct vision, reconstruct the nasal tip cartilages and resect duplicated anatomic structures. An iliac bone graft, appropriately shaped as the keel of a boat, is often the procedure of choice to restore the nasal dorsum and reduce the illusion of hypertelorism in patients with only mildly increased interorbital distances. The midline nasal incision is carefully approximated in a two-layer fashion (Fig. 99-18).

SOFT TISSUE CLEFTS

As emphasized by Tessier[12] and by Kawamoto,[23] orbital hypertelorism is often associated with an unending

variety of orbital-facial clefts. Soft tissue reconstruction is often indicated, and a variety of local flaps have been described (Fig. 99-19). Skin expansion[10] offers the possibility of delivering an increased amount of skin in a preliminary procedure, and it can then be used to provide additional soft tissue coverage in the repair of clefts in the nasal, maxillary, and medial canthal regions. The entire nasal dorsal aesthetic unit can also be used as a flap donor site in the reconstruction of alar, lobular, and columellar clefts.[24]

LONGITUDINAL STUDIES

In a longitudinal cephalometric study of patients after orbital hypertelorism correction, McCarthy et al[25] reported a series of 18 patients aged 3 to 21 years at the time of surgery. The amount of bone resected in the nasoglabellar region averaged 22.1 mm. A remarkable degree of skeletal (orbital) stability was demonstrated (Figs. 99-20 and 99-21); only three patients showed lateral drift or relapse of the orbits. Of the three, two had undergone surgery at the age of 4 years and the remaining patient at the age of 10 years. Long-term nasomaxillary form was acceptable, except in those patients who had previously undergone repair of an associated cleft palate or orbitofacial cleft.

In a subsequent study by the same group[26] of 20 patients who underwent corrective orbital hypertelorism surgery before the age of 5.3 years (see Fig. 99-21), it was reported that the procedure could be safely performed with satisfactory aesthetic results. There was minimal evidence of long-term (>7 years) clinical or skeletal (orbital) relapse. Nasomaxillary development proceeded as expected. Three patients were considered surgical failures; two patients were undercorrected, and in another patient it was thought that there was inadequate exenteration of the ethmoid cells and midline structures. In another study reviewing nine patients with orbital hypertelorism and orbitofacial clefts who underwent facial bipartition repair between 1.5 and 8.0 years, there was no evidence of interference with normal sagittal growth of the maxilla when the patients were observed for a mean of 7 years.[11]

These studies stand in contrast to another report[27] of patients undergoing hypertelorism correction that suggested such surgery may interfere with anterior facial growth, and it was recommended that repair be deferred until late adolescence. Moreover, it is the chapter author's opinion that the most satisfactory results are obtained in the older patient (i.e., adolescent or older).

In a serial computed tomographic study[17] of the geometric changes in the orbits after surgical translocation, the changes in the distance between the globes correlated most accurately with the documented geometric changes in the lateral orbital walls.

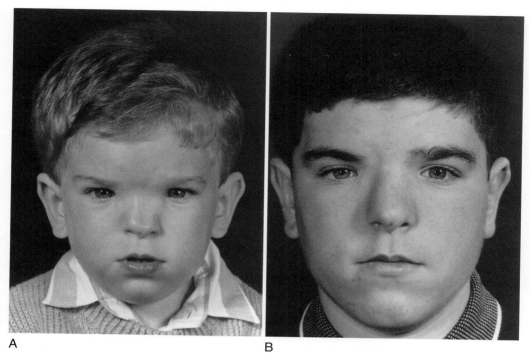

FIGURE 99-18. Example of nasal bone grafting and medial canthopexy alone in the correction of minor forms of orbital hypertelorism. *A,* A 4-year-old boy with midline (zero) cleft, nasal duplication and bifidity, and orbital hypertelorism. *B,* Ten years after open rhinoplasty, resection of duplicated nasal structures, nasal tip plasty, bone grafting of the nasal dorsum, and bilateral medial canthopexy.

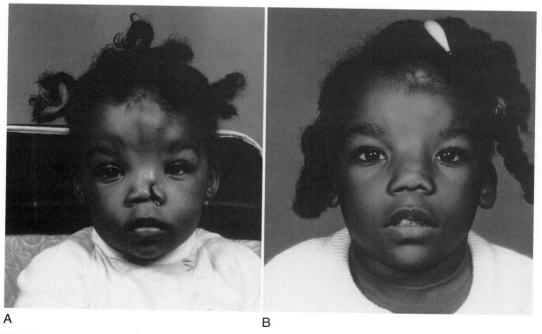

FIGURE 99-19. Surgical correction of a nasal cleft and frontal encephalocele. *A,* A 2-year-old girl with a cleft involving the alar rim, nasal bone, medial canthus, and frontal bone (Tessier, No. 1). Note the frontal encephalocele and medial canthal dystopia. *B,* Appearance several years after repair of the alar defect with local flaps and closure of the frontal bone defect with an autogenous bone graft. (From McCarthy JG, Thorne CHM, Wood-Smith D: Principles of craniofacial surgery: orbital hypertelorism. In McCarthy JG, ed: Plastic Surgery. Philadelphia, WB Saunders, 1990:2974.)

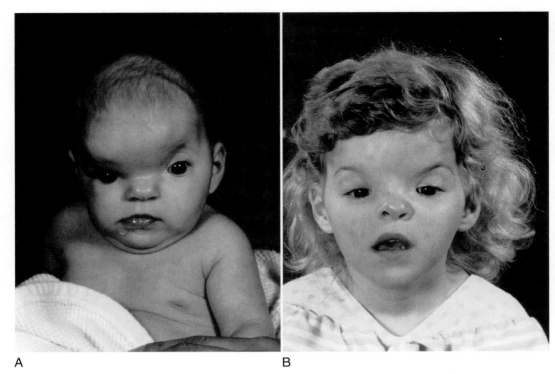

FIGURE 99-20. Early correction of orbital hypertelorism. *A,* A newborn with craniofrontonasal dysplasia, frontal bossing, orbital dystopia, and orbital hypertelorism. *B,* Appearance at age 5 years after two-stage cranial vault remodeling and correction of orbital hypertelorism and orbital dystopia (the right orbit was translocated in a superior and medial direction).

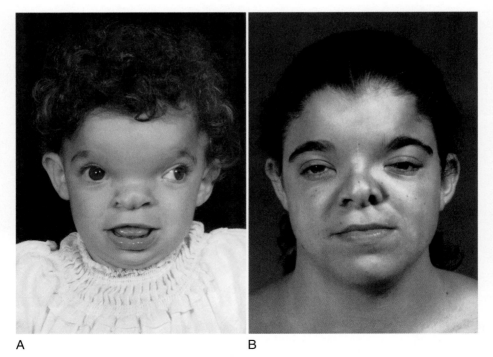

FIGURE 99-21. *A,* A 5-year-old girl with craniofrontonasal dysplasia, orbital hypertelorism, and nasal clefting before a bipartition procedure (see Fig. 99-16). *B,* At age 14 years (almost 10 years after the bipartition procedure).

A well-defined midline space must also be made by bone resection and ethmoid sinus exenteration to provide space for the medially translocated orbits and their contents.

REFERENCES

1. Converse JM, Ransohoff J, Mathews ES, et al: Ocular hypertelorism and pseudohypertelorism. Advances in surgical treatment. Plast Reconstr Surg 1970;45:1.

2. Converse JM, Smith B: An operation for congenital and traumatic hypertelorism. In Troutman RC, Converse JM, Smith B, eds: Plastic and Reconstructive Surgery of the Eye and Adnexa. London, Butterworths, 1962.

3. Tessier P, Guiot G, Rougerie J, et al: Cranio-naso-orbito-facial osteotomies. Hypertelorism [in French]. Ann Chir Plast 1967;12:103.

4. Tessier P: Orbital hypertelorism. I. Successive surgical attempts. Material and methods. Causes and mechanisms. Scand J Plast Reconstr Surg 1972;6:135.

5. Tessier P, Guiot G, Derome P: Orbital hypertelorism. II. Definite treatment of orbital hypertelorism (OR.H.) by craniofacial or by extracranial osteotomies. Scand J Plast Reconstr Surg 1973;7:39.

6. Tessier P: Experiences in the treatment of orbital hypertelorism. Plast Reconstr Surg 1974;53:1.

7. Schmid E: Surgical management of hypertelorism. In Longacre JJ, ed: Craniofacial Anomalies: Pathogenesis and Repair. Philadelphia, JB Lippincott, 1968.

8. McCarthy JG: A study of gustatory and olfactory function in patients with craniofacial anomalies. Plast Reconstr Surg 1979;64:52.

9. van der Meulen JC: Medial faciotomy. Br J Plast Surg 1979;32:339.

10. Ortiz Monasterio F, Molina F: Orbital hypertelorism. Clin Plast Surg 1994;21:599.

11. Ortiz Monasterio F, Molina F, Sigler A, et al: Maxillary growth after early facial bipartition. J Craniofac Surg 1996;7:440.

12. Tessier P: Anatomical classification of facial, craniofacial and laterofacial clefts. J Maxillofac Surg 1976;4:69.

13. Holmes AD, Meara JG, Kolker AR, et al: Frontoethmoidal encephaloceles: reconstruction and refinements. J Craniofac Surg 2001;12:6.

14. Choy AE, Margolis S, Breinin GM, McCarthy JG: Analysis of preoperative and postoperative extraocular muscle function in surgical translocation of bony orbits: a preliminary report. In Converse JM, McCarthy JG, Wood-Smith D, eds: Symposium on Diagnosis and Treatment of Craniofacial Anomalies. St. Louis, CV Mosby, 1979:128.

15. Hansman CF: Growth of interorbital distance and skull thickness as observed in roentgenographic measurements. Radiology 1966;86:87.

16. Munro IR: Improving results in orbital hypertelorism correction. Ann Plast Surg 1979;2:499.

17. Hoffman WY, McCarthy JG, Cutting CB, et al: Computerized tomographic analysis of orbital hypertelorism repair: spatial relationship of the globe and the bony orbit. Ann Plast Surg 1990;25:124.

18. Ortiz Monasterio F, Medina O, Musolas A: Geometrical planning for the correction of orbital hypertelorism. Plast Reconstr Surg 1990;86:650.

19. Converse JM, Wood-Smith D, McCarthy JG, et al: Craniofacial surgery. Clin Plast Surg 1974;1:499.

20. Converse JM, McCarthy JG: Orbital hypertelorism. Scand J Plast Reconstr Surg 1981;15:265.

21. Zide B, McCarthy JG: The medial canthus revisited—anatomical basis of medial canthopexy. Ann Plast Surg 1983;11:1.

22. Posnick JC: Monobloc and facial bipartition osteotomies. A step-by-step description of the surgical technique. J Craniofac Surg 1996;7:229.

23. Kawamoto HK: The kaleidoscopic world of rare craniofacial clefts: order out of chaos (Tessier classification). Clin Plast Surg 1976;3:529.

24. van der Meulen JC, van Adrichem LNA, Vaandrager J: The nasal dorsum as a donor site for the correction of alar, lobular and columellar malformations. Plast Reconstr Surg 2001;107:676.

25. McCarthy JG, Coccaro PJ, Wood-Smith D, Converse JM: Longitudinal cephalometric studies following surgical correction of orbital hypertelorism: a preliminary report. In Converse JM, McCarthy JG, Wood-Smith D, eds: Symposium on Diagnosis and Treatment of Craniofacial Anomalies. St. Louis, CV Mosby, 1979:229.

26. McCarthy JG, La Trenta GS, Breitbart AS, et al: Hypertelorism correction in the young child. Plast Reconstr Surg 1990;86:214.

27. Mulliken JB, Kaban LB, Evans CA, et al: Facial skeletal changes following hypertelorbitism correction. Plast Reconstr Surg 1986;77:7.

Reconstruction: Facial Clefts

DAVID J. DAVID, MD, FRCS

Rare craniofacial clefts are a heterogeneous group of deformities lumped together by surgeons because of the extreme challenge they present for treatment. It has been common in the recent literature to include craniofacial microsomia in this group, as well as Treacher Collins syndrome, although the etiology of each group may be quite different. Facial duplications and some manifestations of syncephalic twins find a place in this group as well.

Jacques van der Meulen[1] quotes *Dorland's Medical Dictionary* (1981) to define a cleft as "a fissure or elongated opening, especially one occurring in the embryo or derived from a failure of parts to fuse during embryonic development." Tessier[2] has the view that the margins of the cleft should show hypoplasia and deficiency of tissue. Some of the conditions traditionally included under the "rare" cleft heading, such as syncephalic twins and facial duplications, may not fulfill these definitions.

It has been difficult to study the conditions effectively from the point of view of their incidence, etiology, pathology, and pathogenesis because of their rarity, variability, and complexity. Surgical interventions have often taken precedence over the establishment of carefully considered protocol management. In view of this, an emphasis is placed on those aspects of the current state of knowledge that enable providers to establish reasonable treatment protocols spanning the growth period of patients based on the natural history of the individual disease processes.

CLASSIFICATION
Types of Classifications

Review of the literature shows that embryologic explanations in terms of fusion[3] and merging[4] of the facial processes do not seem to fit the rare craniofacial clefts into these schemes. For these, other explanations have been suggested, such as amniotic bands[5] and other forms of external damage to the developing facial processes.[6,7] Johnston[8] postulated defects in the neural crest cell migration.

Classifications have reflected the controversies in the causation of these interesting defects. The purely anatomic approach of Tessier,[9,10] later reported and commented on by Kawamoto,[11] has gained much current use because of its simplicity. David et al[12] reported the range of craniofacial clefts, which had been studied with three-dimensional computed tomography (CT), noting the extent of the defects throughout the whole craniofacial skeleton and some variations from the original Tessier classification.

Pfeifer[7,13] and Mazzola[14] introduced an embryologic emphasis into an otherwise anatomically divided face in their classifications. This combination of topography and embryology gives a pointer to variations in the causes and natural history of clefts in the various facial regions and therefore to possible variations in the treatment regimens.

Karfik[15] produced a classification of rare craniofacial clefts and indeed other facial disorders that have an embryologic component as well as being anatomic (Table 100-1). This is an attempt at a holistic approach and "lumping" of all craniofacial disorders into the classification.

van der Meulen et al,[1,16] first in 1983 and later in 1990, have produced an impressive holistic thesis concerning the morphogenesis of craniofacial malformations that generates a classification inclusive of malformations of the brain and cranium (cerebrocranial dysplasias), facial defects involving the brain and the eyes and cranium (cerebrocraniofacial dysplasias), and defects of the face and cranium only (craniofacial dysplasias). The three groups are divided into early and late developmental defects. This point of development occurs when the fusion processes of the face are completed at the 17-mm crown-rump length stage of embryonic development. They replace the term *cleft* with *dysplasia*, a more general term meaning abnormality in development, enabling them to base their classification wholly on the embryology of the brain, face, and cranium (Table 100-2). This classification seeks to explain the developmental mysteries of the deformities of anencephaly through to lymphangioma by facial clefting and craniosynostosis. As a scientific working thesis to be subjected to verification and development, this approach and this particular classification have much merit. As the basis of a meaningful form of communication between clinicians, it has to compete with the more simplistic topographic-anatomic classifications that are usually confined to specific regions or well-recognized disease processes.

TABLE 100-1 ✦ KARFIK FACIAL CLEFT CLASSIFICATION

Group A: Rhinencephalic Disorders

Axial (A1)	Prolapse	Meningocele
		Glioma
		Dermoid cyst
		Teratoma
	Clefts	Medial nasal (double nose)
		Median cleft of upper lip and premaxilla
	Defects	Coloboma of nostril
		Partial of nose
		Total of nose
		Septal
		Atresia nasi
Para-axial (A2)	Clefts	Coloboma, iridic or palpebral
		Total or partial para-axial
		Cleft lip, typical
		Lacrimal duct dystopia

Group B: Branchiogenic Disorders

Lateral otocephalic (B1)	Clefts	Macrostomia
		Lateral cervical fistula
	Dysostosis	Mandibular (e.g., Pierre Robin)
		Mandibulofacial (e.g., Treacher Collins)
	Defects	Partial or total auricular
		Atresia
Medial axial (B2)	Clefts	Tongue
		Lower lip
		Mandible
		Fissura colli medialis
		Fissura thoracis medialis

Group C: Ophthalmo-orbital Disorders

Malformation	Eyeball
	Microphthalmia
	Anophthalmia
	Lids
	Blepharophimosis
	Epicanthus
	Ptosis
	Agenesis
Defect	Orbital
Clefts	Upper lid coloboma
	Commissural

Group D: Craniocephalic Disorders

Malformation	Head and face (e.g., Apert and Crouzon diseases)
Defect	Scalp
	Skull

Group E: Atypical Facial Disorders

Oblique facial clefts
Dysembryoma, parasitic
Hemifacial atrophy
Hyperplasia
Neoplasm, congenital
Teratoma

From Kawamoto HK: Rare craniofacial clefts. In McCarthy JG, ed: Plastic Surgery. Philadelphia, WB Saunders, 1990:2933.

TABLE 100-2 ♦ CLASSIFICATION OF CRANIOFACIAL MALFORMATIONS

Cerebrocranial dysplasias
  Anencephaly
  Microcephaly
  Others
Cerebrofacial dysplasias
  Rhinencephalic dysplasias
  Oculo-orbital dysplasias
Craniofacial dysplasias
  With clefting
    Lateral nasomaxillary cleft
    Medial nasomaxillary cleft
    Intermaxillary clefting
    Maxillomandibular cleft
  With dysostosis (craniofacial helix)
    Sphenoidal
    Sphenofrontal
    Frontal
    Frontofrontal
    Frontonasoethmoidal
    Internasal
    Nasal
    Premaxillomaxillary and intermaxillopalatine
    Nasomaxillary and maxillary
    Maxillozygomatic
    Zygomatic
    Zygo-auromandibular
    Temporo-aural
    Temporo-auromandibular
    Mandibular
    Intermandibular
  With synostosis
    Craniosynostosis
      Parieto-occipital
      Interparietal

    Craniofaciosynostosis
      Interfrontal
      Sphenofrontoparietal
      Frontoparietal
      Frontointerparietal
    Faciosynostosis
      Frontomalar
      Vomeropremaxillary (Binder)
      Perimaxillary (posterior) (clefting)
      Perimaxillary (anterior) (pseudo-Crouzon)
      Perimaxillary (total) (Crouzon)
    With dysostosis and synostosis
      Crouzon
      Acrocephalosyndactyly (Apert)
      Triphyllocephaly (cloverleaf skull)
    With dyschondrosis
      Achondroplasia
Craniofacial dysplasias with other origin
  Osseous
    Osteopetrosis
    Craniotubular dysplasia
    Fibrous dysplasia
  Cutaneous
    Ectodermal dysplasia
  Neurocutaneous
    Neurofibromatosis
  Neuromuscular
    Robin syndrome
    Möbius syndrome
  Muscular
    Glossoschisis
  Vascular
    Hemangioma
    Hemolymphangioma
    Lymphangioma

From van der Meulen JC, Mazzola R, Stricker M, et al: Classification of craniofacial malformations. In Stricker M, van der Meulen JC, Raphael B, et al, eds: Craniofacial Malformations. Edinburgh, Churchill Livingstone, 1990:154.

Subclassifications

Median facial clefts have been subjected to special attention. Those conditions, which have forebrain malformations and agenesis or hypodevelopment of the midline structures of the face, were classified as early as 1832 by Geoffroy St. Hilaire[17] and include patients with single or dual orbits. Kundrat[18] used the term *arhinencephaly* to describe the less severe conditions with absence of the rhinencephalon and hypotelorism with absence of midline facial structures. DeMyer and Zeman[19] produced a classification based on the gradation of severity relating the facial deficiency to the underlying brain deficiency (Fig. 100-1).

Attempts have also been made to classify those median facial cleft conditions that coexist with hypertelorism. Tessier,[20,21] Converse et al,[22] and van der Meulen et al[16] have made the distinction between those situations in which only the interorbital distance is increased and those in which there is an increase in divergence of the orbital axis from the midsagittal

plane. DeMyer[23] and Greig[24] used the term *ocular hypertelorism,* giving the impression that this was a primary disease process. Tessier[21] was at pains to point out that orbital hypertelorism is a physical finding associated with other cranial and facial malformations. DeMyer[23] described median cleft face syndrome, consisting of orbital hypertelorism, V-shaped frontal hairline, cranium bifidum occultum, median cleft of the upper lip, median cleft of the premaxilla, median cleft of the palate, and primary telecanthus. Sedano et al[25] used the term *frontonasal dysplasia* for this condition. Frontoethmoidal meningoencephalocele is a unique condition believed to have an etiology and natural history different from the craniofacial clefts.[26]

CLASSIFICATION OF FRONTOETHMOIDAL MENINGOENCEPHALOCELE

Meningoencephaloceles may be broadly subdivided into occipital, parietal, basal, and sincipital. The last group has been further classified by Suwanwela and

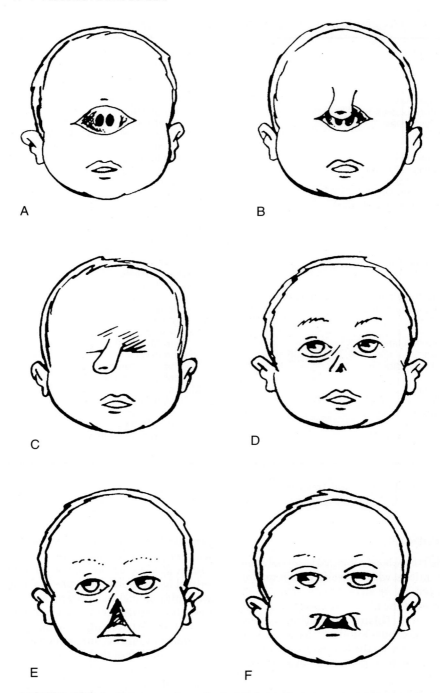

FIGURE 100-1. Spectrum of cerebrofacial dysplasias: *A,* cyclopia; *B,* synophthalmus; *C,* ethmocephaly; *D,* cebocephaly; *E,* without premaxilla; *F,* with premaxilla. (From van der Meulen J, Mazzola R, Stricker M, Raphael B: Classification of craniofacial malformations. In Stricker M, van der Meulen J, Raphael B, Mazzola R, eds: Craniofacial Malformations. Edinburgh, Churchill Livingstone, 1990:157.)

Suwanwela,[27] on the basis of a paper by Meyer,[28] into frontoethmoidal-nasofrontal, frontoethmoidal-nasoethmoidal, frontoethmoidal-naso-orbital, interfrontal, and craniofacial clefts.

The bone defects associated with sincipital meningoencephaloceles have been included in many attempts to classify craniofacial clefts. Two of the most significant endeavors are Tessier's anatomic classification[9,10] and Mazzola's morphologic classification[14] based on embryologic considerations.

CRANIOFACIAL MICROSOMIA

A number of morphologic classifications deal with various bone and soft tissue manifestations of this disease, considered by most authors to be a clefting condition.[29-34]

Tessier Classification

In 1973, Tessier presented a classification of rare craniofacial clefts; a more detailed description was published in 1976,[9,10] and almost contemporaneously, Kawamoto[11] published on the subject. David et al[12] described the range of clefts with the morphologic aid of three-dimensional reconstruction from CT.

The rarity and large variety of craniofacial clefts have prevented the establishment of a concise, meaningful, and comprehensive classification system. On the basis of his personal experience, which included clinical, radiologic, and surgical observations of 336 patients, Tessier devised an ordered numbering system to identify the consistent anatomic pathways of soft tissue and skeletal clefts (Fig. 100-2). The appealing simplicity of the Tessier system has both improved communication between observers of craniofacial clefts and provided better appreciation of the reconstructive surgery required to restore normality.

The application of three-dimensional reconstructions of high-resolution CT data has enhanced our knowledge of the extent of the disordered craniofacial morphology of patients with craniofacial clefts. Since the original report, the author has added another 116 patients to the study.[12] It is this classification that is used to describe the phenotypic features of these conditions.

MORPHOLOGY

Using the Tessier Classification as a Guide

Since 1975, the Australian Craniofacial Unit has assessed 828 patients with rare craniofacial clefts that could be classified by the Tessier system (Table 100-3). Multiple examples of each of the Tessier clefts were available for review, and relevant data have been

TABLE 100-3 ✦ POPULATION OF PATIENTS WITH TESSIER CRANIOFACIAL CLEFTS PRESENTING TO THE AUSTRALIAN CRANIOFACIAL UNIT, 1975-2002

Hemifacial microsomia/Goldenhar syndrome	321
Treacher Collins syndrome	73
Rare craniofacial clefts (excluding those above)	219
Encephaloceles	
nasofrontal	125
naso-orbital	22
nasoethmoidal	53
Holoprosencephaly	13
Arrhinencephaly	2
Total	828

included in the following section to elucidate each of the Tessier types (number 0 to number 14).

NUMBER 0

Soft Tissue Characteristics. The midline soft tissue anomaly may range from a mild broadening of the philtrum (Fig. 100-3A) to a true median cleft lip. The columella and nasal tip are typically bifid and broadened with a midline depression. The alae nasi are intact but laterally displaced. The nose appears shortened in the vertical dimension.

Skeletal Characteristics. Midline facial clefting produces a characteristic hypertelorism that may or may not be associated with a characteristic keel shape of the maxillary alveolus, and there is sometimes an anterior open bite. Vertical hypoplasia in the region of the cleft and its margins produces a reduction in median and paramedian midfacial height (Fig. 100-3B). The cartilaginous and bony nasal septum is thickened, and the nasal bones and nasal processes of the maxilla are broad, flattened, and displaced laterally from the midline. The midline cleft is manifested superiorly as enlargement and inferior prolapse of the ethmoid and sphenoid sinuses, orbital hypertelorism, and symmetric widening of the anterior cranial fossa (Fig. 100-3C). The body of the sphenoid is anatomically normal, although it is broadened with displacement of the pterygoid plates away from the midline. The extension of this cleft into the cranium constitutes a number 14 cleft.

NUMBER 1

Soft Tissue Characteristics. Above the cleft lip, the clefting of the alar dome is associated with deviation to the opposite side of the shortened and broadened columella and nasal tip. Extension of the soft tissue cleft onto the nasal dorsum can be manifested as a series

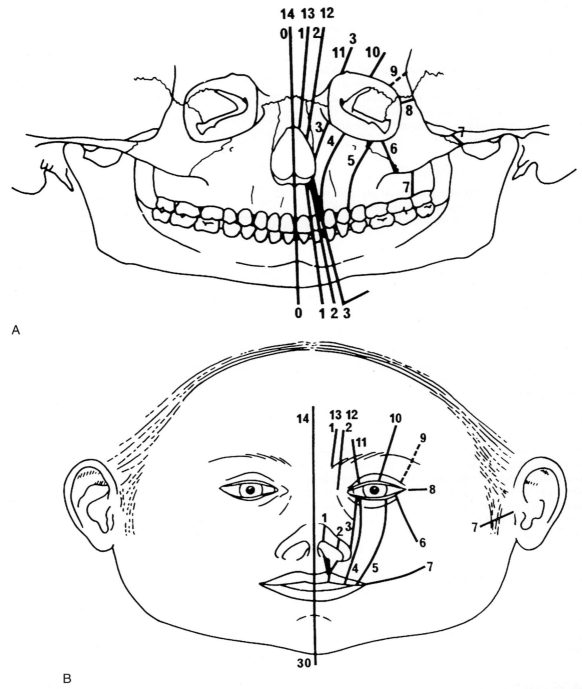

FIGURE 100-2. Tessier classification of craniofacial clefts: *A,* soft tissue; *B,* skeletal. (From David DJ, Moore MH, Cooter RD: Tessier clefts revisited with a third dimension. Cleft Palate J 1989;26:163-184.)

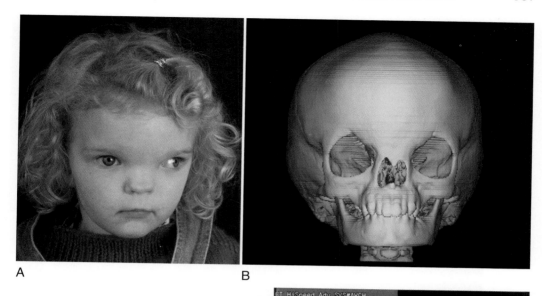

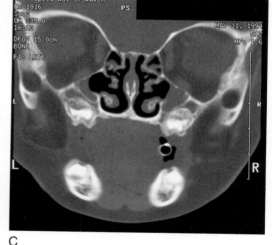

FIGURE 100-3. *A*, A 5-year-old girl with untreated midline craniofacial cleft of the Tessier number 0-14 type. *B*, The CT reconstruction shows the increased distance between the orbits and the broadened shape of the piriform aperture and indicates the bifid nature of the septum. *C*, The coronal two-dimensional CT reformat shows the depressed cribriform plate, the widened nasoethmoid region, and the bifid septum.

of vertical soft tissue furrows and ridges (Fig. 100-4*A*). Vertical inner canthal dystopia and severe telecanthus mark the superior aspect of the number 1 facial cleft. A cranial soft tissue extension characterized by a tongue-like projection of the frontal hairline delineates the number 13 cleft.

SKELETAL CHARACTERISTICS. Skeletal clefting of the maxilla may extend posteriorly to form a complete cleft of the hard and soft palate. The maxilla is hypoplastic in all three dimensions. There is a keel-shaped alveolus and anterior open bite (Fig. 100-4*B*). Normal septation is preserved between the nasal cavity and the hypoplastic maxillary antrum on the affected side (Fig. 100-4*C*). Distortion of the nasal skeleton produces gross flattening of the nasal dorsum. There is asymmetry of the pterygoid plates, of the

greater and lesser wings of the sphenoid, and of the floor of the anterior cranial fossa (Fig. 100-4*D* and *E*). The distortion of the cranial base may result in a mild plagiocephaly.

NUMBER 2

SOFT TISSUE CHARACTERISTICS. Above the cleft of the lip and palate is a true broad cleft of the nostril that is medial to the intact but laterally displaced tail of the alar cartilage. A shallow soft tissue groove extends superiorly to the asymmetrically widened nasal root (Fig. 100-5*A*). The lacrimal system, palpebral fissures, and eyebrows remain intact.

SKELETAL CHARACTERISTICS. The alveolar cleft extends posteriorly as a complete unilateral cleft of

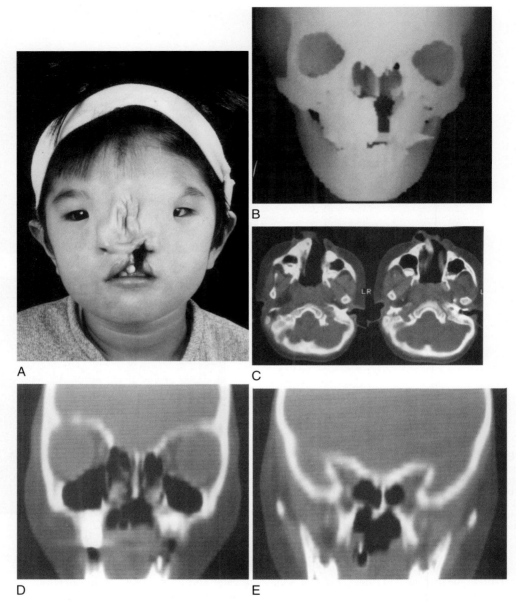

FIGURE 100-4. *A,* A 4-year-old Malay Chinese girl with the left-sided craniofacial clefts of the Tessier number 1-13 type. *B,* Alveolar clefting between the central and lateral incisor extends into the piriform margin. *C,* Normal septation between the nasal cavity and the hypoplastic cleft maxilla. *D* and *E,* Coronal two-dimensional CT reformats confirm cleft-side maxillary hypoplasia, inferior orbital dislocation, pterygoid plate asymmetry, and anterior and middle cranial fossa floor asymmetry. (From David DJ, Moore MH, Cooter RD: Tessier clefts revisited with a third dimension. Cleft Palate J 1989;26:163-184.)

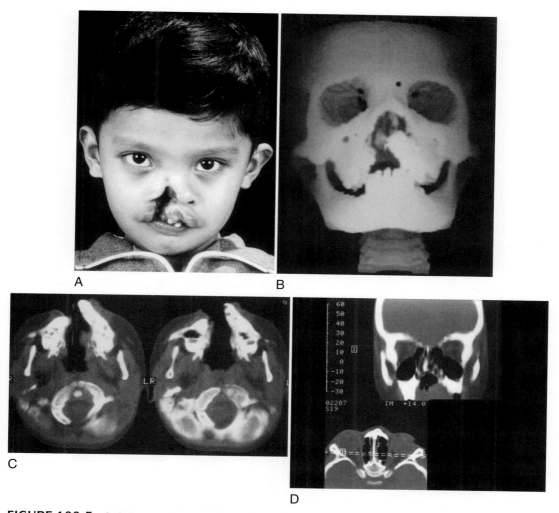

FIGURE 100-5. *A,* A 4-year-old Malaysian boy with an unrepaired right-sided cleft of the Tessier number 2 type. *B,* Cleft marginal hypoplasia produces a characteristic keel-shaped alveolus and hypoplastic maxilla. *C,* Axial two-dimensional CT scan shows the alveolar cleft and inferior displacement of the cleft-side maxilla. *D,* Coronal two-dimensional CT reformat through the posterior orbits demonstrates the asymmetry extending from below in the maxilla, through the ethmoids, to the anterior cranial fossa. (From David DJ, Moore MH, Cooter RD: Tessier clefts revisited with a third dimension. Cleft Palate J 1989;26: 163-184.)

the hard and soft palate. The nasal septum is intact but deviated to the opposite side. The nasal cavity remains separated from the normally pneumatized although hypoplastic maxilla on the cleft side (Fig. 100-5*B* and *C*). Above the nasomaxillary notching, the ethmoid sinus is less well developed, and there is no pneumatization of the frontal sinus on this side. Anterior rotation of the greater and lesser wings of the sphenoid occurs on the cleft side in relation to the narrower orbit and smaller ethmoid sinus. There is mild asymmetry of the anterior cranial fossa, which is narrower on the cleft side (Fig. 100-5*D*). The cranium is brachycephalic with marked occipital flattening.

NUMBER 3

SOFT TISSUE CHARACTERISTICS. There is hypoplasia of the soft tissue margins of the cleft in the vertical dimension. This produces extreme soft tissue deficiency between the alar base and the cleft of the medial aspect of the lower eyelid (Fig. 100-6*A*). The inferior lacrimal punctum is evident at the lateral margin of the lower eyelid cleft. The lacrimal drainage system ends at an

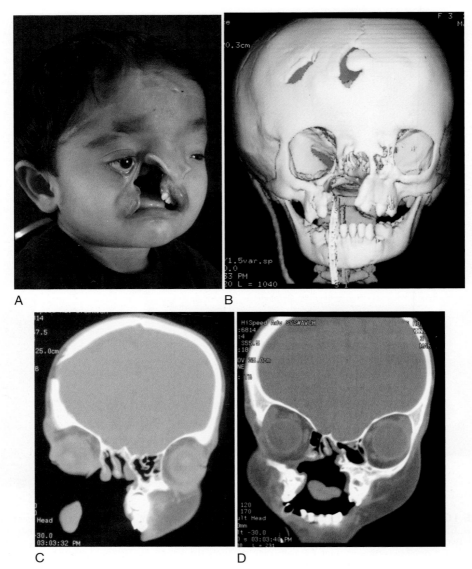

FIGURE 100-6. *A,* A 4-year-old Malaysian girl with an isolated unrepaired right-sided Tessier number 3 cleft. *B,* Three-dimensional CT reconstruction shows the anatomy of the skeletal number 3 cleft. *C,* Axial two-dimensional CT scan demonstrates the hypoplastic cleft right maxilla with associated relative absence of pneumatization. *D,* Coronal two-dimensional CT reformat shows the clefting process and the distortion of the anterior cranial fossa.

opening directly onto the cheek without communication into the nasal cavity. The globe is normal in size, but it is displaced inferiorly and laterally.

SKELETAL CHARACTERISTICS. The nasal septum shows the characteristic distortion seen in typical cleft lip and palate. There is absence of septation between the nasal cavity on the cleft side and the maxilla. The maxilla is hypoplastic in three dimensions, with no pneumatization (Fig. 100-6*B* and *C*).

Superior extension of the skeletal clefting into the medial portion of the orbital floor and into the inferior orbital rim in the region of the frontal process of the maxilla allows direct communication between the orbit above and the nasomaxillary region below. There is mild narrowing of the ethmoid sinus and of the body of the sphenoid on the cleft side. Both the orbit and the floor of the anterior cranial fossa are inferiorly displaced (Fig. 100-6*D*).

NUMBER 4

Soft Tissue Characteristics. There is severe vertical soft tissue deficiency in a number 4 cleft, with the medial margins of the cleft lip extending directly into the medially placed cleft of the lower eyelid (Fig. 100-7A). Within the medial segment of the right-sided cleft lip, muscle elements are apparently absent. Muscle bunching is noted in the ipsilateral lateral lip segment, as is seen in a typical unilateral cleft lip. The anatomically normal nasal ala is superiorly displaced in association with a severe deficiency in the overall nasal length. Marked dystopia of the right globe results in its inferior displacement into the medially deficient orbital floor and inferior rim. Both globes are otherwise normal. In some instances, however, the globe is affected, being small or having some form of coloboma.

Skeletal Characteristics. The complete palatal cleft passes through the maxilla medial to the infraorbital foramen and extends to the medial portion of the inferior orbital rim without evidence of an intact maxillary sinus (Fig. 100-7B to E). Bone septation persists medially, thereby separating the nasal cavity from the orbit, maxillary sinus, and mouth, which are contiguous. Marked midfacial hypoplasia is present. The cleft is manifested as asymmetry of the body of the sphenoid; it is smaller on the right, with asymmetric placement of the pterygoid plates relative to the midline (Fig. 100-7C). The orbital floor cleft has no communication with the inferior orbital fissure. The cleft does not extend to the skull base, but there is marked facial asymmetry associated with plagiocephaly (Fig. 100-7F).

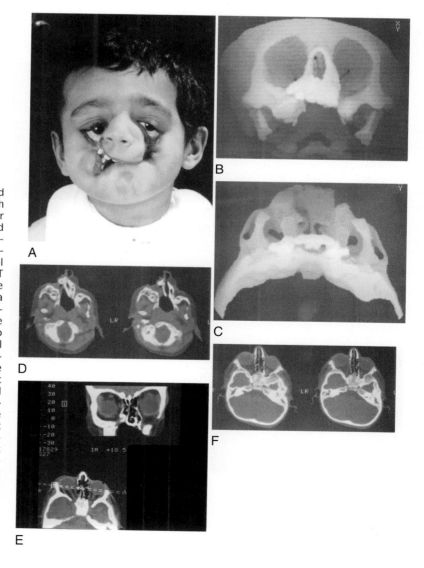

FIGURE 100-7. *A,* A 2-year-old Malaysian boy of Indian descent with unrepaired clefts of the Tessier number 4 type on the right side and number 5 on the left side. *B,* Three-dimensional CT reconstruction exposes the asymmetric midfacial skeletal clefting. *C,* Three-dimensional CT reconstruction is tilted to view the pterygoid plates and posterior maxilla from behind. The marked cleft-induced asymmetry extends from the anterior maxilla (upper border) to the pterygoid plates and cranial base (lower border). *D,* Axial two-dimensional CT scan outlines the course and relation of the cleft through the lower midface. *E,* Coronal two-dimensional CT reformat emphasizes the cleft extension into the medial portion of the orbit on the right (Tessier number 4). *F,* Axial two-dimensional CT scan at the midorbit level confirms the asymmetry extending from the orbits anteriorly through the base of the skull and sphenoid body to the occiput posteriorly. (From David DJ, Moore MH, Cooter RD: Tessier clefts revisited with a third dimension. Cleft Palate J 1989;26: 163-184.)

NUMBER 5

SOFT TISSUE CHARACTERISTICS. There is a vertical soft tissue deficiency between the lateral portion of the lip and the lower eyelid cleft. The left side of the nose shows vertical shortening, and the left alar base is displaced superiorly (Fig. 100-8A).

Facial asymmetry secondary to the skeletal abnormality is reflected by a vertical orbital dystopia. However, both globes are normal but, as in number 4, may not be so, and there is no abnormality of the upper eyelids, eyebrow, forehead, or frontal hairline.

SKELETAL CHARACTERISTICS. The skeletal clefts vary from a narrow skeletal furrow that traverses the anterior maxillary wall as on the right (Fig. 100-8B) to a broad cleft of the maxilla lateral to the infraorbital foramen and maxillary sinus. This latter cleft enters the inferolateral orbital rim and floor without posterior communication with the inferior orbital fissure on the left side (Fig. 100-8C). Medial collapse

of the lateral maxillary segments is present bilaterally, with reduction in the transverse dimensions of the maxillary arch. Manifestations of the skeletal disturbance in the sphenoid include a shortening and thickening of the lateral orbital walls in the region of the greater wing and mild asymmetric placement of the pterygoid plates relative to the midline. The right-sided pterygoid plates are smaller and closer to the midline (Fig. 100-8D and E). There is minimal asymmetry of the cranial base and calvaria.

NUMBER 6

SOFT TISSUE CHARACTERISTICS. The soft tissue furrow, which is more apparent on the right, radiates from the oral commissure toward the lateral two thirds of the lower eyelid. The antimongoloid obliquity of the palpebral fissures is associated with laterally placed lower eyelid clefts and some ectropion (Fig. 100-9A). A left-sided anophthalmia is accompanied by adjacent

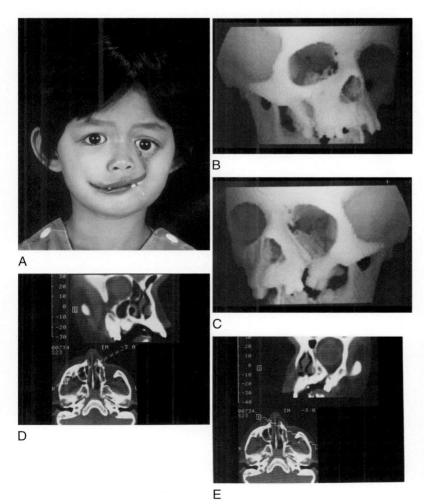

FIGURE 100-8. *A,* A 5-year-old Malaysian boy with bilateral facial clefting of the Tessier number 5 type, which is worse on the left side. *B* and *C,* Oblique three-dimensional CT reconstructions show the anterior boundaries of the bilateral number 5 clefts from the premolar alveolar cleft to the orbital floor above. *D* and *E,* Oblique two-dimensional CT reformats demonstrate some of the techniques available for tracking the clefts posteriorly through the face. (From David DJ, Moore MH, Cooter RD: Tessier clefts revisited with a third dimension. Cleft Palate J 1989;26:163-184.)

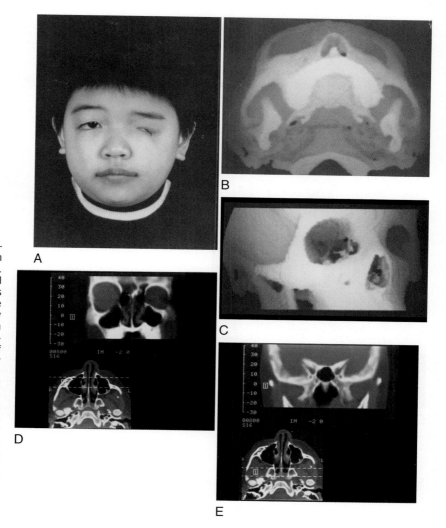

FIGURE 100-9. *A,* An 8-year-old Malaysian Chinese boy with bilateral Tessier number 6 clefts. *B,* Worm's-eye three-dimensional CT reconstruction demonstrates the skeletal hypoplasia in the region of the zygomaticomaxillary suture, which is more marked on the left side. *C,* Oblique three-dimensional CT reconstruction of the midface shows the posterior maxillary and orbital hypoplasia. *D,* Broad coronal two-dimensional CT reformat exposes the posterior maxillary hypoplasia cleft extension into the lateral orbit. *E,* Coronal two-dimensional CT reformat visualizes more posteriorly the middle cranial fossa asymmetry. (From David DJ, Moore MH, Cooter RD: Tessier clefts revisited with a third dimension. Cleft Palate J 1989;26:163-184.)

soft tissue hypoplasia and is reflected in a short palpebral fissure, enophthalmos, and minor ptosis of the eyebrow.

SKELETAL CHARACTERISTICS. No abnormality is present in the alveolar arch except for some tilting of the occlusal plane secondary to hypoplasia of the left side of the maxilla. There is a vertical bony groove in the region of the zygomaticomaxillary suture that ends in the inferolateral portion of a small bony orbit. More laterally, the remainder of the zygomatic body and arch is normal in both shape and dimension (Fig. 100-9B). The lateral orbital floor is down-slanting but intact, and it lacks direct communication with the temporal or infratemporal fossa. The hypoplasia of the left side of the maxilla and orbit is associated with a reduction in the transverse and anteroposterior dimensions of the anterior cranial fossa; mild asymmetry of the middle cranial fossa and calvaria

is present (Fig. 100-9C to E). No significant asymmetry of size, shape, or position is present in the sphenoid.

NUMBER 7

SOFT TISSUE CHARACTERISTICS. A soft tissue furrow extends from the macrostomia laterally and superiorly across the cheek toward the preauricular hairline (Fig. 100-10A). The lower eyelids are intact. The anatomy of the external ear is normal, and there are no preauricular tags.

SKELETAL CHARACTERISTICS. Bone clefting is through the pterygomaxillary junction with hypoplasia of the alveolar process in the molar region, thereby producing a posterior open bite. The maxilla is hypoplastic, although the maxillary sinuses are symmetrically pneumatized. The hypoplastic zygomatic

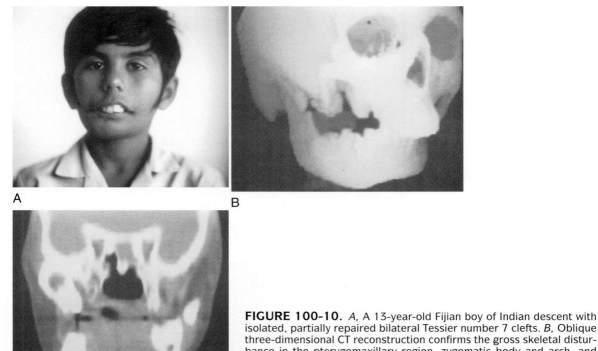

FIGURE 100-10. *A,* A 13-year-old Fijian boy of Indian descent with isolated, partially repaired bilateral Tessier number 7 clefts. *B,* Oblique three-dimensional CT reconstruction confirms the gross skeletal disturbance in the pterygomaxillary region, zygomatic body and arch, and temporomandibular articulation. *C,* Coronal two-dimensional CT reformat exposes the abnormal pterygoid plates and mandibular condyles and demonstrates the tilt of both the cranial base above and the mandible below. (From David DJ, Moore MH, Cooter RD: Tessier clefts revisited with a third dimension. Cleft Palate J 1989;26:163-184.)

body arches upward, but then it takes a downward course and is severely malformed and displaced. The zygoma is continuous posteriorly with an apparently normal zygomatic process of the temporal bone (Fig. 100-10*B*). The mandibular condyle and coronoid process are hypoplastic and asymmetric. There is no antegonial notching of the mandible. Marked cranial base asymmetry, with tilting and asymmetric positioning of the temporomandibular articulations, is present. The anatomy of the sphenoid is abnormal, especially on the right, where there is no recognizable medial or lateral pterygoid plate (Fig. 100-10*C*).

NUMBER 8

SOFT TISSUE CHARACTERISTICS. The classic soft tissue deformities of the mouth, auricle, and periorbital tissues are seen in the number 8 cleft (Fig. 100-11*A*). Secondary to the bone deficiency in the lateral orbital wall and floor, there is soft tissue continuity between the orbit, temporal fossa, and infratemporal region. Preauricular hairline indicators delineate the number 8 cleft as the first of the "northbound" clefts.

SKELETAL CHARACTERISTICS. Complete absence of the bony lateral orbital wall and rim constitutes the skeletal element of the number 8 cleft. The lateral border of the orbit is formed by the greater wing of the sphenoid; small spicules of bone, which represent the rudimentary zygoma, may be found in Treacher Collins syndrome (Fig. 100-11*B* and *C*). The symmetry of the facial anomalies is reflected in the apparently normal, symmetric anterior and middle cranial fossa (Fig. 100-11*D*). Figure 100-11*D* demonstrates the type number 8 cleft through the lateral canthus.

NUMBER 9

SOFT TISSUE CHARACTERISTICS. The superolateral bone deficiency of the orbits may allow a lateral displacement of the globes (Fig. 100-12*A*). In this example, microphthalmos is present. The lateral third of the upper eyelid and the outer canthus are distorted, thus preventing apposition to the globe. The upper eyelid does not have a true cleft. A soft tissue furrow radiates superiorly and posteriorly from the outer canthus into the temporoparietal hair-bearing scalp, which is bordered along its superior margin by the prolongation of the lateral third of the eyebrow. The

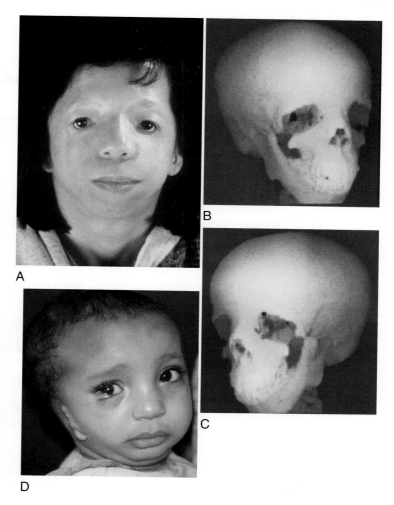

FIGURE 100-11. *A,* A 29-year-old Hong Kong Chinese woman with Treacher Collins syndrome (Tessier number 6, 7, and 8 clefts). *B* and *C,* Three-dimensional CT reconstructions expose the true extent of the bone deficiency in the frontozygomatic region, the lateral orbital wall being formed by the hypoplastic greater wing of sphenoid. *D,* A 1-year-old Arabic child with Goldenhar syndrome and the number 8 cleft extending through the lateral canthus in a horizontal fashion. (*A–C* from David DJ, Moore MH, Cooter RD: Tessier clefts revisited with a third dimension. Cleft Palate J 1989;26:163-184.)

temporal hairline projects forward bilaterally toward the scarred area of the repaired number 9 clefts. There is no demonstrable facial nerve function in the forehead or upper eyelids.

SKELETAL CHARACTERISTICS. Skeletal clefting extends superiorly and posteriorly through the upper part of the greater wing of the sphenoid to the upper portion of the squamous temporal and adjacent parietal bones. The skeletal disturbance is more severe on the right side, where a bone defect is noted in the upper temporal squama (Fig. 100-12*B* and *C*). There is asymmetric hypoplasia of the greater wing of the sphenoid with associated posterior and lateral rotation of the lateral orbital wall (Fig. 100-12*D*). Pneumatization of the body of the sphenoid is symmetric and normal. Mild cranial base asymmetry is reflected in the pterygoid plates. The left pair is more laterally displaced from the midline. Skull vault plagiocephaly is evident with an apparent reduction in the anteroposterior dimension of the anterior cranial fossa.[35]

NUMBER 10

SOFT TISSUE CHARACTERISTICS. The palpebral fissure is grossly elongated with an amblyopic eye displaced inferiorly and laterally. There is also a divergent squint of the right eye. The eyebrow is deficient medially and becomes thinned out laterally (Fig. 100-13*A*), where it is contiguous with a broad downward and forward projection of the frontotemporal hairline (this may be seen in both the number 9 and number 10 clefts). A broad frontal encephalocele bulges forward from the middle third of the right side of the forehead, supraorbital ridge, and orbital roof.

SKELETAL CHARACTERISTICS. The bone cleft, through which the frontal encephalocele presents, involves the anterior half of the orbital roof, the supraorbital rim, and two thirds of the vertical height of the frontal bone lateral to the supraorbital nerve (Fig. 100-13*B*). The bony orbit is inferiorly displaced and widened with the lateral orbital wall shortened and

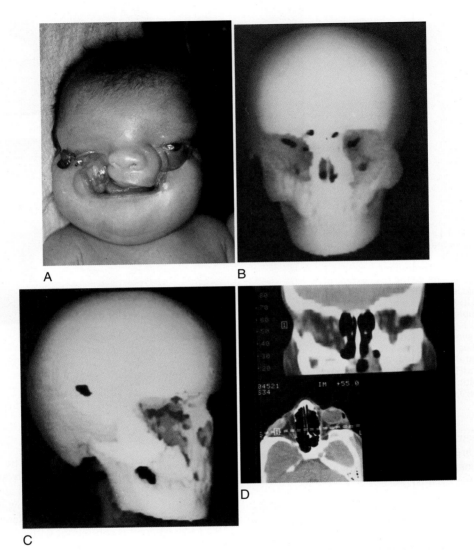

FIGURE 100-12. *A,* A newborn Hong Kong Chinese girl with bilateral Tessier number 9 clefts extending into the temporal bone. There is a confluence of clefts: types 4-6 on the right side and types 4 and 5 on the left. *B* and *C,* Bone clefting radiates superiorly and posteriorly from the upper lateral orbit. *D,* Gross bone deficiency in the region of the lateral orbital walls, with apparent posterior and lateral rotation of the axes of the orbits. (From David DJ, Moore MH, Cooter RD: Tessier clefts revisited with a third dimension. Cleft Palate J 1989;26:163-184.)

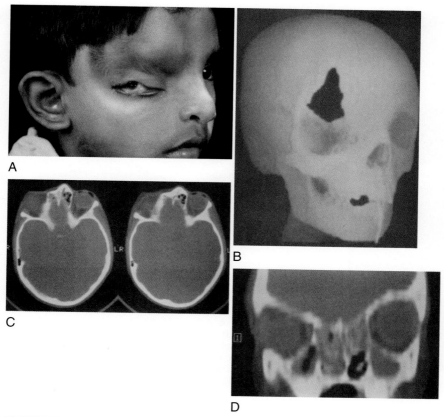

FIGURE 100-13. *A,* An 8-year-old Malaysian boy of Indian descent with multiple craniofacial clefts, including a Tessier number 10 cleft on the right side. *B,* Frontal, supraorbital, and orbital roof bone cleft lateral to the supraorbital nerve. *C,* Axial two-dimensional
CT scans through the orbits show the widening and lateral displacement of the cleft-side
orbit. *D,* Asymmetry and inferior displacement of the cleft-side orbit and anterior cranial
fossa are evident on a coronal two-dimensional CT reformat. (From David DJ, Moore
MH, Cooter RD: Tessier clefts revisited with a third dimension. Cleft Palate J 1989;26:163-
184.)

laterally deviated (Fig. 100-13*C*). Similar distortion of
the anterior cranial fossa is evident, being broader and
more flattened on the affected side (Fig. 100-13*D*). The
calvaria above the level of the cleft and the cranial base
below are symmetric.

NUMBER 11

SOFT TISSUE CHARACTERISTICS. The soft tissue features include a cleft of the medial portion of the upper
eyelid, an irregularity in hair orientation at the medial
end of the eyebrow, and a long tongue-like projection
of the frontal hairline onto the forehead (Fig. 100-
14*A*).

SKELETAL CHARACTERISTICS. There is a mild
flattening of the frontal process of the maxilla and
extensive pneumatization of both the ethmoid and
frontal sinuses, both of which are more prominent on
the cleft side (Fig. 100-14*B*). No bone clefting of the

supraorbital rim or frontal bone is evident. The
cranial base and sphenoid architecture, including the
pterygoid processes, are symmetric and normal (Fig.
100-14*C*). In this example, no associated number 3
cleft was found.

NUMBER 12

SOFT TISSUE CHARACTERISTICS. There is a lateral
displacement of the inner canthus with a mild thinning, aplasia, or irregularity of the medial end of the
eyebrow. There are no eyelid clefts (Fig. 100-15*A*). The
soft tissue contour of the forehead is normal, with only
a short downward prolongation of the paramedian
frontal hairline to mark the superior extent of the soft
tissue cleft.

SKELETAL CHARACTERISTICS. Flattening of the
frontal process of the maxilla, an increase in the
transverse dimension of the ethmoid sinus, and a

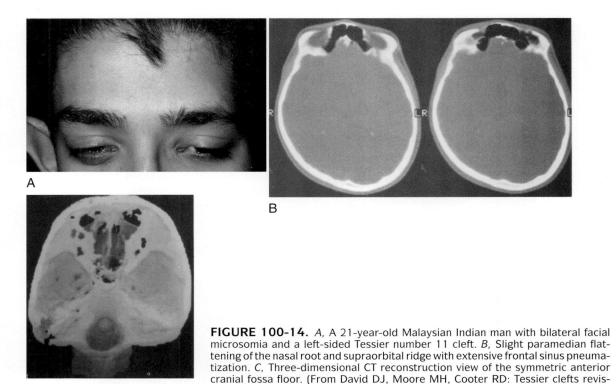

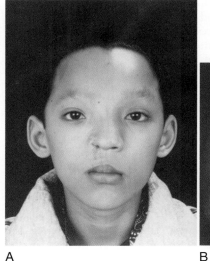

FIGURE 100-14. *A,* A 21-year-old Malaysian Indian man with bilateral facial microsomia and a left-sided Tessier number 11 cleft. *B,* Slight paramedian flattening of the nasal root and supraorbital ridge with extensive frontal sinus pneumatization. *C,* Three-dimensional CT reconstruction view of the symmetric anterior cranial fossa floor. (From David DJ, Moore MH, Cooter RD: Tessier clefts revisited with a third dimension. Cleft Palate J 1989;26:163-184.)

laterally convex bowing of the medial orbital wall produce orbital hypertelorism (Fig. 100-15*B*). Superiorly, there is a minor flattening of the frontal bone medially, and the nasofrontal angle is somewhat obtuse. The extensive pneumatization of the sinuses on the cleft side extends backward through the frontal and ethmoid sinuses and into the sphenoid sinus. The anatomy of the sphenoid, including the pterygoid processes, is otherwise normal. The anterior and middle cranial fossa floors are both broadened on the cleft side with minor widening of the cribriform plate.

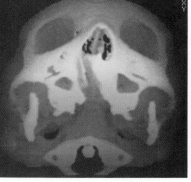

FIGURE 100-15. *A,* An 11-year-old Malaysian boy with right-sided Tessier number 2-12 clefts. *B,* Worm's-eye three-dimensional CT reconstruction shows the mild flattening and widening of the frontal process of the maxilla and underlying ethmoids on the cleft side. (From David DJ, Moore MH, Cooter RD: Tessier clefts revisited with a third dimension. Cleft Palate J 1989;26: 163-184.)

NUMBER 13

SOFT TISSUE CHARACTERISTICS. There is a large lipoma of the dorsum of the nose that extends onto the lower frontal bone above, and a characteristic hypertelorism is more marked on the cleft side. The cleft extends medially to the undisturbed eyebrow to end in a short paramedian frontal widow's peak (Fig. 100-16A).

SKELETAL CHARACTERISTICS. The bone cleft begins in the region of the nasal bone and extends superiorly through the full height of the frontal bone. Posteriorly, the cleft extends through the cribriform plate and ethmoid sinus as far as the lesser wing and body of the sphenoid. The pterygoid processes are anatomically normal, but they are displaced laterally from the midline on the cleft side. There is orbital hypertelorism below and asymmetry of the floor of the anterior cranial fossa above (Fig. 100-16B and C). There is also asymmetric distortion of the sphenoid bones (Fig. 100-16D).

NUMBER 14

SOFT TISSUE CHARACTERISTICS. The severe orbital hypertelorism is associated with a broad flattening of the glabella and extreme lateral displacement of the inner canthi. The periorbita, including the eyelids and eyebrows, are otherwise normal (Fig. 100-17A). A long midline projection of the frontal hairline marks the superior extent of the soft tissue features of this midline cranial cleft.

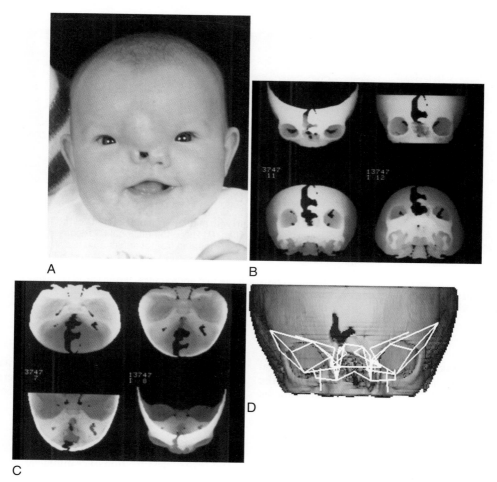

A

B

C

D

FIGURE 100-16. *A,* A 3-month-old Australian girl with right-sided Tessier number 1-13 cleft. *B* and *C,* Three-dimensional CT reconstruction sequence graphically demonstrates the superficial and deep dimensions of the Tessier number 13 cleft. *D,* A wire frame model of the sphenoid shows how the keystone to the craniofacial skeleton is distorted. (*A–C* from David DJ, Moore MH, Cooter RD: Tessier clefts revisited with a third dimension. Cleft Palate J 1989;26:163-184.)

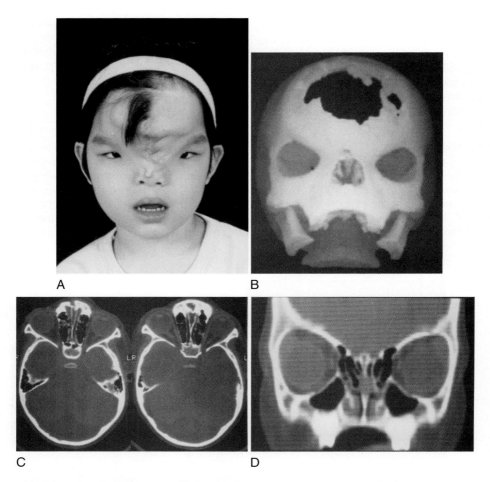

FIGURE 100-17. *A,* A 4-year-old Malaysian girl with midline craniofacial clefts of the Tessier number 0-14 type that were previously operated on. *B,* Three-dimensional CT reconstruction reveals the orbital hypertelorism below and extensive median frontal defect above. *C,* Marked widening and extensive pneumatization of the ethmoid sutures, with associated bifid perpendicular plate. *D,* Coronal two-dimensional CT reformat exposes the inferior prolapse of the widened ethmoid sinus with a characteristic harlequin appearance. (From David DJ, Moore MH, Cooter RD: Tessier clefts revisited with a third dimension. Cleft Palate J 1989;26:163-184.)

SKELETAL CHARACTERISTICS. The median frontal defect delineates the region through which the frontal encephalocele herniates. The lateral segments of the frontal bone sweep upward from the region of the intact glabella and are flattened laterally (Fig. 100-17*B*). No pneumatization of the frontal sinus is evident. The crista galli and the perpendicular plate of the ethmoid are bifid (Fig. 100-17*C*). Just as the ethmoid, including the cribriform plate, is widened and caudally displaced, the sphenoid sinus is broadened and extensively, but symmetrically, pneumatized. The lateral rotation of the greater and lesser wings of the sphenoid results in a relative shortening of the anteroposterior dimension of the middle cranial fossa. The floor of the anterior cranial fossa is up-slanting from its medial aspect to its lateral aspect, with a harlequin appearance on the coronal scan (Fig. 100-17*D*).

DISCUSSION

The Tessier classification of craniofacial clefts offers a numbering system that centers on the orbit and delineates consistent anatomic pathways for craniofacial clefts. The radiographic imaging techniques available to Tessier were far less sophisticated than those available today. His original assessments of the skeletal abnormalities were largely based on clinical impression and two-dimensional radiographs. Computed three-dimensional imaging has added an appropriate tool for visualizing the anatomy of craniofacial clefts. Nylon models generated from the scans provide a permanent, nearly perfect record of the skeletal anomaly.

The availability of two- and three-dimensional CT reconstructions of each cleft type has further defined the patterns of skeletal disturbance. As an adjunct to the standard three-dimensional images, serial coronal, oblique, and sagittal two-dimensional reformats provide a finer radiographic probe to "track" the cleft through the depth of the craniofacial skeleton. CT imaging allows the delineation of even marginal skeletal distortions and of any associated abnormalities within adjacent soft tissues.

The clinical documentation of a complete series of Tessier clefts has both confirmed and added to many of Tessier's descriptions. Among the superficial indicators of clefting were irregularities in the frontal and temporal hairline. These hairline indicators represented the most superior markers of soft tissue disturbance in the lateral and superior cranial clefts (numbers 7 through 14).[36] On occasion, as with the number 11 cleft (see Fig. 100-14A), the hairline marker was the most prominent soft tissue finding.

As part of his numeric cleft classification, Tessier suggested that the anterior components of clefts that traverse both the cranium and the face occur along regular axes such that the sum of their designated numbers would total 14. Although some clefting patterns in the author's series conform to this rule, multiple clefts of the cranium and face were not uncommon. The extensive radiologic examination of this series not only demonstrated the three-dimensional extent of the clefts but also revealed a previously unsuspected spectrum of cleft combinations. Thus, the idea of "time zones," postulated vascular causation, and global absolutes such as the association of anophthalmia with particular clefts were not always confirmed in this series.[9]

This review again distinguishes between the median and paramedian craniofacial clefts and the group of frontoethmoidal meningoencephaloceles. The frontoethmoidal meningoencephalocele is associated with a craniofacial skeleton that is normal in content but displaced in position by the soft tissue encephalocele. Craniofacial clefts associated with encephaloceles show skulls that are markedly deficient in three dimensions, both in their soft tissue and in skeletal makeup.[26] Frontoethmoidal meningoencephaloceles also lack the frontal hairline indicator seen with the midline cranial clefts.[36]

In addition to the documentation of the superficial craniofacial skeletal distortion associated with craniofacial clefts, the two- and three-dimensional CT images reveal previously unrecognized associated cranial base dysmorphology. From the close examination of the sphenoid, which is the keystone of the cranial base, the majority of facial clefts in the author's series were seen to have some distortion in the cranial base (Fig. 100-18). These were manifested as asymmetries in the shape or size of the greater or lesser sphenoid wings and were frequently reflected in the pterygoid processes, which were often unequally displaced from the midline or asymmetric in their anatomy. The sphenoid, and in particular its pterygoid processes, which collapse into or away from medially or laterally located clefts, may be the posterior extension of the cleft. Such medial or lateral displacement and distortion of the pterygoid plates could then be markers of the axis about which the clefts are centered. Correspondingly, asymmetries of the anterior and middle cranial fossa and calvarial distortions above could often be identified even in isolated facial clefts, without evidence of associated cranial clefts. Tessier selected the orbit as the axis about which the numbering of clefts was centered. He speculated that all facial clefts had their origins in the cranial base.[10] However, the speculation of such principles of embryologic causation based on small series is a tenuous proposition that could be open to criticism. One thing is clear from the Adelaide series, and that is that the majority of the rare clefts are multiple and run into each other.

The data reported demonstrate that the visible components of craniofacial clefts do not necessarily reflect their true extent. It is valuable to maximize the amount of diagnostic information available before operation if one is to attempt complete correction of the abnormality.

The rarity of severe craniofacial clefts has made the collection and complete anatomic documentation of a large series difficult.

Craniofacial Microsomia

The morphology of craniofacial microsomia has been expressed by various authors. David et al[33] proposed an alphanumeric approach (SAT classification) to make some sense of the wide range of deformities that can be part of this particular disease.

The alphanumeric coding system was based on the universally accepted TNM classification of malignant tumors.[37,38] The derivation of SAT is as follows: S, skeletal; A, auricle; and T, soft tissue. In this system, S has five levels; S1, S2, and S3 are adapted from the grades of mandibular deformity proposed by Pruzansky,[29] and patients with orbital involvement may be allocated to levels S4 and S5 after Lauritzen et al[39] (Fig. 100-19). A normal auricle is represented by A0; A1, A2, and A3 follow the grades of microtia described by Meurman[40] (Fig. 100-20). The soft tissue category has three levels, from minimal deformity (T1) to severe (T3), similar

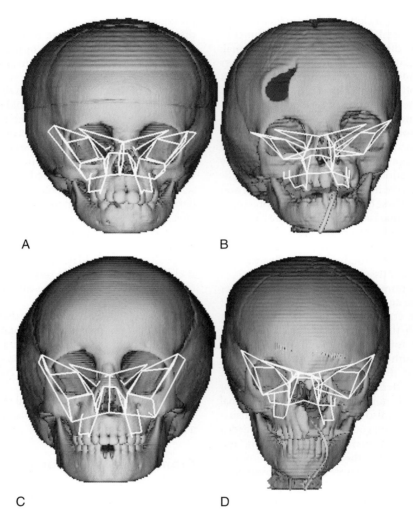

A

B

C

D

FIGURE 100-18. Osseous landmarks of the sphenoid are used for analysis of the abnormality. Overlaid on three-dimensional CT reconstructions are lines connecting the landmarks to form a "wire frame" for visualization. *A,* A normal, dry skull at the age of 12 months showing the symmetry of the landmarks. *B,* Comparison of patient at the age of 12 months with a Tessier number 10 cleft showing the asymmetry in the height of the lesser wings. *C,* A normal, dry skull at the age of 4 years. *D,* Comparison of a patient at the age of 4 years with multiple Tessier clefts (numbers 0-14, 1-13, 2-12) showing the asymmetry in the height of the lesser wings and the pterygoid processes.

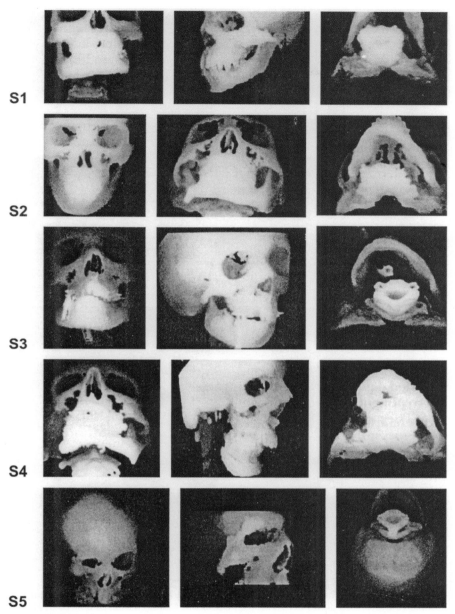

FIGURE 100-19. The S levels of skeletal deformity in the SAT system, from the minimal deformity S1 to the severe malformation S5. (From David DJ, Mahatumarat C, Cooter D: Hemifacial microsomia: a multisystem classification. Plast Reconstr Surg 1987;80:525-533.)

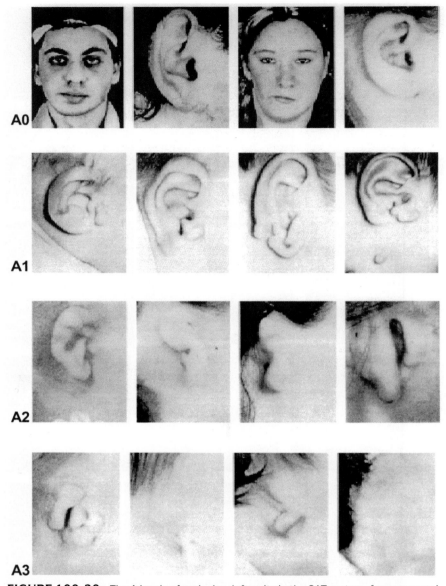

FIGURE 100-20. The A levels of auricular deformity in the SAT system, from a normal ear A0 to the severe deformity A3. (From David DJ, Mahatumarat C, Cooter D: Hemifacial microsomia: a multisystem classification. Plast Reconstr Surg 1987;80:525-533.)

to the grading of Murray et al[41] (Figs. 100-21 and 100-22 and Table 100-4).

Midline Agenesis

PREMAXILLA

Patients may have premaxillary aplasia, hypotelorism, severe midline cleft of lip and palate, flat nose, or absent columella and philtrum. These children are severely retarded and usually do not survive long. Other patients may present with similar but less severe facial features with the exception that there is a hypoplastic premaxilla (Fig. 100-23).

NOSE

Arrhinia with bilateral proboscis can have a cartilaginous or bony block centrally, small hyperteloric orbits, small globes, and absence of hair, but the patients managed by the Australian Craniofacial Unit

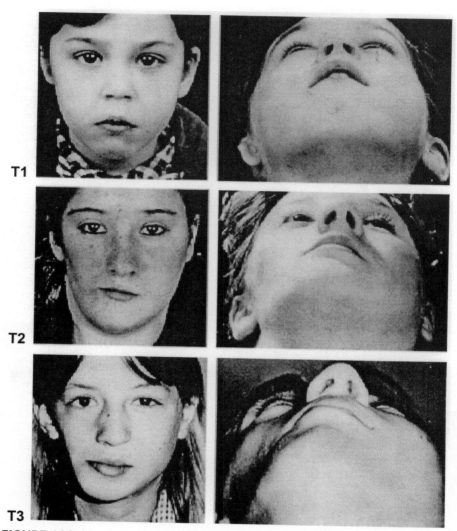

FIGURE 100-21. The T levels of soft tissue deformity in the SAT system range from T1 to T3. (From David DJ, Mahatumarat C, Cooter D: Hemifacial microsomia: a multisystem classification. Plast Reconstr Surg 1987;80:525-533.)

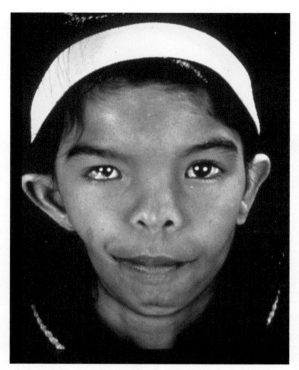

FIGURE 100-22. A patient with craniofacial micro-somia with a paramedian cleft. Note the widening of the right medial canthus.

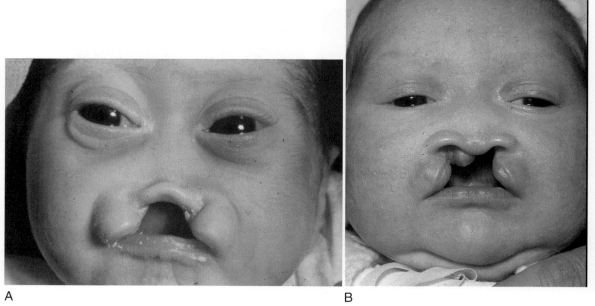

A

B

FIGURE 100-23. *A,* Holoprosencephaly with absence of midline structures and nonviability. *B,* A patient with midline craniofacial cleft with hypotelorism and a hypoplastic premaxilla with a small segment of nasal septum. This child went on to have severe maxillary hypoplasia but normal mental development.

TABLE 100-4 ✦ SAT CLASSIFICATION OF CRANIOFACIAL MICROSOMIA[33]

Skeletal Categories

S1	Small mandible with normal shape
S2	Condyle, ramus, and sigmoid notch identifiable but grossly distorted; mandible strikingly different in size and shape from normal
S3	Mandible severely malformed, ranging from poorly identifiable ramal components to complete agenesis of ramus
S4	An S3 mandible plus orbital involvement with gross posterior recession of lateral and inferior orbital rims
S5	The S4 defects plus orbital dystopia and frequently hypoplasia and asymmetric neurocranium with a flat temporal fossa

Auricle Categories

A0	Normal
Al	Small, malformed auricle retaining characteristic features
A2	Rudimentary auricle with hook at cranial end corresponding to the helix
A3	Malformed lobule with rest of pinna absent

Soft Tissue Categories

T1	Minimal contour defect with no cranial nerve involvement
T2	Moderate defect
T3	Major defect with obvious facial scoliosis, possibly severe hypoplasia of cranial nerves, parotid gland, muscles of mastication; eye involvement; clefts of face or lips

Soft tissue: The signs range from minor skin tags to major absence of soft tissue developed from the mesoderm of the first and second arches, muscles of mastication, parotid gland, and elements of the external ear and the number 7 cleft manifested as a macrostomia.

have normal intelligence (Fig. 100-24). The proboscis contains the same tissues to be found in the normal nose. With the absence of the heminose, there is no pneumatization of the maxillary, ethmoid, and frontal sinuses (Fig. 100-25). There is no nasolacrimal apparatus, and there may be canthal dystopia and telecanthus.

Duplications

Duplications of the face are rare and range from two complete faces on a single head (diprosopus) to simple nasal duplication. Verdi et al[42] reported this spectrum of abnormalities. Fearon and Mulliken[43] noted that duplications of the maxilla are frequently accompanied by cleft lip and palate, multiple uvulae, and other craniofacial anomalies. Chen and Noordhoff[44] suggested a classification for duplication of the stomodeal structures. Sjamsudin et al[45] described a patient with maxillary duplication (Fig. 100-26).

Frontoethmoidal Meningoencephalocele

BONE DEFECTS

The description *frontoethmoidal* is most appropriate because it describes the site of the cranial end of the defect, which is always in the position of the foramen

cecum at the junction of the frontal and ethmoid bones (Fig. 100-27). The posterior margin of the defect is formed by the crista galli. This is often distorted, and the cribriform plate is usually tilted downward, as a deep central trough, the anterior end of which is well below the planum sphenoidale; the cribriform plate forms an angle of 45 to 50 degrees with the orbitomeatal plane. The cranial exit holes vary in size and shape. The nasofrontal defects tend to be round and central. The naso-orbital defects are usually bilobed. The nasoethmoidal type can be bilobed, lozenge shaped, or round.

The morphology of the facial bone defects shows more variation. In the nasofrontal type, the holes are *usually* at the junction of the frontal and nasal bones (Fig. 100-28); the nasal bones are attached to the inferior margin of the defect, which varies in shape.

In the nasoethmoidal type, the facial defects lie between the nasal bones and the nasal cartilages (Fig. 100-29), the nasal bones being above and the nasal cartilages below. The nasal bones are deformed and often broadened, with crimped margins. The frontonasal angle is obliterated, producing an overhanging ledge. If the facial defect is confined to the nasal pyramid and is small and oval, the medial walls of the orbit are not involved. If, however, the meningoencephalocele is larger and the facial defect extends more

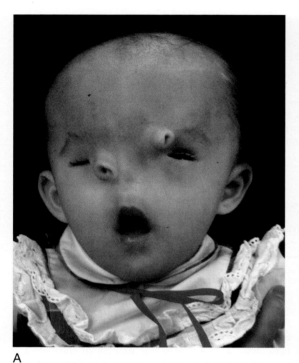

A

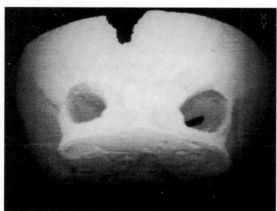

B

FIGURE 100-24. Arrhinia with probosces. *A,* Clinical view. *B,* Three-dimensional reconstruction shows total absence of nasal cavity and origin of the probosces.

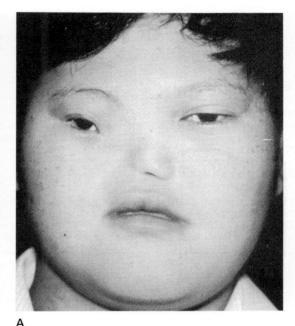

A

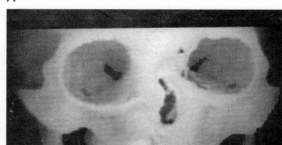

B

FIGURE 100-25. Nasal aplasia (unilateral). *A,* Clinical view; note canthal dystopia. *B,* Three-dimensional reconstruction shows absence of nasal cavity on affected side. (From van der Meulen J, Mazzola R, Stricker M, Raphael B: Classification of craniofacial malformations. In Stricker M, van der Meulen J, Raphael B, Mazzola R, eds: Craniofacial Malformations. Edinburgh, Churchill Livingstone, 1990:191.)

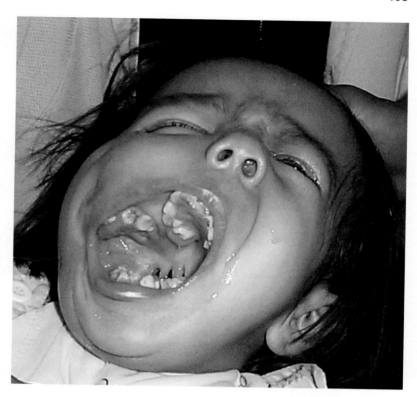

FIGURE 100-26. A patient with maxillary duplication. The pair of bifid uvulae, each associated with its own maxillary arch, is clearly visible.

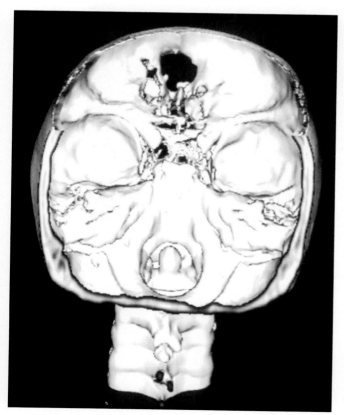

FIGURE 100-27. A CT scan of a patient with frontoethmoidal meningoencephalocele viewed from the aspect of the anterior cranial fossa. The exit hole is at the site of the foramen cecum at the junction of the frontal and ethmoid bones.

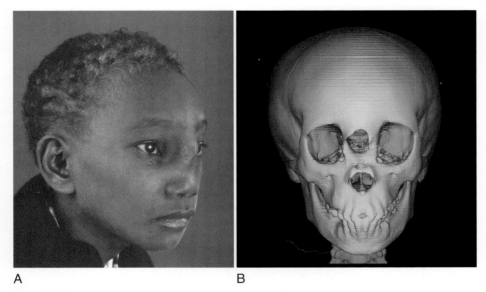

FIGURE 100-28. *A,* A frontoethmoidal meningoencephalocele of the nasofrontal type. *B,* Three-dimensional reconstruction shows the exit foramen above the nasal bones.

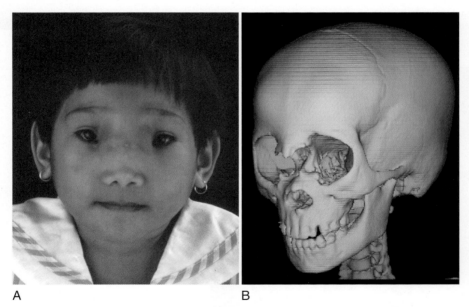

FIGURE 100-29. *A,* A frontoethmoidal meningoencephalocele of the nasoethmoidal type. *B,* Three-dimensional reconstruction shows the distorted nasal bones above the crescentic deformities in the medial orbital walls and the depressed piriform aperture inferiorly.

laterally, the anterior margins of the medial orbital walls are eroded and crescent shaped.

The naso-orbital meningoencephaloceles present on the face through holes in the medial orbital wall (Fig. 100-30), in the frontal process of the maxilla and the lacrimal bones. The bony track can be long and shaped like an inverted Y. The inverted Y may be asymmetric (see Fig. 100-5). These encephaloceles come through the frontal process of the maxilla onto the face, leaving the nasal bones intact anteriorly and the lacrimal bones and lateral plate of the ethmoid intact posteriorly. However, during the passage of the cerebral hernia through the substance of the ethmoid, the lateral plate of that bone is pushed laterally, forming a bony tunnel.

ETIOLOGY

Multiple, interacting genetic and environmental influences are most likely to be at work in the area of rare craniofacial clefts and the associated conditions. Aside from Treacher Collins syndrome, Goldenhar syndrome, and Cohen syndrome (craniofrontonasal dysplasia), heredity appears to play only a small role in the formation of the rare craniofacial clefts. However, the rarity of afflicted patients and the limited opportunity afforded to clinicians to study them and their families over time and in detail may conceal the subtleties of the genetic influences producing variable expressivity as well as variable penetrance and the influence of a multitude of environmental factors that may come to bear on the development of the individual child (Fig. 100-31).

Genetics

OROFACIAL CLEFTING IS CAUSED BY A COMBINATION OF THE EFFECTS OF MULTIPLE GENES. Cleft lip with or without cleft palate (CL/P) is found in isolation (i.e., nonsyndromal) at relatively high frequency in the general population. Notably, it has been reported that 25% to 35% of patients with CL/P (and 10% to 20% of patients with cleft palate only) also have a family history of clefting, highlighting the critical genetic contribution to this malformation in a significant proportion of individuals. Despite this fact, numerous studies have clearly shown that simple mendelian inheritance (i.e., single gene) models are often insufficient to explain this pattern of inheritance. Consequently, inheritance is generally regarded as being multigenic, that is, it is estimated that as many as 20 genes can interact in a combinatorial manner to cause clefts.

INHERITANCE OF CLEFTING CAN BE EXPLAINED AT THE MOLECULAR LEVEL. The protein products of many thousands of genes are needed to specify the development of the human face. In simple mendelian disorders (i.e., those inherited diseases that are caused by a mutation in a single gene), the protein encoded by the causative gene may be significantly affected in one of a number of a ways:

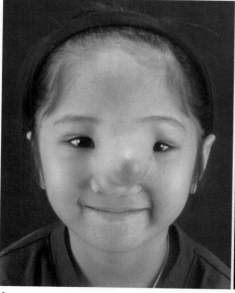
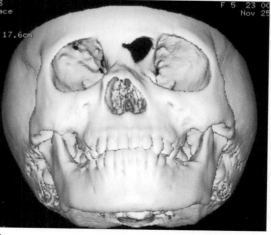

A   B

FIGURE 100-30. *A,* A frontoethmoidal meningoencephalocele of the naso-orbital type. *B,* Three-dimensional reconstruction shows the exit foramen in the region of the left lacrimal bone.

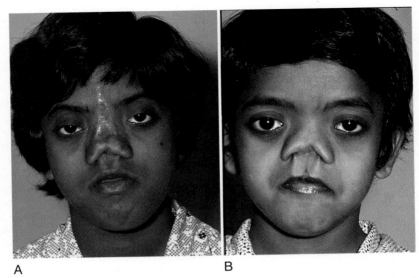

A   B

FIGURE 100-31. Malay siblings with identical deformities; *A* is the sister and *B* the brother. The deformity consists of a mild hypertelorism, a midline craniofacial cleft reflected through the nose and upper lip, and a midline diastasis of the maxilla with a V deformity.

1. it may not be produced at all;
2. its amino acid content may be altered such that it affects its normal functioning within the cell; or
3. it may be reduced or increased in amount relative to the amount required to carry out its function, thus affecting cellular functions that are dependent on it.

However, it is clear that not all changes in gene sequence cause clinically important phenotypes. In fact, much of the normal phenotypic variability between individuals in the population is attributed to natural, nonpathologic variations in gene sequence found throughout the human genome. It then follows that the difference between a change in a gene that causes a mendelian disorder and a change in the same gene that has no obvious effect on phenotype is simply a measure of the effect of that change on the normal function of the gene product (or at least the ability of the cells and tissues to compensate for the change in protein function). However, changes in DNA and protein sequences do not necessarily have a deleterious effect on cellular function.

When clefts occur, the growth and fusion of the palatal shelves during development are compromised by the combinatorial effect of a mixture of gene variants that individually may have no clinical significance. Thus, the overall impact of any single genetic change will depend on the combination and relative impact of the other changes present in any given individual.

For example, a particular change with a minor contributory effect in one family member may in fact be absent in another affected member because of the presence of additional minor changes. A single major gene effect has nevertheless been suggested to account for as many as 10% to 50% of familial orofacial clefts.

The Current State of Genetic Studies. Traditional genetic linkage studies of simple mendelian disorders rely on large multigenerational families with many affected members or, alternatively, numerous small families with a suspected common molecular cause to track down the location of the gene causing the disease. Clearly, in some families with a history of CL/P, the disorder is indeed monogenic (i.e., caused by a single gene, for example, X-linked recessive cleft palate). However, most families do not fall in this category. The limited numbers of individuals affected by clefting in different families and the possible effects of variations in many genes reduce the power of linkage studies to pinpoint the contributory genetic factors. The uncertainty as to which model of inheritance to best use for these analyses has compounded this issue. In studies using cohorts of patients of different ethnic origin, for example, or population founder effects, a model of inheritance that gives significant results in one patient may not in another. As a result, significant linkage has been obtained in only a few studies.

Until now, existing molecular technologies have precluded genome-wide scans for associations with clefting. Consequently, the majority of studies have focused on the careful selection of candidate genes to investigate the association of variations in gene sequences with orofacial clefting. These approaches have similarly met with only limited success, with important loci for nonsyndromic patients suggested to reside at 2p13, 4q31, 6p23, 17q21-q24, and 19q13.2. The most consistent of these (but still not found in every study) is the weak but significant association between DNA sequence polymorphisms at the transforming growth factor-α (*TGFA*) locus on chromosomes 2p13 and nonsyndromic CL/P. It has, however, been suggested that the *TGFA* locus only modifies expression (severity) of the CL/P trait, which is controlled by a major (necessary) locus elsewhere. A candidate for the major locus is the *EDN1* gene on chromosome 6p23. Other loci, such as the retinoic acid receptor-α (*RARA*) gene (at 17q) and the *BCL3* gene (at 19q), have also been implicated in certain CL/P families.

Unfortunately, the designs of many association studies have been potentially susceptible to population structure problems because they do not control for the effect of stratification. Such problems can be overcome to some degree with family-based study designs. Nonparametric linkage methods (e.g., affected sib pair studies) have recently been touted as perhaps being more appropriate than traditional pedigree-based methods. However, several hundred affected sibling pairs are likely to be required for linkage to CL/P susceptibility loci to be detected. To date, no study has collected such numbers.

Evaluation of the history of the pregnancy, clinical appearance of the child (and the parents), and scrutiny of the family history may help in classifying an isolated instance of CL/P, but some may remain unsolved. The following environmental or nongenetic factors may then be considered.

Environmental Factors

Although considerable advances have been made in understanding the etiology of hemifacial microsomia,[46] little is known at this stage about the etiology and pathogenesis of rare craniofacial clefts. They are rare, not often managed in a scientific context, and infrequently studied during long periods of development. There are no suitable animal models for study, and most of the conclusions about etiology have been extrapolated from information about cleft lip and palate.

EXPOSURE TO RADIATION

The dose necessary to produce teratogenic effects in humans during pregnancy is relatively high. Although Poswillo[47] and others demonstrated that cleft lip and palate can be induced by exposing experimental animals to radiation, there is no evidence that it produces an increase in cleft lip and palate, let alone the rare craniofacial clefts.

MATERNAL ENVIRONMENT

INFECTIONS IN PREGNANCY. Although some effort has been made to relate infections with viruses, bacteria, and protozoa to facial clefting, there are no convincing correlations. Similarly, there is no convincing evidence of adverse effects on facial development of maternal metabolic dysfunction.

DRUGS AND CHEMICALS. These have been significantly implicated in the teratogenic effect on facial development. The categories include anticonvulsants, antimetabolic agents, steroids, and tranquilizers. These could act individually or in combination on possibly genetically predisposed individuals.

PATHOGENESIS
Clefts

There is a presumption that the rare clefts are, with respect to their pathogenesis, similar to cleft lip and palate. The fusion theory of facial clefting postulates a failure of the processes to make contact. It is possible that the processes could meet but not fuse if epithelial cell death over the contact area does not occur.

The mesodermal penetration theory postulates that there is a problem with the dorsoventral flow of the neural crest cells. Johnston[48] damaged the neural crest cells before migration and produced a cleft. Poswillo[49] built on this concept to form his theories of cleft production in Treacher Collins syndrome and hemifacial microsomia. Vascular disturbance produced by failure of appropriate vascularization[50] from the stapedial artery-external carotid artery system has been blamed for the damage to the neural crest cells. Poswillo[46] suggested that localized hemorrhage best accounts for the variety and range of deformities found in craniofacial microsomia.

The genetic nature of Treacher Collins syndrome is well established as a dominant disorder of craniofacial development that results from mutation of the *TCOF1* gene on chromosome 5.[51,52] The *TCOF1* gene encodes a large protein called Treacle, the precise function of which remains undetermined. A mouse model of Treacher Collins syndrome has been generated by ablation of the murine equivalent of the human *TCOF1* gene. These studies have revealed an essential role for the Treacle protein in survival of cells derived from the cephalic neural crest.[53] The genetic component of craniofacial microsomia is less evident, and that of the rare clefts is obscure. One factor that is constantly observed in the natural history of all three is that the facial deformities proceed throughout growth with a tendency for the deformity to progress during that period.

Clefts and Craniosynostosis

Craniofrontonasal syndrome as reported by Cohen[54] features, among other things, coronal synostosis and hypertelorism with bifid nose (Fig. 100-32). This syndrome occurs sporadically, and symptoms in females are worse than in males. X-linked dominant inheritance is postulated. The gene has been mapped to Xp22.[55]

AMNIOTIC BANDS

Amniotic disruption has been implicated in some patients with craniofacial clefting and amniotic bands, with deformities of the extremities (Fig. 100-33).[56] The lines of cleavage are said to be nonembryologic. Torpin[57] has implicated maternal trauma and premature amnion rupture in the production of the syndrome. The amniotic rupture syndrome has a reported incidence of 1:5000 to 1:15,000.[58] These patients may have visceral defects as well. MacKinnon and David[59] have seen it in association with craniosynostosis as well.

Frontoethmoidal Meningoencephalocele

This condition differs from the midline clefts. There is little or no evidence of sibling affection.[60] The geo-graphic peculiarities in the distribution of frontoethmoidal meningoencephaloceles are well documented[26]; they are common in Malaysia, Thailand, and Burma and rare in Europe, North America, and Australia. In both Thailand and Malaysia, it is the Thais and Malays who are affected, not the Chinese, in spite of the presence in both countries of large Chinese ethnic minorities. The apparent increase in paternal age of the patients makes some suggestion of an autosomal dominant gene mutation, but much more study of larger population groups is necessary.

The working thesis of the pathogenesis of the craniofacial deformity in frontoethmoidal meningoencephalocele is that the meningoencephalocele is a "blowout" of the intracranial contents, through a midline tunnel from the anterior cranial fossa at the site of the foramen cecum into the facial skeleton. The skeletal deformities are related to the space-occupying effects of the hernia of extruded brain and not intrinsic to the tissues themselves. Complete removal of the dysplastic tissue should allow the developing brain and eyes to mold the orbital skeleton, and the forces generated by the nasal airway, speech, and mastication will remodel the facial deformity, a view shared by Naim-Ur-Rahman.[61]

MANAGEMENT PRINCIPLES

Management by a multidisciplinary team during the growth period, that is, up to 18 years or beyond, is invariably necessary. Whereas individual surgical techniques are important, it is necessary to manage all

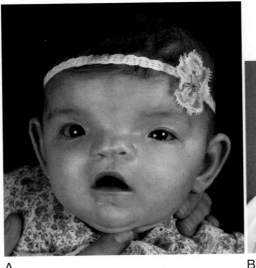
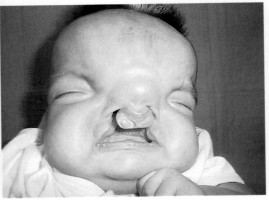

A   B

FIGURE 100-32. *A,* A child with craniofrontonasal dysplasia and a midline craniofacial cleft with a tendency to bifid nose. *B,* A more severe craniofrontonasal dysplasia with gross hypertelorism and associated bilateral cleft lip and palate.

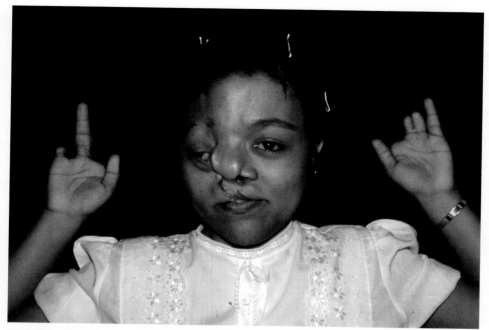

FIGURE 100-33. A patient with right-sided Tessier cleft numbers 3, 4, 10, and 12 with bilateral, asymmetric upper limb ring constrictions and amputations. Severe right-sided orbital dystopia poses a significant reconstructive problem. (From Coady MSE, Moore MH, Wallis K: Amniotic band syndrome: the association between rare facial clefts and limb ring constrictions. Plast Reconstr Surg 1998;101:640-649.)

aspects of the patient's care within a structure that enables protocol management to be instituted, audited, and developed. There are six general principles that should be adhered to by any organization managing craniofacial clefts:

1. *Multidisciplinary care.* These complex problems cannot be solved in the short term or by a single discipline acting alone. Even if there are no other systemic effects of the disease, the brain, eyes, hearing and respiratory function, dental function, facial and jaw function, and hence speech and development are likely to be affected.
2. Management must be delivered during the *growth period* of the child, which is from birth until late teens. Treatment interventions must be prioritized and delivered at a time in growth when they produce the best results, least harm, and least suffering. Treatment should be harmonious with the natural history of the disease process during growth.
3. *Protocol* management enables a predictable treatment regimen to be offered on the basis of the current knowledge of the natural history of the disease and, in most instances, the stage of growth and development. Protocol

development can be based on outcome studies, comparative studies, and prospective trials. Patients either start the protocol at birth and continue through to the completion of growth or enter later, whether or not they have received any treatment to date.
4. *Best practice,* in the context of health care delivery, concerns the highest standards of performance in delivering safe, high-quality care as determined on the basis of available evidence and by comparison among similar health care providers.
5. *Research and development* are conducted both clinically and in the basic sciences involved in the investigation and treatment of facial clefts. Best practice cannot be attained nor protocols developed without the research component. Because these conditions occur infrequently, multicenter studies are necessary.
6. *Infrastructure support* then becomes mandatory for these conditions to be fulfilled. This involves commitment by an institution, systems to support the multidisciplinary assessment and treatment of patients, long-term follow-up, funding for research and development, and appropriate data storage and transfer facilities.

Investigation

Special investigations are always based on a complete history and a thorough medical examination. A wide range of anomalies may accompany severe craniofacial anomalies. Radiology is the mainstay of the investigations. Cephalometric radiology, usually biplanar, enables data to be collected about positions of bones relative to the cranial base compared with normal population figures. If repeated throughout growth, cephalometric radiology with subsequent analysis tracks the growth with age and provides a useful measure of the changes made from treatment.

Three-dimensional cephalometric data enable investigators to more accurately appreciate the bone deformities associated with the rare craniofacial clefts. Soft tissue analyses are also important in assessment of patients, none more than the brain setting data, which give a good indication of any brain deformity. Other more detailed soft tissue information is best studied with magnetic resonance imaging.

From the three-dimensional cephalometric data, an accurate nylon model of the skull can be reproduced. It serves as a record of the deformity and as a model for surgical planning (Fig. 100-34).[62,63] Dental models are produced from impressions of the teeth and are used in conjunction with the cephalometric data and the nylon models of the skull to assist in surgical planning.

Special investigations associated with neurology, ophthalmology, otorhinolaryngology, and speech pathology are necessary to complete the picture before a treatment program is planned.

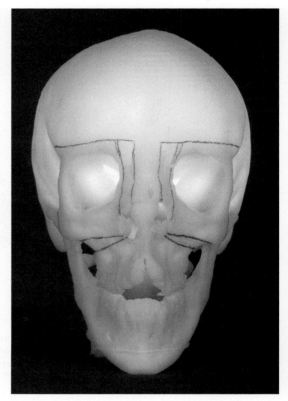

FIGURE 100-34. A nylon model constructed from a three-dimensional CT scan of a patient with a midline cleft demonstrates not only the deformity but how the model can be used for surgical planning.

Treatment

RARE CLEFTS

In spite of the convenience and current popularity of Tessier's classification of rare clefts as a form of communication, when it comes to treatment, three separate groups emerge:

1. the midline and paramedian clefts causing, among other deformities, the orbital dystopias;
2. the oro-naso-ocular clefts, which may produce spectacular complex deformities of the midface;
3. the lateral clefts, including craniofacial microsomia and Treacher Collins syndrome, which may produce gross mandibular deformities.

The Australian Craniofacial Unit protocols that have been developed in each of these categories are based on the natural tendency of the cleft to recur during growth and a knowledge of the changes that take place in the craniofacial skeleton during this period (Table 100-5). The majority of these deformities occur as multiple manifestations of the Tessier anatomic types (Table 100-6).

FRONTOETHMOIDAL MENINGOENCEPHALOCELE

It is believed that this deformity is caused by an extrusion of brain matter through the area of the foramen cecum, passing along various pathways onto the face and into the orbit, producing deformity of the developing skeleton by pressure and by occupying space. The management of patients with frontoethmoidal meningoencephalocele is based on this concept.[64,65]

Surgical Techniques

AIRWAY MANAGEMENT

Soft Tube Nasopharyngeal Intubation

Maintaining the airway for adequate oxygenation is a problem in a number of clefting conditions, the worst of which is severe Treacher Collins syndrome. Prolonged nasopharyngeal intubation for up to 6 months[72,73] may give the patient enough time for growth to obviate tracheostomy. If genuine choanal atresia exists, this will need to be dealt with surgically;

Text continued on p. 422

TABLE 100-5 ✦ AUSTRALIAN CRANIOFACIAL UNIT TREATMENT PROTOCOLS

Protocols have been developed for treatment of rare craniofacial clefts, frontoethmoidal meningoencephalocele,[64,65] and facial duplications.

Rare Clefts

The Median and Paramedian Clefts Causing Orbital Dystopia (Tessier Numbers 0-14, 1-13, 2-12, 10)

Birth to 1 year
Preservation of essential functions: airway management; establishment of feeding, sight (e.g., protecting eyes or exposing them for the development of vision), and hearing; covering of exposed brain.
The soft tissue elements of the cleft lip and palate are closed according to an established protocol. The one used at the Australian Craniofacial Unit is the lip and anterior palate at 3 months and the soft palate at 6 months.
For those conditions with craniosynostosis (Cohen syndrome), the cranial component is corrected by fronto-orbital advancement and excision of the fused sutures at 3 to 6 months of age.

5 years
As most of the orbital growth is complete by this time, orbital translocation can be planned. However, if a box osteotomy is contemplated, the developing teeth near the orbital floor need to be noted and the operation delayed until they can be preserved. In the experience of the Australian Craniofacial Unit, even correction of hypertelorism by facial bipartition before this age risks recurrence of the medial bone deformity. There is no harm in waiting longer.
Correction of severe hypertelorism is facilitated by introduction of tissue expanders, laterally, deep to the periosteum of the zygomatic arch.[66]
Temporary nasal reconstruction is performed at the time of correction of the hypertelorism, in the knowledge that it will need to be repeated.

5 to 10 years
On the basis of the cleft lip and palate model, orthodontic management is commenced when enough permanent teeth have erupted to expand the arch and align the teeth. Alveolar bone grafting is performed at this stage and extended to correct the more extensive defects in the maxilla that may be present in these cases.

10 years to the completion of growth
Maintenance of the orthodontic situation with retainers
Maintenance of function where necessary (such as eyelid reconstruction to preserve the globe, maintenance of hearing)

At the completion of growth
Orthodontic preparation for and execution of midface surgery—this may be at any level or in any combination, with or without bone grafting or mandibular surgery. The pattern is determined by the deformity and after consideration at a planning meeting.
After this establishment of the facial platform, other secondary surgery is performed, including definitive nasal reconstruction (Fig. 100-35).

The Oro-Naso-Ocular Clefts (Tessier Numbers 3, 4, 5, 6)

Birth to 1 year
As a consequence of the dramatic appearance of these children, vigorous counseling is often necessary to avoid their being branded mentally retarded, which they rarely are.
Lifesaving maneuvers include establishment of airway and effective feeding.
Function-enhancing and function-preserving maneuvers usually focus on the eyes, which are often unsupported inferiorly and inadequately covered by lids, giving rise to all the dangers of exposure keratitis and corneal damage.
During the first year, the lip and palate are repaired as usual. The eyelids should be reconstructed to protect the globes, which may need support from a small bone graft in the orbital floor.

1 to 5 years
General support and attention are given to function, sight, speech, hearing, and psychosocial development.

5 to 10 years
When enough permanent teeth have erupted to start expansion of the arches and alignment of the dentition, as for alveolar bone grafting in ordinary cleft lip and palate, bone grafting of the whole of the maxillary cleft can be undertaken. The timing is determined by plain radiologic examination.
The procedure is facilitated in those severe cases by the use of subperiosteal tissue expansion to achieve tension-free musculoperiosteal cover of the bone graft.

10 years to the completion of growth
Maintenance of the orthodontic situation.
At the completion of growth, any osteotomies and further bone grafting, soft tissue augmentation, and nasal reconstruction are undertaken.

Continued

TABLE 100-5 ✦ AUSTRALIAN CRANIOFACIAL UNIT TREATMENT PROTOCOLS—cont'd

Lateral Clefts

Craniofacial Microsomia

This protocol is based on the multisystem classification as well as the growth-time concept.[33]

Birth to 1 year
In rare cases in which airway is compromised, this must take priority.
Establishment of feeding
Assessment and establishment of hearing
Repair of cleft lip and palate
In those severe cases with an empty eye socket, expansion by an intraorbital tissue expander[67]

2 years
Speech assessment and therapy as required

5 years to teenage years
The correction of orbital dystopia can be done, but it is best left until a time closer to the definitive repair of the facial skeleton.
Growth-enhancing or growth-controlling maneuvers are established according to the degree of the deformity. These include (1) orthodontic activators (Harvold); (2) costochondral graft and joint reconstruction, when no joint is present; and (3) bone distraction, when a joint is present. *Note:* In the author's opinion, although these techniques are widespread and popular, their place in the protocol for management of hemifacial microsomia is as yet unproven. The most likely place is for the lengthening of the S2 mandible in the growth phase, although this can be achieved more quickly by subsigmoid osteotomy alone.

Teenage years to maturity
Orthodontic treatment is finished in mild cases, or preparation is made for surgery in more severe cases.

At the completion of growth
Definitive surgical correction ranges from genioplasty alone in the least severe cases to bimaxillary surgery and composite free flap reconstruction of the mandible and soft tissue (Fig. 100-36).
Reconstruction of the ear (middle and pinna) can be by autogenous cartilage or prosthesis with osseointegrated implantation (Fig. 100-37).

Treacher Collins Syndrome (Tessier Numbers 6, 7, 8)

The disorder is caused by a dominant gene (*TCOF1*) with incomplete penetrance and variable expressivity.
The shape of the facial bones will always tend to revert to the pathologic form, even if the position has been corrected.[68]

Birth to 1 year
Emphasis is placed on the patient's total care, which varies with the severity of the disease. It includes multidisciplinary assessment, development of a treatment plan, and parental counseling.
Airway maintenance
Management of feeding (related to the airway)
Early assessment of the auditory mechanism and an appropriate hearing aid

1 to 5 years
Maintenance of vital functions (especially the airway). The palate cannot be closed until the airway is consistently patent.
In severe cases of airway compromise, distraction osteogenesis is used.[69]
Orbital and bone deformities may be addressed.

5 years to teenage years
Orbital bone grafting may need to be repeated (because of resorption) in severest deformities.
The mandible may need redistraction to help a deteriorating airway.
Orthodontic management of the dentition proceeds through this time.

At the completion of growth
Correction of the mandibular and nasomaxillary deformities can be done when growth is sufficiently advanced.
External ear reconstruction is performed with middle ear reconstruction if there is enough normal anatomy. The same timing and principles apply as for hemifacial microsomia.

Tessier Cleft Number 7

Birth to 1 year
Repair of the cleft lip including macrostomia; repair of the palate may need to be delayed if the mandible is small and the airway compromised.
Airway management, as for severe Treacher Collins syndrome, when the airway management protocol should be implemented; if necessary, the mandible is advanced by distraction osteogenesis.

1 to 5 years
Maintenance of airway
Development of speech

5 to 10 years
Bone graft of the maxilla if necessary

10 years to maturity
Orthodontic preparation of the dental arches for orthognathic surgery at the completion of growth

Tessier Clefts Number 9 and Number 10

These clefts are rare and are almost always seen in combination with other clefts.
The number 10 cleft, in its severest manifestation, has a defect in the frontal bone with an associated encephalocele and pressure on the orbital contents. This needs to be dealt with in infancy; the rest of the protocol is as for orbital dystopia.
The number 9 cleft, in its severest manifestation, has exposed dura in the temporal region that needs to be covered urgently. Bony orbital reconstruction is then performed at 5 years plus.

Frontoethmoidal Meningoencephalocele

Birth to 1 year
Many manifestations have severe intracranial anomalies that forbid a surgical result.
The intracranial and extracranial deformity is assessed by computed tomography and magnetic resonance imaging.
Transcranial removal of the dysfunctional brain and removal of the component extruding onto the face and into the orbit, together with closure of the cranial base defect, allow growth in response to the developing brain and eye and the functions of mastication and respiration.

1 to 5 years
As above, but more emphasis is placed on orbital and nasal reconstruction.

5 years to maturity
Orbital osteotomies can be performed at this stage. Rarely is the whole orbit moved because the pathologic process is medial and true hypertelorism with a widened lateral canthal distance is rare.[70]

Maturity
Definitive nasal reconstruction and jaw surgery can be done. Those patients with long faces and malocclusions can have midface osteotomies.[71]
During all phases, the patient may need treatment of hydrocephalus or other intracranial problems that are associated with this deformity.

Facial Duplications

Birth to 1 year
Soft tissue defects are closed to reconstitute the oral sphincter and to protect the eyes; where possible, scars are put as far medial as possible in the lines between cosmetic units.[16]
Removal of useless soft tissue remnants can be performed during this time as well.

5 years to maturity
When the permanent dentition has declared itself by eruption or radiologically, it is possible to decide which bone and teeth to preserve. Sometimes in these rare conditions, elements from both parts of the reduplication can be used. Shaping and growth-enhancing maneuvers (orthodontics, bone distraction) can be used during this time.

At the completion of growth
Definitive osteotomies and soft tissue transfers and augmentations can be performed.

TABLE 100-6 ✦ BREAKDOWN BY TESSIER ANATOMIC TYPES OF THE RARE CRANIOFACIAL CLEFTS SEEN AT THE AUSTRALIAN CRANIOFACIAL UNIT[*]

T0	T1	T2	T3	T4	T5	T6	T7	T8	T9	T10	T11	T13	T14	T0-14	T1-13	T2-12	Multiple
10	1	1	22	11	5	1	6	3	1	5	1	2	1	62	6	9	72

*Excluding hemifacial microsomia, Goldenhar syndrome, Treacher Collins syndrome, and holoprosencephaly or arrhinencephaly.

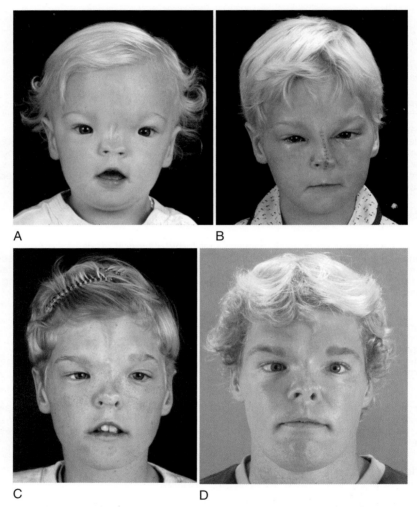

FIGURE 100-35. Median and paramedian clefts causing hypertelorism. *A,* At 20 months. *B,* At 5 years. *C,* At 12 years. *D,* At 19 years. The definitive nasal reconstruction consisted of a costochondral bone graft fixed with a single screw once the midface platform had been established at the end of growth.

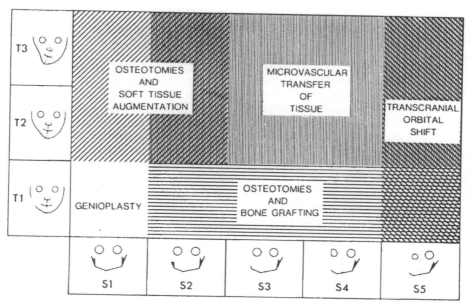

FIGURE 100-36. Craniofacial microsomia. The surgical treatment plan is based on skeletal and soft tissue deformities. (From David DJ, Mahatumarat C, Cooter D: Hemifacial microsomia: a multisystem classification. Plast Reconstr Surg 1987;80:525-533.)

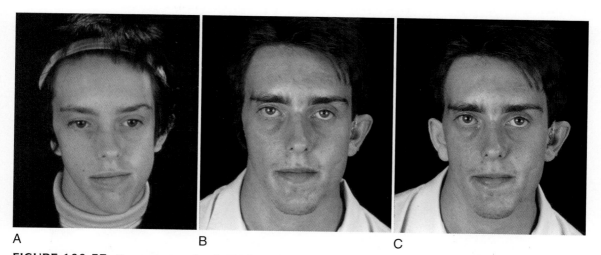

A   B   C

FIGURE 100-37. Ear reconstruction for craniofacial microsomia with osseointegration to support a prosthesis. *A,* At the completion of growth and before definitive surgical intervention. *B,* After bimaxillary surgery to centralize the face. *C,* With the osseointegrated platform and the attached ear in place.

however, the condition is often overdiagnosed and confused with the constricted nasal airway associated with a small maxilla. Attempts to widen the choanae in these circumstances only produce soft tissue damage and scarring.

Treatment of Choanal Atresia

The upper airway obstruction due to choanal atresia is often found in patients with hypertelorism and Treacher Collins syndrome (Fig. 100-38).[74] Correction is by removal of bone transnasally, which is usually performed by the otorhinolaryngologist, or transpalatally in patients with severe defects in which the palatal shelf is connected to the clivus. For both procedures, long-term nasopharyngeal splinting is required to establish the airway.

Tonsilloadenoidectomy, Palatal Split Sequence

Conservative management of sleep apnea should first be attempted with continuous positive airway pressure or trials of nasopharyngeal soft tube intubation. Combined adenotonsillectomy may be useful. If deterioration continues, the palate is split and the posterior free margin resected; the raw edges are then sealed with a continuous absorbable suture. All possible efforts should be made to avoid tracheostomy.

Mandibular Distraction for Recalcitrant Airway Obstruction

When the pathologic process is in the mandible, distraction can be undertaken as the next part of the *airway* protocol.[69] In Treacher Collins, Nager, and similar syndromes, the initial results are pleasing from the airway point of view. However, over the years, relapse occurs, and the airway obstruction returns (Fig. 100-39).

FUNCTION-ENHANCING TECHNIQUES
Closure of Clefts

LATERAL CLEFTS. The lateral cleft Tessier number 7, often associated with hemifacial microsomia, produces a macrostomia, may be bilateral, and is associated with a cleft lip and palate of the regular type. Under these circumstances, the planning of the reconstruction of the orbicularis oris can be difficult. The cleft lip element is preferably repaired by a modification of the Millard rotation advancement.

The lateral cleft requires dissection through three layers of skin and subcutaneous fat, muscle, and mucosa. Once the landmarks on the lip elements and the site of the modiolus have been determined, the modiolus is constructed by interdigitating muscle. If the cleft extends out into the lateral cheek, this muscle must also be dissected and united. The mucosa is easily united, and the skin and subcutaneous tissue can be closed with Z-plasties placed in appropriate anatomic lines (Fig. 100-40).

NASO-ORO-OCULAR CLEFTS. There can be no set operation because there is no standard deformity in any of the dimensions. Closure of the cheek and eyelid components is usually involved.

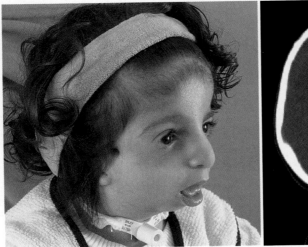
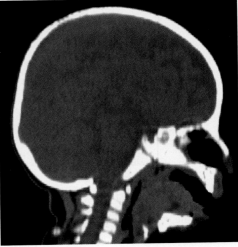

A   B

FIGURE 100-38. *A,* A patient with severe Treacher Collins syndrome. *B,* The CT scan demonstrates the solid block of bone between the hard palate and the base of skull; the fusion occurs just anterior to the spheno-occipital synchondrosis, producing complete choanal atresia.

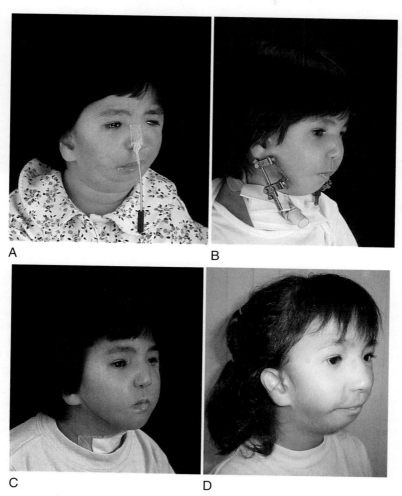

FIGURE 100-39. A patient with Nager syndrome. *A,* Demonstrating the severe problem with feeding and airway obstruction. *B,* During external distraction. *C,* Five weeks after distraction with tracheostomy removed and significant mandibular advancement achieved. *D,* Five years later. The failure of the mandible to grow and the relative relapse are obvious.

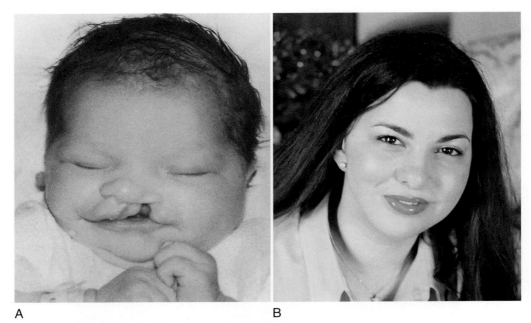

A   B

FIGURE 100-40. *A,* A patient with Goldenhar syndrome with bilateral macrostomia and complete cleft of the lip and palate. *B,* The Z-plasty technique was used to close the macrostomia. The end result is seen at the age of 18 years, after bimaxillary surgery and soft tissue augmentation with a de-epithelialized groin flap secured by microvascular anastomosis.

Oro-ocular (Tessier Number 4 and Number 5). In this deformity, there is a decrease in the distance between the lower eyelid and the alar base. Even though the cleft is lateral to the nasolacrimal drainage system, it is often affected and frequently dysfunctional. The stump of the medial canthal ligament is present and can act as a point of stabilization in the lower lid reconstruction. There is the possibility of a cleft in the upper lip lateral to Cupid's bow.

Although the principle of "first the skeleton, then the soft tissue" still applies, it refers to the more mature individual. In the younger patient, the orbital floor defect and the orbital rim can be reconstructed. A small fragment of bone can be put over the anterior maxillary defect, but the area is small and the bone will disappear. The cleft maxilla and developing alveolus is a bag of developing teeth and should be minimally disturbed at this stage.

Reconstruction of the soft tissue involves closure of the eyelid defect (reconstruction of the orbicularis oculi) and repair of the lip (reconstruction of the orbicularis oris). Tessier (as reported by Kawamoto[75]) has described some useful skin flaps. Stricker et al[76] have opted for a cheek rotation flap in patients with extreme skin shortage. This technique is preferable, together with the eyelid on the flap. If necessary, a tissue expander may be placed to achieve maximum effect with minimal scaring (Fig. 100-41).

Naso-oro-ocular (Tessier Number 3 and Number 4). Like all the other rare clefts, this problem is never solved by the initial soft tissue operation, and a final result is possible only after protocol management during years of growth. This most difficult cleft presents a number of specific challenges, such as

1. the decreased vertical distance between the alar base and the medial canthus;
2. the disrupted nasolacrimal duct and sac, which may leave remnants that become infected;
3. the absence of nasal bone, nasal lining, and a suitably strong site for insertion of the newly reconstructed lower part of the medial canthal attachment of the lower lid; and
4. the need to reconstruct the affected side of the nose (Fig. 100-42).

The decreased distance between the medial canthus and the alar base can be lengthened by Z-plasties of various configurations. The orbital floor and rim are reconstructed with bone graft; the nasal lining is formed by mobilizing mucosa from the septum or the lateral nasal wall. For the patient with severe defects, rotation advancement of the cheek, including the lateral lower lid element, is achieved by taking the flap through the lateral canthus and conjunctiva below the tarsal plate. In this way, maximum use is made of the high-quality lateral cheek skin, especially when prior

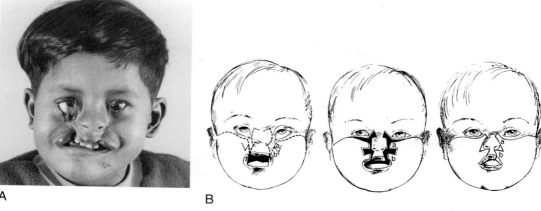

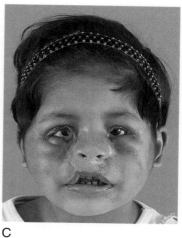

FIGURE 100-41. Soft tissue reconstruction of an oro-ocular cleft (Tessier number 4 and number 5) bilaterally. *A,* Correction of the nasomaxillary dysplasia by rotation and advancement of cheek flaps (after van der Meulen). *B,* van der Meulen's techniques in diagrammatic form. *C,* A variation on the right side included attachment of the lower lid to the cheek rotation flap after tissue expansion. (From Stricker M, van der Meulen J, Raphael B, Mazzola R: Surgery. In Stricker M, van der Meulen J, Raphael B, Mazzola R, eds: Craniofacial Malformations. Edinburgh, Churchill Livingstone, 1990:518.)

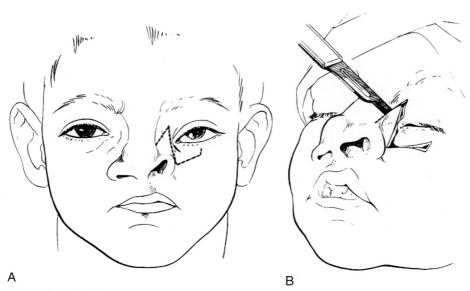

FIGURE 100-42. Treatment of the number 3 cleft. *A,* Marking of the Z-plasty used to correct the medial canthal dystopia and to increase the vertical height. *B,* Development of the Z-plasty. (Courtesy of Dr. P. Tessier.)

tissue expansion is used (see later).[66] It is often necessary to combine this procedure with a forehead flap to reconstruct the nose and interdigitate with the lateral rotation flap (Fig. 100-43). The use of a tissue expander under the forehead skin can maximize the tissue available and minimize the scar.

The ultimate aim is to dissect the margins of the cleft, line them with periosteum, bone graft the gaps, and cover with muscle where appropriate. In wide clefts, this cannot be done at an early stage effectively, and it must wait until bone growth and orthodontic manipulation are complete (see protocol). This early closure aims to protect the eye, to maximize function of the mouth and nose, and to improve cosmesis, knowing the protocol will need to be followed to produce an optimal result.

Midline Clefts. The principal functional goal in this area is to design a functioning and aesthetically acceptable nose. It is not urgent to treat milder clefts with little functional deficit. Waiting until appropriate skeletal maturity has occurred so the underlying skeleton can be repositioned before nasal reconstruction is undertaken is to be preferred. The repair of the central lip and palate is similar in principle, and often in technique, to that used for cleft lip and palate deformity.

Surgery for correction of the orbital dystopia resulting from the midline clefts involves the following: removal of abnormal midline structures, such as cysts or dysplastic brain, as in frontoethmoidal meningoencephalocele; reduction of the interorbital space by medial translocation of the orbits, in part, as a "box," or as part of a facial bipartition; maintenance of separation of the cranial and nasal cavities; reconstruction of the nose; and soft tissue adaptation or augmentation.

Most rare clefts are multiple and of almost an infinite variety of expressions, making formula operations impractical and surgical planning a necessity (Fig. 100-44).[59] The individual techniques are discussed under osteotomies.

Correction of Eyelid Deformities

Treacher Collins Syndrome. The coloboma of the lower lid is a deficiency that affects all layers of the lid. A multilayered repair is necessary.

Z-plasty with Muscle Flap (Fig. 100-45). This repair is used when there is marked tissue deformity. The Z is marked out on the lower lid, and the two flaps are raised from the underlying muscle. The lower lid margin of the coloboma, consisting of the tarsoconjunctival layer, is cut at right angles and sutured. The orbicularis muscle is elevated as a separate flap along the lid margin and by overlapping provides support for the lid. The skin flaps are then transposed and sutured into position.

Transposition of a Musculocutaneous Flap from Upper to Lower Lid (Fig. 100-46). More severe deformities may need transposition of a flap of upper lid skin and orbicularis muscle into an incision made in the lower lid. The ptosed lateral canthal attachment can be fixed in a superior position to the reconstructed orbital rim.

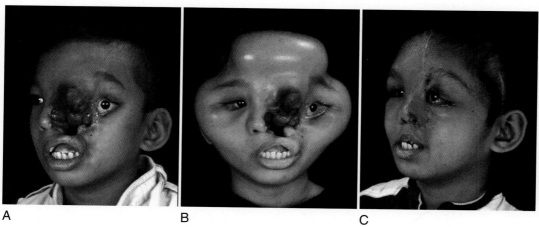

A   B   C

FIGURE 100-43. Primary correction of the left-sided 1-13, 2-12, 3 Tessier clefts. *A,* Preoperative frontal view. *B,* The bilateral malar and forehead tissue expanders are shown fully inflated before removal of the expanders, reduction of the frontal encephalocele and bone grafting, correction of the orbital dystopia by means of facial bipartition, left heminose reconstruction by means of a forehead flap, left medial canthopexy, and advancement of bilateral cheek flaps. *C,* After correction of the hypertelorism and cheek, nose, and lip reconstruction.

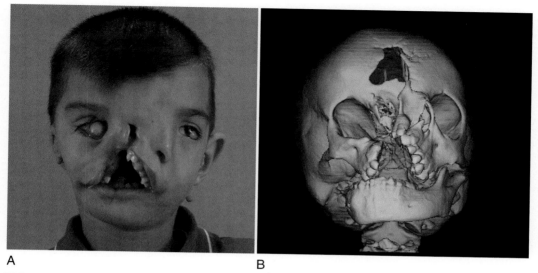

A   B

FIGURE 100-44. A patient with complex, multiple midline craniofacial clefts combined with all the elements of Goldenhar syndrome and a significant suggestion of facial duplication; he is an otherwise highly intelligent, active child. There can be no formula surgery for such a patient. *A,* Frontal view. *B,* The three-dimensional CT reconstruction shows the frontal defect, the gross orbital dystopia, the maxillary cleft, and the right-sided absence of mandible and temporomandibular joint.

Transposition Flap of Full-Thickness Upper Eyelid to Lower Eyelid (Fig. 100-47).[77] The coloboma is released as described, revealing the lower lid defects. A flap of upper eyelid is now raised; instead of just skin and muscle, the full thickness of the lid is used, including enough tarsal plate and conjunctiva to close the lower lid defect. The flap is based laterally, and the inferior edge must be continuous with the incision on the lower lid. With the wide exposure thus provided at the lateral canthus, the lateral canthal ligament can be isolated. Even though it is hypoplastic, it can be transposed upward and attached to the reconstructed lateral orbital rim.

This technique is almost always associated with the bone reconstruction of the orbit in Treacher Collins syndrome (see next section).

TESSIER NUMBER 3, 4, AND 5 CLEFTS. Whenever this type of reconstruction is planned, any associated global dystopia should be corrected at the same time, with construction of an intact orbital floor and support for the eye. Minor lid colobomas can be closed directly.[78]

With the larger defects seen in the Tessier number 4 and number 5 clefts, there is usually a medial element and even an intact lacrimal drainage system. There are a number of published techniques for reconstruction in this area; however, the defects are rarely the same. The principle is to move more normal lateral tissue medially and place the scars in or as close to the natural

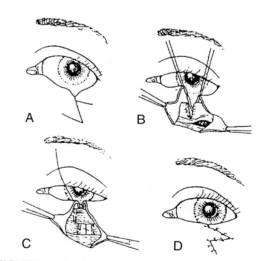

A   B

C   D

FIGURE 100-45. The correction of the eyelid coloboma in Treacher Collins syndrome. *A,* The proposed Z-plasty is marked out in the lower eyelid, and the skin flaps are cut and elevated from the underlying muscle. *B,* The margins of the coloboma are transected through all layers, tarsoconjunctival and muscle, at right angles to the lower lid. *C,* The tarsoconjunctival layer is sutured with a running pull-out nylon suture. The muscle layer is elevated as a separate layer and overlapped along the line of the bed margin, thus giving support for the lid. *D,* The skin flaps are transferred and sutured into position with fine interrupted sutures of 6-0 nylon. (From David DJ: Treacher Collins syndrome. In Muir IFK, ed: Current Operative Surgery: Plastic and Reconstructive Surgery. London, Baillière Tindall, 1985:109.)

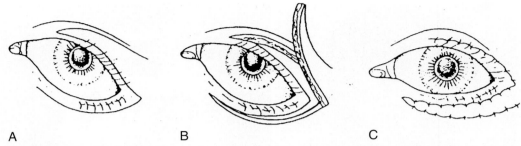

FIGURE 100-46. Transposition of a musculocutaneous flap from the upper to the lower lid. *A,* The upper eyelid is marked out, based laterally; the lateral canthus will be transposed upward as this flap is transposed downward. *B,* The lower eyelid is released horizontally through all layers but the tarsoconjunctival layer. If the eyelid is very depressed, the technique in *C* should be used. *C,* The upper eyelid musculocutaneous flap is transposed into the lower lid defects made by the upward movement of the lateral canthus, which is fixed into a drill hole in the lateral orbital margin. The skin is sutured with fine 6-0 nylon. (From David DJ: Treacher Collins syndrome. In Muir IFK, ed: Current Operative Surgery: Plastic and Reconstructive Surgery. London, Baillière Tindall, 1985:109.)

crease lines as possible, a concept elegantly outlined by van der Meulen.[16]

The lateral lid elements are left attached to a cheek rotation flap, which extends through the lateral canthus, upward and backward to the preauricular crease line. The lateral lower lid elements are sutured to the medial, and the conjunctiva is mobilized to be sutured to the skin margin laterally. If the defect is large, it may be useful to employ a tissue expander under the lateral skin to make the rotation easier.

The more medially placed cleft through the region of the nasolacrimal apparatus poses a particular reconstructive problem. The lack of nasal lining and nasolacrimal bone is difficult to correct. The correction of the lid coloboma is, however, performed in the same fashion as mentioned previously, except there is no medial element, the lower lid component of the superficial portion of the medial canthal ligament is absent, and the lid remnant needs to be rotated without

tension and attached firmly in the region of the medial canthus. This is best accomplished with the aid of tissue expansion of the cheek flap. The lateral cheek can then be used to interdigitate with the deficient lateral nasal elements to lengthen the nose and keep the scar in the natural crease between nose and cheek.

Tissue expanders can be used in repair of a cleft, to expand the orbit, in bone grafting of the maxilla, in reconstruction of the nose, and in severe hypertelorism to relax the periosteum laterally. The expander can be introduced deeply under the periosteum to give enough relaxation of these constricting tissues to facilitate orbital translocation and to minimize relapse.[66]

GROWTH-ENHANCING TECHNIQUES

These maneuvers are performed during development to encourage growth of affected areas of the facial skeleton and, by so doing, minimize secondary deformi-

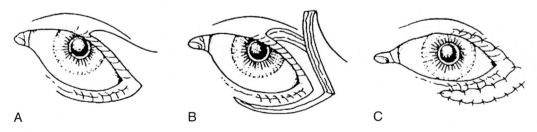

FIGURE 100-47. Transposition flap of full-thickness upper eyelid to lower eyelid. *A,* The upper eyelid is outlined; the superior position of the base of the flap is the point to which the lateral canthus will be elevated. *B,* Full-thickness incision through the lower lid will reveal the tissue deficiency. The upper lid is of full thickness with a tarsal plate and conjunctival island on the musculocutaneous flap. Care is taken to leave a superior rim of tarsal plate with its attached levator mechanism. *C,* The defect in the tarsal plate is closed with 6-0 nylon. The lateral canthus is transposed upward and fixed into the lateral orbital wall by a suture plane through one or two drill holes. The upper lid flap is now sutured in the lower lid defect in layers. (From David DJ: Treacher Collins syndrome. In Muir IFK, ed: Current Operative Surgery: Plastic and Reconstructive Surgery. London, Baillière Tindall, 1985:109.)

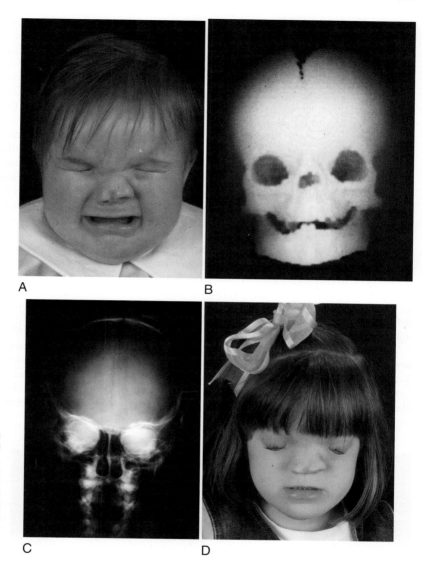

FIGURE 100-48. A child with bilateral anophthalmia and midline nasal cleft. *A,* At 7 months of age. *B,* The three-dimensional CT reconstruction shows the constricted orbits. *C,* Tissue expanders have been inserted and inflated during several years. The radiograph shows dilute contrast medium to demonstrate the degree of expansion. *D,* At 6 years of age.

ties that can develop in adjacent structures. They are rarely an end in themselves but set up a situation for successful reconstruction after growth.

Orbital Expansion[67]

The orbit does not expand adequately in patients with anophthalmia because of lack of an organ exerting the necessary pressure on the developing bone. Surgical expansion of the orbit is accomplished by osteotomies.[79-82] Anterior projection of the conjunctival sac and expansion of the sac precede serial insertion of prostheses of increasing diameter. This is a cumbersome method superceded by intraorbital tissue expansion. A 5-mL spherical tissue expander* is introduced into the back of the orbit after periorbital dissection through a partial coronal scalp flap, the contents are pushed forward, and the tube is run through a perforation in the lateral orbital wall. The injection port is located in a convenient position over the temporoparietal region; 2 to 3 mL is injected at the time, and tiny increments of expansion are made monthly up to approximately 5 years of age. The position is checked by plain radiology after injection of a small amount of contrast medium. In this way, the orbit can be expanded and the lateral hourglass deformity in the temporal region obviated (Fig. 100-48).

---

*Laboratoires Sebbin, 95650 Boissy l'Aillerie, France.

When the expander is removed, the space is filled with costal cartilage to maintain the forward projection of the conjunctival sac, which itself must then be expanded by mucosal grafts supported by a conformer. Small eyelids remain a problem. Lateral extension of the palpebral fissure produces lids with no lashes laterally. In the microphthalmic orbit, the globe is retained; in cryptophthalmia, the remnants can be discarded.

Costochondral Graft

In severe craniofacial microsomia in which the temporomandibular joint is absent, construction by costochondral grafting occurs at approximately 5 years of age.[83,84] Ross[85] can provide a new growing unit within the existing functional matrix.

When this procedure is proposed in the growing child, it must be planned with a view to future orthodontic control and manipulation of facial growth. The new position of the mandible will be determined by an acrylic occlusal wafer (Fig. 100-49) that serves as a splint. The orthodontist supervises hygiene and alterations to the splint with growth.

The graft is obtained by harvesting the sixth or seventh rib from the contralateral chest wall. More than 1 cm of costal cartilage needs to be attached to the bone; care is necessary to preserve the periosteum and perichondrium at the junction. Enough rib and extra cartilage are harvested to fashion a zygomatic arch and glenoid fossa.

The superior approach is made through a coronal scalp flap, and the hypoplastic coronoid and condylar processes of the mandible are freed of their attachments. This enables the lower jaw to be repositioned into the wafer without contralateral osteotomy. The arch is reconstructed with rib, and the superior part of the joint is a disk of cartilage set into the rib in the position of the joint. It is fixed with wire. A submandibular incision is made to assist in freeing up part of the dissection and positioning the graft, which is located superiorly by a loosely placed nylon suture between the two parts of the cartilaginous joint and below by three screws into the mandible triangulated if possible for stability (Fig. 100-50).

This technique provides the possibility of growth enhancement for a long time, enabling dentition to develop more normally and facial distortion to be minimized.[85] Almost invariably, further surgery is required at the completion of growth.

Bone Distraction

This popular and interesting technique of producing new bone in the mandible is now widely used. It is as yet difficult to determine how it is more beneficial to the patient when it is introduced into the protocol for growth enhancement compared with acute airway

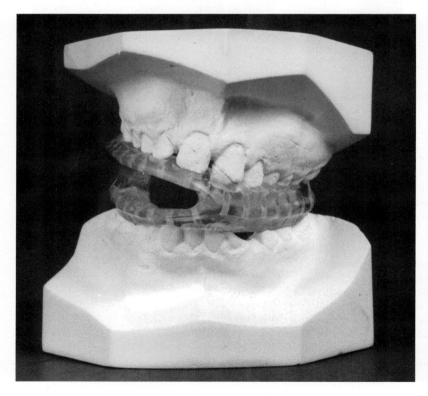

FIGURE 100-49. An appliance designed to facilitate the gradual eruption of the maxillary teeth. The acrylic is shaved progressively as eruption occurs. (From David DJ, Abbott JR, Jay M, et al: Deformities. In David DJ, Simpson DA, eds: Cranio-Maxillo-Facial Trauma. Edinburgh, Churchill Livingstone, 1995:604.)

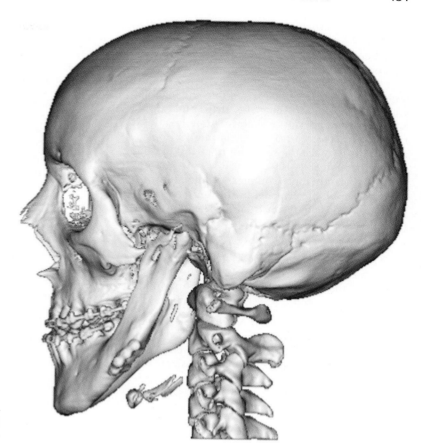

FIGURE 100-50. A three-dimensional CT scan of a costochondral graft in situ with rigid screw fixation.

problems. The disadvantages of this technique include length of time for the procedure, discomfort, expense, and need for repeated procedures; it does not obviate definitive surgery at the end of growth.

Orthodontics

The orthodontist encourages the eruption of teeth as described for hemifacial microsomia; expands segments of the cleft maxilla in preparation for alveolar bone grafting; and uses active appliances to centralize the bite, strengthen muscles, and encourage bone growth.[30]

Early Excision of "Tumor" in Frontoethmoidal Meningoencephalocele

During growth, especially in infancy, removal of the dysplastic brain emerging through the base of skull in the region of the foramen cecum and spilling into the nose and orbit and onto the face will enhance the achievement of a more normal craniofacial configuration. In severe instances, medial movement of the superomedial part of the orbit is all else that may be necessary, together with canthopexy and nasal reconstruction with a bone graft.

BONE GRAFTING, OSTEOTOMIES, AND FREE FLAPS

Each deformity is unique, and the precise operation or combination of operations needs to fit into the management protocol with respect to timing and sequence. A multidisciplinary surgical planning meeting should precede the surgery to decide the exact operative plan.

Bone Grafting

The preferred donor sites for the harvesting of bone are the calvaria, the rib cage, and the iliac crest.

ORBIT

Laterally in Treacher Collins Syndrome (including bone flaps). The cranial vault has become the favored donor site, and the technique has been described by Tessier.[86] The calvaria must be sufficiently thick for the outer table to be harvested. This is not often true in children. A full-thickness calvarial "bone flap" is removed from one or both parietal regions. The flap is split; half is used to repair the orbit, and the other half is replaced.

Reconstruction is achieved by a combination of onlay and inlay grafts. The superolateral margins of the orbit are overhanging and need to be reshaped by excision of a crescent of bone or by burring. Careful dissection is necessary to separate the periorbitum and the fascia over the temporalis muscle and the fascia over the masseter muscle. If the bone defect is much larger than expected, bone is laid into the inferolateral defect to support the globe; strips build up the lateral wall and inferior orbital rim extending posteriorly to form the zygomatic arch. Fixation is by plates and screws to make the structure rigid and to minimize resorption (Fig. 100-51).

A significantly more complex technique involves the transfer of preshaped calvaria on a musculoperiosteal pedicle to reconstruct the lateral orbitozygomatic complex (Fig. 100-52).[87,88]

Centrally (in Tessier Clefts Number 4 and Number 5). The grafts placed in infancy always need replacing later. A wide dissection is necessary to define the margins of the cleft. The floor is inserted first and the rim fashioned on top.

Medially (in Tessier Cleft Number 3). The floor medial to the infraorbital nerve, part of the lacrimal bone, frontal process of the maxilla, and part of the nasal bone may be involved. Iliac bone is easier to work with because of the need for three-dimensional fashioning of the graft. Before this maneuver can be successful, nasal lining needs to be secured as well as adequate skin cover. The bone graft is used as the fixation point for the medial canthopexy (Fig. 100-53).

ANTERIOR MAXILLA. In infancy, the distance between the orbital rim and the alveolus is small; the apposition of a small graft to the anterior maxilla helps support the soft tissue repair. When this is done at an older age, either as a primary repair or as a repeated performance, the graft should be fixed with a screw and covered with mobilized periosteum and muscle. In severe defects, the tension in this covering can be released by inserting a deeply placed tissue expander beforehand.[66]

ZYGOMA. Onlay bone grafts to augment the cheeks are frequently needed in reconstruction of these deformities. Introduced through the mouth or through a coronal flap from above, the graft must be rigidly fixed to facilitate graft survival. Hip and rib are more flexible than calvarial bone.

MAXILLARY ALVEOLUS. The indications for alveolar bone grafts are before eruption of an adjacent tooth,

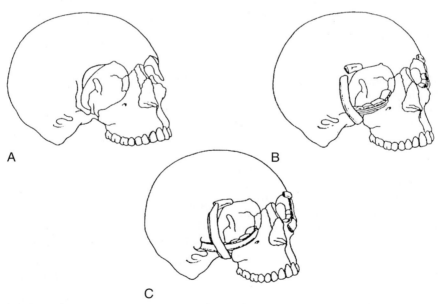

FIGURE 100-51. *A,* The supralateral orbital margins are usually overhanging, and these can be reshaped by cutting a crescent of bone from this region with an osteotome if the bone fragment is to be preserved and used elsewhere or a dental burr if the deformity is slight. *B,* Bone is layered into the inferior orbital defect to build up the floor and thus the support for the globe. Layers of rib or calvarial bone can then be used to reconstruct the lateral orbital wall. Bone grafts should be securely wired into place. *C,* A groove is fashioned in the temporal bone, into which the onlay arch graft is placed. Further strips can be layered on top of these basic elements if necessary. (From David DJ: Treacher Collins syndrome. In Muir IFK, ed: Current Operative Surgery: Plastic and Reconstructive Surgery. London, Baillière Tindall, 1985:112.)

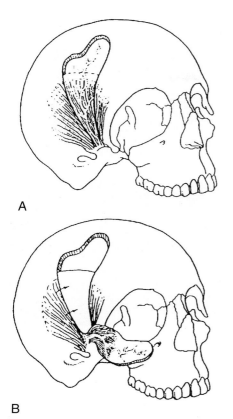

FIGURE 100-52. *A,* The approach is made through the bicoronal scalp flap, exposing the temporalis muscle and overlying galea in a plane just deep to the hair follicles. The area of calvarial bone to be used is marked out and included in the flap. *B,* The bone flap is raised in continuity with the central part of the temporalis muscle, in which is included the main trunk of the superficial temporal vessels. The bone part of the flap can be either full thickness or partial thickness of the calvaria. (From David DJ: Treacher Collins syndrome. In Muir IFK, ed: Current Operative Surgery: Plastic and Reconstructive Surgery. London, Baillière Tindall, 1985:113.)

before maxillary osteotomy, and as a pre-prosthetic measure. The technique is described elsewhere in this publication and remains the same for those clefts that traverse the alveolus in unusual positions (Fig. 100-54). The surgery is preceded by orthodontic expansion of the maxillary elements and uprighting of the teeth adjacent to the cleft. The bone of choice is cancellous bone from the iliac crest covered by gingival periosteum.

NOSE. Definitive nasal reconstruction is usually the final step in a long management process. There needs to be provision of adequate lining, and there are many techniques, including mobilization and rearrangement of the available mucosa, transposition of flaps from adjacent skin, and inversion of the flap being used for skin cover.

Likewise, there are various designs of bone grafts; a two-part graft with a columellar strut may help provide forward projection of the tip of the graft (Fig. 100-55). This projection can be just as well achieved by fixing the dorsal strut of the costochondral graft to the nasofrontal region with a single screw or sometimes two screws (Fig. 100-56). The remnants of the tip can be repositioned over the cartilaginous tip or cartilage grafts positioned to form a tip.

The lateral part of the nasal pyramid can be formed by thin triangles of cortical bone between the strut and the piriform margin. Nasal, paranasal, and frontal skin is used to complete the covering integument. In the author's hands, the best technique is the use of pre-expanded forehead skin. The expander is placed superficial to the galea, and expansion is begun after 2 to 3 weeks; expansion is completed during the next 3 weeks and then left for another 3 weeks for consolidation. The transposition of the flap is then planned in reverse; there is always a third stage to tidy up and reshape the nose.

In patients with lateral nasal proboscis and heminose,[89] the skeletal anomalies are corrected with appropriate osteotomies (see next), and a dummy external nose is made in one procedure. The nasal skeleton is constructed with a rib graft. The proboscis is dissected, leaving an attached subcutaneous pedicle to allow relocation inferiorly by tunneling the pedicle and setting it into an inferiorly based flap in the region of the new nostril base (Fig. 100-57).

Osteotomies

Osteotomies of the craniofacial skeleton in patients with craniofacial clefts are usually performed at the end of growth for the particular region. The deformities are widely variable, so matching the osteotomy to the deformity is a matter of individual planning

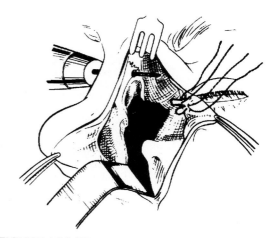

FIGURE 100-53. Transnasal approach for the medial canthopexy. (Courtesy of Dr. P. Tessier.)

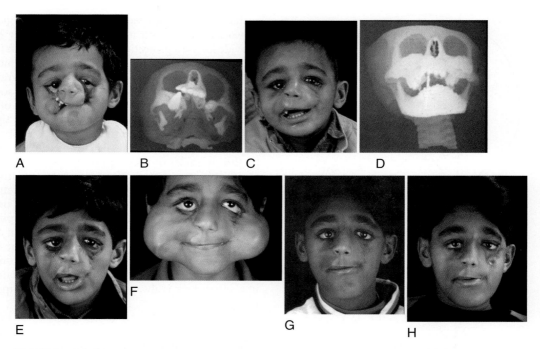

FIGURE 100-54. The sequence of events in the management of a patient with bilateral Tessier 4-5 clefts indicating the extent of the bone grafting necessary to reconstruct the alveolar, orbital, and maxillary defects. Tissue expansion helps to cover the grafted area adequately with periosteum. *A,* The defect before surgery. *B,* The significant distortion of the bony skeleton demonstrated by three-dimensional CT. *C,* After bone grafting and cheek flap rotation. *D,* The postoperative three-dimensional CT scan indicating the extent of bone grafting of the orbits and maxilla. *E,* The situation in early teenage years with some resorption of bone. *F,* Further tissue expansion before bone grafting and soft tissue revision. *G,* Postoperative result. *H,* At the completion of growth.

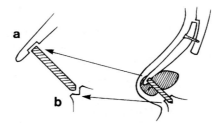

FIGURE 100-55. Nasal columella support. If the surgeon contemplates the need for a columella support, it is formed from cortical bone, which may be embedded in a small groove (a) at the lower end of the graft. The base of the supporting strut is firmly embedded in a hole (b) prepared at the level of the anterior nasal spine. The screw fixation technique has obviated the need for this more cumbersome and less rigid form of reconstruction. (From David DJ, Abbott JR, Jay M, et al: Deformities. In David DJ, Simpson DA, eds: Cranio-Maxillo-Facial Trauma. Edinburgh, Churchill Livingstone, 1995:581.)

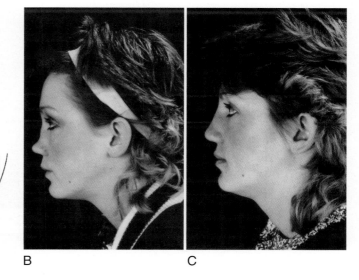

FIGURE 100-56. Nasal bone grafts. *A,* Diagrammatic representation of the bone graft overlying the freshly rasped nasal bones as far as possible. This is fixed with a countersunk screw or, if required for stability, two screws. *B,* A typically depressed nasal septum. *C,* Appearance after bone grafting. (From David DJ, Abbott JR, Jay M, et al: Deformities. In David DJ, Simpson DA, eds: Cranio-Maxillo-Facial Trauma. Edinburgh, Churchill Livingstone, 1995:579.)

in the context of the protocol management for the disease.

ORBITAL. The orbit can be moved in three dimensions and in segments to suit correction of the individual deformity. In many instances, a frontal craniotomy is needed to secure the dura and to remove brain and meningeal hernias, cysts, and tumors associated with the deformities. This frontal craniotomy is performed by the neurosurgeon.

Fronto-orbital. The osteotomy is used to advance, equalize, or re-form (as in the Tessier number 10 cleft) the fronto-orbital region. It extends through the region of the frontozygomatic suture, through the lesser

wing of sphenoid, and across the orbital roof to the area of the foramen cecum. The horizontal glabellar cut connects with the anterior fossa and the medial orbital wall. This bar can be removed and replaced with calvarial graft, cut asymmetrically or fashioned to suit the reconstructive needs (Fig. 100-58).

Partial Orbital (Fig. 100-59). The four quadrants of each orbit can be moved separately or in combination. The upper two quadrants require a craniotomy as described. The approach is made through a coronal flap; for the lower cuts, the upper buccal sulcus is used, with either a subciliary or transconjunctival approach to the lower eyelid.

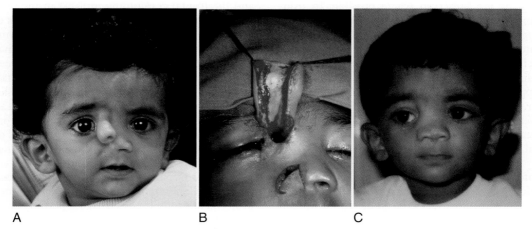

FIGURE 100-57. *A,* A 10-month-old Indian boy with right nasal agenesis and proboscis. *B,* The proboscis being de-epithelialized and tunneled under the right nasal skin. *C,* The completed heminasal reconstruction.

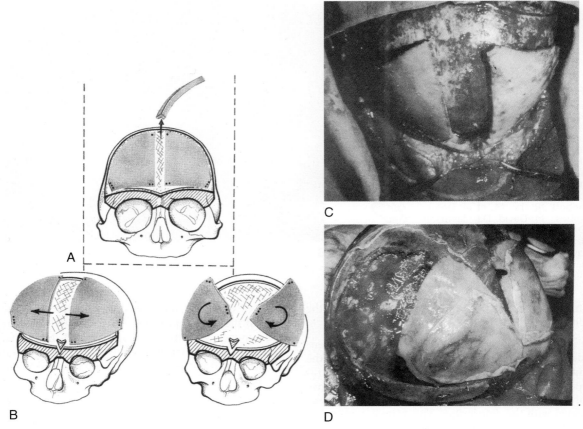

FIGURE 100-58. Segmental forehead remodeling (bilateral) by lateral displacement of frontal plates *(A)* and rotation of frontal plates *(B)*. *C* and *D,* Operative views. (From van der Meulen J, Mazzola R, Stricker M, Raphael B: Classification of craniofacial malformations. In Stricker M, van der Meulen J, Raphael B, Mazzola R, eds: Craniofacial Malformations. Edinburgh, Churchill Livingstone, 1990.)

The midline structures of the area of the cribriform plate are preserved where possible. In frontoethmoidal meningoencephalocele, the exit holes through the facial skeleton are so variable that the osteotomy cuts have to be designed on an individual basis; however, they usually involve moving the superomedial quadrants medially. The same principles can be applied to expanding the orbit by translating quadrants of the orbit in patients with micro-orbitism. Converse[90] expanded the orbit in all directions, and Marchac[81] described a technique moving the superolateral segment.

Total Orbital. In reality, this means moving the anterior two thirds of the orbital pyramid, that is, the part of the orbit that takes the globe with it when it is translocated. The mobilization is in part achieved through a transcranial approach. Additional incisions in the eyelids and upper buccal sulcus may be needed. The upper osteotomy is made 1 cm above the supra-orbital rim; a frontal bar is often left between this cut and the frontal craniotomy to assist in the location and fixation of the segments. The lower cut is made across the anterior maxilla just beneath the infraorbital foramen. Care must be taken to ensure that the patient is mature enough for the developing teeth to have cleared this area. The posterior lateral orbital cuts are made vertically through the lateral wall flush with the temporal fossa. This osteotomy is continued across the orbital roof and inferiorly into the inferior orbital fissure. The medial wall is cut at about the level of the anterior ethmoidal foramen; if the medial canthal ligament is intact, it should be left intact.

If the orbit is being moved upward, a measured amount of bone is removed from the frontal bone. The orbit is gently mobilized and fixed superiorly; the inferior defect is grafted. When the orbit is being translocated medially, the midline structures are maintained if possible (Fig. 100-60)[22] or removed if necessary (Fig. 100-61).[2]

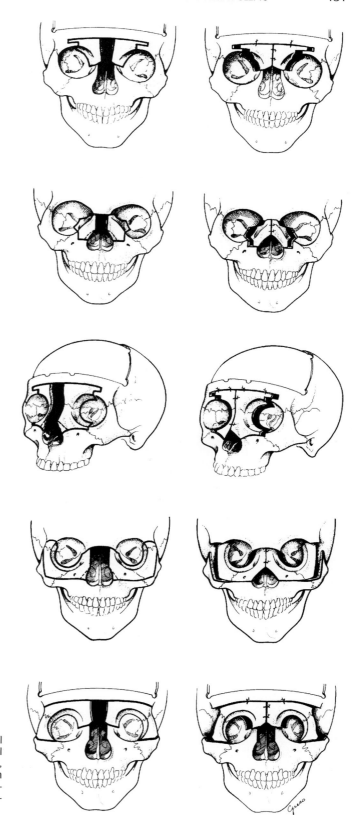

FIGURE 100-59. Reduction of the interorbital distance by various types of partial orbital osteotomies. (From Stricker M, van der Meulen J, Raphael B, Mazzola R: Surgery. In Stricker M, van der Meulen J, Raphael B, Mazzola R, eds: Craniofacial Malformations. Edinburgh, Churchill Livingstone, 1990:401.)

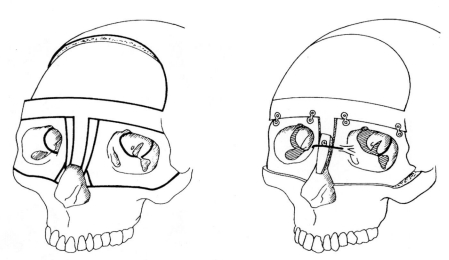

FIGURE 100-60. Hypertelorism correction according to Converse et al.[22] Midline structures are preserved wherever possible. The cuts are made behind the axis of the globe so that the globe is translocated with the orbital box. (From David DJ, Abbott JR, Jay M, et al: Deformities. In David DJ, Simpson DA, eds: Cranio-Maxillo-Facial Trauma. Edinburgh, Churchill Livingstone, 1995.)

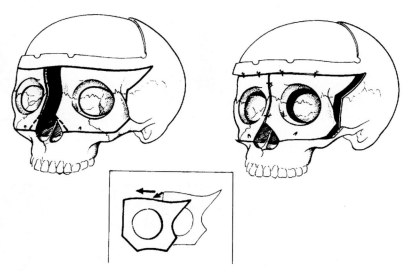

FIGURE 100-61. Medial translocation of the two orbits by the original Tessier procedure. (From van der Meulen J, Mazzola R, Stricker M, Raphael B: Classification of craniofacial malformations. In Stricker M, van der Meulen J, Raphael B, Mazzola R, eds: Craniofacial Malformations. Edinburgh, Churchill Livingstone, 1990.)

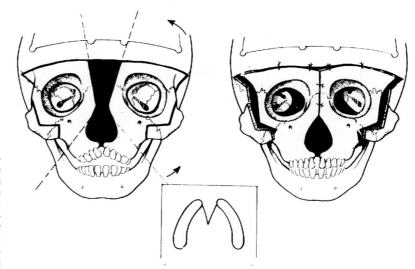

FIGURE 100-62. Medial translocation of the two orbits by the "medial fasciotomy" procedure (van der Meulen). (From van der Meulen J, Mazzola R, Stricker M, Raphael B: Classification of craniofacial malformations. In Stricker M, van der Meulen J, Raphael B, Mazzola R, eds: Craniofacial Malformations. Edinburgh, Churchill Livingstone, 1990.)

Facial Bipartition (Fig. 100-62). In some of the more dramatic central clefts, the face is already divided by the cleft; another indication is the central cleft with the V deformity of the alveolus.

The "box" osteotomy is now in continuity with the maxilla, which needs to be disconnected at the pterygomaxillary junction. Rotation and translocation can be planned into the reconstruction. For patients with wide hypertelorism, it is preferable to insert tissue expanders deep to the periosteum over the zygomatic arch to overcome the soft tissue tightness that prevents easy movement and maintenance of the reconstruction.[91]

MIDFACE

Le Fort III. This operation detaches the facial bones from the cranial base. The osteotomy passes through the glabella, across the orbital floor to the inferior orbital fissure, through the lateral orbital wall to the frontozygomatic suture or there about. The posterior disconnection is between the maxillary tuberosity and the pterygoid plates and laterally through the zygomatic arch. The gaps are bone grafted, and the new position is supported with miniplate fixation and orthodontic occlusal control (Fig. 100-63).

Le Fort II. There are many variations of midface osteotomies—Le Fort II, perialar, and combinations (Fig. 100-64).

Le Fort I. This is the most common and most useful of the midface osteotomies (Fig. 100-65). It has been and remains convenient to describe midface osteotomies by reference to the fracture pattern described by Le Fort; there are many variations that must be made to suit the variability of the conditions being treated.[92,93] The surgery is planned at a meeting at which, at least, patient, surgeon, and orthodontist

are present. Radiologic examination, cephalometric data, dental casts, and (for complex defects) nylon models of the skull generated from CT data are used to assist in the planning. Where possible, the maxilla should have been expanded, the teeth aligned, and the segments united with bone grafting according to protocol. In this way, the osteotomy can be designed, the position of translocation determined, and an occlusal wafer manufactured to enable this movement to be accurately made at operation. Custom-made arch bars are fitted before surgery and used to secure the wafer and intermaxillary fixation if necessary.

The patient is usually anesthetized by a nasoendotracheal tube; an epinephrine and local anesthetic

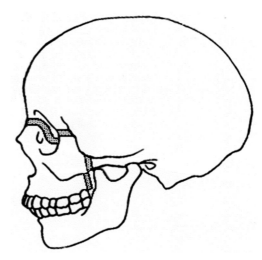

FIGURE 100-63. The Le Fort III osteotomy is shown on a lateral skull view. The stippled areas indicate the osteotomy lines and where bone grafts are usually placed.

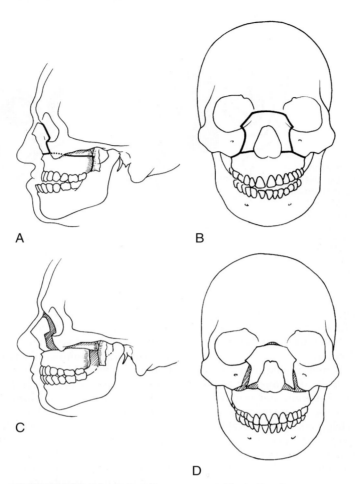

A

B

C

D

FIGURE 100-64. Le Fort II osteotomy. *A,* The Le Fort II osteotomy can be performed in combination with other osteotomies, with either the zygoma or a Le Fort I section. *B,* It is important to have the upper part of the osteotomy behind the nasolacrimal apparatus to protect it and to swing the osteotomy down medial and inferior to the infraorbital foramen to the line recommended for the Le Fort I osteotomy. *C,* The gaps are bone grafted and secured with miniplate fixation. *D,* There is often a step in the infraorbital rim that needs to be grafted or smoothed over. The step at the glabella can be burred down and the gap grafted. Canthopexy and the addition of bone graft for nasal support are further options. It is best not to detach the canthal ligaments if they are reasonably well seated. (From David DJ, Abbott JR, Jay M, et al: Deformities. In David DJ, Simpson DA, eds: Cranio-Maxillo-Facial Trauma. Edinburgh, Churchill Livingstone, 1995.)

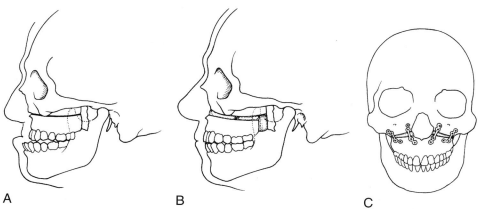

A   B   C

FIGURE 100-65. Le Fort I osteotomy. *A,* The horizontal osteotomy is placed above the tooth roots along the anterior wall of the maxillary sinus and carried through the buttresses at the piriform margin and zygomatic and pterygoid regions. *B,* Bone grafts are placed in the horizontal aspects of the cut if the advancement is more than a few millimeters. The author has never placed these grafts between the maxillary tuberosity and the pterygoid plates, although many surgeons follow this practice. *C,* Four miniplates of the softer variety (without memory) are placed at the zygomatic and piriform buttresses. These can easily be bent to shape. (From David DJ, Abbott JR, Jay M, et al: Deformities. In David DJ, Simpson DA, eds: Cranio-Maxillo-Facial Trauma. Edinburgh, Churchill Livingstone, 1995.)

solution is injected subperiosteally and under the nasal mucosa of the septum and lateral nasal wall. If it is well placed, this produces a degree of hydrodissection as well as vasoconstriction.

An upper buccal sulcus incision is made down to the periosteum, which is elevated toward the orbital rim, exposing but preserving the infraorbital nerve; the incision is extended onto the malar body, and the nasal mucosa is elevated in continuity with the maxillary dissection. The osteotomy is made with a reciprocating saw from the buttress at the piriform aperture, across the anterior maxilla, to the malar buttress; the covering nasal mucosa and lateral periosteum are protected by malleable metal retractors during this procedure. Separation of the pterygoid and the maxillary tuberosity is achieved with a curved osteotome. The vomer is sectioned, releasing the nasal septum from the palate. The next maneuver is a downfracture that exposes the lateral maxillary wall and allows the posterior osteotomy to be completed under direct vision. Small bone nibblers can be used to remove bone precisely in the region of the posterior lateral part of the maxillary antrum where the maxillary artery is at risk. Mobilization should produce the translocation without tension. Fixation is achieved with titanium miniplates that do not have "memory." These plates are placed at the four buttresses.

SEGMENTAL MAXILLARY. The work of Wassmund[94] and Schuchardt[95] has been developed to include a wide range of individual osteotomies, culminating in the orthodontic-distraction-surgical combination of moving small tooth-bearing segments of the deformed and cleft maxilla as reported by Yeow et al[96] (Fig. 100-66).

MANDIBULAR. Osteotomies may be carried out on the alveolar process of the mandible, on the body or ramus, and on the chin or in combinations of all of these structures.

Sagittal Split Osteotomy of the Ramus (Fig. 100-67). Trauner and Obwegeser[97] applied the principle of a sagittal osteotomy that produces an overlap of fragments in the retromolar region; Dal Pont[98] extended the area of contact along the lateral cortical plate of the mandible. With this technique, corrections in the anteroposterior plane are well tolerated, asymmetry less so as lateral stress is placed on the temporomandibular joint. The mandible can also be rotated after sagittal split osteotomy. This maneuver is said to be limited by the pull of muscles opposing the correction. This tendency has been minimized by the use of rigid interfragment fixation.

The intraoral incision is small, 3 cm in length, and runs lateral to the anterior line of the ramus to the region of the second molar tooth. The cut goes down to the periosteum; the lateral and medial aspects of the ramus are exposed. The osteotomy starts above the lingula and extends horizontally to the anterior border and down medial to the oblique line. Laterally, its course to the lower border is backward for retropositioning of the mandible or forward to the lower border to get a longer lateral fragment to facilitate mandibular advancement.[99] The fragments

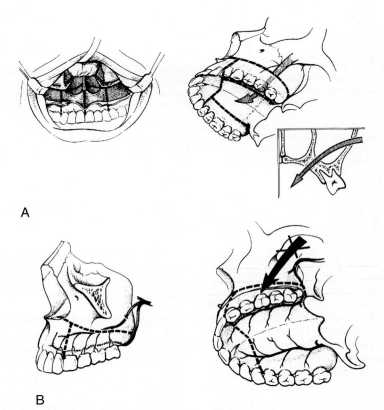

A

B

FIGURE 100-66. Partial osteotomies. *A,* Techniques described by Bell, Epker, and Schendl. *B,* Vascular distribution in relation to the techniques. (From Stricker M, van der Meulen J, Raphael B, Mazzola R: Surgery. In Stricker M, van der Meulen J, Raphael B, Mazzola R, eds: Craniofacial Malformations. Edinburgh, Churchill Livingstone, 1990: 406.)

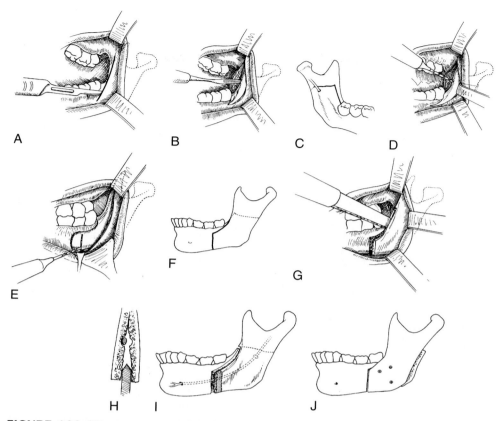

FIGURE 100-67. Sagittal split osteotomy technique. *A,* Intraoral incision just lateral to the anterior border of the mandibular ramus, extended to the bone over the external oblique ridge. *B,* Elevation of the flaps medially and laterally. *C,* Schematic view of the osteotomy as if seen from the medial aspect. *D,* Medial cut being made with a side-cutting burr. The soft tissues are protected by the channel retractor. *E,* Vertical component of the lateral cut. *F,* Schematic representation of the line of the split. *G,* Cleaving or splitting of the fragments. *H,* Separation of the lateral fragment (proximal segment) away from the neurovascular bundle. *I,* Osteotomy segments in new position. *J,* Positioning of the screws for rigid fixation. (From David DJ, Abbott JR, Jay M, et al: Deformities. In David DJ, Simpson DA, eds: Cranio-Maxillo-Facial Trauma. Edinburgh, Churchill Livingstone, 1995.)

are secured by three interfragment screws, two above and one below the neurovascular bundle.

Vertical Subsigmoid Ramus Osteotomy (Fig. 100-68). This osteotomy is used when there is significant asymmetry with tilting of the occlusal plane. Where there is a necessity for lateral movement of the mandibular segment with this osteotomy, the condylar fragment can remain enlocated, unrotated and unangulated in the new position.

Because rigid fixation and minimal use of intermaxillary fixation are advantageous, and because a satisfactory technique for achieving this from an intraoral approach has yet to be devised, an external approach through a submandibular incision is recommended. The platysma is incised at a lower level than the skin and lifted superiorly to avoid the mandibular branch

of the facial nerve. The lower border of the mandible is approached by blunt dissection, and the muscles and periosteum are elevated from the body up to the sigmoid notch on both surfaces of the ramus; care is taken to dissect posterior to the lingula. Malleable retractors protect the soft tissue, and the osteotomy is made with a reciprocating saw. For complete mobilization, the coronoid process occasionally has to be sectioned. When the osteotomies have been completed on both sides, the distal segment is related to the maxilla by a preshaped acrylic wafer shaped according to the treatment plan. Care is taken to have the posterior segments unangulated and the condyles correctly placed in the glenoid fossa. The fragments can then be rigidly fixed with plates, screws, and interpositional bone grafts. The jaw is supported for a few days with rubber band intermaxillary fixation.

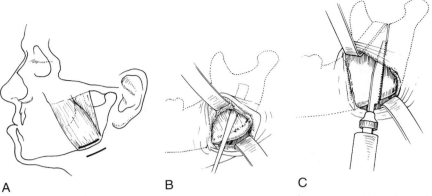

A   B   C

FIGURE 100-68. External approach to the subsigmoid osteotomy. *A,* Incision is made below the angle of the mandible specifically to avoid the mandibular branch of the facial nerve. The masseter is divided from the inferior border. *B,* Subperiosteal dissection on both sides of the mandible posterior to the entry of the neurovascular bundle. *C,* Adequate protection with retractors allows the osteotomy to be safely performed with a reciprocating saw. (From David DJ, Abbott JR, Jay M, et al: Deformities. In David DJ, Simpson DA, eds: Cranio-Maxillo-Facial Trauma. Edinburgh, Churchill Livingstone, 1995.)

Inverted L Osteotomy of the Ramus (Fig. 100-69). This osteotomy is used in patients with severe mandibular hypoplasia, such as in Treacher Collins syndrome, in which the temporomandibular joint is functional and significant forward projection needs to be achieved. The osteotomy of the ramus is made above the entry of the neurovascular bundle and carried to the lower border as in the vertical subsigmoid osteotomy, thus leaving the temporomandibular joint, coronoid process, and posterior part of the ramus in position. The body and angle together with the nerve and blood supply are advanced and rotated. An interpositional bone graft is fixed with miniplates. The surgical approach is similar to that for the subsigmoid osteotomy.

Genioplasty (Fig. 100-70)

This useful technique can be performed alone or to complement other craniofacial osteotomies. A horizontal osteotomy below the level of the mental nerve foramina can be used to reposition the chin in three dimensions. The downward movement is supported by an intervening bone graft. The surgical approach is through the buccal sulcus. The initial incision passes obliquely down to the bone, leaving some muscle on the dental side. Subperiosteal dissection should leave the soft tissue adherent to the chin point; the mental foramina are located and cleared by at least 5 mm.[100] The osteotomy is made with a reciprocating saw, giving wide clearance to the tooth roots. The muscle

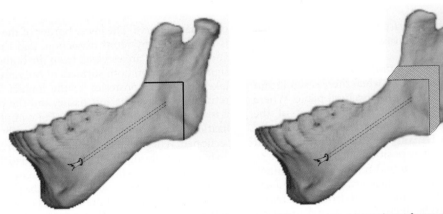

FIGURE 100-69. Inverted L osteotomy. The inverted L ramus osteotomy is performed above the entrance of the neurovascular bundle. After the muscles are freed, the distal segment can be distracted and bone graft inserted into the gaps. Plate fixation is preferred. There may be both onlay and inlay components in the bone grafting.

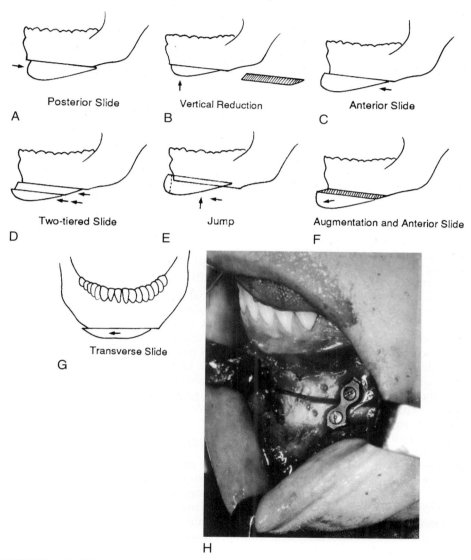

FIGURE 100-70. Genioplasty. *A* to *G,* A variety of repositioning osteotomies can be performed on the chin with use of similar basic technique: retrusion, vertical reduction, advancement, "jumping," side-to-side, and bone grafting as onlay or inlay. *H,* Reduction genioplasty.
The osteotomy is placed inferior to the mental foramina, and the fragments are fixed with a
pair of two-hole titanium plates. (From David DJ, Abbott JR, Jay M, et al: Deformities. In
David DJ, Simpson DA, eds: Cranio-Maxillo-Facial Trauma. Edinburgh, Churchill Livingstone,
1995.)

attachments to the chin point are retained for all but the "jump" type of advancement, in which the distal segment is advanced and jumped entirely on top of the proximal segment. With the other osteotomies, the attachments are left to ensure the blood supply to the fragment and to move the soft tissue attachments with the bone. In reducing the chin, it is important that the segment removed is from the body of the chin, not the chin point. If the point is resected, the soft tissue may fall away from its bony support, producing the "witch's chin" appearance.[101] The fragments can be positioned according to the surgical plan and fixed with plates and screws.

Bone Distraction

This subject is covered extensively elsewhere in this volume. However, it is relevant to include a discussion of its current place in treatment.[102] The state of knowledge with respect to bone distraction of the craniofacial skeleton is as follows:

- New bone can be generated.
- New soft tissue cannot be produced.
- It needs to be repeated during growth.
- It takes a long time.
- It does not obviate future surgery.
- It produces discomfort for the patient.
- It is expensive.

Bone distraction is clearly of benefit for bilateral mandibular distraction of the Treacher Collins or similar cleft mandible when there is airway obstruction.[69] The rationale in hemifacial microsomia is not so clear because there is no obvious advantage to the patient at any stage or in any degree of the disease over the traditional maneuvers. Prospective comparative studies are anticipated with less intrusive intraoral distractors to lengthen the ramus in the type 2 bone deformity during growth compared with lengthening osteotomy alone and active appliance alone.

Vascularized Tissue Transfer

In view of the problems that have arisen with reconstruction of the complex deformities associated with the rare clefts, vascularized bone transfers and composite bone, muscle, and skin flaps are routinely included in the treatment armamentarium. These flaps were initially vascularized by pedicles dissected in continuity from parent arteries and veins. Transfers are now more often accomplished by microvascular techniques.

The range of these techniques has been described well in this volume and in David and Simpson[99] and van der Meulen.[16] The most common use is that of the vascularized groin flap, transferring bone or soft tissue for reconstruction in severe instances of hemifacial microsomia (Fig. 100-71).

SPECIAL TECHNIQUES

OSSEOINTEGRATION. Because titanium and hydroxyapatite can become integrated into bone, forming a permanent structure, there are a number of ancillary techniques, like osseointegration, for teeth and other extraoral prostheses that are often used in the reconstruction of craniofacial clefts (Fig. 100-72). An alternative to autogenous reconstruction of the ear is to use an artificial device supported by an osseointegrated framework. This is most useful for patients with severe hemifacial microsomia.

RESULTS AND COMPLICATIONS

Results

There is a significant difference in presenting the short-term outcome of individual operations and the results of the completed management program, which often extends over 2 decades. The outcomes need to be considered in separate categories because of the various disease processes involved.

RARE CLEFT, CENTRAL WITH ORBITAL DYSTOPIA

Initial operations often involve osteotomies and nasal reconstruction (Fig. 100-73). Tissue expanders may be inserted. The Converse method preserving the cribriform plate and vertical plate of the ethmoid may be used. For some patients, this may be followed by a Le Fort I osteotomy, bone grafts, and physical rehabilitation (Figs. 100-74 and 100-75). Long-term follow-up indicates that many patients remain stable.

LATERAL CLEFTS

The number 9 cleft is rare and poses the problem of exposure of the temporal dura (Fig. 100-76). The soft tissues should be repaired in infancy, for some patients as a matter of some urgency.[35] The facial cleft, lip, and palate are then repaired in early childhood. Tissue expanders, bone grafting, and orthodontic alignment may also be undertaken.

The results of treatment of Treacher Collins syndrome are twofold (Figs. 100-77 and 100-78). Patients with relatively minor defects with well-formed external ears, minor orbitozygomatic clefting, and reasonable jaw harmony have a good long-term prognosis, the reconstructions being well maintained. Patients with more severe defects are often very likely to have relapse. Appearance may be improved but rarely totally transformed. This makes the emphasis on hearing, speech, and subsequent psychosocial development in these children even more important.

Text continued on p. 454

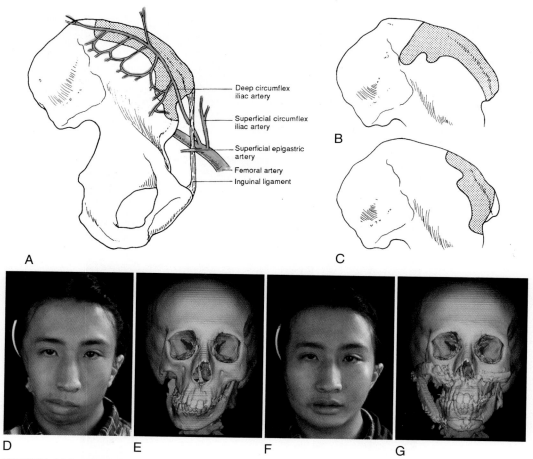

FIGURE 100-71. Fashioning the deep circumflex iliac artery flap (full or split thickness) for mandibular reconstruction from the contralateral ilium. *A,* The bone with vessels superimposed. *B* and *C,* Alternative methods. *D,* A patient with severe craniofacial microsomia. *E,* The three-dimensional CT reconstruction demonstrates the orbitozygomatic deformity as well as the absent joint and ramus of mandible. *F,* After bimaxillary surgery, zygomatic and joint reconstruction, and free flap reconstruction of the right mandible and soft tissue. *G,* The three-dimensional representation of the bone reconstruction. (*A* to *C* from David DJ, Abbott JR, Jay M, et al: Deformities. In David DJ, Simpson DA, eds: Cranio-Maxillo-Facial Trauma. Edinburgh, Churchill Livingstone, 1995.)

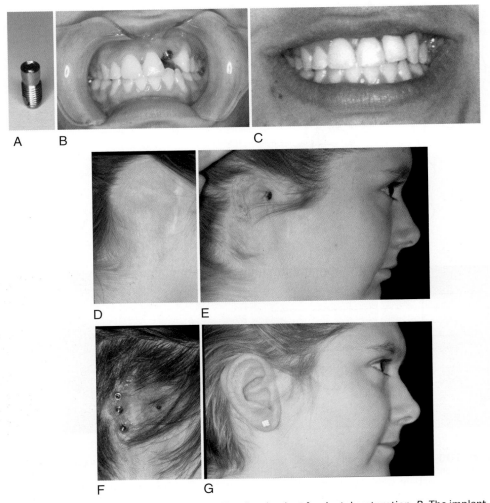

FIGURE 100-72. Osseointegration. *A,* Titanium implant for dental restoration. *B,* The implant placed into the previously bone-grafted alveolar gap. *C,* Full dental restoration in a patient with unilateral cleft lip and palate. *D,* A patient with hemifacial microsomia with absent ear. *E,* The external canal prepared. *F,* The implants in place. *G,* The ear attached.

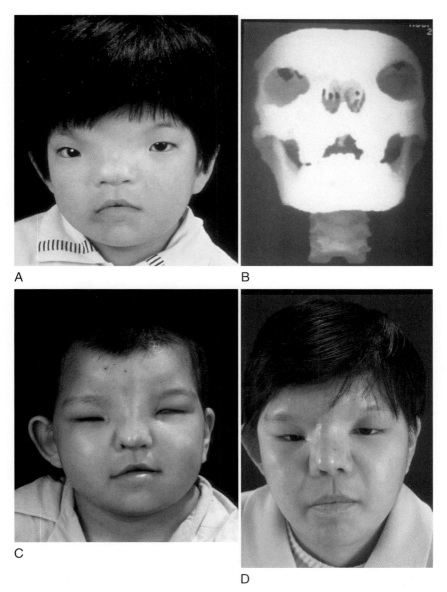

FIGURE 100-73. *A,* A patient with a midline craniofacial cleft with hypertelorism and V-shaped maxillary deformity. *B,* The three-dimensional CT reconstruction. *C,* After correction of the hypertelorism and nasal reconstruction at 8 years of age. *D,* After Le Fort I osteotomy, bone graft of cheeks, and further nasal reconstruction 12 years later.

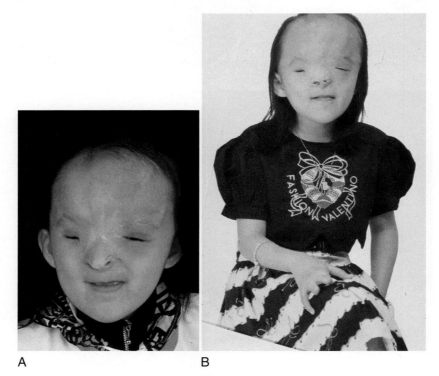

FIGURE 100-74. The long-term follow-up of the patient shown in Figure 100-24. *A,* After correction of hypertelorism and nasal reconstruction. *B,* As a teenager. This child has minimal vision and considerable physical disadvantages but has become a popular singer on Malaysian television.

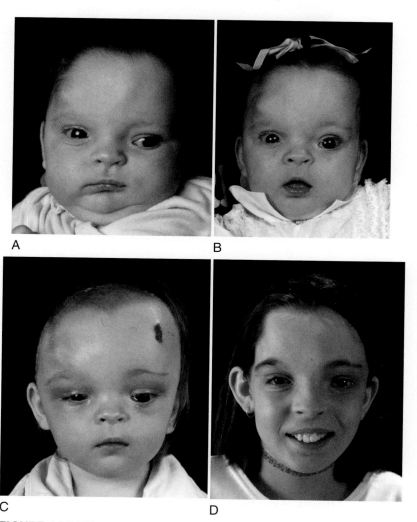

FIGURE 100-75. A child with a Tessier number 10 cleft and orbital dystopia. *A*, Shortly after birth. *B*, Preoperatively. *C*, Postoperatively. *D*, As a teenager at the end of growth.

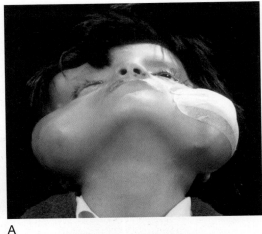

A

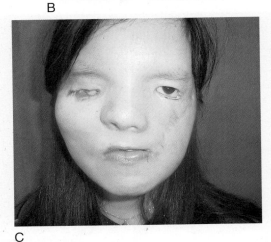

B

C

FIGURE 100-76. The long-term follow-up of the patient with a Tessier number 9 cleft shown in Figure 100-12. Surgical interventions included tissue expansion *(A)* and maxillary surgery *(B)*. *C,* At the end of treatment as a young adult.

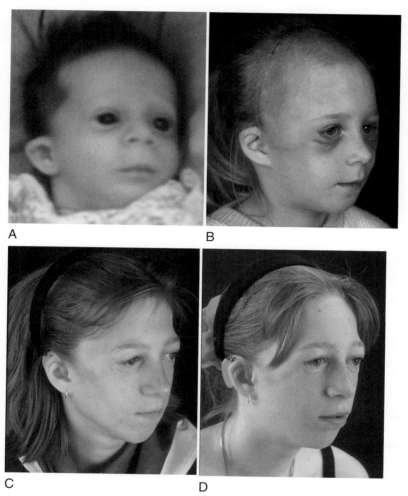

FIGURE 100-77. A child with a relatively mild expression of Treacher Collins syndrome. *A*, Shortly after birth. *B*, After correction of the eyelid colobomas and bone grafting of the orbitomalar complex. *C*, In early teenage years. *D*, After orthodontics and genioplasty.

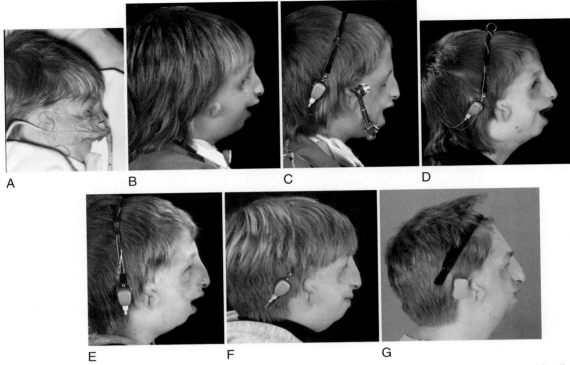

FIGURE 100-78. A patient with severe Treacher Collins syndrome. *A,* As an infant with severe airway and feeding problems. *B,* With a tracheostomy. *C,* Showing distraction of the mandible. *D,* After distraction, when the airway was improved. *E* and *F,* Showing gradual relapse with time. *G,* In late teenage years, almost complete relapse is obvious.

The results of the protocol management of craniofacial microsomia are more optimistic. A tentative thesis is that there is not the continuous genetic drive, and once growth is complete, stability is possible (Figs. 100-79 and 100-80). For patients undergoing joint reconstruction, the costochondral graft growth is unpredictable. Soft tissue reconstruction with microvascular anastomosis is effective but may sag and need repositioning. Adequate ear reconstruction remains a challenge; the unaesthetic result and malposition are the most common problems.

ORO-NASO-OCULAR CLEFTS

For patients with oro-ocular (Tessier number 4 and number 5) clefts, even in some severe instances, it may be possible to obtain acceptable results (Fig. 100-81). There is always residual scarring; however, the single most difficult long-term problem is the lower eyelid shape and function. For patients with bilateral defects, the nose is often short and remains difficult to lengthen.

The more medial clefts involving the lateral nasal lining (oro-naso-ocular, Tessier number 3) require nasal lining in the reconstruction. The lacrimal drainage apparatus is always compromised and rarely satisfactorily corrected. The medial canthal ligament is absent, and the medial lid attachment may take a number of attempts before a successful result is achieved (Fig. 100-82).

MULTIPLE AND COMPLEX CLEFTS

Nowhere is it more important to have a systematic, long-term, and persistent approach to the management of these children. Given the opportunity, they are usually highly motivated. Vast improvements in function and aesthetics are possible, but normality is never attained (Fig. 100-83). Consequently, the emphasis on personal development must be maintained throughout treatment to facilitate coping and achievement. From the beginning, eyes are often exposed and corneas damaged; eyelid function and form remain a constant problem throughout life.

FRONTOETHMOIDAL MENINGOENCEPHALOCELE

The results often depend on the severity of the deformity, particularly the extent of the cerebral

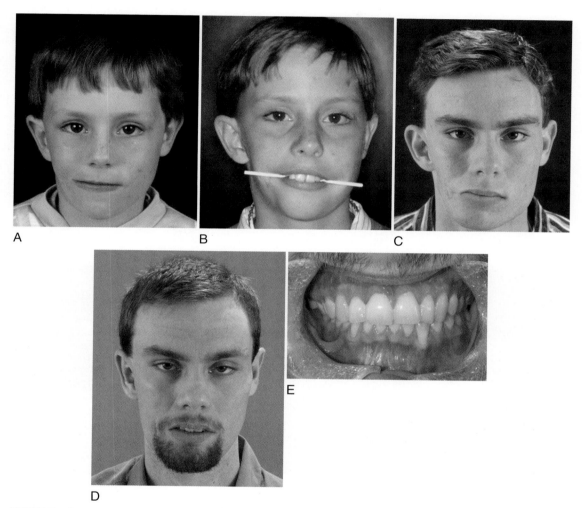

A

B

C

D

E

FIGURE 100-79. The long-term result of management of a patient with craniofacial microsomia, skeletal S2 deformity (see Fig. 100-36). *A,* As a child after closure of an extensive right macrostomia. *B,* Demonstrating the tilted occlusal plane. *C,* At the completion of growth after use of an active appliance. *D,* Four years after bimaxillary surgery and soft tissue augmentation with a de-epithelialized free groin flap. *E,* The occlusion at completion of treatment.

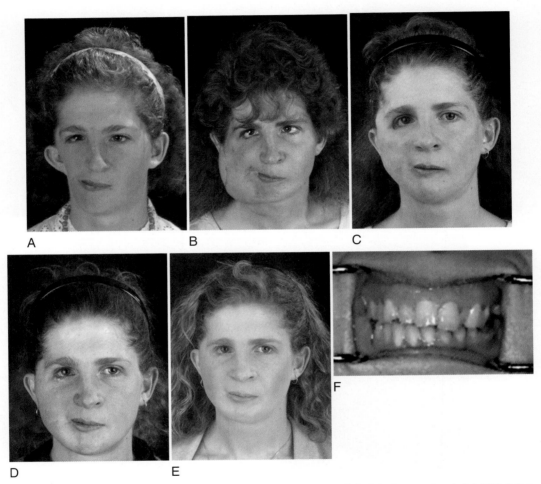

FIGURE 100-80. The result of management of a patient with craniofacial microsomia, skeletal S5 deformity (see Fig. 100-36). *A,* After closure of the macrostomia and presenting as a young adult. *B,* After bimaxillary surgery associated with correction of right orbital dystopia and fronto-orbital advancement with insertion of a circumflex iliac plus soft tissue free flap. *C,* After trimming of the flap. *D,* Early postoperative result. *E,* Five years later. *F,* The occlusion at completion of treatment.

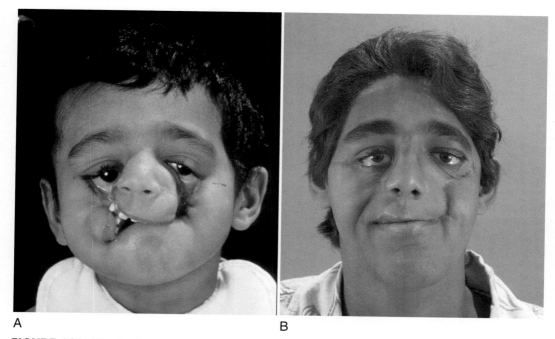

A   B

FIGURE 100-81. The long-term result of the management of bilateral Tessier number 4 and number 5 clefts (see Fig. 100-54). *A,* Preoperatively. *B,* Now in his 20s; there has been some tissue relapse on the left side.

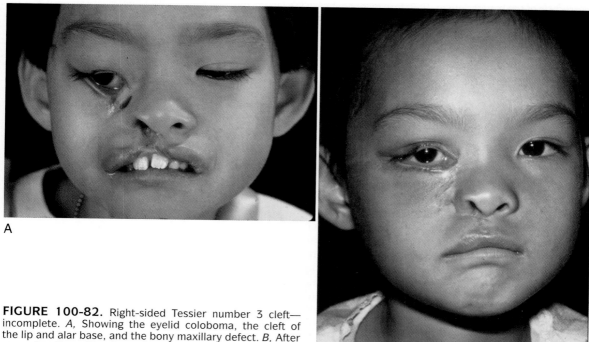

A

FIGURE 100-82. Right-sided Tessier number 3 cleft—incomplete. *A,* Showing the eyelid coloboma, the cleft of the lip and alar base, and the bony maxillary defect. *B,* After reconstruction with primary bone grafting and a cheek rotation flap.

B

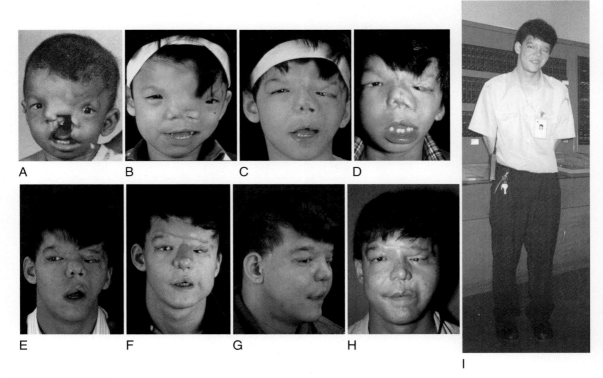

FIGURE 100-83. A cluster of craniofacial clefts producing gross hypertelorism, nasal and maxillary disruption, and left frontal bone distortion. *A,* Before any treatment. *B,* On presentation to the Australian Craniofacial Unit. *C,* After correction of the hypertelorism. *D,* Before orthodontics in the late mixed dentition. *E,* After bimaxillary surgery. *F,* After further soft tissue augmentation by free flap. *G,* After further nasal reconstruction. *H,* After final nasal and cheek surgery and finishing orthodontics at the end of growth. *I,* Working in his job as a switchboard operator.

abnormality. The earlier the displaced dysplastic mass is removed, the better the chance for the developing facial skeleton to remold. Repeated surgery is necessary for nasal reconstruction. The frontal sinus rarely develops after surgery, and aesthetic contouring of the frontal bone may be necessary.

The results of the nasofrontal variety are more predictable, the face usually being of proper proportions and the eyes unaffected (Fig. 100-84). Intellectual development may be within normal limits.

The patient with the nasoethmoidal type of defect with the characteristic long face, tortuous lacrimal ducts, and variable orbital involvement may have more long-term problems. Nasal reconstruction needs to be repeated with growth. Epiphora is common and long standing but will recover if left alone, although it may take years. A Le Fort I maxillary osteotomy with impaction at maturity sometimes helps to correct the length of the face (Fig. 100-85).

If there is only a small volume of dysplastic brain involved in the naso-orbital type, the reconstructive task is simpler and its outcome more stable (Fig. 100-86).

Complications

There are many real and potential complications resulting from the long-term management of craniofacial clefts. Aspects of these have been reported in the literature since the early years of the craniofacial discipline.[103-105]

The potential for complications across this range of diseases is significant. It is the author's belief that in spite of the many good reports cited, many major complications as well as the minor ones go unreported, especially by occasional operators. In general terms, complications can be described as follows.

NEUROSURGICAL

DURAL DAMAGE. Although it is not as common as in the craniosynostoses, dural damage occurs often enough to be of concern. It can result in persistent cerebrospinal fluid leak, potential for infection, or more rarely the interesting complication of growing fracture. Prevention is the best strategy, achieved by suture or patching with fascia lata or pericranium. If a growing fracture occurs, this is treated

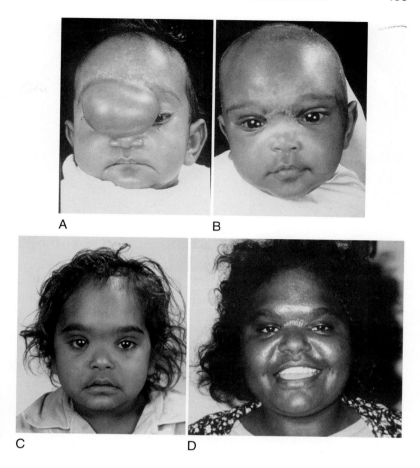

FIGURE 100-84. A nasofrontal variety of frontoethmoidal meningoencephalocele. *A,* Before treatment. *B,* After transcranial correction. *C,* At 7 years of age. *D,* As a teenager.

by dural repair and bone grafting of the overlying skull defect.

PERSISTING CEREBROSPINAL FLUID FISTULA. This occurs most commonly with correction of hypertelorism and frontoethmoidal encephaloceles. In most instances, the leak ceases within a few days. If it persists after 10 days, spinal taps to reduce the pressure will often be effective. Failing that, a nuclear scan will identify the area of the leak and it can be repaired.

INTRACRANIAL HEMATOMA. This is uncommon. However, intracerebral bleeding associated with vascular lesions that are part of the midline cysts has caused concern and may lead to intraventricular bleeding.

ACUTE HYDROCEPHALUS. For almost all patients with frontoethmoidal meningoencephalocele, there is some degree of intracranial disorganization. Excision of the contents of the meningoencephalocele may cause

an acute rise in intracranial pressure that must be relieved as a matter of urgency.

CEREBRAL ISCHEMIA, GLIOSIS, AND EPILEPSY. In patients with midline clefts with hypertelorism, especially those associated with cysts, there is abnormal venous drainage from the anterior part of the cerebral hemispheres. Hemorrhage can be troublesome from this area, and its subsequent control can produce some infarction of the anterior poles, subsequent gliosis, and the consequences, which may include epilepsy.

ORBITAL AND OCULAR

BLINDNESS. In contrast with frontofacial advancement in patients with craniosynostosis, blindness is uncommon in patients with clefts from either damage to the globe or traction on the optic nerve. Presurgical damage to eyes from exposure or colobomas demands proper assessment in advance and appropriate protective measures to preserve the globe where possible.

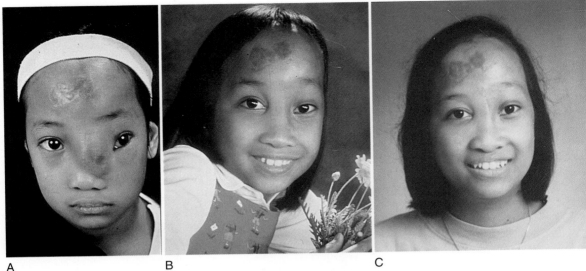

FIGURE 100-85. A nasoethmoidal variety of frontoethmoidal meningoencephalocele. *A,* Before surgery. *B,* Shortly after correction by the transcranial method and nasal reconstruction. *C,* As a young adult 10 years postoperatively.

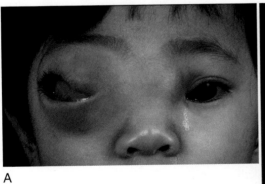

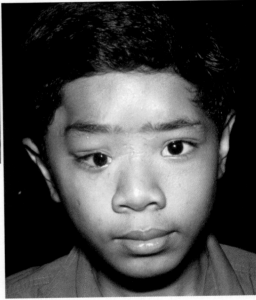

FIGURE 100-86. A naso-orbital variety of frontoethmoidal meningoencephalocele. *A,* Showing gross distortion of the right orbit and displacement of the globe. *B,* After transcranial correction, removal of the encephalocele, and repositioning of the globe. The patient is shown 10 years postoperatively.

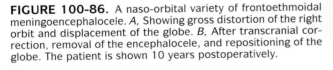

DIPLOPIA. This can result from malposition of the whole orbit, malposition of the globe within the orbit, or extraocular muscle damage. In the more gross orbital deformities, binocular vision is rarely present at the time of surgery. The chances of dystopia can be minimized by preservation of a frontal bar as a reference point for orbital repositioning. After direct trauma or nerve damage, extraocular muscle function usually recovers spontaneously if left for 12 months. Sixth nerve paresis has occurred most commonly in instances of severe hypertelorism having medial orbital translocation. Muscle surgery may ultimately be needed.

ENOPHTHALMOS. Enophthalmos does not occur commonly with the rare clefts but is common after correction of the naso-orbital variety of frontoethmoidal meningoencephalocele in which dysplastic brain has enlarged the orbit. In spite of extensive bone grafting, it may persist.

CANTHAL DYSTOPIA. The most significant postoperative problem is at the medial canthus in those clefts with a medial lid coloboma or deficient ligament. Wedge excisions and advancement of the lower lid, Z-plasties, and the Mustardé "jumping man" technique[106] can be used to correct this difficult problem.

EPIPHORA. Rarely is an adequate drainage system damaged; more often, it is not present or functional (frontoethmoidal meningoencephalocele and Tessier number 3 cleft). In frontoethmoidal meningoencephalocele, waiting for more than 1 year gives time for a dysfunctional drainage system to regain function. Lester-Jones glass tubes or plastic tubes are often necessary to facilitate drainage; they rarely produce totally acceptable results.

CORNEAL EXPOSURE AND KERATITIS. Intraoperative precautions must be taken, such as temporary tarsorrhaphy, insertion of ointment, or shields. Longer term precautions are necessary to prevent exposure and its consequences because of lack of lid function.

ANOSMIA

Patients with midline clefts and frontoethmoidal meningoencephalocele often have a reduced sense of smell, and this should be recorded preoperatively. Whenever the area of the cribriform plate is dissected, the sense of smell is at risk. Midline preserving operations for hypertelorism should be used if possible.[107]

BLOOD LOSS

The situation of most concern is transcranial surgery in infancy, for which all the monitoring and replacement techniques need to be employed by experienced staff. Starting blood replacement at the commencement of surgery will prevent tragedy in the more severe instances.[108]

OTHER COMPLICATIONS

All of the problems associated with craniofacial surgery can and do occur during the management of craniofacial clefts. These are well reported.[104,105,109,110] They include infection; vascular compromise to hard and soft tissue; anesthetic and postoperative airway complications; relapse; failed bone grafting; and complications associated with relatively new technology such as plates and screws, distraction devices, and foreign body inserts.

Experience of more than a quarter of a century reinforces the view that craniofacial surgery should be done in major centers by experienced, organized professionals whose job it is to deliver health care to the facially deformed.

CONCLUSION

The etiology and pathogenesis of rare craniofacial clefts at the time of writing remain obscure. As a range of conditions have traditionally been included under the same umbrella, classifications that are meaningful with respect to causation and outcome of treatment have not been forthcoming. The most popular (Tessier) morphologic classification frequently does not match its symbols to clinical reality. In spite of this, advances are being made on a number of fronts, namely, genetic studies, histochemical studies, epidemiologic studies, animal studies testing potential teratogens, and clinical outcome studies.

Almost every surgical and technological modality currently in use by craniofacial surgeons is employed in the management of the craniofacial clefts and associated anomalies. What is not as clear is that it is widely accepted that management should be by multidisciplinary teams organized with appropriate infrastructure, treating a critical number of patients during a growth period of time, using agreed protocols. It follows from real acceptance of this that treatment outcomes can be measured so that protocols can be developed and new technologies introduced rationally. Equally important is the possibility of multicenter scientific studies pooling data that are very difficult to assemble in dealing with such rare anomalies.

REFERENCES

1. van der Meulen JC, Mazzola R, Vermey-Keers C, et al: A morphogenetic classification of craniofacial malformations. Plast Reconstr Surg 1983;71:560-572.
2. Tessier P, Guiot G, Derome P: Orbital hypertelorism. II. Definite treatment of orbital hypertelorism (OR.H.) by craniofacial or by extracranial osteotomies. Scand J Plast Reconstr Surg 1973;7:39-58.
3. His W: Die Entwicklung der menschlichen und thierischen Physiognomien. Arch Anat Physiol Anat Abt 1892;384-424.

4. Patten BM: The normal development of the facial region. In Pruzansky S, ed: Congenital Anomalies of the Face and Associated Structures. Springfield, Ill, Charles C Thomas, 1961:11-45.

5. Morian R: Über die schrage Gesichtsspalte. Arch Klin Chir 1887;35:245.

6. Politzer G: Neue Untersuchungen über die Entstehung der Gesichtsspalten. Monatsschr Ohrenheilkd Laryngorhinol 1937;71:63-73.

7. Pfeifer G: Die Entwicklungsstörungen des Gesichtsschädels als Klassifikationsproblem. Zahn Mund Kieferheilkd 1967;48:22-40.

8. Johnston MC: The neural crest in abnormalities of the face and brain. In Bergsma D, ed: Morphogenesis and Malformations of Face and Brain. New York, Liss, 1975:1-18.

9. Tessier P: Anatomical classification of facial, cranio-facial and latero-facial clefts. J Maxillofac Surg 1976;4:69-92.

10. Tessier P: Anatomical classification of facial, craniofacial and lateroface clefts. In Tessier P, ed: Symposium on Plastic Surgery in the Orbital Region. St. Louis, CV Mosby, 1976:189-198.

11. Kawamoto HK: The kaleidoscopic world of rare craniofacial clefts: order out of chaos (Tessier classification). Clin Plast Surg 1976;3:529-572.

12. David DJ, Moore MH, Cooter RD: Tessier clefts revisited with a third dimension. Cleft Palate J 1989;26:163-184.

13. Pfeifer G: Systematik and Morphologie der kraniofazialen Anomalien. Fortschr Kiefer Gesichtschir 1974;18:1-14.

14. Mazzola RF: Congenital malformations in the fronto-nasal areas; their pathogenesis and classification. Clin Plast Surg 1976;3:573.

15. Karfik V: Proposed classification of rare congenital cleft malformations in the face. Acta Chir Plast 1966;8:163-168.

16. van der Meulen JC, Mazzola B, Stricker M, et al: Classification of craniofacial malformations. In Stricker M, van der Meulen JC, Raphael B, et al, eds: Craniofacial Malformations. Edinburgh, Churchill Livingstone, 1990:149-309.

17. Geoffroy St. Hilaire I: Histoire générale et particulière des anomalies en l'organisation chez l'homme et les animaux . . . ou traité de tératologie. Baillière, Paris, 1832.

18. Kundrat H: Arhinencephalie als typische Art von Missbildung. Graz, Leuschner & Lubensky, 1882.

19. DeMyer W, Zeman W: A lobar holoprosencephaly (arhinencephaly) with median cleft lip and palate: clinical, electroencephalographic and nosologic considerations. Confinia Neurol 1963;23:1.

20. Tessier P, Guiot G, Rougerie J, et al: Osteotomies cranionasoorbito faciales—hypertelorism. Ann Chir Plast 1967;12:103-118.

21. Tessier P: Orbital hypertelorism. 1. Successive surgical attempts, material and methods, causes and mechanisms. Scand J Plast Reconstr Surg 1972;6:135-155.

22. Converse JM, Ransohoff J, Mathews ES, et al: Ocular hypertelorism and pseudohypertelorism. Plast Reconstr Surg 1970;45:1-13.

23. DeMyer W: The median cleft face syndrome. Differential diagnosis of cranium bifidum occultum, hypertelorism and medial cleft nose, lip and palate. Neurology 1967;17:961-971.

24. Greig DM: Hypertelorism: a hitherto undifferentiated congenital craniofacial deformity. Edin Med J 1924;31:560.

25. Sedano HO, Cohen MM Jr, Jirasek J, et al: Frontonasal dysplasia. J Pediatr 1970;76:906-913.

26. David DJ, Sheffield L, Simpson DA, White J: Fronto-ethmoidal meningoencephaloceles: morphology and treatment. Br J Plast Surg 1984;37:271-284.

27. Suwanwela C, Suwanwela N: A morphological classification of sincipital encephalomeningoceles. J Neurosurg 1972;36:201-211.

28. Meyer von E: Über eine basale Hirnhernie in der Gegend der Lamina cribrosa. Virchows Arch Pathol Anat 1890;120:309.

29. Pruzansky S: Not all dwarfed mandibles are alike. Birth Defects 1969;2:120.

30. Harvold EP, Vargervik K, Chierici G: Treatment of Hemifacial Microsomia. New York, Liss, 1983.

31. Munro IR, Lauritzen CGK: Classification and treatment of hemifacial microsomia. In Caronni EP, ed: Craniofacial Surgery. Boston, Little, Brown, 1985:391-400.

32. Murray JE, Kaban LB, Mulliken JB, et al: Analysis and treatment of hemifacial microsomia. In Caronni EP, ed: Craniofacial Surgery. Boston, Little, Brown, 1985:377-390.

33. David DJ, Mahatumarat C, Cooter RD: Hemifacial microsomia—a multisystem classification. Plast Reconstr Surg 1987;80:525-535.

34. Vento AR, LaBrie RA, Mulliken JB: The O.M.E.N.S. classification of hemifacial microsomia. Cleft Palate Craniofac J 1991;28:68-76.

35. David DJ, Moore MH, Cooter RD, Chow SK: The Tessier number 9 cleft. Plast Reconstr Surg 1989;83:520-527.

36. Moore MH, David DJ, Cooter RD: Hairline indicators of craniofacial clefts. Plast Reconstr Surg 1988;82:589-593.

37. Copeland MM: American Joint Committee on Cancer Staging and End Results Reporting: objectives and progress. Cancer 1965;18:1637.

38. Spiessl B, Scheibe O, Wagner G, eds: TNM Atlas: Illustrated Guide to the Classification of Malignant Tumors. Berlin, Springer-Verlag, 1982.

39. Lauritzen C, Munro IR, Ross RB: Classification and treatment of hemifacial microsomia. Scand J Plast Reconstr Surg 1985;19:33-39.

40. Meurman Y: Congenital microtia and meatal atresia. Arch Otolaryngol 1957;66:443.

41. Murray JE, Kaban LB, Mulliken JB: Analysis and treatment of hemifacial microsomia. Plast Reconstr Surg 1984;74:186-199.

42. Verdi GD, Hersh JH, Russell LJ: Partial duplication of the face: case report and review. Plast Reconstr Surg 1991;87:759-762.

43. Fearon JA, Mulliken JB: Midfacial duplication: a rare malformation sequence. Plast Reconstr Surg 1987;79:260-264.

44. Chen YR, Noordhoff MS: Duplication of stomatodeal structures: report of three cases with literature review and suggestion for classification. Plast Reconstr Surg 1989;84:733-740.

45. Sjamsudin J, David DJ, Singh GD: An Indonesian child with orofacial duplication and neurocristopathy anomalies. J Craniomaxillofac Surg 2001;29:195-197.

46. Poswillo D: The pathogenesis of the first and second branchial arch syndrome. Oral Surg Oral Med Oral Pathol 1973;35:302-328.

47. Poswillo D: The aetiology and surgery of cleft palate with micrognathia. Ann R Coll Surg Engl 1968;43:61-88.

48. Johnston MC: Facial malformation in chick embryos resulting from removal of neural crest. J Dent Res 1964;43:822.

49. Poswillo D: The pathogenesis of the Treacher Collins syndrome (mandibulofacial dysostosis). Br J Oral Surg. 1975;13:1-26.

50. McKenzie J, Craig J: Mandibulo-facial dysostosis (Treacher Collins syndrome). Arch Dis Child 1955;30:391

51. The Treacher Collins Syndrome Collaborative Group: Positional cloning of a gene involved in the pathogenesis of Treacher Collins syndrome. Nat Genet 1996;12:124-129.

52. Edwards SJ, Gladwin AJ, Dixon MJ: The mutational spectrum in Treacher Collins syndrome reveals a predominance of mutations that create a premature-termination codon. Am J Hum Genet 1997;60:515-524.

53. Dixon J, Brakebusch C, Fassler R, Dixon MJ: Increased levels of apoptosis in the prefusion neural folds underlie the craniofacial disorder, Treacher Collins syndrome. Hum Mol Genet 2000;9:1473-1480.

54. Cohen MM Jr: Craniofrontonasal syndrome. In Cohen MM Jr, MacLean RE, eds: Craniosynostosis: Diagnosis, Evaluation and Management, 2nd ed. New York, Oxford University Press, 2000:380-384.

55. Feldman GJ, Ward DE, Lajeunie-Renier E, et al: A novel phenotypic pattern in X-linked inheritance: craniofrontonasal syndrome maps to Xp22. Hum Mol Genet 1997;6:1937-1941.

56. Coady MS, Moore MH, Wallis K: Amniotic band syndrome: the association between rare facial clefts and limb ring constrictions. Plast Reconstr Surg 1998;101:640-649.

57. Torpin R: Fetal Malformations Caused by Amnion Rupture During Gestation. Springfield, Ill, Charles C Thomas, 1968.

58. Byrne J, Blanc WA, Baker D: Amniotic band syndrome in early fetal life. Birth Defects 1982;18:43-58.

59. MacKinnon CA, David DJ: Oblique facial clefting associated with unicoronal synostosis. J Craniofac Surg 2001;12:227-231.

60. Suwanwela C, Sukabote C, Suwanwela N: Frontoethmoidal encephalo-meningocele. Surgery 1971;69:617-625.

61. Naim-Ur-Rahman: Nasal encephalocele: treatment by transcranial operation. J Neurol Sci 1979;42:73-85.

62. Abbott JR, Netherway DJ, Wingate P, et al: Craniofacial imaging, models and prostheses. Aust J Otolaryngol 1994;1:581-587.

63. Abbott JR, Netherway DJ, Wingate PG, et al: Computer generated mandibular model: surgical role. Aust Dent J 1998;43:373-378.

64. David DJ: New perspectives in the management of severe craniofacial deformity. Ann R Coll Surg Engl 1984;66:270-279.

65. Lodge M, Abbott A, David D, et al: Fronto-ethmoidal meningo-encephalocoeles compared with rare facial clefts. In Marchac D, ed: Craniofacial Surgery. Proceedings of the VIth International Congress of the International Society of Craniofacial Surgery. Bologna, Italy, Monduzzi Editore, 1995:197-200.

66. Menard RM, Moore MH, David DJ: Tissue expansion in the reconstruction of Tessier craniofacial clefts: a series of 17 patients. Plast Reconstr Surg 1999;103:779-786.

67. Dunaway DJ, David DJ: Intraorbital tissue expansion in the management of congenital anophthalmos. Br J Plast Surg 1996;49:529-535.

68. David DJ: Treacher Collins syndrome. In Muir IFK, ed: Current Operative Surgery: Plastic and Reconstructive Surgery. London, Baillière Tindall, 1985:103-118.

69. Moore MH, Guzman-Stein G, Proudman TW, et al: Mandibular lengthening by distraction for airway obstruction in Treacher Collins syndrome. J Craniofac Surg 1994;5:22-25.

70. David DJ, Simpson DA: Fronto-ethmoidal meningoencephaloceles. Clin Plast Surg 1987;14:83-89.

71. Jackson IT, Tanner NS, Hide TA: Frontonasal encephalocele—"long nose hypertelorism." Ann Plast Surg 1983;11:490-500.

72. Allen TH, Steven IM: Prolonged endotracheal intubation in infants and children. Br J Anaesth 1990;81:474-481.

73. Allen TH, Steven IM: Prolonged nasotracheal intubation in infants and children. Br J Anaesth 1972;44:835-840.

74. Schafer ME: Upper airways obstruction and sleep disorders in children with craniofacial anomalies. Clin Plast Surg 1982;9:555-567.

75. Kawamoto HK: Rare craniofacial clefts. In McCarthy JG, ed: Plastic Surgery. Philadelphia, WB Saunders, 1990:2966.

76. Stricker M, van der Meulen J, Raphael B, et al: Surgery. In Stricker M, van der Meulen JC, Raphael B, et al, eds: Craniofacial Malformations. Edinburgh, Churchill Livingstone, 1990:389-550.

77. Jackson IT: Reconstruction of the lower eyelid defect in Treacher Collins syndrome. Plast Reconstr Surg 1981;67:365-368.

78. Mustardé JC: Congenital deformities in the orbital region. Proc R Soc Med 1971;64:1121-1134.

79. Converse JM, Wood-Smith D, McCarthy JG, et al: Bilateral facial microsomia. Plast Reconstr Surg 1974;54:413-423.

80. Tessier P: Le telorbitisme, hypertelorisme orbitaire (oculaire). In Tessier P, et al, eds: Chirurgie plastique orbito-palpebrale. Paris, Masson, 1977.

81. Marchac D, Cophignon J, Achard E, et al: Orbital expansion for anophthalmia and micro-orbitism. Plast Reconstr Surg 1977;59:486-491.

82. van der Meulen JC, Vaandrager JM: Surgery related to the correction of hypertelorism. Plast Reconstr Surg 1983;71:6-19.

83. Munro IR, Chen YR, Park BY: Simultaneous total correction of temporomandibular ankylosis and facial asymmetry. Plast Reconstr Surg 1986;77:517-529.

84. Crawley WA, Serletti JM, Manson PN: Autogenous reconstruction of the temporomandibular joint. J Craniofac Surg 1993;4:28-34.

85. Ross RB: Costochondral grafts replacing the mandibular condyle. Cleft Palate Craniofac J 1999;36:334-339.

86. Tessier P: Autogenous bone grafts taken from the calvarium for facial and cranial applications. Clin Plast Surg 1982;9:531-538.

87. McCarthy JG, Zide BM: The spectrum of calvarial bone grafting: introduction of the vascularized calvarial bone flap. Plast Reconstr Surg 1984;74:10-18.

88. van der Meulen JC, Hauben DJ, Vaandrager JM, Birgenhager-Frenkel DH: The use of a temporal osteoperiosteal flap for the reconstruction of malar hypoplasia in Treacher Collins syndrome. Plast Reconstr Surg 1984;74:687-693.

89. Trott JA: Lateral nasal proboscis and heminose. In Caronni EP, ed: Craniofacial Surgery: Proceedings of the 2nd International Congress of the International Society of Craniofacial Surgery. Bologna, Italy, Monduzzi Editore, 1989:381-384.

90. Converse JM, Telsey D: The tripartite osteotomy of the midface for orbital expansion and correction of the deformity in craniostenosis. Br J Plast Surg 1971;24:365-374.

91. Moore MH, Trott JA, David DJ: Soft tissue expansion in the management of the rare craniofacial clefts. Br J Plast Surg 1992;45:155-159.

92. Souyris F, Caravel JB, Raynaud JF: Ostéotomie intermédiaire de l'étage moyen de la face. Ann Chir Plast 1973;18:149-154.

93. Popescu VC: Advancement of the middle third of the face without bone in a case of Crouzon's disease. J Maxillofac Surg 1974;2:219-223.

94. Wassmund M: Lehrbuch der praktischen Chirurgie des Mundes und der Kiefer. Leipzig, Meusser, 1935.

95. Schuchardt K: Plastiche Operationen in Mund und Kiefer Bereich. Berlin, Urban & Schwarzenberg, 1959.

96. Yeow VK, Chen YR, Su CP: Combining single- and double-tooth osteotomies with traditional orthognathic surgery. J Craniofac Surg 1999;10:447-453.

97. Trauner R, Obwegeser H: The surgical correction of mandibular prognathism and retrognathism with consideration of genioplasty. Parts I and II. Oral Surg Oral Med Oral Pathol 1957;10:677-689, 787-792.

98. Dal Pont G: Retromolar osteotomy for correction of prognathism. J Oral Surg 1961;19:42-47.

99. David DJ, Abbott JR, Jay M, et al: Deformities. In David DJ, Simpson DA, eds: Craniomaxillofacial Trauma. Edinburgh, Churchill Livingstone, 1995:545-648.

100. Ousterhout DK: Sliding genioplasty, avoiding mental nerve injuries. J Craniofac Surg 1996;7:297-298.

101. Gonzalez-Ulloa M: Ptosis of the chin: the witches' chin. Plast Reconstr Surg 1972;50:54-57.

102. David DJ: The argument against bone distraction (its place in the management of craniofacial deformity). In Arnaud E, Diner PA, eds: Proceedings of the 4th International Congress of Maxillofacial and Craniofacial Distraction, Paris, 2003. Bologna, Italy, Monduzzi Editore, 2003:335-339.

103. Matthews D: Craniofacial surgery—indications, assessment and complications. Br J Plast Surg 1979;32:96-105.

104. Whitaker LA, Munro IR, Jackson IT, Salyer KE: Problems in craniofacial surgery. J Maxillofac Surg 1976;4:131-136.

105. Whitaker LA, Munro IR, Salyer KE, et al: Combined report of problems and complications in 793 craniofacial operations. Plast Reconstr Surg 1979;64:198-203.

106. Mustardé JC: Repair and Reconstruction in the Orbital Region. Edinburgh, Churchill Livingstone, 1980.

107. Converse JM, Wood-Smith D, McCarthy JB: Report on a series of 50 craniofacial operations. Plast Reconstr Surg 1975;55:283-293.

108. Sweeney DB, Sainsbury DA: Anaesthesia for cranio-maxillary-facial surgery. Curr Anaesth Crit Care 1992;3:11-16.

109. Munro IR, Sabatier RE: An analysis of 12 years of cra-niomaxillofacial surgery in Toronto. Plast Reconstr Surg 1985;76:29-35.

110. David DJ, Cooter RD: Craniofacial infection in ten years of transcranial surgery. Plast Reconstr Surg 1987;80:213-223.

Reconstruction: Craniosynostosis

JOSEPH G. MCCARTHY, MD ✦ LARRY H. HOLLIER, JR., MD

HISTORY

The development of surgical procedures for the treatment of the patient with craniosynostosis represents one of the most interesting chapters in the history of surgery. Late in the 19th century, sporadic cases of strip craniectomies were reported by several surgeons.[1,2] With the development of radiography to document suture synostosis, the technique had found wide application by neurosurgeons by the 1920s. It was recognized that the procedure yielded best results when it was performed by the age of 3 months. The technique, however, was beleaguered by an unusually high rate of sutural resynostosis. In a review of more than 500 patients with craniosynostosis who had undergone strip craniectomies, it was noted that only 52% had achieved satisfactory craniofacial form[3]; the best postoperative results were observed in patients with isolated sagittal synostosis.

The development of craniofacial surgical techniques by Tessier in the 1960s (i.e., midface or Le Fort III advancement and fronto-orbital advancement) stimulated the international surgical community in the problems of craniosynostosis. In the 1970s, the Tessier techniques developed for the adult and adolescent patients were applied to children and infants—fronto-orbital advancement/cranial vault remodeling[4,5] and midface advancement.[6] This period also saw refinements in midface advancement—the monobloc advancement.[7] Distraction osteogenesis, initially used

in mandibular reconstruction,[8] was used to advance the midface. After preliminary canine experiments,[9] external and internal distraction devices were designed for midface and combined fronto-orbital (monobloc) advancement.[10-12] Distraction may well supplement traditional osteotomy/advancement techniques because it obviates the need for prolonged operations, bone grafts, and complicated fixation; infection rates and overall health care costs are also reduced.

Distraction osteogenesis is also being used to reconstruct the fronto-orbital and cranial vault abnormalities associated with isolated and syndromic craniosynostosis. After osteotomies are made without extensive dural dissection, either metallic or resorbable distraction devices are applied to the cranium, and traditional distraction principles are practiced.

FUNCTIONAL AND ANATOMIC REQUIREMENTS

Much of the focus in cranial vault reconstruction for the patient with craniosynostosis has been directed at the question of diminished intracranial volume and its attendant morbidity. However, studies have demonstrated that there is no consistent correlation between reduced intracranial volume and craniosynostosis.[13] Indeed, in many children with craniosynostosis, intracranial volume measurements are normal or even increased. This is not to say that patients with craniosynostosis do not suffer from an increase in intracranial pressure. In their landmark study, Marchac and Renier[14] demonstrated a 42% incidence of increased intracranial pressure in multisuture (syndromic) synostoses and 13% in single-suture craniosynostoses. Furthermore, cranial vault remodeling does appear to reduce the intracranial pressure in patients so affected. Whereas it is agreed that this is important in preventing the secondary effects of increased pressure, such as visual and developmental abnormalities, controversy still exists as to whether cranial vault reconstruction in the subset of patients without elevated intracranial pressure has any functional significance.

Particularly problematic is the issue of intelligence and neurocognitive development. Some authors report that release of fused sutures and cranial vault remodeling do not affect the mental development of infants.[15,16] Virtanen et al[15] contended that in a series of patients undergoing early operative correction for sagittal synostosis, certain indices of neurocognitive performance were below those of age-matched control subjects and remained delayed throughout the period of examination after surgery.

Other authors contended that although young children with craniosynostosis are often normal from a mental standpoint, there is an increase in frequency of psychomotor problems as they develop.[17] These authors believed that early surgery prevented this problem in their population of patients and consequently recommended cranial vault reconstruction during infancy.[17] One confounding variable is the instrument used to assay the functional effects of surgery. It is thought by many that the standardized intelligence tests so frequently used in assessing young children are not the optimal method for evaluation. Alternative tests, such as those quantitating brain perfusion (positron emission tomographic scans), may be more sensitive in assessing the effects of cranial vault remodeling in craniosynostosis.[18] This subject is discussed later in the chapter.

ROLE OF CRANIOFACIAL GROWTH AND DEVELOPMENT

An important consideration in the planning of surgical reconstruction in the growing child is the role of subsequent craniofacial growth and development—not only the *physical* changes in the brain, cranial vault, orbits, and midface-maxilla but also the *psychosocial* development. It is known that in the first 3 years of life, growth of the brain contributes substantially to enlargement of the cranial vault and skull base.[4] In like fashion, orbital enlargement parallels growth of the globe. However, nasomaxillary growth lags and is not completed until approximately 14 years in the average male.[19]

In the patient with craniosynostosis and fused sutures, the growth potential of these structures is significantly impaired, and failure of cranial vault, orbital, and midface development can result in serious functional sequelae—intracranial hypertension, hydrocephalus, exorbitism and corneal exposure, sleep apnea and respiratory insufficiency, and malocclusion. Moreover, multiple studies have documented the significant harm on psychosocial development because of difficulties in peer interactions and school activities.[20,21]

In the 1970s, McCarthy,[4] Marchac,[5] and Whitaker[22] postulated that by releasing the constricting forces associated with sutural synostosis in the child younger than 1 year, one could take advantage of the rapidly enlarging brain and eye to achieve satisfactory cranial vault and orbital volume and shape. Subsequent studies,[23] however, demonstrated that although these goals could be attained in the upper third of the craniofacial skeleton, the midface hypoplasia associated with the craniofacial synostosis syndromes could not be prevented. Hence, McCarthy[6] reported on a series of Le Fort III midface advancements in patients as young as 4 years. The procedures resulted in significant improvement in midface morphologic appearance, occlusion, and upper airway function. It is understood, however, that secondary midface advancement or distraction is required in adolescence when craniofacial development is completed.

RECONSTRUCTIVE MODALITIES: ISOLATED CRANIOSYNOSTOSIS

Craniectomies and Cranial Vault Remodeling

SCAPHOCEPHALY (SAGITTAL SYNOSTOSIS)

Sagittal synostosis is the most common of the isolated (nonsyndromic) single-suture synostoses. There is a distinct male predisposition for this condition, with the male-to-female incidence approaching 4:1.[24]

The condition results from fusion of the midline sagittal suture. As a result, there is a diminished transverse growth of the cranial vault with an exaggeration of the anteroposterior growth. The resultant head shape is described as scaphocephalic or dolichocephalic. There is also often prominent bossing of the frontal or occipital calvaria, depending on the location of the sutural fusion. For example, if the more anterior portion of the sagittal suture fuses, there is compensatory growth in the region of the metopic suture resulting in frontal bossing. Conversely, if the most posterior portion of the sagittal suture is involved, compensatory occipital growth results in the deformity's being more prominent posteriorly.

Although it is universally agreed that surgical intervention is necessary, the timing and the type of procedure remain controversial. The earliest procedures performed for scaphocephaly involved a strip craniectomy of the region of the fused sagittal suture. However, rapid refusion of the suture typically followed, prompting surgeons to apply toxic materials or physical barriers to the edges of the ostectomized calvaria to prevent this phenomenon.[25] Others attempted a more extensive craniectomy in an effort to prevent refusion, with some advocating complete removal of the vertex of the cranium.[26] Others have proposed combining strip craniectomy with barrel stave osteotomies to expand the temporal and parietal regions.[27] With these techniques, however, there is a consensus that success is dependent on early craniectomy, generally within the first 3 to 4 months of life. Many patients, however, do not present to the surgeon at such a young age.

Critics of strip craniectomy argue for more extensive remodeling of the skull at the time of surgery, even in younger patients.[28,29] In one retrospective study of 118 patients operated on for sagittal synostosis, cranial vault remodeling procedures were associated with an excellent aesthetic result in 80% of the patients, compared with approximately 40% when only strip craniectomy was used.[29] Although the group undergoing cranial vault remodeling experienced a greater blood loss and a longer operative time, there was no significant difference between complications experienced in either group and the time of hospitalization was the same.

It is, however, agreed that in older patients (beyond 12 months of age) and in those with significant dysmorphology, cranial vault remodeling is necessary. The "hung span" technique[30] is favored in this situation, and it is also the procedure of choice in patients with scaphocephaly previously operated on unsuccessfully.

Techniques

One of the most important considerations in the surgical correction of sagittal synostosis is whether surgical attention is to be focused preferentially on the frontal or occipital aspect of the cranium or on both. If only the frontal or occipital region exhibits significant bossing, the supine or prone operating table position, respectively, is adequate. However, if both areas are significantly involved and a total or circumferential cranial vault remodeling is to be undertaken, it is necessary to place the patient in the modified prone or "sphinx" position in which the neck must be hyperextended. Preoperative evaluation should include the range of motion of the neck and radiographic studies to rule out any cervical spine abnormalities. The support under the malar eminences must be adequately padded to prevent pressure necrosis, and care should be taken to avoid pressure on the eyes. More-

over, an important consideration in this table position is venous air embolism. Because of the "head up" orientation, it is possible that the multiple venous channels exposed in the ostectomized cranium may act as a conduit for the inflow of air, particularly in the hypovolemic patient. The patient should be monitored with either a precordial Doppler probe to detect intracardiac air or with end-tidal carbon dioxide monitoring. It is prudent, when placing a patient in a sphinx position, to have a central venous catheter inserted to the level of the atrium in the event that aspiration of intracardiac air is necessary at any time during the procedure.

PI PROCEDURE. The basic underlying pathologic process in scaphocephaly is an increase in the anteroposterior dimension of the skull with a diminished transverse diameter. Perhaps the most commonly used technique to correct this deformity is the pi procedure (Fig. 101-1).[31] The technique is so named because the ostectomy is in the shape of a pi. This leaves a stable central strut that is secured to the frontal segment with resorbable plates and screws after slowly advancing it anteriorly, compressing the brain, and diminishing the anteroposterior length. Simultaneous with this maneuver, there is an expansion of the dura laterally, thus expanding the transverse dimension in the temporal and parietal regions. The bone previously removed is remodeled and replaced in situ. There have been modifications of this procedure designed to address clinical variance of the scaphocephaly. The pi procedure is used for situations in which frontal bossing is the most pronounced. In situations in which occipital bossing is the primary problem, the reversed pi is used in similar fashion.[32] When the bossing in either the frontal or the occipital region is particularly severe, the Y variant of this procedure may be used in which the projecting frontal or parietal regions are removed for remodeling.[32] Each of these described techniques shares the common characteristic of a stable strut that can be advanced to the stable portion of the frontal or occipital skull to diminish the anteroposterior length of the cranial vault.

An alternative method of addressing the deformities associated with sagittal synostosis relies more extensively on direct remodeling of the involved calvaria rather than on expansion of the dura. In this technique, all segments of the skull involved in the deformity are removed. The bossing of the frontal or occipital segment is corrected by longitudinal osteotomies centered around the apex of the concavity and outfractured to restore normal contour. In the remaining temporal bone, barrel stave osteotomies are made and the intervening segments outfractured to correct temporal narrowing. To reduce the excessive anteroposterior dimension, Persing et al[33] advocated removal of triangular wedges from the frontal bone segment

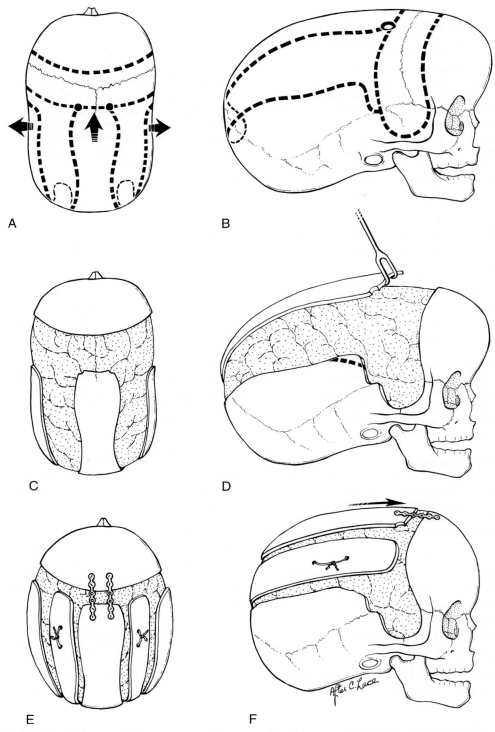

FIGURE 101-1. The pi procedure. *A* and *B*, Superior and lateral views of the lines of osteotomy. Note that it is similar to the Greek letter π. *C*, After removal of the bone flaps. Note that a bone flap has been removed from over the anterior aspect of the sagittal sinus. *D*, The hook demonstrates advancement of the central bony strut. *E* and *F*, Appearance after replacement of the bone flaps and advancement of the central strut with fixation by resorbable plates and screws. (Adapted from C. Luce.)

just above the supraorbital rim to allow the forehead to be inclined posteriorly. The frontal and occipital bone segments are secured to one another by a recontoured and shortened central strip of bone overlying the sagittal suture that is wired and slowly cinched down. This technique, as in the pi procedure, increases the bitemporal and biparietal dimensions. The previously removed bone flaps are recontoured and replaced.

HUNG SPAN TECHNIQUE. The hung span technique[30] is designed primarily to increase intracranial volume in patients with scaphocephaly by widening the biparietal dimension and by reducing the anteroposterior dimension. It is so named after the engineering technique used in building bridges and is indicated when primary procedures have failed or there is evidence of increased intracranial pressure in a patient with sagittal synostosis. In this technique, parieto-occipital bone flaps are elevated and removed, maintaining a central strut overlying the sagittal sinus (Fig. 101-2). Barrel staves are made in an inferior direction in the remaining parietal bone and outfractured. This establishes the amount of temporoparietal widening that will be achieved (see Fig. 101-2). At this point, long polylactic acid (resorbable) plates are shaped to the desired lateral contour (hung span) and fixed to the stable position of the frontal and occipital bone. The staves, which have been outfractured, are secured to the rigid plate (Fig. 101-2E). If anteroposterior shortening is desired, an oblique osteotomy is made along the region of the lambdoid suture bilaterally to allow mobilization of the occipital region while not completely detaching it (Fig. 101-2C). A section of the central strut is then resected anteriorly and the strut advanced while the intracranial pressure is monitored (Fig. 101-2D). When the desired anteroposterior shortening is achieved, the strut is fixed to the frontal bone with a plate. The parietal bone flaps are recontoured and replaced in their original positions and secured with Vicryl sutures or resorbable plates and screws (Fig. 101-3).

Unlike the pi procedure, the hung span technique does not rely solely on a reduction in the anteroposterior dimension to maintain the correction of the abnormal skull shape. It provides a rigid scaffolding for the widened cranial vault, independent of any anteroposterior reduction that is accomplished. As such, it is useful for the older patient with residual or recurrent scaphocephaly after previously unsuccessful surgical correction. The rapidly growing brain of the young child is not required to maintain the correction. It is also indicated in patients with elevated intracranial pressure in whom an increase in cranial volume is of primary importance. It is not always necessary that the anteroposterior dimension of the skull be reduced to achieve the desired shape.

BRACHYCEPHALY

Brachycephaly is a term applied to the cranial morphologic appearance resulting from bilateral coronal synostosis: the skull is foreshortened in the anteroposterior dimension and widened bitemporally. There is also an increase in the vertical dimension of the skull known as turricephaly. Unlike unicoronal synostosis, bilateral coronal involvement is associated with a higher incidence of increased intracranial pressure and associated morbidity.[14]

These patients have an appearance similar to the syndromic craniosynostoses, such as Apert and Crouzon syndromes, in which bicoronal craniosynostosis is also frequently a component. However, unlike in Apert syndrome and the other acrocephalosyndactylies, there is no associated involvement of the extremities. Moreover, unlike in most of the syndromic cases, midface involvement is unusual and midface advancement is not indicated. Finally, although inheritance of this condition is possible, it is generally not transmitted in autosomal dominant fashion as are the syndromic craniosynostoses.

Correction of this deformity is similar to correction of the cranial vault shape in syndromic cases and is discussed later in further detail (see Fig. 101-5). In addition, the incidence of postoperative cranial vault problems requiring secondary surgery is higher than that observed in the other isolated craniosynostoses.[34,35]

PLAGIOCEPHALY (UNICORONAL SYNOSTOSIS)

Plagiocephaly is a generic term designating an asymmetric or oblique head. Most commonly, however, it refers to a skull deformity associated with unicoronal synostosis. Affected patients usually present with flattening of the forehead ipsilateral to the fused suture, and there is contralateral bossing of the forehead. The nasal radix or root of the nose tends to be deviated toward the ipsilateral side, and the external ear on the affected side is anteriorly displaced. The classic "harlequin" sign seen on posteroanterior skull radiograph is an oblique line through the orbit due to elevation of the greater wing of the sphenoid secondary to the sutural fusion.

Before any reconstructive procedure, one must confirm that the skull asymmetry is indeed due to a sutural fusion and that the affected suture is the coronal. Plagiocephaly secondary to lambdoid synostosis, although exceedingly rare, occurs and can lead to confusion.[36] In these patients, the changes noted in the forehead are markedly less pronounced. The ipsilateral occipital mastoid region is flattened with the contralateral occiput exhibiting bossing. The diagnosis should be confirmed with the radiographic evaluation of the sutures.

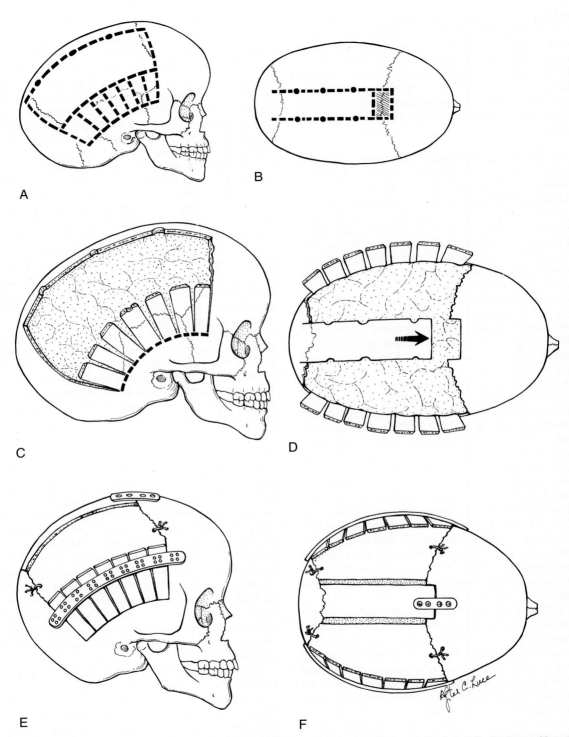

FIGURE 101-2. The hung span technique. *A* and *B,* Lateral and superior views of the lines of osteotomy. Note the barrel stave osteotomies in the temporoparietal area and the central strut of bone overlying the sagittal sinus. The anterior aspect is resected *(shaded area). C* and *D,* Lateral and superior views after removal of the bone flaps and out-fracturing of the barrel staves. Note the projected advancement and insetting of the central strut *(arrow). E* and *F,* A long (180 mm) resorbable plate is used to maintain the outfractured barrel staves in position, and a smaller plate is used to secure the advanced central strut.

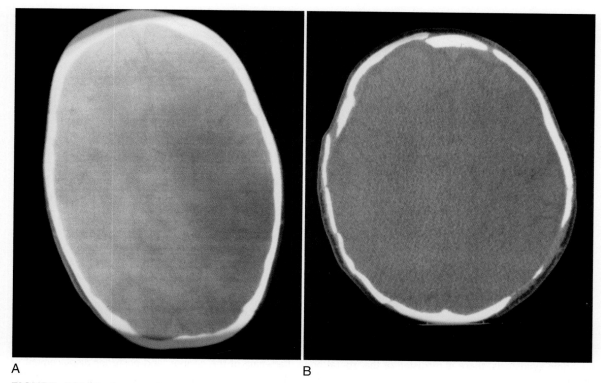

FIGURE 101-3. Computed tomographic scans illustrating the hung span technique. *A,* Preoperative axial cut. *B,* Postoperative axial cut demonstrating reduction in the anteroposterior and increase in the transverse dimensions. (From McCarthy JG, Bradley JP, Stelnicki E, et al: Hung span method of scaphocephaly reconstruction in patients with elevated intracranial pressure. Plast Reconstr Surg 2002;109:2009-2018.)

In the differential diagnosis, one must rule out positional molding as the cause of the asymmetry; this has been confused with lambdoid synostosis in children subjected to operations erroneously. In fact, lambdoid (sutural) synostosis is rare. Positional molding or deformational plagiocephaly has been seen with increasing frequency since initiation of the "Back to Sleep" campaign by the American Academy of Pediatrics that emphasized the importance of placing children in the supine position during sleep in an effort to lessen the incidence of sudden infant death syndrome.[37] Viewed from above, these children have a head shape best described as a parallelogram, whereas those with lambdoid synostosis have a trapezoidal head shape (Fig. 101-4).[38] Most cases of deformational plagiocephaly may be treated by positioning of the child away from the area of flattening or, in particularly severe cases, by orthotic cranioplasty with molding helmets.[39] The latter therapy, however, is most effective only when it is instituted within the first few months of life.

Techniques

In the preoperative work-up for cranial vault reconstruction for unicoronal synostosis, one must make particular note of any evidence of head tilt. Not infrequently, these patients have a paresis of the superior oblique muscle on the side affected by the synostosis.[40] This extraocular muscle functional deformity is due, in part, to the recessed position of the brow on the affected side. If a head tilt is noted preoperatively, a formal ophthalmologic examination is mandatory because many of the affected patients may require extraocular muscle surgery postoperatively.

The procedure most commonly used to address unicoronal synostosis is a bifrontal advancement and forehead remodeling.[4,5] Unilateral procedures to advance the supraorbital rim and remodel the forehead on the side of the stenosed suture have been attempted but give inferior results.[41] This observation, however, would be expected; although the suture is fused on only one side, the compensatory changes affect the entire forehead and supraorbital rim—it is truly a bilateral deformity.

When designing the supraorbital bar (Fig. 101-5), one must keep in mind that the supraorbital rim on the affected side is elevated while the rim on the contralateral side is depressed. The tenon of the frontal bar should be designed tongue-in-groove style to allow

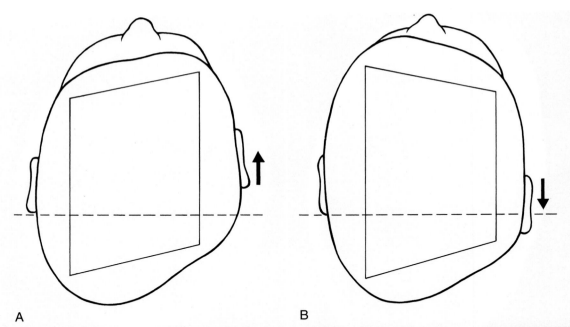

A   B

FIGURE 101-4. The difference between the cranial vault deformity associated with a deformational (nonsynostotic) deformity *(left)* and a lambdoid synostosis *(right)*. Note that in the deformational plagiocephaly, there is a frontal bossing with anterior shearing of the auricular helix and flattening of the occiput on the affected side *(arrow)*. With a unilateral lambdoid synostosis, there is retrusion of the frontal bone, flattening of the occiput, and posterior displacement of the auricular helix on the affected side *(arrow)*. (Adapted from Huang M, Gruss J, Clarren S, et al: The differential diagnosis of posterior plagiocephaly: true lambdoid synostosis versus positional molding. Plast Reconstr Surg 1996;98: 765-774.)

a gradual inferior movement of the bar with advancement of the supraorbital segment on the affected side.

With respect to the forehead, the deformity often appears most pronounced on the side contralateral to the stenosed suture. The bossing in this region can be quite marked. It is often easiest to divide the forehead in the midline and to perform multiple radial osteotomies with "greenstick" outfracturing to correct the convexity. The osteotomy to remove the frontal bone flap is generally made posterior to the fused suture.

The greater wing of the sphenoid, which is thickened and elevated on the affected side, is usually removed with a rongeur to the level of the supraorbital fissure after the frontal bone flap has been elevated.

If the frontal bone flap is severely deformed, a cranial bone graft of adequate size and contour can be harvested from either parietal area. The frontal bone flap can then be placed in the donor site (Fig. 101-6).

TRIGONOCEPHALY (METOPIC SYNOSTOSIS)

The severity of the deformity (trigonocephaly) associated with metopic synostosis varies greatly. In its mildest expression, trigonocephaly is characterized by a simple ridge in the midline of the forehead with otherwise normal morphologic appearance. In its most severe expression, the forehead is keel shaped with recession of the supraorbital rims, a decrease in the bitemporal distance, and orbital hypotelorism. There is also bossing in the region of the parietal bones. Although most of the cases are sporadic, there can be an association with genetic abnormalities and syndromes, such as Opitz C and fronto-ocular syndrome.[42-44] Metopic synostosis represents only 10% of the single-suture nonsyndromic craniosynostoses.[45-47]

Techniques

An important preoperative consideration in patients with trigonocephaly associated with metopic synostosis is the high incidence of cognitive and behavioral abnormalities. Sigoti et al[48] demonstrated that fully one third of the children in their series with metopic synostosis demonstrated learning disabilities or behavioral problems such as attention deficit disorder. Indeed, midline anomalies of the central nervous system, such as dysgenesis or complete agenesis of the corpus callosum, are also associated with metopic synostosis.[49,50] A complete neuropsychological assessment is recommended before any surgical procedure.

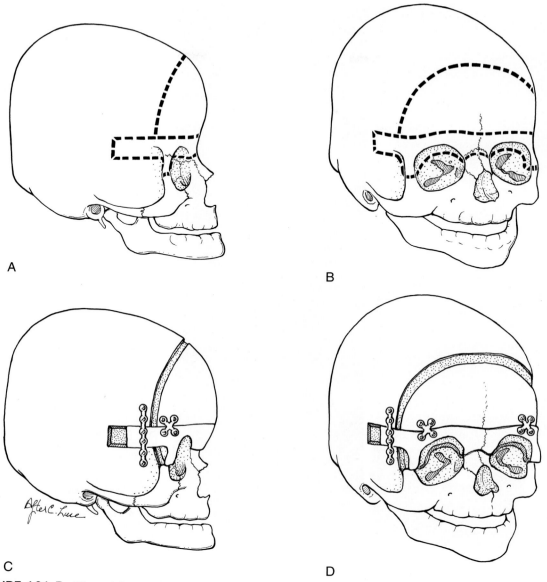

FIGURE 101-5. Bilateral fronto-orbital advancement and cranial vault remodeling. *A* and *B,* Lateral and oblique views of the lines of osteotomy. *C* and *D,* Lateral and oblique views after advancement of the fronto-orbital segment and repositioning of the frontal bone flap. Resorbable plates and screws are used for fixation. The position of the tenon denotes the amount of skeletal advancement that was achieved. (Adapted from C. Luce.)

The parents should be made aware of these associations and the need for long-term follow-up in these children to detect these problems if they develop over time.

The clinically relevant deformities associated with metopic synostosis and trigonocephaly relate to the forehead and the periorbital region. The forehead exhibits bitemporal narrowing and prominence in the midline. The periorbital region exhibits a decreased interorbital distance and deficient projection of the lateral supraorbital rims. Consequently, most surgical procedures designed to correct trigonocephaly use a supraorbital bar remodeling as well as a recontouring of the bifrontal craniotomy flap.

The supraorbital bar is most frequently advanced laterally to improve the projection in this region with a greenstick fracture made in the midline to diminish the keel-shaped appearance. The necessity for expansion of the supraorbital bar in the midline to treat the hypotelorism present in most patients is

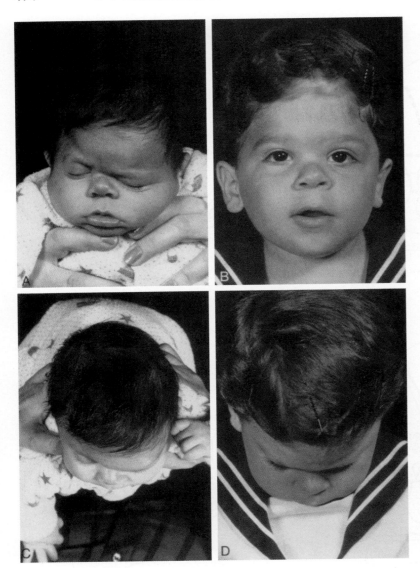

FIGURE 101-6. Newborn boy with plagiocephaly-unilateral coronal synostosis. *A,* Preoperative frontal view. Note the right-sided plagiocephaly and recession of the brow. There is frontal bossing with inferior displacement of the globe on the opposite side. *B,* Appearance after the technique illustrated in Figure 101-5. *C,* Preoperative superior view. *D,* Postoperative superior view. (From McCarthy JG, ed: Plastic Surgery. Philadelphia, WB Saunders, 1990: 3033.)

controversial. McCarthy et al[51] have advocated a step-cut osteotomy in the midline for correction of this problem in severe cases (Figs. 101-7 and 101-8). However, other authors have noted that there is a gradual normalization of the intercanthal distance in children with metopic synostosis with growth, even when this has not been addressed specifically at the time of the fronto-orbital remodeling.[34,35,52-54]

With respect to the forehead deformity, it is best treated by dividing the bifrontal flap in the midline and rotating each segment 90 degrees to achieve the best fit for optimal forehead contour. Barrel stave osteotomies with greenstick fractures may also help improve the bitemporal narrowing.

RECONSTRUCTIVE MODALITIES: SYNDROMIC CRANIOSYNOSTOSIS

Within this category are included Crouzon, Apert, Pfeiffer, Saethre-Chotzen, and Carpenter syndromes. As a group, these conditions share much in common from the standpoint of both appearance and function. With the exception of Crouzon syndrome, these syndromes are associated with limb abnormalities, most commonly syndactyly of the fingers. With the exception of Carpenter syndrome, these conditions are autosomal dominant in their inheritance pattern, although the majority of cases occur through spontaneous mutation. From the standpoint of the cranial

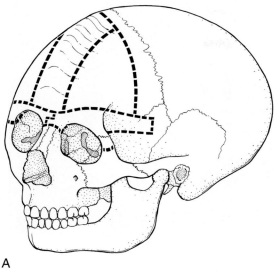

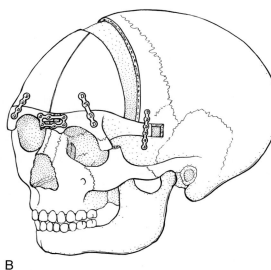

FIGURE 101-7. Surgical correction of metopic synostosis. *A,* Lines of osteotomy. Note the area of resection of the central forehead. *B,* After advancement and "expansion" of the fronto-orbital segment by a step osteotomy and replacement of the frontal bone flaps. Some of the tenon has been resected.

vault, most patients present with a turribrachycephalic deformity, or a decrease in the anteroposterior dimension and an increase in the superoinferior dimension. Although any or all of the cranial vault sutures may be involved, most commonly there is minimally a bicoronal synostosis as a component to the deformity. It is also thought that there is an extensive involvement of the cranial base sutures in these conditions, resulting in often profound midface hypopla-

sia with the attendant problems of exorbitism and malocclusion.

Preoperative Considerations

There are myriad factors to be considered in the preoperative work-up of a patient with syndromic craniosynostosis. Most common among these is the question of intracranial hypertension. In a classic study, Renier et al[55] demonstrated that 42% of children in their series presenting with untreated multiple-suture synostosis had documented evidence of an elevated intracranial pressure. In patients with Crouzon syndrome, as many as 66% were found to have intracranial hypertension.[47]

The etiology of the intracranial hypertension in patients with craniosynostosis is not entirely clear. Volumetric studies of the cranial vault have not demonstrated a consistent correlation between intracranial volume reduction and intracranial hypertension. However, Renier et al[55] found that after fronto-orbital advancement and cranial vault remodeling, intracranial pressure was reduced to within normal limits in 93% of patients.

Demonstration of papilledema as an indicator of intracranial hypertension has been found to be unreliable in young children. Tuite et al[56] found that in children older than 8 years, papilledema was 100% accurate as an indicator of intracranial hypertension. However, in children younger than 8 years, it was found in only 22% of the patients with a documented elevation of intracranial pressure.[56] There is currently no noninvasive study that is completely reliable for the detection of intracranial hypertension preoperatively. The radiographic findings of a "copper beaten" skull are nonspecific although frequently associated with patients demonstrating elevated intracranial pressure. Attempts have been made to correlate transcranial Doppler sonographic waveforms with intracranial pressure.[57,58] Although definite changes are demonstrated on the transcranial Doppler study with increase in intracranial pressure, no quantitative assessment is as yet possible. If, however, a diagnosis of intracranial hypertension is made in a patient with craniosynostosis, cranial vault remodeling is indicated regardless of the patient's age to prevent possible ocular damage and neurologic injury. During the surgical procedure, these patients may demonstrate increased bleeding and a tense dura, making the operation more difficult and increasing the likelihood of complications. In the preoperative period, the patients should be typed and crossmatched in anticipation of significant blood loss and consideration given to intraoperative hypotension to minimize blood loss. In addition, hyperventilation and diuresis aid in diminishing the intracranial pressure and decreasing the tension on the dura, minimizing the chance of dural laceration.

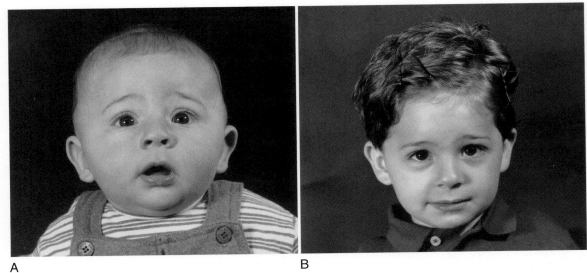

A   B

FIGURE 101-8. Surgical correction of trigonocephaly. *A,* A 9-month-old boy with trigonocephaly and decreased bitemporal distance. *B,* Appearance of the correction by the technique illustrated in Figure 101-7.

An important concern in syndromic craniosynostosis is hydrocephalus. This has been demonstrated in up to 10% of the patients.[59] If hydrocephalus is thought to be of significant severity to warrant ventriculoperitoneal shunting, an important question is the timing of this procedure. When it is performed before cranial vault remodeling, it is possible that the expansile force of the dura in maintaining the reconstructed cranial vault shape may not be present. There is a potential that this reduction of ventricular pressure could account for relapse in the reconstructed and expanded cranial vault, although this has never been demonstrated conclusively.

Another preoperative consideration in syndromic craniosynostosis is the status of the airway. There is clearly an association between syndromic craniofacial synostoses and airway obstruction. In a series of 40 patients, Lo and Chen[60] demonstrated a 40% incidence of airway obstruction, with 12% of these patients representing a severe problem. There was no significant difference in the severity of airway compromise between patients with either Apert or Crouzon syndrome. The problem is primarily attributed to the midface hypoplasia and reduction in nasopharyngeal dimensions, although lower airway obstruction, choanal atresia, and tonsillar hypertrophy must also be considered. The parents must be specifically questioned with respect to airway symptoms such as snoring or noisy breathing preoperatively. When in question, a preoperative endoscopy and a sleep study can be helpful in documenting the presence and site of an airway compromise. The anesthesiologist must be warned of the potential difficulty with intubation and

be prepared for alternative means of establishing an airway, including elective tracheostomy in the most severe cases.

The patients may also present with exorbitism in association with the retruded frontal bone and the midface hypoplasia. Care must be given to ensure corneal protection intraoperatively because the globes are at high risk for corneal exposure. In addition, one must take care to avoid placing pressure on the globes throughout the procedure by the position of the reflected coronal flap.

CLOVERLEAF SKULL DEFORMITY

The cloverleaf skull deformity or Kleeblattschädel is a rare condition that can be observed in all of the syndromic or multiple-suture synostoses. These patients present at birth with a trilobar cranial vault deformity due to stenosed sutures, and they often demonstrate evidence of severe intracranial hypertension with ocular exposure and airway compromise. Immediate consideration must be given to stabilizing the airway and protecting the globes.[61]

The cranial vault deformity is most frequently addressed urgently with radical craniectomy.[62,63] When it is performed in the neonatal period, nearly complete reossification of the skull can be expected subsequent to this procedure. Other authors have described monobloc advancement or distraction for these severe conditions, techniques addressing both the cranial vault and the midface simultaneously.[64,65] Despite these efforts, the morbidity after surgical reconstruction in the Kleeblattschädel syndrome is high, and the surgical results are frequently disappointing.[63]

Other Cranial Vault Remodeling Procedures

Although the syndromic craniofacial synostoses can be associated with a range of cranial vault shapes, the most consistent is turribrachycephaly. As with many of the craniosynostoses, an advancement of the fronto-orbital bar and remodeling of the cranial vault (see Fig. 101-5) are indicated in these patients.[4,5] However, this does little to correct the associated turricephaly found in many of the patients. A variety of different techniques have been described to address this problem.[33,66-68] Lauritzen et al[68] described the "dynamic cranioplasty" technique for the treatment of turricephaly. The technique provides a transverse tension with bone flaps based in the temporoparietal region but allows anterior and posterior expansion with a superiorly hinged frontal flap and an inferiorly based occipital flap. Cohen et al[66] described correction of this condition by removing the frontal bone flap and performing an osteotomy low in the temporal skull and continuing posteriorly and superiorly toward the occipital calvaria. The bone flap is elevated but not detached, and it is displaced inferiorly, compressing the brain. The inferior border of the flap, which overlaps the temporal bone, is fixed in position with screws or sutures. This diminishes the vertical dimension of the cranial vault and allows frontal advancement. Despite these techniques, recurrent turricephaly in syndromic patients remains a vexing problem, and secondary cranial vault procedures are often indicated, especially in the patient with Apert syndrome.[34,35,67]

Midface Distraction or Advancement

Another surgical consideration in syndromic craniosynostosis is the position of the midface. In the majority of the patients, some degree of midface hypoplasia is evident. Although it typically progresses over time, exorbitism and airway compromise secondary to midface hypoplasia may be present even in the neonatal stage in severe cases. This may represent a surgical emergency and require tracheostomy and tarsorrhaphy for immediate treatment with subsequent fronto-orbital advancement and cranial vault remodeling. However, monobloc frontofacial advancement has been described for severe cases in the first year of life, but it may be associated with a high morbidity at this age.[69]

Even when it is not present in the neonatal period, progressive midfacial hypoplasia is often manifested with growth in the syndromic craniosynostoses, especially in Crouzon syndrome. Midface advancement or distraction (Le Fort III osteotomy) is performed to correct this situation. Although the safety of this procedure in the preschool-aged patient has been clearly demonstrated, it must be emphasized to the parents that the patients will probably require midface advancement at the cessation of craniofacial growth.[23] In recent years, midface distraction has evolved as the treatment of choice in the preschool-aged patient.

SUBCRANIAL LE FORT III OSTEOTOMY

The subcranial Le Fort III osteotomy, originally described by Gillies and Harrison[70] but popularized by Tessier,[71] is performed through a coronal incision. The supraorbital rims, medial and lateral walls of the orbit, and roof are exposed in a subperiosteal plane. The deep temporal fascia is incised approximately 15 mm above the supraorbital rim, and surgical access is gained to the space that lies between the superficial and deep layers of the deep temporal fascia. With dissection in this space, access is gained to the arch of the zygoma, and the wound is connected to the previous dissection carried along the outer aspect of the lateral orbital wall. It is then possible to expose the body and arch of the zygoma in a subperiosteal plane. Likewise, the floor of the orbit can also be exposed through this incision, but additional access is gained by transconjunctival or transcutaneous eyelid incisions. The dissection can also be extended along the lateral aspect of the maxilla toward the pterygomaxillary junction.

The osteotomy is commenced in the lateral orbital wall at its junction with the cranium (Fig. 101-9). The lateral orbital wall is sectioned in a full-thickness fashion, and with a combination of mechanical saw and osteotome, the osteotomy is extended along the floor of the orbit. The zygoma is sectioned at its junction with the arch.

Through the temporal fossa, the osteotomy is extended across the lateral aspect of the maxilla to and through the pterygomaxillary fossa with a curved osteotome. The same procedure is repeated on the contralateral side.

The osteotomy through the nasofrontal junction is reserved toward the end because penetration of the nasal cavity usually elicits some element of bleeding. This persists until the midface segment is completely osteotomized and mobilized. The osteotomy begins just anterior to the nasofrontal suture, with care being taken to avoid injury to the cribriform plate and possible cerebrospinal fluid fistula. The osteotomy is carried posterior to the lacrimal fossa, down the medial orbital wall, and across the medial aspect of the floor of the orbit to join the previously executed osteotomy. The nasal septum is sectioned with an osteotome. Eyelid incisions are usually not necessary for this maneuver.

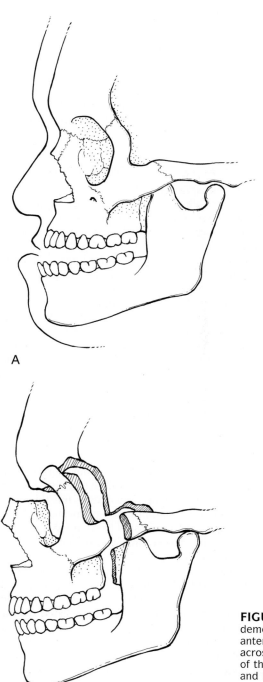

A

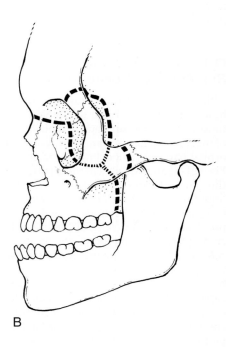

B

C

FIGURE 101-9. The subcranial Le Fort III osteotomy. *A,* Lateral view demonstrating the pathologic process. Note the midface hypoplasia, anterior crossbite, and anterior open bite. *B,* The lines of osteotomy: across the nasofrontal junction, through the medial orbital wall, floor of the orbit, full thickness of the lateral orbital wall, zygomatic arch and retromaxillary area, and pterygomaxillary junction. *C,* Mobilization of the osteotomized segment and the resulting skeletal defects. (Adapted from C. Luce.)

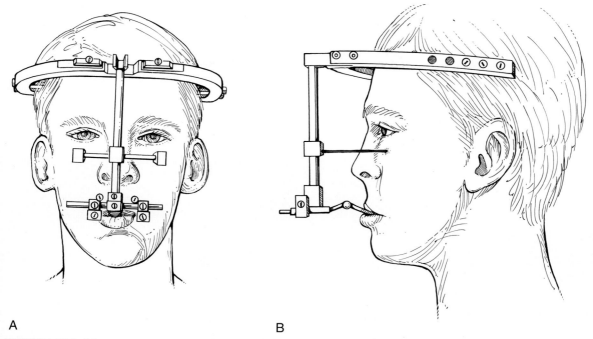

A   B

FIGURE 101-10. The external halo midface distraction device. *A,* Frontal view. *B,* Lateral view. Note that the halo is secured to the cranium with large screws, to the infraorbital-zygomatic area with wires to skeletal screws, and to the maxillary occlusion with wires to a dental splint.

There are two methods of advancing the midface segment: distraction and advancement with bone grafting.

Midface Distraction Devices

There are two types of midface distraction devices: the halo or external traction device[12] and the buried craniofacial device.[72] The external halo device (Fig. 101-10) has the advantage of securing attachment to the cranium with the application of distraction forces at the level of both zygomatic bodies as well as at a preoperatively designed maxillary splint. The buried devices (Fig. 101-11) are secured with screws to the cranium and to the zygomatic body. The activation components penetrate the scalp and are the only portion of the device that is observable. These devices require a second operation for removal, whereas the halo device can be removed in the office.

Whichever method is chosen, device activation is delayed for 3 to 5 days and proceeds at the rate of 1 mm/day. In the growing child, one wants to over-correct at the occlusal level with a resulting overjet of 3 to 4 mm. The overall vector is usually along the occlusal plane; however, in many syndromic patients, the face is short in the vertical dimension, and a small inferior component to the vector may be helpful. The external or halo device has the benefit of allowing changes in the vector during the course of distraction. As with the standard Le Fort III advancement,

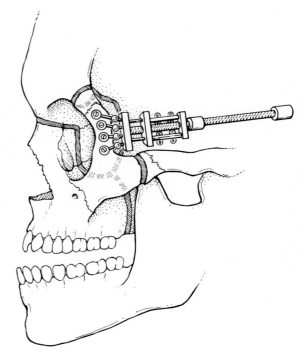

FIGURE 101-11. A buried midface distraction device. The lines of osteotomy (subcranial Le Fort III) are designated. Note that the device is secured with multiple screws attached to the device on either side of the osteotomy. The activating component is passed through a separate incision in the scalp to allow easy access for activation.

the endpoint is ultimately based on the patient's appearance, not the occlusion, especially in the growing child.

A preliminary study has indicated that midface movement is generally greater with the technique of distraction compared with standard advancement and grafting, and airway improvement is therefore more predictable (Fig. 101-12).[73]

Midface Advancement with Bone Grafting

The traditional Le Fort III osteotomy[71] is associated with an immediate intraoperative advancement. The occlusion is used to establish a new position for the midface segment by the establishment of temporary intermaxillary fixation (Fig. 101-13). The general vector of the advancement is anteroinferior. After

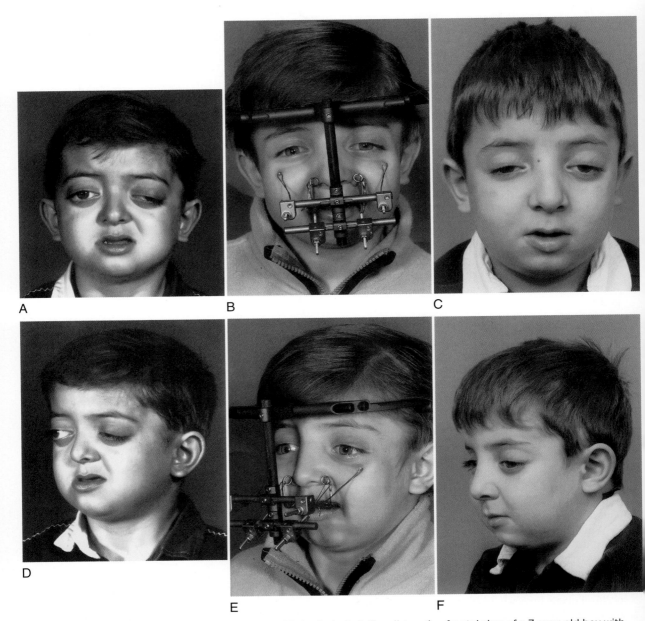

FIGURE 101-12. Midface distraction (external halo device). *A,* Pre-distraction frontal view of a 7-year-old boy with Crouzon syndrome, exorbitism, and midface hypoplasia. *B,* External halo device in position (see Fig. 101-10). *C,* Post-distraction frontal view showing augmentation of the midface and correction of the exorbitism. *D,* Pre-distraction oblique view. *E,* External halo device in position. *F,* Post-distraction oblique view.

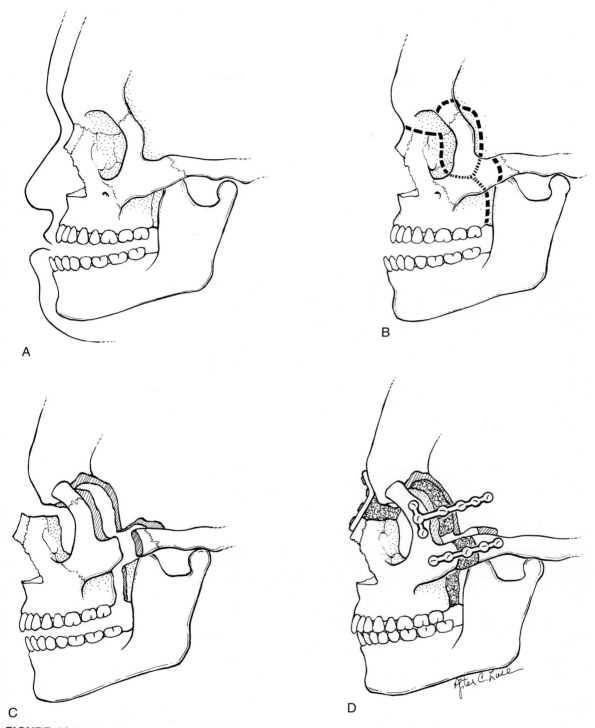

FIGURE 101-13. Subcranial Le Fort III advancement osteotomy with bone grafting. *A,* Lateral view demonstrating the pathologic process. Note the midface hypoplasia, anterior crossbite, and anterior open bite. *B,* The lines of osteotomy: across the nasofrontal junction, through the medial orbital wall, floor of the orbit, full thickness of the lateral orbital wall, zygomatic arch and retromaxillary area, and pterygomaxillary junction. *C,* Mobilization of the osteotomized segment and the resulting skeletal defects. *D,* Autogenous bone grafts are placed in the nasofrontal junction, lateral orbital wall, zygomatic arch, and pterygomaxillary fissure defects. Fixation is obtained by miniplates. (Adapted from C. Luce.)

intermaxillary fixation is established, there are residual defects in the lateral orbital wall and nasofrontal junction that are filled with cranial, iliac, or rib autogenous bone grafts. Rigid skeletal fixation is achieved with the plates and screws across the lateral orbital wall and cranium and across the nasofrontal junction. Additional plates and screws are constructed across the body of the zygoma and the zygomatic arch. The wounds are irrigated with saline, and the coronal incision is closed as previously described (Figs. 101-14 and 101-15).

LE FORT III COMBINED WITH LE FORT I ADVANCEMENT OSTEOTOMY

The combined Le Fort III-Le Fort I advancement osteotomy (with bone grafts and rigid skeletal fixa-

tion) allows differential movement of the individual osteotomized skeletal segments (Fig. 101-16). It is especially indicated in the patient with a significant deficiency of the orbitozygomatic region and only a minimal anterior crossbite.

LE FORT II OSTEOTOMY

The Le Fort II osteotomy[74] is similar to the Le Fort III osteotomy except that the zygomas are not mobilized (Fig. 101-17). It finds little indication in patients with craniosynostosis who routinely have zygomatic recession and require advancement of these structures. The line of osteotomy runs from the nasofrontal junction and is extended along the medial orbital wall to the floor of the orbit, across the inferior orbital rim at a

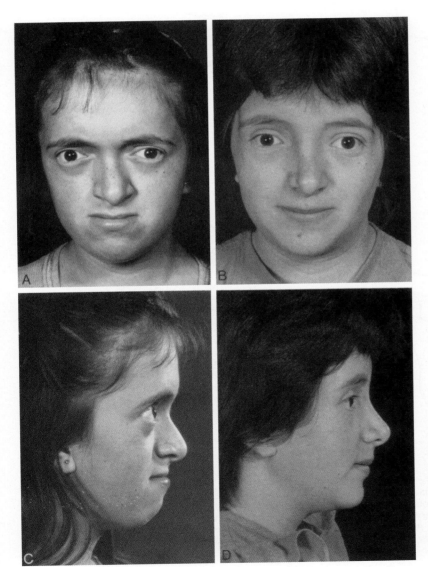

FIGURE 101-14. Adolescent girl with Crouzon disease. *A,* Preoperative frontal view. Note the midface hypoplasia, exorbitism, and microgenia. *B,* Postoperative frontal view. *C,* Preoperative profile. *D,* Postoperative profile after the technique illustrated in Figure 101-13 as well as horizontal osteotomy of the mandible (genioplasty) and nasalplasty. (From McCarthy JG, ed: Plastic Surgery. Philadelphia, WB Saunders, 1990:3040.)

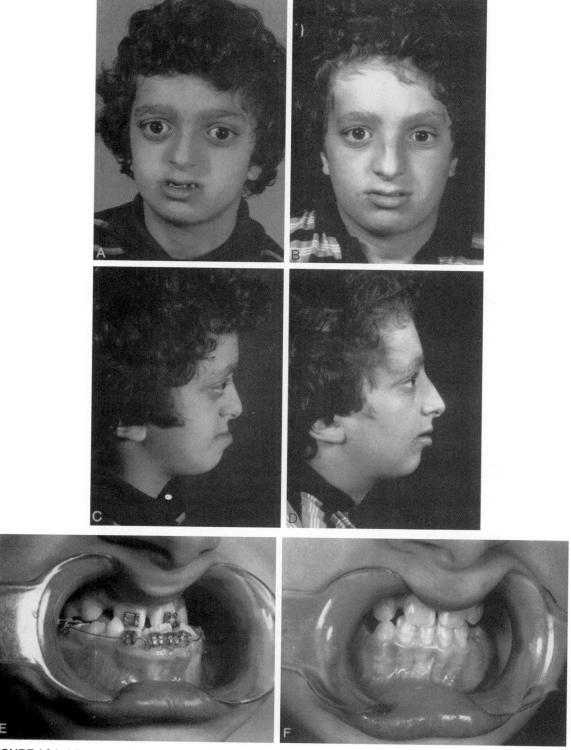

FIGURE 101-15. Le Fort III advancement in a 9-year-old boy. *A* and *C,* Preoperative views. Note the midface hypoplasia, exorbitism, and lip relationships. *B* and *D,* Appearance after Le Fort III advancement. *E,* Preoperative occlusion with an anterior crossbite. *F,* Postoperative occlusion. (From McCarthy JG, ed: Plastic Surgery. Philadelphia, WB Saunders, 1990:3041.)

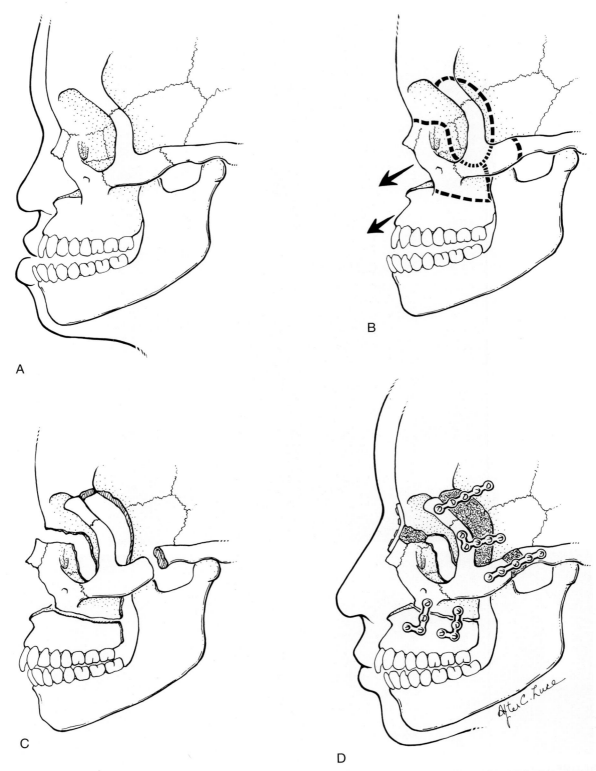

FIGURE 101-16. Combined Le Fort III-Le Fort I osteotomy. *A,* Lateral view of the preoperative deformity demonstrating that the hypoplasia in the orbital-maxillary area is different from that at the maxillary occlusal plane. *B,* Lines of osteotomy with the arrows designating the direction of movement of the skeletal segments. *C,* View after mobilization of the osteotomized segments. *D,* Appearance after placement of interposition bone grafts and the establishment of rigid skeletal fixation. (Adapted from C. Luce.)

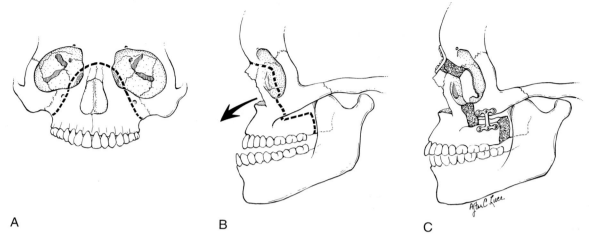

FIGURE 101-17. The LeFort II advancement osteotomy. *A* and *B,* Frontal and lateral views of the lines of osteotomy. The arrow designates the projected vector of advancement. *C,* Lateral view after advancement with interposition bone grafts at the nasofrontal junction, anterior maxilla-zygoma, and pterygomaxillary regions. Rigid skeletal fixation is established with plates and screws at the nasofrontal junction and the zygomatic-maxillary region. (Adapted from C. Luce.)

position lateral to the infraorbital foramen, and across the anterolateral aspect of the maxilla to and through the pterygomaxillary fissure. The septum is also divided as in the Le Fort III osteotomy (Fig. 101-18).

MONOBLOC OSTEOTOMY

The monobloc procedure[7] is performed through a combined craniofacial approach because the fronto-orbital segment is advanced with its midface counterpart as a single piece, hence the term monobloc (Fig. 101-19). There may or may not be associated cranial vault remodeling.

The procedure begins with an anterior craniotomy that is designed to improve forehead contour and to protect the frontal lobes of the brain when the orbital roof osteotomy is made. After the anterior craniotomy is completed and the frontal bone flap is placed on the operating table, a classic fronto-orbital osteotomy is made except that the roofs of the orbit are not osteotomized. A supraorbital rim of approximately 15 mm in height is osteotomized and extended in a tongue-in-groove fashion into the temporal area. The osteotomy is extended down the lateral orbital wall in a full-thickness fashion as previously described. It is then extended across the anterolateral aspect of the maxilla to and through the pterygomaxillary fissure. The nasal septum is osteotomized through the craniotomy, and the entire monobloc is advanced and liberated.

Monobloc Distraction

Monobloc distraction can be performed with either an external[65] or internal[72,75] device as described before

for subcranial Le Fort III distraction (Fig. 101-20). The halo frame device allows the application of pulling forces (vectors) at the fronto-orbital and occlusal levels (see Fig. 101-10).

Monobloc Advancement with Bone Grafting

After the monobloc segment is mobilized, a preoperatively constructed splint is placed to establish temporary intermaxillary fixation. The preoperative plan is realized by the placement of autogenous bone grafts in the lateral orbital wall defects and rigid skeletal fixation (plates and screws) across the cranial tenons, lateral orbital walls, and zygomatic arches (Figs. 101-21 and 101-22).

The technique has been criticized for a high infection rate,[76] but technical refinements have lowered the rate.[77] There is also the possibility that monobloc distraction will lower the rate of ascending infection because there is not the immediate formation of an intracranial dead space.[73]

DEVELOPING TECHNIQUES

Distraction Osteogenesis

Since its introduction by Ilizarov and its subsequent application to the craniofacial skeleton by McCarthy[8] in 1992, distraction osteogenesis has been used more frequently in craniofacial reconstructive surgery.[8,78] With respect to surgery for craniosynostosis, there are several advantages of using distraction to remodel the cranial vault. Because the bone segments need not be completely detached from the underlying dura, they remain better vascularized and undergo

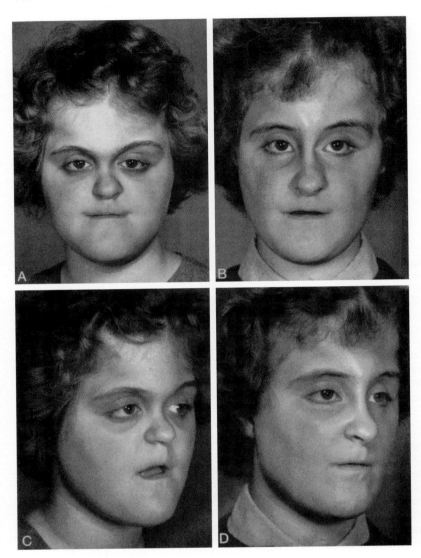

FIGURE 101-18. Female patient with craniosynostosis associated with vitamin D-resistant rickets. *A* and *C*, Preoperative views. Note the midface hypoplasia and foreshortened nose. *B* and *D*, After Le Fort II advancement as illustrated in Figure 101-17. (From McCarthy JG, Reid CA: Craniofacial synostosis in association with vitamin D-resistant rickets. Ann Plast Surg 1979;4:149.)

less remodeling and resorption from the remodeling. In addition, by remaining attached to the underlying dura and being gradually advanced, no dead space results from the fronto-orbital advancement, thus diminishing the possibility of infection. Finally, in reoperative cases, the ability to gradually stretch the overlying deficient soft tissues is advantageous and should diminish the incidence of relapse in these situations.

Although this has been performed in clinical cases, its widespread application is limited because of the lack of development of devices designed to achieve cranial vault remodeling by this technique.[79] The ideal device would be one that is capable of being placed entirely beneath the skin and activated transcutaneously. It

would provide sufficient force to advance the cranial vault segments against significant resistance but would ultimately be resorbable, obviating the need for secondary surgery for removal. A variety of devices including those activated by transcutaneous magnet are currently in the process of development but have not yet been placed into widespread clinical use.[80] Moreover, the principle of contraction or "reverse distraction" has been applied to correct the scaphocephaly deformity by cranial compression in infants with sagittal synostosis.[81]

It is also possible to distract the midface without osteotomies in immature animals,[9] and the same principle has been successfully applied in boys aged 12 and 13 years.[82]

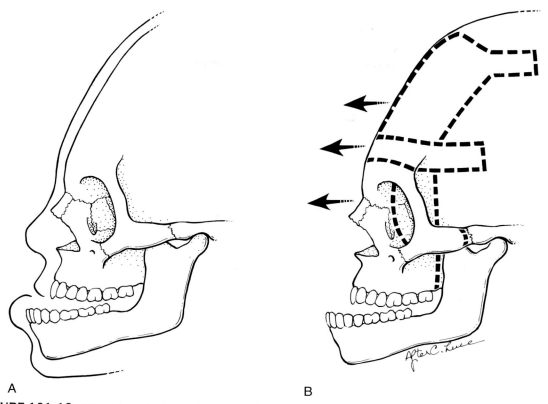

FIGURE 101-19. Monobloc osteotomy. *A,* Preoperative lateral view demonstrating severe midface hypoplasia with associated retrusion of the supraorbital rim and frontal bone. There is also an anterior crossbite. *B,* Lines of osteotomy. Note the projected vectors of advancement.

Minimally Invasive Surgery

There has been considerable interest in the use of minimally invasive techniques across the surgical specialties. In plastic surgery, the most widespread application of endoscopy and minimally invasive dissection has been in brow lifting because of the ability to avoid the coronal incision with its attendant scarring and blood loss. The same is true for craniosynostosis. Indeed, endoscopic craniectomy with cranial vault remodeling by precise postoperative helmet molding therapy has been reported in a limited number of patients with isolated or nonsyndromic craniosynostosis, and it has been demonstrated that it can be performed safely with minimal blood loss and acceptable aesthetic results.[27,83] The obvious concern with such a technique is the possibility of inadvertent damage to the sagittal sinus or other structures with subsequent difficulty in controlling the resultant hemorrhage because of the limited nature of the incisions.

In the future, endoscopic surgery will be greatly facilitated by the application of distraction devices to advance hypoplastic skeletal segments. In a canine study, midface advancement was achieved by endoscopic Le Fort III osteotomy and the application of external distraction devices.[9]

Yet another application of these techniques has been in fetal surgery. The primary limitation in fetal surgery has been premature labor resulting in significant morbidity to the neonate.[84] The ability to operate on the fetus through minimal hysterotomies has the advantage of minimizing the stimulation to the uterus and diminishing the incidence of preterm labor. With respect to surgery for craniosynostosis, it has been demonstrated in an animal model that endoscopic craniectomy is safe and successful in correcting a surgically formed model of craniosynostosis.[85] As of yet, there have been no reported cases of this in humans, but as was shown in the animal study, the potential benefit of performing such procedures in utero would be to minimize the secondary or pathologic compensatory craniofacial changes associated with craniosynostosis. The animals in the study had significant improvements not only in cranial vault shape but in overall morphologic features of the orbits and the cranial base.[85]

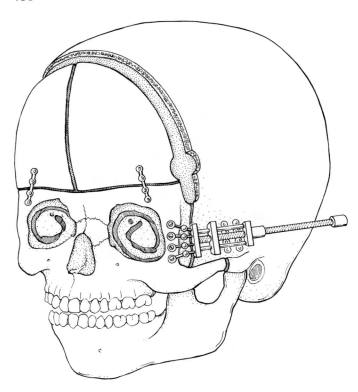

FIGURE 101-20. Monobloc distraction. Note that the distraction device is secured across the osteotomy in the lateral orbital wall. The activation component is passed through the scalp for easy access. Rigid skeletal fixation has also been used to secure the repositioned frontal bone flaps. Distraction is illustrated with an internal device, but it can also be done with the external halo device (see Fig. 101-10).

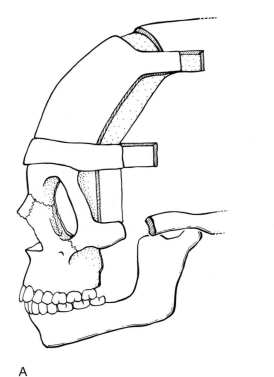

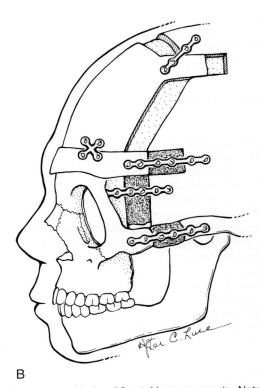

A

B

FIGURE 101-21. *A,* Lateral view after mobilization of the monobloc, supraorbital and frontal bone segments. Note the resulting skeletal defects. *B,* Lateral view demonstrating interposition bone grafts with the establishment of rigid skeletal fixation with plates and screws. (Adapted from C. Luce.)

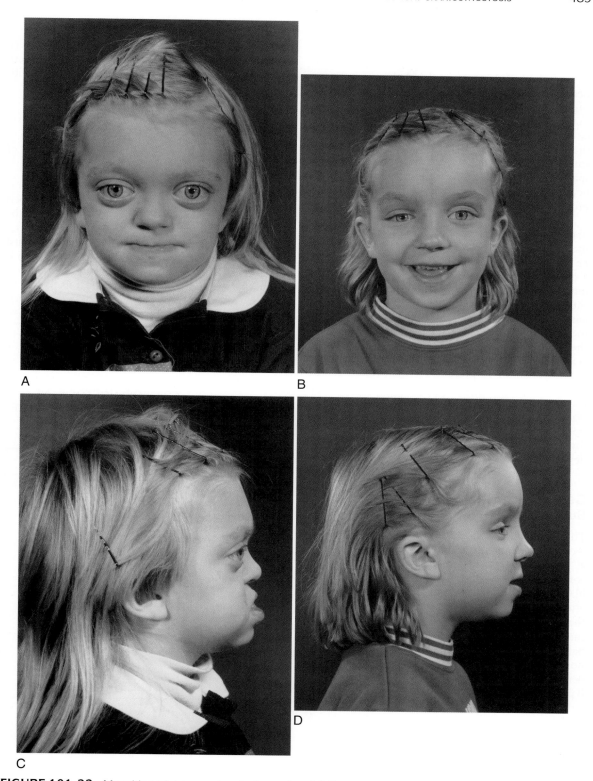

FIGURE 101-22. Monobloc advancement, osteotomy. *A* and *C*, Preoperative views of a 7-year-old girl with Crouzon syndrome. Note the exorbitism as well as retrusion of the forehead and midface. *B* and *D*, Postoperative view with restoration of facial contour and correction of the exorbitism (see Fig. 101-21).

Virtual Reality Surgery

Surgery for craniosynostosis has always relied in great part on the surgeon's eye to position the reconstructed bone fragments in the optimum position. Because of swelling and other variables at the time of surgery, this is fraught with potential error. The ability to move bone fragments to a position determined to be optimal preoperatively would be ideal. In addition, the ability to segment large bone fragments into smaller pieces, optimally moving each fragment in space independently of one another, would also be beneficial, particularly in midface reconstructive procedures.

Cutting et al[86] have developed and used a system that allows just such a procedure. With their technique, the optimal position of the bone fragments to be advanced is determined preoperatively by use of a normative database and onlaying this to a three-dimensional computer representation of the patient's skull. Intraoperatively, diodes are affixed to the skull base as a reference point and to each individual fragment to be repositioned. Readings are taken before the osteotomy, and once it is performed, the fragment is advanced with use of the computer to guide the optimal position. At present, excellent results can be achieved with this procedure, but there is a sharp learning curve.[86] Initial problems with devascularization of the multiple fragments and subsequent infection have been addressed by limiting the extent of dissection of the individual fragments to avoid devascularization.

Gene Therapy and Biochemical Sutural Manipulation

There has been an increasing interest in the biomolecular mechanisms of craniosynostosis. Mulliken et al[87] have demonstrated the association of bilateral coronal synostosis with abnormalities in the fibroblast growth factor receptor genomic sequences in affected patients. It has been shown in animal models that the underlying dura controls sutural fusion rather than the suture itself.[88] Sutures that normally remain patent will fuse when placed over the dura of sutures normally undergoing early fusion. It has been further demonstrated that transforming growth factor (TGF)-β plays a critical role in suture fusion. Sutures undergoing fusion exhibit intense immunoreactivity for TGF-β isoforms when tested immunohistochemically.[89] In addition, it has been shown that neutralizing antibodies to TGF-β2 prevent osseous obliteration of the suture.[90] As the mechanisms of premature sutural fusion are further elucidated, it is possible that direct chemical or indirect genetic manipulation of chemical expression may prevent or ameliorate the problem of craniosynostosis.

TREATMENT ALGORITHM

At the Institute of Reconstructive Plastic Surgery at the New York University Medical Center, there are several treatment periods for the patient with craniosynostosis:

1. Infancy—younger than 1 year
2. Early childhood—younger than 6 years
3. Period of mixed dentition/early adolescence
4. Late adolescence or adulthood (completion of craniofacial growth and development)

The referenced treatment algorithm must be individualized for each patient with craniosynostosis (Table 101-1). First of all, functional issues must be addressed before those of appearance. Second, anticipated craniofacial growth (or lack of growth) must be considered. For example, if midface distraction is recommended for a 6-year-old, the parents must understand that a secondary procedure most likely will be required after facial growth (i.e., that of the mandible) is complete.

TABLE 101-1 ✦ TREATMENT ALGORITHM: CRANIOSYNOSTOSIS, NEW YORK UNIVERSITY INSTITUTE OF RECONSTRUCTIVE PLASTIC SURGERY

Infancy (younger than 1 year)

Ventriculoperitoneal shunt
Tracheostomy
Gastrostomy
Strip craniectomy
Fronto-orbital advancement
Cranial vault remodeling

Early Childhood (younger than 6 years)

Secondary fronto-orbital advancement/cranial vault remodeling
Tonsillectomy/adenoidectomy
Midface distraction/advancement
External canthopexy
Orthodontic therapy

Period of Mixed Dentition/Early Adolescence

Orthodontic therapy

Late Adolescence/Adulthood

Midface distraction/advancement
Orthognathic jaw surgery (including genioplasty)
Rhinoplasty
External canthopexy

RESULTS

When assessing the results of reconstructive surgery for correction of the various craniosynostoses, one must distinguish between syndromic and nonsyndromic cases because the degree of deformity and the results are vastly different. The most widely accepted method of quantifying results is the scale established by Whitaker et al[91] in 1987. The authors graded results according to the need for additional surgery: patients assigned to category I needed no further surgical refinements; patients assigned to category IV required a repeated operation of a magnitude similar to the initial procedure. In their review of 20 years of experience with craniosynostosis surgery, McCarthy et al[34,35] clearly demonstrated the improved results obtained in the nonsyndromic or isolated cases. The best results obtained were found in metopic synostosis, with virtually all patients doing well and requiring no repeated operations. The most unfavorable results in the nonsyndromic craniosynostoses were found in patients with sagittal synostosis requiring total cranial vault remodeling. However, in comparison of syndromic with nonsyndromic cases, almost 37% of syndromic patients required major secondary procedures, whereas 13% of nonsyndromic patients did. Despite these findings, approximately 74% of syndromic patients were thought to have satisfactory craniofacial form (category I-II), whereas approximately 88% of nonsyndromic patients had this result. Approximately 65% of the syndromic patients either required Le Fort III midface advancement or had the procedure recommended.

In a similar study, Williams et al[92] reported total reoperation rates for nonsyndromic and syndromic synostoses of 5.9% and 27.3%, respectively. The incidence of complications is also significantly different between the syndromic and nonsyndromic cases. McCarthy et al[34,35] found an overall complication rate of 11% in the syndromic patients versus 5% in nonsyndromic patients. With respect to infectious complications, a combined review from two craniofacial centers totaling 567 intracranial procedures found an overall infection rate of 2.5%.[93] No infections were encountered in infants younger than 13 months, and there were no cases of meningitis. Eighty-five percent of the infections occurred in patients undergoing reoperations. The authors did not find that tracheostomies were a risk factor for infection, and there was no difference in infection rates when the scalps were shaved or not.

Another serious complication of cranial vault surgery is hemorrhage. Numerous authors have evaluated this complication in craniofacial surgery.[94-96] Transfusions are required for the majority of cranial vault remodeling procedures. As such, all patients should be typed and crossmatched for blood preoperatively, and this blood should be available in the operating room. Severe complications occur when intraoperative blood loss goes unrecognized and the patient's hemodynamic status is compromised.[95] In an analysis of 73 patients undergoing craniosynostosis surgery, Eaton et al[96] found the mean intraoperative transfusion to be approximately 72% of the estimated red cell match. They did not, however, find that there was significant transfusion-associated morbidity in these patients when management was appropriate.

REFERENCES

1. Lane LC: Linear craniectomy for relief of mental imbecility due to premature sutural close and microcephalus. JAMA 1892;18:49.
2. Lannelongue OM: De la craniectomie dans la microcephalie. Compt Rend Acad Sci 1890;110:1382.
3. Shillito J, Matson DD: Craniosynostosis: a review of 519 surgical patients. Pediatrics 1968;41:829-853.
4. McCarthy JG, Coccaro PJ, Epstein F, Converse JM: Early skeletal release in the infant with craniofacial dysostosis: the role of the sphenozygomatic suture. Plast Reconstr Surg 1978;62:335-346.
5. Marchac D, Cophigon J, Hirsch JF, Renier D: Fronto-cranial remodeling for craniosynostosis with mobilisation of the supra-orbital bar. Neurochirurgie 1978;24:23-31.
6. McCarthy J, Grayson B, Bookstein F, et al: LeFort III advancement osteotomy in the growing child. Plast Reconstr Surg 1984;74:343-354.
7. Ortiz-Monasterio F, del Campo AF, Carrillo A: Advancement of the orbits and the midface in one piece, combined with frontal repositioning, for the correction of Crouzon's deformities. Plast Reconstr Surg 1978;61:507-516.
8. McCarthy J, Schreiber J, Karp N, et al: Lengthening the human mandible by gradual distraction. Plast Reconstr Surg 1992;89:1-8.
9. Staffenberg D, Wood R, McCarthy J, et al: Mid-face distraction advancement in the canine without osteotomies. Ann Plast Surg 1995;34:512-517.
10. Molina F: Distraction of the maxilla. In McCarthy JG, ed: Distraction of the Craniofacial Skeleton. New York, Springer-Verlag, 1999:308.
11. Cohen S, Boydston W, Hudgins R, Burstein F: Monobloc and facial bipartition distraction with internal devices. J Craniofac Surg 1999;10:244-251.
12. Polley J, Figueroa A: Management of severe maxillary deficiency in childhood and adolescents through distraction osteogenesis with an external adjustable rigid distraction device. Plast Reconstr Surg 1997;8:181-185.
13. Gault D, Renier D, Marchac D, et al: Intracranial volume in children with craniosynostosis. J Craniofac Surg 1990;1:1-3.
14. Marchac D, Renier D: Intracranial pressure in craniosynostosis. J Neurosurg 1982;57:370-377.
15. Virtanen R, Korhonen T, Fagerholm J, Viljanto J: Neurocognitive sequelae of scaphocephaly. Pediatrics 1999;103:791-795.
16. Kapp-Simon K, Figueroa A, Jocher C, Schafer M: Longitudinal assessment of mental development in infants with nonsyndromic craniosynostosis with and without cranial release and reconstruction. Plast Reconstr Surg 1993;92:831-839.
17. Renier D, Marchac D: Discussion of "longitudinal assessment of mental development in infants with nonsyndromic craniosynostosis with and without cranial release and reconstruction," by Kapp-Simon K, et al. Plast Reconstr Surg 1993;92:840-841.

18. Adams K, Gilman S, Koeppe R, et al: Neuropsychological deficits are correlated with frontal hypometabolism in positron emission tomography studies of older alcoholic patients. Alcohol Clin Exp Res 1993;17:205-210.

19. Akguner M, Barutcu A, Karaca C: Adolescent growth patterns of the bony and cartilaginous framework of the nose: a cephalometric study. Ann Plast Surg 1998;41:66-69.

20. Barritt J, Brooksbank M, Simpson D: Scaphocephaly: aesthetic and psychosocial considerations. Dev Med Child Neurol 1981;23:183-191.

21. Barden R, Ford M, Wilhelm W, et al: The physical attractiveness of facially deformed patients before and after craniofacial surgery. Plast Reconstr Surg 1998;82:229-235.

22. Whitaker L, Schut L, Kerr L: Early surgery for isolated craniofacial dysostosis. Improvement and possible prevention of increasing deformity. Plast Reconstr Surg 1977;60:575-581.

23. McCarthy J, LaTrenta G, Breitbart A, et al: The LeFort III advancement osteotomy in the child under seven years of age. Plast Reconstr Surg 1990;86:633-646.

24. Ocampo R, Persing J: Sagittal synostosis. Clin Plast Surg 1994;21:563.

25. Paul R, Sugar O: Zenker solution in the surgical treatment of cranial synostosis. J Neurosurg 1972;6:604-607.

26. Epstein N, Epstein F, Newman G: Total vertex craniectomy for the treatment of scaphocephaly. Childs Brain 1982;9:309-316.

27. Jimenez D, Barone C: Endoscopic craniectomy for early surgical correction of sagittal synostosis. J Neurosurg 1998;88:77-81.

28. Panchal J, Marsh J, Parks T, et al: Sagittal craniosynostosis outcome assessment for two methods and timing of intervention. Plast Reconstr Surg 1999;103:1574-1584.

29. Maugans T, McComb J, Levy M: Surgical management of sagittal synostosis: a comparative analysis of strip craniectomy in calvarial vault remodeling. Pediatr Neurosurg 1997;27:137-148.

30. McCarthy JG, Bradley JP, Stelnicki E, et al: Hung span method of scaphocephaly reconstruction in patients with elevated intracranial pressure. Plast Reconstr Surg 2002;109:2009-2018.

31. Jane JA, Edgerton M, Futrell J, Park T: Immediate correction of sagittal synostosis. J Neurosurg 1978;49:705-710.

32. Volmer D, Jane J, Park T, Persing J: Variants of sagittal synostosis: strategies for surgical correction. J Neurosurg 1984;61:557-562.

33. Persing J, Jane J, Edgerton M: Surgical treatment of cranial synostosis. In Persing J, Edgerton M, Jane J, eds: Scientific Foundations and Surgical Treatment of Cranial Synostosis. Baltimore, Williams & Wilkins, 1989:190.

34. McCarthy J, Glasberg S, Cutting C, et al: Twenty year experience with early surgery for craniosynostosis. Part I. Isolated craniofacial synostosis—results and unsolved problems. Plast Reconstr Surg 1995;96:272-283.

35. McCarthy J, Glasberg S, Cutting C, et al: Twenty year experience with early surgery for craniosynostosis. Part II. Craniofacial synostosis syndromes and pansynostosis—results and unsolved problems. Plast Reconstr Surg 1995;92:284-295.

36. Rekate H: Occipital plagiocephaly: a critical review of the literature. J Neurosurg 1998;89:24-30.

37. Turk A, McCarthy J, Thorne C, Wisoff J: The "back to sleep campaign" and deformational plagiocephaly: is there a cause for concern? J Craniofac Surg 1996;7:12-18.

38. Huang M, Gruss J, Clarren S, et al: The differential diagnosis of posterior plagiocephaly: true lambdoid synostosis versus positional molding. Plast Reconstr Surg 1996;98:765-774.

39. Kelly K, Littlefield T, Pomatto J, et al: Importance of early recognition and treatment of deformational plagiocephaly with orthotic cranioplasty. Cleft Palate Craniofac J 1999;36:127-130.

40. Gosain A, Steele M, McCarthy J, Thorne C: A prospective study of the relationship between strabismus and head posture in patients with frontal plagiocephaly. Plast Reconstr Surg 1996;97:881-891.

41. Sgouros S, Goldin J, Hockley A, Wake M: Surgery for unilateral coronal synostosis (plagiocephaly): unilateral or bilateral correction? J Craniofac Surg 1996;7:284-289.

42. Schneider E, Bogdanow A, Goodrich J, et al: Fronto-ocular syndrome: newly recognized trigonocephaly syndrome. Am J Med Genet 2000;93:89-93.

43. Bohring A, Silengo M, Lerone M, et al: Severe end of Opitz trigonocephaly (C) syndrome or new syndrome? Am J Med Genet 1999;85:438-446.

44. Lajeunie E, LeMerrer M, Arnaud E, et al: Trigonocephaly: isolated, associated and syndromic forms. Genetics study in a series of 278 patients. Arch Pediatr 1998;5:873-879.

45. Pyo D, Persing J: Craniosynostosis. In Aston S, Beasley R, Thorne CH, eds: Grabb and Smith's Plastic Surgery, 5th ed. Philadelphia, Lippincott-Raven, 1997.

46. Albin R, Hendee R, O'Donnell R, et al: Trigonocephaly: refinements and reconstruction. Experience with 33 patients. Plast Reconstr Surg 1985;76:202-211.

47. Renier D: Intracranial pressure in craniosynostosis: pre and postoperative recording. Correlation with functional results. In Persing J, Edgerton M, Jane J, eds: Scientific Foundations in Surgical Treatment of Craniosynostosis. Baltimore, Williams & Wilkins, 1989.

48. Sigoti E, Marsh J, Marty-Grames L, Noetzel M: Long term studies of metopic synostosis: frequency of cognitive impairment and behavioral disturbances. Plast Reconstr Surg 1996;97:276-281.

49. Zampino G, DiRocco C, Butera G, et al: Opitz C trigonocephaly syndrome and midline brain anomalies. Am J Med Genet 1987;73:484-488.

50. Sabri M, al Saleh Q, Farah S, et al: Another Arab patient with overlap of Varadi-Patt/Opitz trigonocephaly syndrome. Am J Med Genet 1997;68:54-57.

51. McCarthy J, Bradley J, Longaker M: Step expansion of the frontal bar: correction of trigonocephaly. J Craniofac Surg 1996;7:333-335.

52. Moriyama E, Beck H, Iseba K, et al: Surgical correction of trigonocephaly: theoretical basis and operative procedures. Neurol Med Chir (Tokyo) 1998;38:110-115.

53. DiRocco C, Velardi F, Ferrario A, Marchese E: Metopic synostosis: in favor of a simplified surgical treatment. Childs Nerv Syst 1993;12:654-663.

54. Fearon J, Kolar J, Munro I: Trigonocephaly associated hypotelorism: is treatment necessary? Plast Reconstr Surg 1996;97:503-509.

55. Renier D, Sainte-Rose C, Marchac D, Hirsch J: Intracranial pressure in craniosynostosis. J Neurosurg 1982;57:370-377.

56. Tuite G, Chong W, Evanson J, et al: The effectiveness of papilledema as an indicator of raised intracranial pressure in children with craniosynostosis. Neurosurgery 1996;38:272-278.

57. Hassler W, Steinmetz H, Gawlowski J: Transcranial Doppler ultrasonography in raised intracranial pressure and an intracranial circulatory arrest. J Neurosurg 1988;68:745-751.

58. Nagai H, Moritake K, Takaya M: Correlation between transcranial Doppler ultrasonography and regional cerebral blood flow in experimental intracranial hypertension. Stroke 1997;28:603-607.

59. Golabi M, Edwards M, Ousterhout D: Craniosynostosis and hydrocephalus. Neurosurgery 1987;21:63-67.

60. Lo L, Chen Y: Airway obstruction in severe syndromic craniosynostosis. Ann Plast Surg 1999;43:258-264.

61. O'Keefe M, Algawi K, Fitzsimmon S, et al: Ocular complications of cloverleaf skull syndrome. J Pediatr Ophthalmol Strabismus 1998;35:292-293.

62. Turner P, Reynolds A: Generous craniectomy for Kleeblattschädel anomaly. Neurosurgery 1980;6:555-558.

63. Resnick D, Pollack I, Albright A: Surgical management of the cloverleaf skull deformity. Pediatr Neurosurg 1995;22:29-37.

64. Cohen S, Boydston W, Burstein F, Hudgins R: Monobloc distraction osteogenesis during infancy: report of a case and presentation of a new device. Plast Reconstr Surg 1998;101:1919-1924.

65. Polley J, Figueroa A, Charbel F, et al: Monobloc craniomaxillo-facial distraction osteogenesis in a newborn with severe craniofacial synostosis: a preliminary report. J Craniofac Surg 1995;6:421-423.

66. Cohen S, de Chalain T, Burstein F, et al: Turribrachycephaly: a technical note. Ann Plast Surg 1995;35:627-630.

67. Sonstein W, Hall C, Argamaso R, Goodrich J: Management of secondary turricephaly in craniofacial surgery. Childs Nerv Syst 1996;12:705-712.

68. Lauritzen C, Friede H, Elander A, et al: Dynamic cranioplasty for brachycephaly. Plast Reconstr Surg 1996;98:7-14.

69. Marchac D, Reiner D, Broumand S: Timing of treatment for craniosynostosis and faciocraniosynostosis: a twenty year experience. Br J Plast Surg 1994;47:211-222.

70. Gillies H, Harrison SH: Operative correction by osteotomy of recessed malar maxillary compound in a case of oxycephaly. Br J Plast Surg 1950-51;3:123.

71. Tessier P: Total osteotomy of the middle third of the face for faciostenosis or for sequelae of LeFort III fractures. Plast Reconstr Surg 1971;48:533-541.

72. Cohen S: Craniofacial distraction with a modular internal distraction system: evolution of design and surgical techniques. Plast Reconstr Surg 1999;103:1592-1607.

73. Fearon J: The LeFort III osteotomy: to distract or not to distract. Plast Reconstr Surg 2001;107:1091-1103.

74. Henderson D, Jackson I: Naso-maxillary hypoplasia—the LeFort II osteostomy. Plast Reconstr Surg 1973;11:77-93.

75. Chin M, Toth BA: Le Fort III advancement with gradual distraction using internal devices. Plast Reconstr Surg 1997;100:819-830.

76. Fearon J, Whittaker L: Complications with facial advancement: a comparison between the LeFort III and monobloc advancements. Plast Reconstr Surg 1993;91:990-995.

77. Posnick J, al-Qattan M, Armstrong D: Monobloc and facial bipartition osteotomies for reconstruction of craniofacial malformations: a study of extra-dural dead space and morbidity. Plast Reconstr Surg 1996;97:1118-1128.

78. Ilizarov G, Deviatov A: Surgical lengthening of the shin with simultaneous correction of deformities. Ortop Travmatol Protez 1969;30:32-37.

79. Sugawara Y, Hirabayasai S, Sakurai A, Harii K: Gradual cranial vault expansion. The treatment of craniofacial synostosis: a preliminary report. Ann Plast Surg 1998;40:564-565.

80. Rinehart G, Forget T, Zografakis J, et al: Cranial vault expansion using transcutaneously activated magnetic implants. Pediatr Neurosurg 1998;28:293-299.

81. Greensmith AL, Furneaux C, Rees M, de Chaloin T: Cranial compression by reverse distraction: a new technique for correction of sagittal synostosis. Plast Reconstr Surg 2001;108:979.

82. Hierl T, Kloppel R, Hemprich A: Midfacial distraction osteogenesis without major osteotomies: a report on the first clinical application. Plast Reconstr Surg 2001;108:1667-1672.

83. Tutino M, Chico F, Ortiz-Monasterio F: Endoscopic dissection of dura and craniotomy with minimal trephines: a preliminary study. J Craniofac Surg 1998;9:154.

84. Harrison M, Adzick N: The biology of fetal wound healing: a review. Plast Reconstr Surg 1991;87:788-798.

85. Stelnicki E, Vanderwall K, Harrison M, et al: The in utero correction of unilateral coronal craniosynostosis. Plast Reconstr Surg 1998;101:287-296.

86. Cutting C, Grayson B, McCarthy J, et al: A virtual reality system for bone fragment positioning in a multisegment craniofacial surgical procedure. Plast Reconstr Surg 1998;102:2436-2443.

87. Mulliken J, Steinberger D, Kunze S, Muller U: Molecular diagnosis of bilateral coronal synostosis. Plast Reconstr Surg 1999;104:1603-1615.

88. Levine J, Bradley J, Roth D, et al: Studies in cranial suture biology: regional dura mater determines overlying sutural biology. Plast Reconstr Surg 1998;101:1441-1447.

89. Roth D, Longaker M, McCarthy J, et al: Studies in cranial suture biology. Part I. Increased immunoreactivity for TGF-beta isoforms (beta 1, beta 2, and beta 3) during rat cranial suture fusion. J Bone Miner Res 1997;12:311-321.

90. Opperman L, Chahabra A, Cho R, Ogle R: Cranial suture obliteration is induced by removal of transforming growth factor beta 3 activity and prevented by removal of TGF-beta 2 activity from fetal rat calvaria in vitro. J Craniofac Genet Dev Biol 1999;19:164-173.

91. Whitaker L, Bartlett S, Schut L, Bruce D: Craniosynostosis: an analysis of the timing, treatment and complications in 164 consecutive patients. Plast Reconstr Surg 1987;80:195-212.

92. Williams J, Cohen S, Burstein F, et al: A longitudinal statistical study of reoperation rates in craniosynostosis. Plast Reconstr Surg 1997;100:305-310.

93. Fearon J, Uyu J, Bartlett S, et al: Infections in craniofacial surgery: a combined report of 567 procedures from two centers. Plast Reconstr Surg 1997;100:862-868.

94. Poole M: Complications in craniofacial surgery. Br J Plast Surg 1988;41:608-613.

95. Jones B, Jani P, Bingham R, et al: Complications in pediatric craniofacial surgery: an initial four year experience. Br J Plast Surg 1992;45:225-231.

96. Eaton A, Marsh J, Pilgram T: Transfusion requirements for craniosynostosis surgery in infants. Plast Reconstr Surg 1995;95:277-283.

Reconstruction: Craniofacial Syndromes

SCOTT P. BARTLETT, MD ✦ JOSEPH E. LOSEE, MD
✦ STEPHEN B. BAKER, DDS, MD

CRANIOFACIAL DYSOSTOSIS

Craniosynostosis can be classified as syndromic or non-syndromic. Patients with nonsyndromic synostosis, also referred to as isolated or simple craniosynostosis, usually have a much better prognosis with regard to surgical outcome. Most of these patients usually require only one early major transcranial operation to obtain a satisfactory correction of the facial dysmorphism.[1-3] Patients with syndromic disease, in contrast, typically require multiple operations during their growth and development.

Patients with syndromic craniosynostosis are said to have craniofacial dysostosis; this implies abnormal craniofacial skeletal development in which synostosis is a component as well as the less understood associated bone dysgenesis. Those with limb anomalies are additionally given the name acrocephalosyndactyly. These patients most often have bicoronal synostosis associated with skull base and midface sutural synostosis or a poorly understood midface growth arrest. However, virtually any premature sutural closure pattern may be seen in these patients, including pancraniosynostosis. The most common syndromes of craniofacial dysostosis or acrocephalosyndactyly include Apert, Crouzon, Carpenter, Saethre-Chotzen, and Pfeiffer syndromes; their distinguishing characteristics are discussed elsewhere in this text. These children have an incompletely understood anomaly of the cranial base synchondroses and facial sutures; turri-brachycephaly and midface hypoplasia often develop despite early surgical release and recontouring that

provides an aesthetically acceptable result.[2,4-9] This implies that the surgical correction is a temporizing or compensatory maneuver for patients in whom the pathophysiologic process behind the deformity is poorly understood.[8]

Dysmorphology

The turribrachycephalic skull is shortened in the anterior-posterior dimension, widened in the medial-lateral dimension, and vertically elongated (Fig. 102-1). The anterior cranial base is shortened; the supraorbital rims are hypoplastic and retruded posterior to the cornea. The superior frontal and squamous temporal bones are protuberant, and this adds to the wide transverse dimension seen as a biparietal convexity (Fig. 102-2). The occiput is flattened, with or without associated lambdoid synostosis, compounding the brachycephaly. The upper frontal bones and forehead bulge as the growing brain attempts to expand through the anterior fontanel and adjacent sagittal and metopic sutures. There is associated symmetric hypoplasia of the orbits, zygomaticomaxillary complex, and maxillae. This midface and cranial base hypoplasia leads to exorbitism and a flattening or concavity of the face with a class III malocclusion, anterior open bite, and upper airway compromise (Fig. 102-3). Associated periocular anomalies may include upper lid ptosis with varying degrees of lateral canthal dystopia. Mild to moderate degrees of orbital hypertelorism may also be seen.

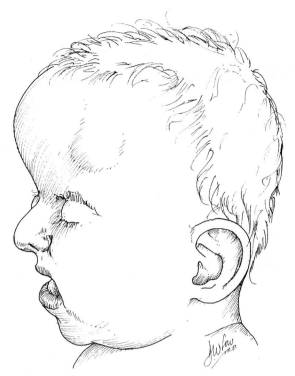

FIGURE 102-1. Lateral view of turribrachycephaly.

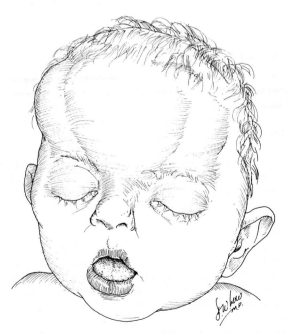

FIGURE 102-2. Anteroposterior view of turribrachy-cephaly.

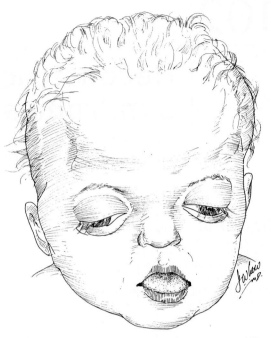

FIGURE 102-3. Anteroposterior view of midface hypoplasia and exorbitism.

Functional Considerations

The functional indications for surgical correction in craniofacial dysostoses are often more significant than those for simple craniosynostoses. When more than one cranial suture is involved and there is a deficiency of midface growth, intracranial volume may be compromised, leading to secondary growth restriction of the brain and an increased incidence of intracranial hypertension.[4,10] Elevated intracranial pressure is the most important functional consideration because of the sequelae of brain dysfunction and visual compromise.[11,12] Renier[12] reported that 42% of untreated children with more than one involved suture and 14% of those with single-suture fusion will demonstrate elevations in intracranial pressure greater than 15 mm Hg.

An increased incidence of hydrocephalus, from 10% to 42%, has also been reported in children with syndromic craniofacial dysostoses.[13-15] Although the hydrocephalus may be due to venous congestion as a result of the cranial base constriction, the etiology is often unclear. Hydrocephalus may respond to vault expansion in some individuals, but in the majority, management by ventriculoperitoneal shunting is the rule. Failure of anteroposterior growth of the orbits from vault and cranial base suture synostosis (and poorly understood cranial base growth restriction) frequently leads to shallow orbits with exorbitism and canthal malposition. The resultant incomplete eyelid closure may lead to exposure keratopathy, corneal ulceration, and even blindness.[16]

In addition to affecting the brain and eye, these syndromes frequently cause respiratory compromise that requires early recognition and treatment to prevent cardiopulmonary and neurologic sequelae.[17] The reported incidence of airway obstruction in syndromic craniosynostosis ranges from 40% to 100%.[18-20] It has been described as a dynamic multilevel airway obstruction that changes in severity with growth.[17] A compromised airway results from reduced nasopharyngeal dimensions; anterior or posterior choanal atresia; decreased pharyngeal height, width, and depth; long and thickened soft palate with abnormal mucopolysaccharide collections; large adenotonsillar lymphoid ring; shortened cranial base with a more acute cranial base angle; and retruded mandible.[17,21,22] A significant portion of these children will additionally have lower airway anomalies that include tracheomalacia, complete cartilaginous tracheas, and granulations.[18-20] Airway obstruction and hypoxia during sleep may present as snoring, mouth breathing, sweating during sleep, noisy respirations, apneic episodes, paradoxical chest movements, persistent restlessness, feeding difficulties, failure to thrive, hypertension, daytime fatigue, and cardiopulmonary or neurologic impairment.[18,23] Even patients with severe respiratory obstruction often do not present to the physician with obvious breathing difficulties while they are awake. It is only during sleep that breathing difficulties become evident. It has been reported that during rapid eye movement sleep, the supporting muscles of the upper airway undergo a decrease in tone, making it vulnerable to collapse.[24] This collapse results in an increase in airway resistance, and this, superimposed on anatomically anomalous and narrowed airways, produces respiratory compromise and obstruction. Complications of persistent airway obstruction include respiratory infections, cor pulmonale, neurologic dysfunction, and brain damage.[18]

Evaluation and Monitoring

The standard of care for children with craniosynostosis resides with the multidisciplinary craniofacial team. The child is evaluated by each of the team members, including geneticist, developmental pediatrician, speech pathologist, ophthalmologist, pediatric dentist, and orthodontist, to name a few, and a comprehensive plan of treatment is formulated and continually revised. With a craniofacial team evaluation, each child undergoes a complete physical examination by the team pediatrician. When appropriate, three-dimensional computed tomographic imaging, cephalograms, magnetic resonance scans, surface anthropometry, preoperative laboratory tests, 8 × 10 black and white photographs, and dental models and splints are obtained and are critical for treatment planning.

The team geneticist is responsible for syndrome clarification. A complete family history, thorough clinical examination, chromosomal analysis, and directed genetic testing (i.e., *TWIST* gene, fibroblast growth factor receptor analysis) are tools used. In addition, the geneticist can assist with issues surrounding family planning, both for the parents and, in the future, for the patient.

The pediatric otolaryngologist performs a formal multilevel evaluation of the airway to diagnose any airway anomalies. Routine studies to assess respiratory function in children with syndromic craniosynostosis demonstrate frequent problems with obstruction that range from mild upper airway obstruction to severe obstructive sleep apnea.[24] The respiratory system can be evaluated by oxygen saturation, 12-lead polysomnography, endoscopy, plain radiography or cephalography, computed tomography or magnetic resonance imaging, and fluoroscopy.[18,23,25]

The pediatric ophthalmologist must monitor for exposure issues, strabismus, and exotropia. A thorough ophthalmoscopic examination for papilledema and later optic atrophy is performed. Reduction of globe herniation with orbital decompression and tarsorrhaphies may be required.

The team pediatric neurosurgeon is responsible for a thorough neurologic evaluation and interpretation of the results of diagnostic studies (computed tomography and magnetic resonance imaging). They are needed to define those infants at risk for hydrocephalus and associated anomalies found in these syndromic children, for example, cranial base–cervical spine anomalies, Chiari malformations, and brain dysmorphism.

The pediatric dentist and orthodontist routinely observe these children closely to monitor and treat the inevitable issues surrounding oral hygiene and malocclusion. In addition, they assist in the preparation and the preoperative planning for procedures aimed at the correction of dentofacial disharmony.

Treatment

The surgical treatment of children with craniofacial dysostosis is one of the more controversial issues in craniofacial surgery. Despite the multiple proposed treatment philosophies, the indications, timing, type, and effectiveness of reconstruction continue to be debated.[4,5,7,10,26-28] Most agree that the goal of surgical correction, in addition to obtaining craniofacial symmetry, proportionality, and balance, is the prevention of recurrent deformities, especially turribrachycephaly.[2-7] It has been written that the postoperative turribrachycephalic cranial vault deformity, observed in many centers, awaits a solution.[15] Experienced surgeons agree, "the problem is notoriously difficult to correct and often requires multiple surgical interventions, which may still not correct the deformity."[8] It has been reported that 35% to 95% of children with syndromic craniosynostosis will require more than one major secondary procedure.[15,29] Permanent correction of the brachycephalic skull by a single subtotal craniectomy and fronto-orbital advancement in infancy is rarely achieved because the progression of the deformity is only temporarily interrupted.[30,31] Despite accomplishment of the limited goal of initial normalization, the infant skull will rarely continue to remain normal as it resumes its abnormal growth pattern, and it will remain wide and acrocephalic whether it has been surgically remodeled or not.[22,30,32,33]

The following text discusses the three most commonly accepted treatment regimens proposed for children with craniofacial dysostoses: the staged approach, total cranial vault remodeling, and posterior followed by anterior vault remodeling.

STAGED APPROACH

This treatment protocol, or a similar version, is the most frequently adopted regimen among craniofacial centers today and is the authors' standard approach to syndromic children with craniofacial dysostosis.[1,3,4,15] Therefore, most of the discussion and detail involves this protocol. The staged approach is performed at intervals coinciding with facial growth, visceral function, and social development.[4]

In the neonatal period and throughout the life of the patient, the functional aspects of care are evaluated and treated as they arise. The airway is evaluated for multilevel disease; if it is necessary to sustain life, a tracheostomy is performed, or an argument is made for early fronto-facial advancement (see discussion that follows).[3] Nutritional issues are infrequently severe enough to necessitate permanent alternative enteral feeding, but if necessary, a gastrostomy is performed. Hydrocephalus, if it is present, is treated with a shunt procedure. If exorbitism is severe, steps are taken to prevent the sequelae of exposure; these include the routine use of lubricants and possible tarsorrhaphy. If multisutural synostosis leads to elevations in intracranial pressure, temporizing early strip craniectomies should be performed in the first months of life. Frontal remodeling and fronto-orbital advancements before 6 months of age may make the patient susceptible to relapse or loss of advancement and, possibly, the early need for repeated cranial vault reshaping.[4] This philosophy of care is not held by all, and some advocate early cranioplasty.[3] If this situation arises, an alternative may be to employ the third protocol to be discussed—posterior followed by anterior cranial vault remodeling.

At 6 to 10 months of age, a formal suture release by frontal cranial vault remodeling and fronto-orbital advancement is performed (Fig. 102-4). A version of the floating forehead technique of fronto-orbital advancement is preferred.[34] The goals of this surgical correction are to increase cranial vault volume, to increase the depth of the orbits, to decrease the

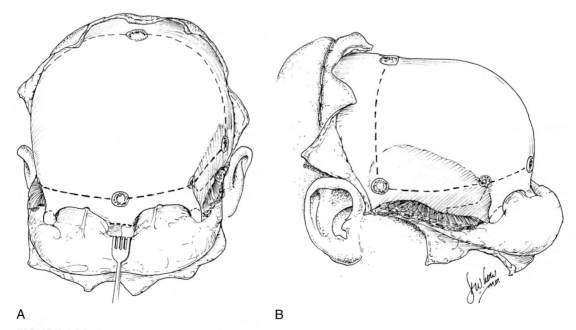

A   B

FIGURE 102-4. *A and B,* Fronto-orbital advancement.

bitemporal width of the cranial base, to increase the anteroposterior length of the skull and cranial base, and to decrease the vertical projection of the cranial vault—correct the turribrachycephaly.

The child is positioned supine with the head placed on a supportive gel ring. The child is orally intubated, if possible, and the anesthesia monitoring devices are placed. A minimum of two peripheral large-bore intravenous catheters are established, along with an arterial line for the continuous monitoring of the blood pressure. A central venous catheter is placed if there is particular concern about air embolus, and a urinary catheter and warming devices are placed. Blood for transfusion should be available and in the operating room. A self-adherent plastic drape is placed over the bridge of the nose and cheeks, down to the ears, separating the oral and nasal cavity from the operative field. The eyes are lubricated and monitored frequently. The head is shaved, a "stealth" zigzag coronal incision is planned, and the proposed incision and forehead are injected with an epinephrine solution. The head is prepared and draped. The incision is made, and the coronal flap is elevated in the subgaleal plane. Just above the supraorbital rims, the subperiosteal dissection is begun. The temporal muscles are dissected out bilaterally. A subperiosteal dissection of the upper two thirds of each orbit is performed. A bifrontal craniotomy is planned, starting 1 cm above the supraorbital rims. At this time, the neurosurgical team takes over, and if possible, a single-piece bifrontal craniotomy is performed. The anterior cranial base and temporal fossae are then epidurally dissected to allow the safe retraction of the frontal and temporal lobes of the brain when the bandeau osteotomy is performed. At this time, the plastic surgical team resumes the operation.

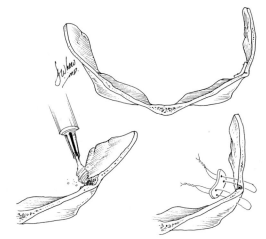

FIGURE 102-6. Cranioplasty of the bandeau osteotomy at the zygomaticofrontal suture.

A standard bandeau osteotomy with temporal tongue-in-groove extensions is performed (Fig. 102-5). The osteotomy is started temporally and continues to the lateral orbital rim. The anterior cranial base (orbital roof) is then osteotomized with a saw, placed intracranially, beginning laterally at the sphenoid wing and coursing toward the nasion. An osteotome is placed intracranially at the sphenoid wing and driven down the lateral orbital wall, completely freeing the bandeau. Malleable retractors are positioned to protect the frontal and temporal lobes and the globe while the osteotomies are performed.

The bandeau is taken to the side table and fashioned (Fig. 102-6). At the new junction of the frontal and temporal segments of the bandeau, an endocranial kerf is made with a contouring burr. The outer cortex is greenstick fractured at the new angle to decrease the bitemporal width, and this is held in place with wires and resorbable plates. At this point, some have advocated bilateral excision of the temporal bones that produce the abnormally wide and convex temporal fossa, inverting and replacing them in a concave versus convex position to correct the widened bitemporal distance.[34] The bandeau osteotomy is replaced in an advanced position (10 to 20 mm) and rigidly fixed in place with a combination of wire and resorbable plate fixation. As a benefit of "rigid fixation," bone grafts at the advanced nasofrontal junction, lateral orbital wall, and temporal fossa are optional and not routinely used. The bifrontal osteotomy flap is then contoured with bone bending forceps, partially osteotomized as necessary, and replaced orthotopically in an advanced position to meet the newly positioned bandeau osteotomy. On occasion, to allow desirable forehead contouring, the bifrontal osteotomy bone flap is sectioned in two pieces,

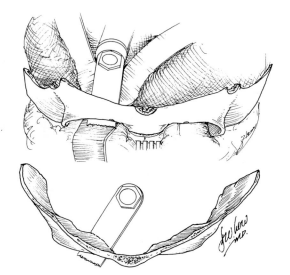

FIGURE 102-5. Bandeau osteotomy.

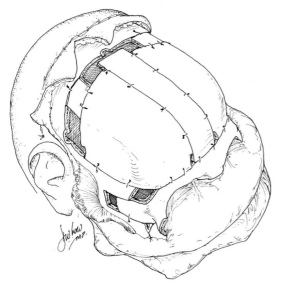

FIGURE 102-7. Completed bone reconstruction of fronto-orbital advancement.

fashioned, replaced in a new orientation by switching the segments or rotating them, and affixed (Fig. 102-7). The temporal muscles are then back-cut and advanced anteriorly to meet the newly advanced bandeau osteotomy and resuspended. The coronal flap is then closed in layers over a drain, with care taken to repair the galeal occipitofrontal aponeurosis.

In childhood, repeated cranial decompression and vault reshaping may be necessary to correct significant visible deformity or if increased intracranial pressure is suspected. This procedure is aimed at the specific portion of the cranial vault that needs expansion. By the age of 5 to 7 years, the cranial vault and orbits have attained approximately 85% to 90% of the adult size. The maxilla has grown to where the secondary teeth have migrated inferiorly. The frontal sinus is still minimally developed and therefore may decrease the incidence of infection. It is at this time that psychosocial issues with peers and schooling develop. It is also when correction of midface hypoplasia is considered. There is no one routine procedure that is employed. Each deformity is evaluated and a tailored approach to surgical correction devised. Midface procedures improve but rarely idealize the occlusion at this stage because growth and development are unpredictable. These children often have class III anterior open bites that are difficult to correct when orbital morphologic appearance is simultaneously adjusted by a monobloc frontofacial advancement; to obtain a normal occlusion, an overcorrection of the orbits may be required and result in an undesirable aesthetic. Many of these children will require orthognathic surgery at skeletal maturity to idealize the mature occlusion. Each child

is evaluated and categorized by the relation of the brow or supraorbital rim, orbits, and midface.

The first type of patient has adequate upper orbital volume with an adequately positioned supraorbital rim that represents an adequate depth of the anterior cranial base. If there is no orbital hypertelorism, a subcranial Le Fort III osteotomy with possible midface distraction is the advancement of choice (Fig. 102-8). A coronal incision is made, and the orbits are circumferentially dissected subperiosteally. The zygoma is divided where the arch joins the eminence. The osteotomy is started with orbital cuts beginning at the zygomaticofrontal suture and down through the lateral orbital wall to the inferior orbital fissure. An osteotomy is then made at the nasofrontal junction, with care taken to avoid the cribriform plate for this structure may be inferiorly displaced in syndromic children. Medial orbital wall osteotomies are started, from the nasion cut, down the medial wall of the orbit and posterior to the identified and protected medial canthal ligament and lacrimal apparatus. These important structures should be undisturbed and advanced with the Le Fort III segment. The orbital floor is then osteotomized with a fine osteotome to connect the medial wall cut to the inferior orbital fissure. An osteotome is then placed into the pterygomaxillary fissure from the coronal approach, and gentle taps separate the maxillary tuberosities from the pterygoid plates. The soft tissues of the retrotuberosity area are digitally released, thus completing the pterygomaxillary disjunction. The disimpaction forceps are placed, and the Le Fort III segment is downfractured. Care is taken because the infraorbital rims are always

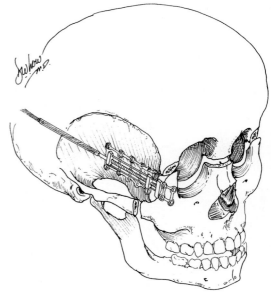

FIGURE 102-8. Subcranial Le Fort III osteotomy.

hypoplastic in these syndromic children and are susceptible to fracture. Fractures must be evaluated for and plated if encountered. If a distraction is to be performed, the buried distractors are now placed.[35,36] If a standard osteotomy is to be performed, the midface is advanced and placed in an occlusal wafer with maxillomandibular fixation. Cranial bone grafts are then placed at the zygomatic arch, lateral orbital wall, posterior maxillary tuberosity, and nasion. Lateral canthopexies and temporal muscle advancements and resuspensions are performed; the incision is closed.

The second type of patient presents with a deficient brow and supraorbital rim indicating deficient anterior cranial base. This, in addition to deficiency of the nose, lower orbits, zygoma, and maxillae, makes these patients candidates for a monobloc frontofacial advancement (Fig. 102-9). A monobloc midface advancement is performed by making a standard bifrontal osteotomy and an intracranial Le Fort III osteotomy. If only the Le Fort III osteotomy is performed in these children, an inadequate correction with excessive lengthening of the nose and flattening of the nasofrontal angle occurs. Concern has been raised about the increased incidence of devastating intracranial infection with the monobloc osteotomy because extradural dead space and an aerocele exist in direct communication with the nasal passages.[3,7,37-40] The reported advantage of distraction osteogenesis when a monobloc advancement is performed is that the large dead space is not formed, and with gradual distraction, the extradural dead space is slowly obliterated by the expanding intracranial contents.[41]

The third type of patient typically has a deficient anterior cranial base, supraorbital rim, and brow in addition to orbital hypertelorism. These dysmorphic features are often seen in children with Apert syndrome. These patients can benefit from a facial bipartition procedure (Fig. 102-10). The facial bipartition osteotomy is performed by vertically splitting the monobloc osteotomy or Le Fort III osteotomy and shifting the facial halves medially to correct the horizontal excess.

The efficacy of midface advancement for the treatment of upper airway obstruction has been called into question because controversial data have been reported in the literature.[24,42] Midface advancement has been touted to be effective, resulting in significant improvement and excellent palliation; slightly effective; and ineffective.[17,20-22,43,44] Lauritzen in 1986 suggested that all severe craniofacial patients with breathing problems first be treated with tracheostomy because Le Fort III midface advancement was ineffective. This suggestion was made despite the author's comments that no definite conclusions about the effectiveness of the advancement could be made; furthermore, it was reported that the net forward shift of the midface advancement was too small, partly owing to inadequate retention. In the current era of rigid internal fixation and distraction osteogenesis, when greater advancements are obtained and maintained, serious question should be raised about this recommendation. Surgical advancement of the retruded midface may improve upper airway caliber, but it has been reported that the greatest success is achieved when midface advancement is performed after skeletal maturity.[42] Given the morbidity and mortality associated with infant tracheostomy, the possibility of surgically expanding the nasopharyngeal space with a midface advancement or distraction, without resorting to tracheostomy, is appealing.[23,45] Permanent tracheostomy represents a significant level of home or institutional care with negative psychosocial and communicative effects on the infant and family; complications may include stoma and subglottic narrowing, bronchitis and pneumonia, obstruction and accidental decannulation, and death.[25,46] Simply stated, tracheostomy places immense burden on care providers and threatens the quality of life for patient and family.[23] Temporizing methods for treatment of upper airway obstruction secondary to midface retrusion have been reported and include positioning, medical therapy, and nasal continuous positive airway pressure.[20,24] However, compliance with nasal continuous positive airway pressure is a problem, and initiation is a major difficulty. The treatment is time-consuming and requires considerable parental dedication. In addition, nasal continuous positive airway pressure is ineffective during periods of acute upper airway infection, which is more common in these children.

At the age of skeletal maturity, attention is turned to the occlusion and craniofacial aesthetics. At the age of 14 to 16 years for girls and 16 to 18 years for boys, orthognathic procedures directed at obtaining class I relations and optimizing facial aesthetics are entertained. A leveling Le Fort I osteotomy is often

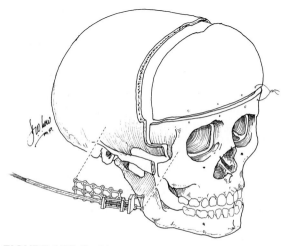

FIGURE 102-9. Monobloc frontofacial advancement.

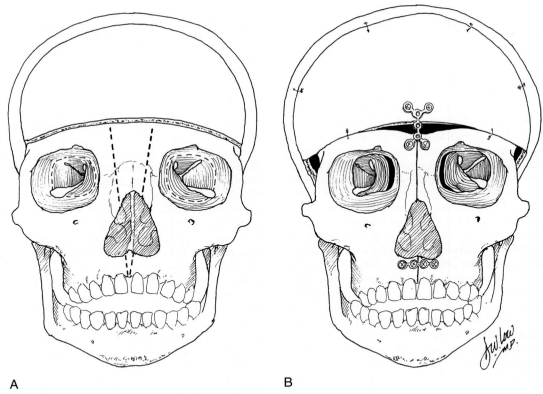

A   B

FIGURE 102-10. *A* and *B,* Facial bipartition procedure.

performed to correct the class III relation. This may be combined with bone graft augmentation of the midface or a genioplasty as the facial dysmorphism dictates. On occasion, a repeated midface advancement may be necessary to complete the reconstructive protocol.

Because of unpredictable growth and development, a subset of patients having undergone fronto-orbital advancement in infancy present with mild to moderate asymmetries of the forehead, temporal skull, and supraorbital rim. These deformities usually do not warrant repeated transcranial correction but often are appearance-related issues for young adults. These patients, in addition, have coronal scars that often were a straight line in design and have widened with growth and over time. At the time of early skeletal maturity, a potential tertiary reconstruction is performed and may include a coronal scar revision (converting the straight line into a zigzag with multiple Z-plasties) and cranioplasty with possible onlay bone grafts, contouring, and the use of bone paste cement.

TOTAL CRANIAL VAULT REMODELING

Persing and Jane[6] have proposed another treatment protocol for the child with bicoronal synostosis and the turribrachycephalic skull. Their expanded surgical procedure of total cranial vault remodeling reshapes the entire skull and enlarges its capacity, particularly posteriorly, allowing simultaneous reduction of height. Their technique of total cranial vault remodeling is modified according to the patient's age and whether the disease is syndromic.

The protocol suggested by Persing and Jane[6] for the syndromic infant younger than 1 year includes a perioperative evaluation that is essentially the same as that in other major centers. However, their approach necessitates the modified prone position (Fig. 102-11), and additional studies are required.[47] Plain radiographs of the skull and cervical spine are taken, including lateral flexion and extension films of the cervical spine, to assess the feasibility of intraoperative positioning in the modified prone position. The plain films are required to rule out craniovertebral anomalies or instabilities that put the patient at risk for spinal cord or brainstem trauma intraoperatively when the patient is placed in the modified prone position of neck hyperextension. Anomalies of the cervical spine have been reported in children with syndromic bicoronal synostosis.[48] The modified prone position is essential for this technique because it allows access to both the anterior and posterior portions of the cranial vault.

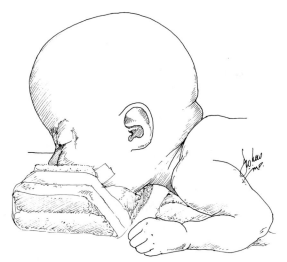

FIGURE 102-11. Modified prone position.

The child is placed prone in a padded headrest, which is the anterior segment of a Philadelphia collar. Cervical spine films are taken again to ensure safety of the spinal cord and brainstem.

The procedure begins with a coronal incision and supraperiosteal subgaleal dissection anteriorly to the supraorbital rims and posteriorly to the semispinalis capitis musculature. A subperiosteal dissection is started at 1 cm above the supraorbital rims and continued subperiorbitally throughout the superior and lateral orbit. Posteriorly, the occipital musculature is elevated subperiosteally to the level of the rim of the foramen magnum. The temporalis muscles are delivered out of the temporal fossa bilaterally. The cranial osteotomies (Fig. 102-12) are performed in such a way as to leave a strip of bone on the vertex adjacent to and protecting the sagittal sinus. Lateral extensions of parietal bone in continuity with this sagittal strip of bone extend from the vertex to the skull base. These bilateral bone extensions or struts left in situ connect the sagittal strip of bone to the skull base and serve as the mechanism to reduce the height of the skull. The bifrontal and biooccipital bone plates are removed as one piece each, and this is done to promote symmetry in the reconstruction. The occipital skull is expanded posteriorly to increase the anteroposterior dimension of the vault. As the height of the skull is reduced, the neurocranial capsule is displaced posteriorly. After the bifrontal and biparieto-occipital craniotomies, epidural dissection is performed posteriorly to a point just above the level of the foramen magnum. Barrel stave osteotomies are made vertically and parallel over the remaining basal parietal and occipital bones. The basal cranial bone is outfractured. The squamous portion of the temporal bone is osteotomized

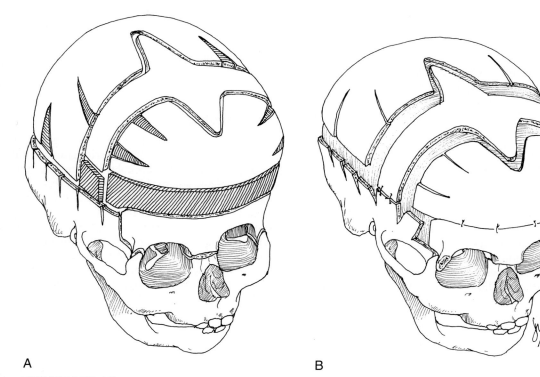

A   B

FIGURE 102-12. *A* and *B,* Total cranial vault reconstruction osteotomies.

and reshaped from a convex to a slightly concave form and rigidly fixed inside the rim of the remaining squamous portion of the temporal bone; this provides correction of and resistance to increased bitemporal width. A standard bandeau osteotomy with half Z-plasty at the zygomaticofrontal suture is performed, advanced, bone grafted at the glabella, and fixed with sutures. An intracranial pressure monitoring device is inserted into the subarachnoid space, and the parietal bone struts that extend from the sagittal strip of bone to the cranial base are cut inferiorly in the parietal region. The height of the skull is decreased as the vertex is shifted inferiorly and posteriorly. The average amount of skull height reduction is 1 to 1.5 cm, and this is done slowly and during the course of an hour while intracranial pressure is monitored. This is performed by placing wire loops through the osteotomized parietal bone struts and the skull base and slowly twisting the wires down. Intracranial pressure, cerebral perfusion pressure, normocapnia, and normotension must be monitored closely by the neurosurgical team. Once skull height reduction is achieved, the bifrontal and biparieto-occipital bone plates are fashioned, radially cut, and contoured. The frontal bone is secured to the supraorbital rim; the occipital bone is fixed to the underlying dura, leaving approximately 1 cm of gap between the barrel staves of the posterior skull base and the parieto-occipital bone flap. The incision is then routinely closed.

Although excellent results have been presented with use of this technique, the long-term follow-up and need for secondary interventions in these patients are unclear. Also, the operative procedure potentially poses a higher risk with regard to blood loss, positioning problems, and neurocranial capsule compression issues. In these very young patients, the authors have not used this protocol routinely except in patients with severe anteroposterior shortening and turricephaly.

POSTERIOR FOLLOWED BY ANTERIOR VAULT REMODELING

This approach of staged posterior followed by anterior vault remodeling is yet another protocol that has been routinely used in children with syndromic craniofacial dysostosis to correct the turribrachycephaly. In unique situations, this approach has been chosen by teams who routinely use one of the preceding protocols. Those who routinely use the staged approach and perform an anterior vault remodeling with fronto-orbital advancement at 6 to 10 months of age may first expand the posterior skull earlier in life (3 to 6 months of age) if increased intracranial pressure or severe progressive turribrachycephaly forces the issue. Those promoting a single-stage total cranial vault remodeling may be forced to adopt the two-stage procedure when craniovertebral anomalies preclude safe positioning in the modified prone position.[6]

The rationale for operating on the posterior vault first is related to the stability of the correction. It is not recommended to commit to early fronto-orbital advancement (age 3 months) when the bone is thin and stabilization may be less adequate and allow relapse over time (which would affect frontal aesthetics). Rather, the posterior vault is expanded, accepting that if relapse occurs in this region, it is less problematic.

TREACHER COLLINS SYNDROME

Treacher Collins syndrome (TCS) is also known as mandibulofacial dysostosis and Franceschetti-Klein syndrome. In 1900, Edward Treacher Collins, a British ophthalmologist, described two patients with TCS, noting the lower eyelid and malar deformities.[49] Even though Treacher Collins was not the first to describe this anomaly, his name became associated with the syndrome.

Franceschetti, Klein, and Zwahlen in 1944 and again in 1949 reported on the defects of the syndrome and first used the term mandibulofacial dysostosis.[50,51] Tessier,[52] in 1969, described TCS as the expression of bilateral 6, 7, and 8 craniofacial clefts. The absent zygoma is the result of the combination of these three clefts. The number 6 cleft represents the defect between the maxilla and zygomatic bone, opening the infraorbital fissure; it also accounts for the eyelid coloboma. The number 7 temporozygomatic cleft results in the ear and oral malformations along with the absence of the zygomatic arch. The number 8 cleft is expressed at the frontozygomatic suture.

Dysmorphology

The cranial base in patients with TCS is generally shorter in all dimensions.[53] The anterior cranial vault is diminished in both bitemporal width and anterior-posterior cephalic length.[54] Franceschetti[50] described the facial profile of patients with TCS as fish-like or bird-like (Fig. 102-13). This angle of facial convexity is due to the severe mandibular retrognathia, the steep mandibular plane angle, and the prominent nasal dorsum. Anterior facial height is often deceptively long because of the anterior open bite, with a normal upper facial height (N-ANS). Posterior facial height is markedly shorter, with a reduced vertical dimension of the posterior choanae.[53] The angle between the S-N plane (anterior cranial base) and the palatal plane is more obtuse than normal.

A hypoplastic or absent zygoma is the most characteristic finding or "central event" in TCS (Fig. 102-14).[54-56] This may vary from a partial clefting to total

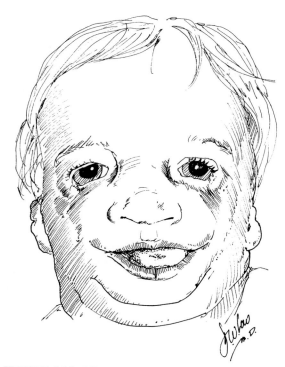

FIGURE 102-13. Treacher Collins syndrome facies.

absence of the zygomaticomaxillary complex. The hypoplastic zygoma may be limited to a small spine attached to the sphenoid tubercle and project forward from the glenoid fossa without any connection to the maxilla, frontal bone, or temporal bone.

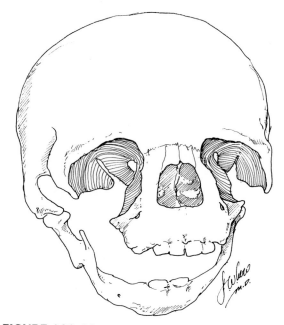

FIGURE 102-14. Skeletal dysmorphology.

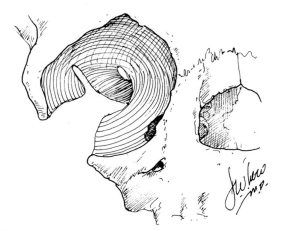

FIGURE 102-15. Orbital dysmorphology.

The orbit is egg shaped; its base is located superomedially, and its axis is oriented inferolaterally (Fig. 102-15).[57] The frontal bone is deformed as evidenced by an overhanging supraorbital rim. The hypoplastic orbital floor is clefted inferolaterally, and this opens directly into an enlarged inferior orbital fissure. This cleft allows the orbital contents to herniate or prolapse into this defect, directly from the orbital cavity to the cheek.[58] The inferior orbital rim is also hypoplastic. The portion of the orbit normally made up by the malar bone, the lateral wall and floor, is undeveloped or absent, and this allows the sphenoid bone to form the lateral orbital rim. This abnormal anatomy results in a decreased lateral wall length and abnormal palpebral fissure and canthal position.

The maxilla is protrusive and overprojected (see Fig. 102-14), deficient in width and posterior height. The maxilla is anteriorly positioned with a high and narrow palate. An occasional posterior cleft is found. The palatal plane is rotated clockwise or upward posteriorly.

The mandible is often micrognathic, having a reduced ramus and body length (Fig. 102-16). In addition, the condyle is often hypoplastic or missing. The lower border of the mandible is uniquely different in patients with TCS.[53] The gonial angle is markedly obtuse with a concave antegonial notch. This "peculiar broad curvature" of the mandible is a distinguishing feature of the syndrome.[57] The chin is retrusive and vertically long and points backward. The hypoplastic mandible can contain all of the normal components. However, any range of deformity can be found, even the occasional mandible lacking the glenoid fossa-temporomandibular joint-ramus complex, corresponding to the type III mandible of hemifacial microsomia.[59] Angle class II malocclusion with an anterior open bite is usually found; however, Angle class III malocclusion has been described. The increased

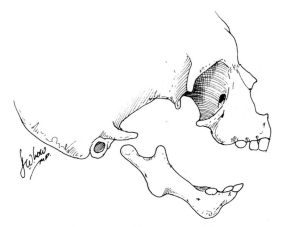

FIGURE 102-16. Mandibular dysmorphology.

lower face height and decreased posterior face height result in a steep mandibular plane angle and an excessively steep clockwise rotation of the occlusal plane.

Colobomas or pseudocolobomas of the lower eyelid are routinely found and are pathognomonic for TCS (Fig. 102-17).[60-62] The medial two thirds of the lower lid is absent of cilia. The inferolateral orbital dystopia results in a classic obliquity and antimongolian slant to the palpebral fissure. The dystopic lateral canthus is without insertion, therefore resulting in a shortened palpebral fissure length (see Fig. 102-15). The eye is often protruding and may herniate with the orbital

contents through the lateral orbital cleft and into the inferior orbital fissure. On occasion, coloboma of the iris, amblyopia and vision loss, strabismus, orbital lipodermoids, cataracts, papillary ectopia, distichiasis, and uveal coloboma have been reported.[63,64] In the most severe forms, true ablepharia with tarsal aplasia, absence of the lacrimal puncta, microphthalmos, and anophthalmos have been found.[57,64]

The cheek and temporal region frequently have long and tongue-shaped sideburns that are often anteriorly displaced and extend into the preauricular region. These are associated with a vertical cheek furrow, oriented in the direction of the corner of the mouth, which is the soft tissue accompaniment of the bony Tessier clefting.[57,58] This soft tissue clefting, along with some element of macrostomia, results in the classic abnormal smile of a child with TCS. Hypoplastic or absent parotid and salivary glands have been reported.[63] The skin of the neck and chin has been described as tight, and the musculoaponeurotic system and subcutaneous tissues are hypoplastic.[55] A fused temporalis, masseter, and pterygoid muscle is found, and this emphasizes the lack of separation between the orbital cavity and temporal and infratemporal fossae (Fig. 102-18).

The external ear, external auditory canal, tympanic membrane, and middle ear space have bilateral and relatively symmetric abnormalities. The external ear is often malformed, malpositioned, or absent. Microtia has been reported to be as high as 85%.[65] The external auditory canals have been reported to be bilaterally stenotic (54%) or atretic (31%).[66] The presence of an external auditory meatus does not mean that middle ear structures will be normal, for most middle ear cavities are bilaterally hypoplastic and dysmorphic, sometimes represented only by a small bony cleft.[65,66] The ossicles are often missing and when present are symmetrically dysmorphic and fused; however, the

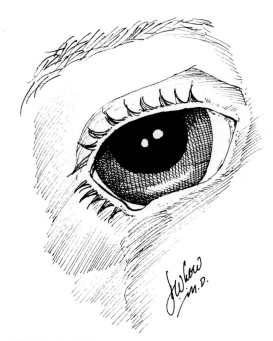

FIGURE 102-17. Lower lid dysmorphology.

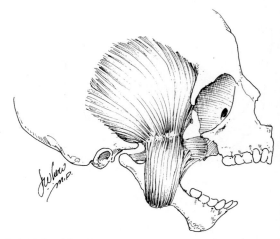

FIGURE 102-18. Musculoaponeurotic dysmorphology.

inner ear is essentially normal.[65-67] The majority of patients (96%) have a unilateral or bilateral moderate or greater degree of hearing loss.[54,66] This hearing loss is conductive but may also have a neurosensory component.[66,67]

In a detailed evaluation, it was found that the nose is the only facial feature more or less normal.[68] The soft tissue measurements as well as the height and width of the nose are satisfactory. The nasal root is often wide and deep, the bridge of the nose mild to moderately wide, and the nasal tip drooping with reduced projection. The nasofrontal angle is often obtuse, and the nasolabial angle is often optimal. The nasal dorsum, on profile, is prominent, and a mid-dorsal hump is often found. This dorsal prominence is accentuated by the malar hypoplasia.

The pharynx is abnormal in its oral, nasal, and hypopharyngeal portions. Macrostomia is often present. Clefts of the palate, and infrequently of the lip, are found.[64] Flexible nasopharyngoscopy has demonstrated pharyngeal hypoplasia with dimensions of the pharynx and nasopharynx 50% smaller than normal.[63,69] A resulting glossoptosis, choanal atresia, and pharyngeal incompetence are common findings.[55,70] The combination of these findings accounts for the often severe degree of respiratory obstruction in these children.

Functional Considerations

For patients with TCS, evaluation of the pharyngeal space is of most concern, with adequacy of the airway given top priority. A combination of maxillary and mandibular hypoplasia, pharyngeal incompetence, choanal atresia or stenosis, and glossoptosis often results in obstruction of the airway. Historically, this situation has led to tracheostomy because sleep apnea and sudden infant death syndrome have been associated with TCS.[60,69,70] In addition to respiratory compromise, maintenance of adequate nutrition may become an issue. The abnormal jaw relations noted before, coexistent clefting in some, difficulty in obtaining labial and dental occlusion, and respiratory dysfunction may dictate the need for alternatives to oral alimentation.

Evaluation and Monitoring

All members of the craniofacial team need to evaluate the infant with TCS. A craniofacial computed tomographic scan with axial, true coronal, and three-dimensional views is needed for evaluation, documentation, and surgical planning.[71] A high-resolution scan of the temporal bone is the single most important study in the surgical otologic evaluation.[65] An experienced pediatric otolaryngologist and formal audiology testing are needed to allow early fitting of

hearing aids. The speech/swallow team is imperative for assistance in the development of communication skills. A pediatric neuro-ophthalmologic assessment to evaluate lid and extraocular muscle function, corneal exposure issues, and visual acuity is useful. Family meetings with the team's geneticist, social worker, and family liaison for the establishment of support networks have proved to be of great value.[54] The compromised respiratory and nutritional reserves often result in a short body stature. However, most children with TCS are of normal intelligence; only 5% of patients are mentally challenged.[63,64] Behavior and intelligence have been documented to improve after successful treatment for sleep apnea.[60]

Treatment

There is much controversy and no clear consensus as to when reconstruction of the patient with TCS should begin. Multiple protocols are published, each with its supporting rationale.[52,54,55,57,60,69,72-74] As with some craniofacial anomalies, it can be argued that the longer one waits to correct the bone deformations, the better the long-term result will be, and ultimately fewer operations will be needed.[75] This must be balanced with the degree of psychological distress the patient and family suffers and the functional demands, such as respiratory or nutritional compromise.[76] The exceptions, of course, are early interventions, such as mandibular lengthening by distraction osteogenesis, performed to prevent tracheostomy and to allow oral alimentation. Tessier[58] has written that it is best to delay major reconstruction until the age of 6 to 10 years because resorption of bone grafts is more severe in TCS than in other malformations, and therefore considerable bone and cartilage are needed for these reconstructions. As with many craniofacial anomalies, most believe that a staged approach to reconstruction is most appropriate. Some procedures, such as mandibular distraction and ear reconstruction, are undertaken during infancy and childhood; others, such as bone reconstruction and orthognathic surgery, are deferred until late adolescence or early skeletal maturity when craniomaxillofacial growth is nearly complete.

Split rib and calvarial bone onlay grafts, full-thickness calvarial bone grafts, and vascularized calvarial osteoperiosteal and osteomuscular flaps have been proposed for bone reconstruction. Other substances including iliac and tibial bone, dermal fat grafts, and various alloplasts have been used with less success.

Controversy surrounds the issue of free calvarial versus vascularized calvarial bone. Those surgeons in favor of free or nonvascularized bone grafts quote studies reporting that rigidly fixed free split- and full-thickness cranial bone grafts can be successfully used for lasting reconstruction.[54,69,72,77] Vascularized pedicles making it impossible to preserve circulation and

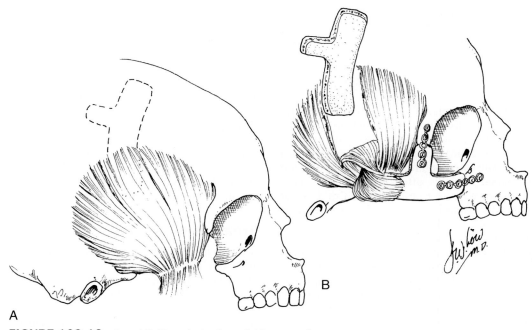

FIGURE 102-19. *A* and *B,* Vascularized cranial bone grafts.

fully contour the bone to match the defect, increases in surgical time, injury to the frontal branch of the facial nerve, and long-term results that differ little are further stated reasons not to use vascularized grafts.

Those in favor of vascularized calvarial bone flaps (Fig. 102-19) claim that free grafts have no growth potential and that the high rate of resorption necessitates multiple repeated operations, hence justifying the added complexity of the reconstruction.[54,78] An experimental study on the long-term remodeling of vascularized and nonvascularized bone grafts demonstrated that the vascularity of a bone graft significantly affects its long-term thickness and remodeling.[79] It concluded that continued bone deposition makes vascularized bone grafts better suited for the long-term maintenance of thickness and contour. Despite this, the majority of surgeons working in this area continue to use nonvascularized constructs.

The zygomatico-orbital complex is best approached and reconstructed by a coronal incision; the orbital floor can additionally be approached through the lower lid incision. These approaches allow the complete circumferential subperiosteal dissection of the orbit and periorbital skeleton. The prolapsed contents of the orbit are separated and retrieved from the inferior orbital fissure or cleft where they may commingle with the soft tissue of the temporal fossa. The inferior orbital fissure is then obliterated with bone grafts (Fig. 102-20A). The inferior and lateral orbital rims are then grafted with bone, and the overhanging superior orbital rim is either osteotomized and repositioned superiorly or contoured with a burr (Fig. 102-20B). The floor and lateral wall of the orbit are then grafted to fill the infraorbital angle, to elevate the orbital contents, and to restore continuity to an overcorrected point of mild

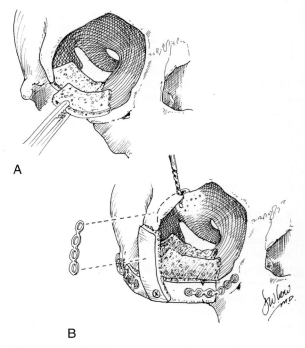

FIGURE 102-20. *A* and *B,* Orbital bone grafting.

exorbitism.[55,60] Bone grafts are best rigidly fixed with plates and screws and, in the young growing patient, absorbable hardware. A lateral canthopexy, to reorient the axis of the orbit and correct the lateral orbital dystopia, is then performed with a nonabsorbable suture or wire. Because postoperative inferior drift is expected, the lateral canthopexy is secured to the newly formed lateral orbital rim in an overcorrected position. In less severe instances of TCS in which there is sufficient soft tissue for adequate coverage, there may be a role for allograft augmentation of the zygomatic complex in lieu of bone grafts. Alternatively, after bone graft reconstruction of the midface and subsequent settling and resorption of the grafts, alloplastic malar augmentation should be entertained.

The degree of mandibular deformity will determine the treatment plan. Type I, IIA, and IIB mandibles (those with present but hypoplastic condyles and a functional albeit hypoplastic glenoid) do not need temporomandibular joint–ascending ramus construction and can be treated with standard osteotomies or distraction osteogenesis. Type III mandibles missing the ramus–temporomandibular joint–glenoid fossa unit require staged surgical construction. Stage 1 reconstruction consists of a costochondral rib graft undertaken during mixed dentition.[54] The glenoid fossa is addressed during the zygomatico-orbital reconstruction.

Mandibular distraction osteogenesis is also being integrated into the treatment protocol. Early distraction of the hypoplastic mandible, in infancy, is often effective in treating upper airway obstruction, preventing tracheostomy, or assisting in early decannulation.[80,81] For the older child, in the mixed dentition phase, distraction is used to bring the shortened posterior mandible down and forward, which theoretically will allow maxillary growth to follow. Whether these interceptive procedures will lessen the need for definitive orthognathic correction once skeletal maturity is achieved is unknown.

A definitive distraction of the mandible or orthognathic surgery is usually performed at early skeletal maturity. Bilateral sagittal split ramus osteotomies and sliding genioplasty in concert with a Le Fort I setback are usually performed.[54,69] The Le Fort I osteotomy is used to correct the vertical, horizontal, and transverse maxillary deformity and to allow rotation of the occlusal plane counterclockwise. It has been argued that no higher Le Fort osteotomy gives technical advantage or aesthetic improvement.[54] However, del Campo[72,82] has described the centrofacial flattening procedure (Fig. 102-21). This procedure employs nasomaxillary osteotomies to reduce the overprojection of the central face. Next, two linear and percutaneous osteotomies on each side of the pyramidal bases are made. The most anterior osteotomy is made just below the junction of the nasal bones and the maxil-

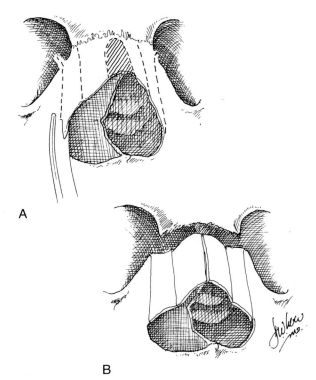

FIGURE 102-21. *A* and *B*, Centrofacial flattening procedure.

lae. The posterior osteotomy, starting at the piriform aperture and ending in the medial wall of the orbit, is made parallel to the first at the lowest limit of the centrofacial pyramidal structure where it joins the flat surface of the cheek. The bone segments are greenstick fractured back and in; this increases the size of the flat surface of the cheek and subsequently narrows the nose. Tessier has described the integral procedure (Fig. 102-22), which is reserved for patients with the most severe forms of TCS with respiratory compromise due to choanal atresia and micrognathia.[52,57,60,76] The integral procedure incorporates a Le Fort II osteotomy that is rotated counterclockwise. This midface rotation intrudes on the nasofrontal angle and impacts the segment into the nasofrontal junction. This results in a lowering of the maxillary tuberosities and opening of the choanae. The procedure is combined with a mandibular advancement and genioplasty. A study of 11 patients who underwent this surgery demonstrated a complete resolution of breathing problems in all subjects.[76]

The external microtic ear is reconstructed with the staged Brent repair by an experienced surgeon, and this technique is covered elsewhere in this text.[83] Although some of the hearing loss in children with TCS is secondary to external auditory canal stenosis,

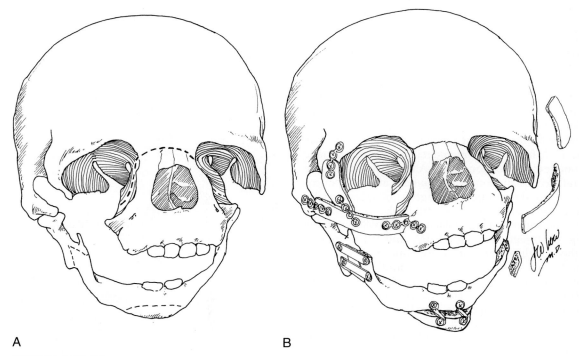

A   B

FIGURE 102-22. *A* and *B,* The integral procedure.

most is due to middle ear abnormalities, and attempt at surgery is generally unsuccessful in providing "non-aided" long-term hearing.[54] The net effect of the deranged middle ear architecture makes surgery for hearing rehabilitation difficult if not impossible.[65] Bone conduction hearing aids are routinely used for patients with TCS, and ever-increasing options for osseointegrated or bone-anchored conduction units are available.

The eyelid deformity is often the most challenging aspect of this anomaly to treat.[60] Posnick[54] has written that "despite several decades of well-intended surgical attempts to correct the soft tissue deficiencies of the eyelid-adnexal regions, few aesthetically pleasing soft tissue eyelid reconstructive results in patients with TCS have been reported." All procedures result in scarring of the lower lids that is noticeable and lessens the final result. However, the upper lid is usually not affected; this provides globe protection and allows correction of lower lid deformities after bone correction has provided a framework for soft tissue repair.[60,69,72] When the lower lid coloboma is a full-thickness defect, the type of reconstruction is dictated by the degree of deformity, and reconstruction must address all layers involved. Lesser coloboma of the lateral lid can be treated with excision of the lower lid lateral to the defect, with reattachment of the remaining medial lid to the lateral canthus and thus avoidance of any scar on the lower lid (Fig. 102-23). For

significant soft tissue deficiencies of the lower lid, a Z-plasty at the border of the coloboma and margin of the lid is required (Fig. 102-24).[57,58,72,74] The skin flaps are elevated from the underlying muscle, the orbital septum is released, and the tarsoconjunctiva is dissected free and sutured in the midline. The preseptal orbicularis is then advanced across the defect and sutured, and the skin flaps are transposed and closed. In patients with severe defects, additional tissue must be recruited. This has been performed in many different ways, including full-thickness skin grafts; slings of temporal muscle fascia, pericranium, or temporoparietal fascia to support the lower lid; bipedicled flaps from the upper lid; tarsoconjunctival flaps; and transpositional flaps from the upper lid (Fig. 102-25).[60] These techniques result in limited success, adnexal scarring, and an "operated on" appearance.[54,69] In addition to these lid reconstructive procedures, the lateral inferior canthal dystopia is corrected, and the axis of the orbit is reoriented with lateral canthopexies. These are performed after the orbital bone reconstruction, when wide undermining of the skeleton has been performed.

Nasal reconstruction is often performed around the time of orthognathic surgery. A rhinoplasty that includes osteotomies with infracture and a reduction of the skeletal and cartilaginous dorsal hump will help correct the central facial dysmorphism of TCS. In addition, standard rhinoplasty techniques, including

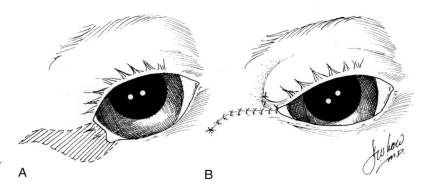

FIGURE 102-23. *A* and *B*, Excision of lower lid coloboma.

cephalic trim of the lower lateral cartilages and columellar strut for tip projection and definition, are usually indicated.[54]

The soft tissues of the cheek and face resulting from the Tessier 6, 7, and 8 clefts are hypoplastic and deficient. This often reveals the irregularities of the bone reconstruction. Dermal grafts, fat injection, free tissue transfer, and bilateral pericranial flaps rotated to cover the zygoma (Fig. 102-26) are options to provide bulk and cushion to soften the contour.[60,69,72]

PIERRE ROBIN SEQUENCE

The triad of glossoptosis, micrognathia, and airway obstruction characterizes Pierre Robin sequence.

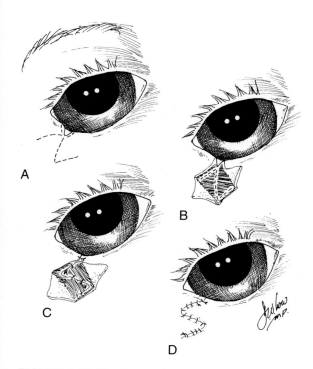

FIGURE 102-24. *A* to *D*, Lower lid Z-plasty.

Although cleft palate is not included in the triad, it is commonly associated with this disorder and may aggravate the obstruction. The reported incidence of the Robin sequence varies between 1 in 5000 and 1 in 50,000.

Several potential causes have been proposed for this disorder.[84] Reduced levels of amniotic fluid may not support the head in utero, and head flexion allows the chin to fall against the chest, impeding mandibular growth. Other causes of intrauterine constraint that cause head flexion will restrict mandibular growth in a similar manner. This type of retrognathia can occur in mandibles with normal intrinsic growth potential.

The triad of findings in Robin sequence is frequently associated with other syndromes. In fact, studies have shown that only 17% of Robin patients are nonsyndromic. Syndromes commonly associated with the Robin sequence include Stickler syndrome (34%), 22q11 deletion (15%), fetal alcohol syndrome (10%), Nager syndrome, Treacher Collins syndrome, and bilateral hemifacial microsomia.[85] In many of the syndromic patients, intrinsic growth deficiency of the mandible has been proposed as the etiology. Other potential causes for micrognathia include neuromuscular disorders of decreased tone leading to an intrauterine flexed head posture and some connective tissue disorders.[86] Although cleft palate is not part of the classic triad of anomalies associated with the Robin sequence, it is commonly associated with this disorder; the hypoplastic mandible pushes the tongue superiorly and prevents fusion of the palate.

Dysmorphology

At the initial evaluation, the anomalies of the Robin sequence may be the only findings present in a syndromic child. It is important to inform the parents that Pierre Robin sequence is merely a descriptive term that denotes the presence of glossoptosis, airway obstruction, and micrognathia. They must realize that in the majority of patients, this is an incomplete diagnosis, and as their child matures, other physical

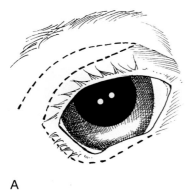
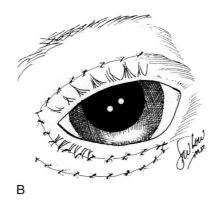

A   B

FIGURE 102-25. *A* and *B*, Lid-switch transpositional flap.

findings may become apparent that will clarify the presence of a specific syndrome.

In normal infants, the respiratory effort is relaxed, noiseless, and barely detectable. In patients with Robin sequence, airway obstruction occurs from the tongue's falling back against the airway. Negative pressure from deglutition and inspiration can impede forward positioning of the tongue, and an abnormal cranial base angulation may narrow the pharynx. Sher[87] has proposed that a compromised genioglossus may aggravate the obstruction. Cozzi and Pierro[88] found that the genioglossus demonstrated variability in muscle tone that could account for severe instances of obstruction with only mild micrognathia. In addition, they found a retrodisplaced mandibular attachment that made the genioglossus less effective in holding the tongue forward. Hotz[89] has proposed that impaction of the tongue in a palatal cleft will reposition the tongue in the airway, aggravating the degree of obstruction. All these factors, if present, increase the work of breathing. This increased respiratory effort is characterized by substernal, suprasternal, and intercostal retractions and results in increased energy expenditure.

Failure to thrive is observed in these patients and is a serious problem that requires supplemental enteric feeds. The physical exertion of breathing can exhaust the child to the point that it compromises the child's ability to feed. The extra work of breathing additionally requires that the child consume more calories to meet these demands. Dietary supplementation can be achieved with a nasoenteric feeding tube, but long-term feeding may require a gastrostomy tube.

The risk of aspiration is increased in patients suffering from airway obstruction. The negative

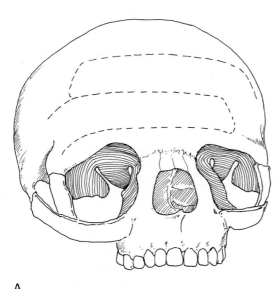
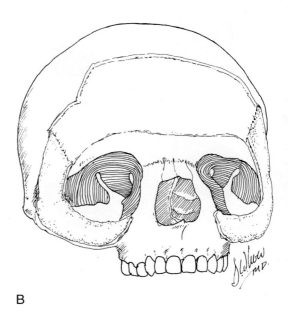

A   B

FIGURE 102-26. *A* and *B*, Pericranial flaps.

intrathoracic pressure generated from inspiration against an obstructed airway makes inspiration of gastric contents a constant hazard. Obstructed breathing can also cause the child to swallow air, which increases the risk of vomiting. Another adverse physiologic sequela of chronic airway obstruction is elevated pulmonary vascular resistance, which may lead to right-sided heart failure.[90]

The mortality associated with the Robin sequence varies from 5% to 30%. In nonsyndromic children with isolated Robin sequence, the mortality has been reported to be 5.9%. In syndromic patients with multiple anomalies, the mortality rises to 22.8%.[91]

Evaluation and Monitoring

On initial evaluation of a patient with micrognathia, it is important to evaluate the patient for glossoptosis and airway obstruction. If all three of these findings are present, the patient can be considered to have Pierre Robin sequence. However, it is important for the parents to realize that less than 20% of Robin patients are nonsyndromic, and the term Pierre Robin sequence is often a temporary label to describe respiratory and feeding problems associated with an undiagnosed syndrome. In the majority of the patients, the final diagnosis will depend on a subsequent evaluation.

The diagnosis of airway obstruction is made on physical examination, blood gas analysis, and thermistor studies. Observation of the infant is important in establishing a diagnosis of airway obstruction. Audible signs of infant apnea are often not present because snoring or stridor is rare. It is important to examine the patient in the supine position because the visual cues of obstruction are not seen when the infant is prone. In the supine position, the obstructing infant will demonstrate substernal, suprasternal, and intercostal retractions with chest wall movement, but one will not hear air movement. Because infants are obligate nose breathers, it is useful to use a stethoscope placed at the nares to listen for air exchange.

Blood gases can be useful in assessing the degree of hypoxia and hypercapnia associated with the obstruction. Obvious changes include carbon dioxide retention with a fall in pH and a compensatory elevation of serum bicarbonate. The serum bicarbonate concentration is more accurate than the PCO_2 to evaluate hypercapnia because crying that occurs with a heel stick can cause hyperventilation, which can rapidly remove carbon dioxide while the sample is being collected. Because the infant's skin can be pink with a PO_2 as low as 45 mm Hg, it may be deceptive as an indicator of hypoxia. Less invasive monitors such as pulse oximeters and apnea monitors are also useful in quantifying the number and severity of obstructive episodes.

Polysomnography has been used to differentiate between central and obstructive apnea. A nine-channel polysomnogram is typically recorded for 24 hours. A nasal thermistor, oral thermistor, and end-tidal carbon dioxide monitor document airflow. Thoracic and abdominal strain gauges record mechanical respiratory effort, and electromyography monitors phrenic nerve activity. Pulse oximetry, electrocardiography, and tachography are the last three recording channels of the polysomnogram. The results of polysomnography reveal central apnea if no muscle effort is associated with the apnea. In contrast, if muscle movement is detected in the absence of airflow, a diagnosis of obstructive apnea is made.

Poor weight gain is the other major morbidity associated with the Pierre Robin sequence. The respiratory efforts in these patients require an enormous energy expenditure that requires additional calorie intake. Unfortunately, the increased respiratory effort results in prolonged feeding times that tire the infant to the point of exhaustion and impair the ability to feed. Decreased calorie intake combined with increased energy expenditure compromises weight gain. Previous studies report that those feeding times of more than 45 minutes are too long and result in failure to thrive. Even marginal airways that allow normal breathing may not allow adequate feeding.

Treatment

Infants with isolated Pierre Robin sequence can often be effectively treated with positioning alone. Prone positioning allows gravity to keep the tongue forward and decreases the chance of its falling into the hypopharynx. There is also evidence that cervical extension may play a role in airway improvement.[92] If positioning is effective, it is usually maintained for 1 to 6 months to allow neuromuscular adaptation and mandibular growth. Although it has not been shown that complete catch-up growth of the mandible occurs, there is evidence of partial catch-up growth, which improves the severity of airway obstruction.

If positioning alone fails to relieve the obstruction, nasopharyngeal tube placement can be effective as a temporary measure. Commonly, an endotracheal tube with a 3.0- to 3.5-cm internal diameter is inserted into the nares until airflow is audible (approximately 8 cm). When the tube is past the choana, misting will be seen on the inside of the tube. The tube is taped at this depth; the end is trimmed, leaving about 2 cm protruding beyond the nares. A 15-mm adapter is attached to the end to prevent proximal migration and to facilitate suctioning. This tube serves as an effective bypass around the obstructed airway. Nasogastric feedings should begin, and after 7 to 14 days of gavage feedings, weight gain should be observed. The nasopharyngeal airway is removed to re-evaluate the severity of apnea; if obstruction persists, a nasoendoscopic evaluation is warranted. Complications of nasopharyngeal tubes include gagging, occlusion, malposition, and soft tissue injury.

Sher[87] evaluated 53 patients with Pierre Robin sequence and found that any patient who required a nasopharyngeal airway for more than 30 days would require surgery. However, only five patients went on to require surgery. It is unlikely that mandibular growth accounts for the fact that the majority of patients with Pierre Robin sequence in Sher's report were successfully treated with a short course of nasopharyngeal support. It was proposed that neurologic development is responsible for the rapid improvement in oropharyngeal function that occurs in the first few weeks of life.[92] This rate of neuromuscular adaptation varies between patients and would explain the different responses among infants treated with positioning and nasopharyngeal airways. The patients who do not demonstrate adequate oropharyngeal adaptation are the children who require surgical intervention.

All surgical procedures used for the treatment of Pierre Robin sequence have the potential for morbidity and should be avoided if conservative measures will provide successful treatment. However, if a surgical procedure is necessary for weight gain and relief of obstruction, it should not be delayed.[93] The difficulty is predicting which patients will require surgical intervention. Specific criteria for surgical intervention versus conservative therapy have been reported (Table 102-1).[94,95] Conservative management is recommended for infants demonstrating improvements in weight gain, strength, and tongue coordination. Surgical treatment is recommended for a patient who suffers from failure to thrive and inability to control tongue movements by 7 days. Surgery is also recommended for any child who cannot be successfully extubated by 3 days.[93]

A syndromic association with Pierre Robin sequence results in an obstruction that is more resistant to conservative therapy. Kirschner[96] has demonstrated that 87.5% of nonsyndromic Pierre Robin patients were successfully managed with conservative

therapy, 6.3% with tongue-lip adhesion, and 6.3% with tracheostomy. In contrast, only 29.4% of syndromic patients could be managed conservatively, whereas 35.3% were treated with tongue-lip adhesion and 35.3% required tracheostomy. Syndromic findings associated with Pierre Robin sequence may include midface hypoplasia or unpredictable mandibular growth, and either of these factors can increase the need for surgical intervention. Syndromic association also increases the mortality in these patients. Caouette-Laberge[91] has reported a mortality of 22.8% for syndromic Pierre Robin patients compared with a mortality of 5.9% for nonsyndromic patients.

When surgery is indicated, it is important to perform a complete diagnostic evaluation to ensure that the appropriate procedure is selected. Multiple factors may contribute to upper airway obstruction (Table 102-2), and no one surgical procedure will effectively treat every patient. Nasoendoscopy is used to evaluate the trachea, adenoids, choana, and oropharynx. Sher[87] performed nasoendoscopy on patients with craniofacial anomalies and obstructive apnea. He also described four mechanisms of obstruction (Table 102-3). This classification is significant in that it helps indicate the appropriate type of surgical treatment. It has been demonstrated that only type I obstruction responds to tongue-lip adhesion.

The tongue-lip adhesion was initially described by Douglas in 1946 and has since undergone several modifications.[97-100] The goal of the tongue-lip adhesion is to relieve the airway obstruction by pulling a low and posteriorly positioned tongue forward. The procedure is performed by suturing the tip of the tongue to the

---

TABLE 102-1 ✦ PHYSIOLOGIC CRITERIA FOR SURGICAL INTERVENTION IN PIERRE ROBIN SEQUENCE[59,60]

Respiratory rate > 60/minute
FiO_2 requirement > 60%
PaO_2 < 65 mm Hg
$PaCO_2$ > 60 mm Hg
Weight gain < 100 g/week
SaO_2 < 70%

TABLE 102-2 ✦ POTENTIAL CAUSES OF UPPER AIRWAY OBSTRUCTION IN PIERRE ROBIN SYNDROME

Structural pharyngeal anomalies
Tracheomalacia
Acute angulation of the basicranium
Lingual anomalies
Subglottic anomalies
Hypotonia

TABLE 102-3 ✦ FOUR TYPES OF AIRWAY OBSTRUCTION IN PIERRE ROBIN SYNDROME[52]

Type I	Posterior movement of tongue to the pharyngeal wall
Type II	Tongue compresses soft palate into posterior pharyngeal wall
Type III	Lateral pharyngeal walls move medially
Type IV	Pharynx constricts in a circular manner

lower lip. A suture runs through the adhesion and connects a button from the posterior tongue to a button on the anteroinferior portion of the lower chin (Fig. 102-27). The buttons and suture serve to relieve tension on the tongue-lip flap during wound healing; these are removed after about 12 days. The adhesion itself is released after 9 months. After the adhesion is performed, the infant should continue use of the nasopharyngeal tube for at least two nights. The most common complication after the tongue-lip adhesion is dehiscence of the adhesion. The button suture has also been reported to cut through the tongue. Although there may be an initial delay in sound production, accelerated speech production occurs after adhesion release, and there are minimal long-term effects on speech.

Since the introduction of mandibular distraction osteogenesis, there has been some thinking that the tongue-lip adhesion is effective only for patients who would have done well without any surgical intervention. This philosophy is reflected in some of the treatment algorithms in which the tongue-lip adhesion is not mentioned as a treatment option.[101] At the Children's Hospital of Philadelphia, this procedure is effective in alleviating airway obstruction and failure to thrive in infants whose conservative therapy has failed.

Kirschner et al[102] reviewed the charts of 107 patients diagnosed with Pierre Robin sequence and found that 33 (30.8%) required surgery. The criteria for surgery at the authors' institution are failure to thrive and continued respiratory difficulty despite the previously mentioned modes of conservative therapy. Respiratory status is based on polysomnography, arterial blood gas values, physical exhaustion, and difficulty with feeding. Of the 33 patients who underwent surgery in Kirschner's study, 29 had a tongue-lip adhesion and 4 required tracheostomy.[102] The tongue-lip adhesion was successful in treating 79.3% of patients who required surgery. Tongue-lip adhesion failed in only 6 of 29 patients, and 5 of these 6 patients were syndromic. The conclusion is that there is a population of patients with Pierre Robin sequence who are refractory to conservative therapy but respond to tongue-lip adhesion and that syndromic patients are more likely to require additional surgery.

Distraction osteogenesis of the mandible has allowed elongation of the mandible beyond that which could be achieved with single-stage osteotomies, and it has been successfully employed for treatment of patients with Pierre Robin sequence. Distraction osteogenesis of the infant mandible for treatment of Pierre Robin sequence is performed under a general anesthetic in the operating room. An appropriate dose of local anesthetic with epinephrine is injected into the area of the planned incision. Mucosal incisions similar to those used for a sagittal split osteotomy are then made. Care must be taken to leave an adequate

amount of soft tissue on the medial side of the incision because the tissue will retract, making closure difficult if the incision is too close to the alveolar ridge. The incision is made to bone, and then a periosteal elevator is used to free the soft tissue from the mandible. Once the bone is visualized, the distractor pins can be applied to the mandible. A saw or osteotome (depending on the density of cortical bone) can be used to cut through the buccal and superior cortical bone. The soft tissue can usually be freed from the lingual cortical bone; however, care must be taken not to injure the lingual nerve. A narrow osteotome is then used to cut as much of the lingual cortex as possible. Because the osteotomies include only the cortical bone, the cancellous bone is greenstick fractured with digital pressure. Avoiding direct contact of the cancellous mandible with a surgical instrument will minimize damage to the tooth buds and inferior alveolar nerve. After the osteotomies are complete, the device is applied to the pins on either side of the mandible (application of the distraction appliances is described elsewhere in this text). Distraction of the mandible can then begin until the desired degree of airway improvement and mandibular elongation has been achieved. In adults, distraction is performed at 1 mm per day; but in infants, distraction can be performed as fast as 2 to 3 mm per day because the bone heals rapidly at this age.[101] The authors use distraction as early as 2 years of age with the goal of achieving early tracheostomy decannulation. A caveat in these patients is that they are too young to be compliant and often place physical stresses on the appliances, leading to premature loosening of the pins and additional surgery.

The treatment protocol used at the Children's Hospital of Philadelphia is as follows. Assuming there are no immediate indications for a tracheostomy, the first surgical procedure performed for Pierre Robin sequence with a type I obstruction is the tongue-lip adhesion. If this procedure fails, mandibular distraction is performed to advance the mandible rapidly and, it is hoped, to improve the airway. Tracheostomy is reserved for patients who are refractory to tongue-lip adhesion or mandibular distraction or who have coexistent associated anomalies, such as tracheomalacia, that are not likely to respond to other therapy.

CONCLUSION

The surgical treatment of children with syndromic craniosynostosis may be the most controversial issue in craniofacial surgery. Many treatment philosophies have been proposed, yet debate continues over the indications, timing, type, and effectiveness of surgery. Surgical correction should be performed as soon as it is technically possible (when the immature bone is able

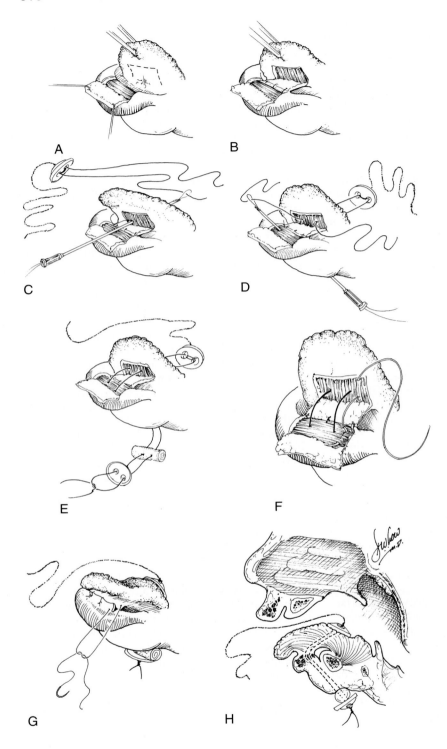

A

B

C

D

E

F

G

H

FIGURE 102-27. *A* to *H,* Tongue-lip adhesion procedure.

to be stabilized enough to prevent relapse) to prevent progression of the deformity and its concomitant morbidity that increases over time. However, the "challenging and often humbling experience" of reconstructing these defects is extremely difficult and requires an interdisciplinary team approach and staged procedures.[55] As with many clefting anomalies, the reconstructive result is often determined by the severity of the deformity. An optimal reconstruction is often difficult or impossible to achieve.[74] Tessier has written that the treatment of Treacher Collins syndrome is one of the most difficult and disappointing endeavors; the immediate results are often promising, but at least partial relapse or deterioration is inevitable so that after several operations, the patient can be improved but still looks like someone with Treacher Collins syndrome.[58] Clearly, this is an area of craniofacial surgery in which innovative new approaches should be developed.

REFERENCES

1. Whitaker LA, Bartlett SP: The craniofacial dysostoses: guidelines for management of the symmetric and asymmetric deformities. Clin Plast Surg 1987;14:73.
2. McCarthy JG, Glasberg SB, Cutting CB, et al: Twenty-year experience with early surgery for craniosynostosis. I. Isolated craniofacial synostosis—results and unsolved problems. Plast Reconstr Surg 1995;96:272.
3. Marchac D: Discussion. Twenty-year experience with early surgery for craniosynostosis. I. Isolated craniofacial synostosis—results and unsolved problems. Plast Reconstr Surg 1995;96:296.
4. Posnick JC: The craniofacial dysostosis syndromes: current reconstructive strategies. Clin Plast Surg 1994;21:585.
5. Posnick JC: Craniofacial dysostosis: staging of reconstruction and management of the midface deformity. Neurosurg Clin North Am 1991;2:683.
6. Persing JA, Jane JA: Treatment of syndromic and nonsyndromic bilateral coronal synostosis in infancy and childhood. Neurosurg Clin North Am 1991;2:655.
7. David JD, Sheen R: Surgical correction of Crouzon syndrome. Plast Reconstr Surg 1990;85:344.
8. Sonstein WJ: Management of secondary turricephaly in craniofacial surgery. Childs Nerv Syst 1996;12:705.
9. Goodrich JT: Evaluation and management of complications in craniofacial surgery. In Goodrich JT, Hall CD, eds: Craniofacial Anomalies: Growth and Development from a Surgical Perspective. New York, Thieme, 1995:194.
10. Marchac D, Renier D: Le front flottant. Traitement précoce des facio-craniosténoses. Ann Chir Plast 1979;24:121.
11. Renier D: Intracranial pressure in craniosynostosis: pre and postoperative recordings—correlation with functional results. In Persing JA, Edgerton MT, Jane JA, eds: Scientific Foundations and Surgical Treatments of Craniosynostosis. Baltimore, Williams & Wilkins, 1989:263.
12. Renier D, Marchac D: Intracranial pressure in craniosynostosis. J Neurosurg 1982;57:370.
13. Fishman MA, Hogan GR, Dodge PR: The concurrence of hydrocephalus and craniosynostosis. J Neurosurg 1971;34:621.
14. Golabi M, Edwards MS, Ousterhout DK: Craniosynostosis and hydrocephalus. Neurosurgery 1987;21:63.
15. McCarthy JG, Glasberg SB, Cutting CB, et al: Twenty-year experience with early surgery for craniosynostosis. II. The craniofacial synostosis syndromes and pansynostosis—results and unsolved problems. Plast Reconstr Surg 1995;96:284.
16. Havlik RJ, Bartlett SP: The treatment of "malignant" exorbitism with an extended supraorbital advancement. Plast Reconstr Surg 1995;95:109.
17. Moore MH: Upper airway obstruction in the syndromal craniosynostoses. Br J Plast Surg 1993;46:355.
18. Lo LJ, Chen YR: Airway obstruction in severe syndromic craniosynostosis. Ann Plast Surg 1999;43:258.
19. Perkins JA, Sie KC, Milczuk H, Richardson MA: Airway management in children with craniofacial anomalies. Cleft Palate Craniofac J 1997;34:135.
20. Mixter RC: Obstructive sleep apnea in Apert's and Pfeiffer's syndromes: more than a craniofacial abnormality. Plast Reconstr Surg 1990;86:457.
21. Ishii K, Kaloust S, Ousterhout DK, Vargervik K: Airway changes after Le Fort III osteotomy in craniosynostosis syndromes. J Craniofac Surg 1996;7:363.
22. Lauritzen C, Friede H, Elander A, et al: Dynamic cranioplasty for brachycephaly. Plast Reconstr Surg 1996;98:7.
23. Cohen SR, Simms C, Burstein FD, Thomsen J: Alternatives to tracheostomy in infants and children with obstructive sleep apnea. J Pediatr Surg 1999;34:182.
24. Gonsalez S, Thompson D, Hayward R, Lane R: Treatment of obstructive sleep apnoea using nasal CPAP in children with craniofacial dysostoses. Childs Nerv Syst 1996;12:713.
25. Cohen SR, Simms C, Burstein FD: Mandibular distraction osteogenesis in the treatment of upper airway obstruction in children with craniofacial deformities. Plast Reconstr Surg 1998;101:312.
26. Hogeman KE, Willmar K: On Le Fort III osteotomy for Crouzon's disease in children: report of a four year follow-up in one patient. Scand J Plast Reconstr Surg 1974;8:169.
27. McCarthy JG, Cutting CB: The timing of surgical intervention in craniofacial anomalies. Clin Plast Surg 1990;17:161.
28. McCarthy JG: Craniosynostosis. In McCarthy JG, ed: Plastic Surgery, vol 4. Philadelphia, WB Saunders, 1990:3013.
29. Whitaker LA, Bartlett SP, Schut L, Bruce D: Craniosynostosis: an analysis of the timing, treatment, and complications in 164 consecutive patients. Plast Reconstr Surg 1987;80:195.
30. Munro IR: Discussion. Dynamic cranioplasty for brachycephaly. Plast Reconstr Surg 1996;98:15.
31. Mulliken JB, Bruneteau RJ: Surgical correction of the craniofacial anomalies in Apert syndrome. Clin Plast Surg 1991;18:277.
32. Friede H, Lilja J, Lauritzen C, et al: Skull morphology after early craniotomy in patients with premature synostosis of the coronal suture. Cleft Palate J 1986;23(suppl 1):1.
33. Posnick JC: Crouzon syndrome: quantitative assessment of presenting deformity and surgical results based on CT scans. Plast Reconstr Surg 1993;92:1027.
34. Marchac D, Renier D, Jones BM: Experience with the "floating forehead." Br J Plast Surg 1988;41:1.
35. Cedars MG, Linck DL 2nd, Chin M, Toth BA: Advancement of the midface using distraction techniques. Plast Reconstr Surg 1999;103:429.
36. Chin M: Le Fort III advancement with gradual distraction using internal devices. Plast Reconstr Surg 1997;100:819.
37. Tessier P: Recent improvements in treatment of facial and cranial deformities of Crouzon's disease and Apert's syndrome. In Tessier P, Callahan A, Mustarde JC, Salyer K, eds: Symposium on Plastic Surgery in the Orbital Region, vol 12. St. Louis, Mosby, 1976.
38. Whitaker LA: Improvement in craniofacial reconstruction: methods evolved in 235 consecutive patients. Plast Reconstr Surg 1980;65:561.

39. Anderl H, Muhlbauer W, Twerdy K, Marchac D: Frontofacial advancement with bony separation in craniofacial dysostosis. Plast Reconstr Surg 1983;71:303.

40. Jackson IT, Adham MN, Marsh WR: Use of the galeal frontalis myofascial flap in craniofacial surgery. Plast Reconstr Surg 1986;77:905.

41. Cohen SR, Boydston W, Burstein FD, Hudgins R: Monobloc distraction osteogenesis during infancy: report of a case and presentation of a new device. Plast Reconstr Surg 1998; 101:1919.

42. Stricker M: Surgery. In Stricker M, van der Meulen J, Raphael B, Mazzola R, eds: Craniofacial Malformations. Edinburgh, Churchill Livingstone, 1990:389.

43. Peterson-Falzone SJ, Pruzansky S, Parris PJ, Laffer JL: Nasopharyngeal dysmorphology in the syndromes of Apert and Crouzon. Cleft Palate J 1981;18:237.

44. Schafer ME: Upper airway obstruction and sleep disorders in children with craniofacial anomalies. Clin Plast Surg 1982;9:555.

45. Simma B, Spehler D, Burger R, et al: Tracheostomy in children. Eur J Pediatr 1994;153:291.

46. Conway WA, Victor LD, Magilligan DJ Jr, et al: Adverse effects of tracheostomy for sleep apnea. JAMA 1981;246:347.

47. Park TS, Haworth CS, Jane JA, et al: Modified prone position for cranial remodeling procedures in children with craniofacial dysmorphism: a technical note. Neurosurgery 1985;16: 212.

48. Hemmer KM, McAlister WH, Marsh JL: Cervical spine anomalies in the craniosynostosis syndromes. Cleft Palate J 1987;24:328.

49. Collins E: Case with symmetrical congenital notches in the outer part of each lower lid with defective development of the malar bones. Trans Ophthalmol Soc UK 1900;20: 190.

50. Franceschetti A, Klein D: The mandibulofacial dysostosis. A new hereditary syndrome. Acta Ophthalmol (Copenh) 1949;27:143.

51. Franceschetti A, Zwahlen P: Un syndrome nouveau: la dysostose mandibulo-faciale. Bull Schweiz Akad Med Wiss 1944;1:60.

52. Tessier P: Vertical and oblique facial clefts (orbitofacial fissures). In Mustarde JC, ed: Plastic Surgery in Infancy and Childhood. Philadelphia, WB Saunders, 1971:94.

53. Roberts F, Pruzansky S, Aduss H: An X-radiocephalometric study of mandibulofacial dysostosis in man. Arch Oral Biol 1975;20:265.

54. Posnick J: Treacher Collins syndrome. In Aston S, ed: Grabb and Smith's Plastic Surgery, 5th ed. Philadelphia, Lippincott-Raven, 1997.

55. Wolfe S: Miscellaneous orbital malformations: Treacher Collins-Franceschetti syndrome. In Wolfe SA, Berkowitz S, eds: Plastic Surgery of the Facial Skeleton. Boston, Little, Brown, 1989:659.

56. Freihofer HP: Variations in the correction of Treacher Collins syndrome. Plast Reconstr Surg 1997;99:647.

57. Raulo Y, Tessier P: Mandibulo-facial dysostosis, analysis: principles of surgery. Scand J Plast Reconstr Surg 1981;15: 251.

58. Tessier P: Surgical correction of Treacher Collins syndrome. In Bell WH, ed: Modern Practice in Orthognathic and Reconstructive Surgery, vol 2. Philadelphia, WB Saunders, 1992:1601.

59. Kaban LB, Moses ML, Mulliken JB: Surgical correction of hemifacial microsomia in the growing child. Plast Reconstr Surg 1980;82:9.

60. Munro I: Craniofacial syndromes. In McCarthy JG, ed: Plastic Surgery, vol 4. Philadelphia, WB Saunders, 1990:3101.

61. Gorlin R: Syndromes of the Head and Neck, 3rd ed. New York, Oxford University Press, 1990.

62. Berry G: Note on a congenital defect (coloboma?) of the lower lid. Ophthalmol Hosp Rep 1889;12:255.

63. Jones K: Treacher Collins syndrome. In Jones K, ed: Smith's Recognizable Patterns of Human Malformation, 5th ed. Philadelphia, WB Saunders, 1997:250.

64. Hertle RW, Ziyland S, Katowitz JA: Ophthalmic features and visual prognosis in the Treacher-Collins syndrome. Br J Ophthalmol 1993;77:642.

65. Jahrsdoerfer RA, Jacobson JT: Treacher Collins syndrome: otologic and auditory management. J Am Acad Audiol 1995;6:93.

66. Pron G, Galloway C, Armstrong D, Posnick J: Ear malformation and hearing loss is patients with Treacher Collins syndrome. Cleft Palate Craniofac J 1993;30:97.

67. Phelps PD, Poswillo D, Lloyd GS: The ear deformities in mandibulofacial dysostosis (Treacher Collins syndrome). Clin Otolaryngol 1981;6:15.

68. Farkas LG, Posnick JC: Detailed morphometry of the nose in patients with Treacher Collins syndrome. Ann Plast Surg 1989;22:211.

69. Dufresne C: Treacher Collins syndrome. In Dufresne C, ed: Complex Craniofacial Problems: A Guide to Analysis and Treatment. New York, Churchill Livingstone, 1992:281.

70. Shprintzen RJ, Croft C, Berkman MD, Rakoff SJ: Pharyngeal hypoplasia in Treacher Collins syndrome. Arch Otolaryngol 1979;105:127.

71. Marsh JL, Celin SE, Vannier MW, et al: The skeletal anatomy of mandibulofacial dysostosis (Treacher Collins syndrome). Plast Reconstr Surg 1986;78:469.

72. Fuente del Campo A, Martinez Elizondo M, Arnaud E: Treacher Collins syndrome (mandibulofacial dysostosis). Clin Plast Surg 1994;21:613.

73. Roncevic R, Roncevic D: Mandibulofacial dysostosis: surgical treatment. J Craniofac Surg 1996;7:280.

74. Jackson IT, Munro IR, Salyer KE, Whitaker LA: Atlas of Craniomaxillofacial Surgery. St. Louis, CV Mosby, 1982.

75. Whitaker L: Personal communications, July 1999.

76. Tulasne JF, Tessier PL: Results of the Tessier integral procedure for correction of Treacher Collins syndrome. Cleft Palate J 1986;23(suppl 1):40.

77. Posnick JC, Goldstein JA, Waitzman AA: Surgical correction of the Treacher Collins malar deficiency: quantitative CT scan analysis of long-term results. Plast Reconstr Surg 1993;92:12.

78. Roddi R, Vaandrager M, van der Meulen JC: Treacher Collins syndrome: early surgical treatment of orbitomalar malformations. J Craniofac Surg 1995;6:211.

79. Gosain AK, Song A, Santoro TD, et al: Long-term remodeling of vascularized and nonvascularized onlay bone grafts: a macroscopic and microscopic analysis. Plast Reconstr Surg 1999;103:1443.

80. Cohen SR, Simms C, Burstein FD: Mandibular distraction osteogenesis in the treatment of upper airway obstruction in children with craniofacial deformities. Plast Reconstr Surg 1998;101:312.

81. Williams JK, Maull D, Grayson BH, et al: Early decannulation with bilateral mandibular distraction for tracheostomy-dependent patients. Plast Reconstr Surg 1999;103:48.

82. del Campo F: Nasomaxillary osteotomies in Treacher Collins treatment. In Montoya AG, ed: Craniofacial Surgery. Bologna, Monduzzi, 1992:155.

83. Brent B: Auricular repair using autogenous rib cartilage grafts: two decades of experience with 600 cases. Plast Reconstr Surg 1992;90:355.

84. Sadewitz VL: Robin sequence: changes in thinking leading to changes in patient care. Cleft Palate Craniofac J 1992;29:246.

85. Shprintzen RJ: The implications of the diagnosis of Robin sequence. Cleft Palate Craniofac J 1992;29:205.

86. Carey JC, Fineman RM, Ziter FA: The Robin sequence as a consequence of malformation, dysplasia, and neuromuscular syndromes. J Pediatr 1982;101:858.

87. Sher AE: Mechanisms of airway obstruction in Robin sequence: implications for treatment. Cleft Palate Craniofac J 1992;29:224.

88. Cozzi F, Pierro A: Glossoptosis-apnea syndrome in infancy. Pediatrics 1985;75:836.

89. Hotz M, Gnoinski W: Clefts of secondary palate associated with the "Pierre Robin syndrome." Swed Dent J Suppl 1982;15:89.

90. Singer L, Sidoti EJ: Pediatric management of Robin sequence. Cleft Palate Craniofac J 1992;29:220.

91. Caouette-Laberge L, Bayet B, Larocque Y: The Pierre Robin sequence: review of 125 cases and evolution of treatment modalities. Plast Reconstr Surg 1994;93:934.

92. Takagi Y, Bosma JF: Disability of oral function in an infant associated with displacement of the tongue. Therapy by feeding in prone position. Acta Paediatr Scand Suppl 1960;49:62.

93. Parsons RW, Smith DJ: Rule of thumb criteria for tongue-lip adhesion in Pierre Robin anomalad. Plast Reconstr Surg 1982;70:210.

94. Freed G, Pearlman MA, Brown AS, Barot LR: Polysomnographic indications for surgical intervention in Pierre Robin sequence: acute airway management and follow-up studies after repair and take-down of tongue-lip adhesion. Cleft Palate Craniofac J 1988;25:151.

95. Augarten A, Sagy M, Yahav J, Barzilay Z: Management of upper airway obstruction in the Pierre Robin syndrome. Br J Oral Maxillofac Surg 1990;28:105.

96. Kirschner RE, McDonald-McGlinn D, Baker SB, et al: Airway management in Pierre Robin sequence: etiology as a predictive factor. Proceedings of the 68th Annual Scientific Meeting of the American Society of Plastic Surgeons, 1999:50-51.

97. Randall P: The Robin anomalad: micrognathia and glossoptosis with airway obstruction. In Converse JM, ed: Reconstructive Plastic Surgery. Philadelphia, WB Saunders, 1977: 2235.

98. Routledge RT: The Pierre Robin syndrome: a surgical emergency in the neonatal period. Br J Plast Surg 1960;13: 204.

99. Parsons RW, Smith DJ: A modified tongue-lip adhesion for Pierre Robin anomalad. Cleft Palate J 1980;17:144.

100. Argamaso RV: Glossopexy for upper airway obstruction in Robin sequence. Cleft Palate Craniofac J 1992;29: 232.

101. Cohen SR, Ross DA, Burstein FD, et al: Skeletal expansion combined with soft tissue reduction in the treatment of obstructive sleep apnea in children: physiologic results. Otolaryngol Head Neck Surg 1998;119:476.

102. Kirschner RE, Low DW, Baker SB, et al: Surgical airway management in Pierre Robin sequence: is there a role for tongue-lip adhesion? Proceedings of the 69th Annual Scientific Meeting of the American Society of Plastic Surgeons, 2000:125-126.

Reconstruction: Craniofacial Microsomia

Joseph G. McCarthy, MD ✦ Barry H. Grayson, DDS

RECONSTRUCTIVE REQUIREMENTS

The evolution or development of surgical techniques for the correction of the skeletal and soft tissue defects of the patient with craniofacial microsomia mirrors the history of plastic surgery: bone grafts, osteotomies, distraction osteogenesis, dermis-fat grafts, local flaps, and microvascular free flaps. It is the challenge posed by the patient, usually a severe asymmetric deformity, and the need to integrate a multidisciplinary treatment team that have attracted the plastic surgeon.

The surgical reconstructive requirements of the patient with craniofacial microsomia vary from patient to patient and are dependent on the individual anatomic and functional deficiencies. They can include soft tissue pathologic processes (skin, subcutaneous fat, parotid, muscles of mastication and facial expression, facial nerve and its branches, and various forms of microtia). The skeletal reconstructive efforts have traditionally been directed at correction of the mandibular deficiency, usually involving the vertical ramus and body as well as the condyle and temporomandibular joint. The Pruzansky classification,[1] subsequently modified by Kaban, Moses, and Mulliken,[2] is helpful in defining the mandibular deformity (Fig. 103-1).

Along with significant mandibular hypoplasia, there is invariably an associated pathologic process involving the maxilla and zygoma. In a small percentage of patients, the fronto-orbital area can be deficient. In summary, the clinician is usually dealing with a combination of skeletal and soft tissue deformities—"bone carpentry" alone is often insufficient in the global treatment of the patient with craniofacial microsomia (see also Chapter 91).

Other variables that must be considered are the functional needs (respiratory, otologic, masticatory) of the patient and the role of subsequent growth and development of the affected and neighboring anatomic parts. The clinician must first consider the functional requirements, especially sleep apnea and other types of respiratory deficiency associated with micrognathia and glossoptosis. With severe respiratory insufficiency, it has been traditional to treat the child with a tracheostomy. Such individuals invariably have feeding problems, and a gastrostomy may also be indicated. A child will occasionally have poor function of the palpebral sphincter, and treatment may be required to protect the cornea. In children with bilateral craniofacial microsomia, the hearing deficits are so severe that speech development is impeded and hearing devices may be required. Cervical vertebral abnormality can be associated with a Chiari malformation,[3] and central nervous system anomaly has also been reported (see also Chapter 91).

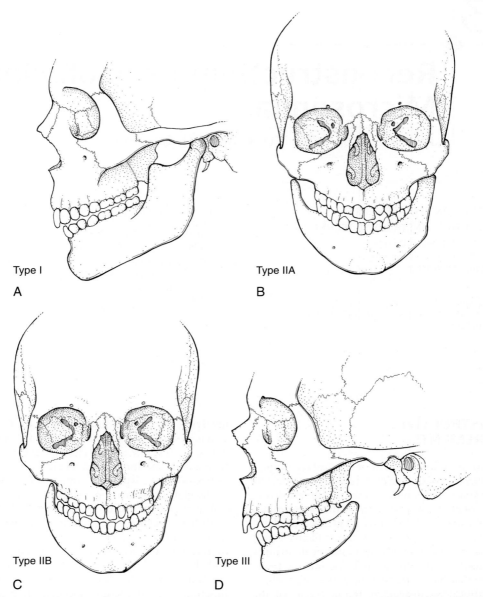

FIGURE 103-1. Pruzansky[1] classification of the mandibular deformity, as modified by Kaban et al.[45] *A,* Type I. The mandibular deficiency is only mild. *B,* Type IIA. The condyle and ramus are small, but the condyle and glenoid fossa are anatomically oriented. However, a flattened condyle can be hinged on a flat, often hypoplastic infratemporal surface. The coronoid process may be absent. *C,* Type IIB. This is similar to type IIA except that the vertical or superoinferior plane of the condyle-ramus is medially displaced. There is not a functioning glenoid fossa. *D,* Type III. There is absence of the ramus, condyle, and coronoid process.

EVOLUTION OF RECONSTRUCTIVE TECHNIQUES

The earlier efforts at correction of the craniofacial asymmetry or deficiency of craniofacial microsomia were directed at restoration of facial contour by a variety of onlay techniques. Whereas skeletal onlay techniques are indicated for true bone deficits, they do not represent the optimal method of correction of the cheek soft tissue deficit, as does a microvascular free flap, for example.

Autogenous rib grafts,[4,5] iliac grafts,[6] grafts harvested from the inferior border of the contralateral mandible,[7] allografts of cartilage or bone,[8] and various allografts[9] have been recommended to augment the deficient craniofacial skeleton. Such techniques, however, fail to align the malpositioned jaws and to restore the occlusion, dental function, and soft tissue contour. The preferred alternative is the use of osteotomies (with or without distraction or bone grafts) to correct jaw asymmetry or deficiency and the associated malocclusion.

The timing of such procedures has been the subject of a long-running controversy, however. The school advocating osteotomies only in the adult or adolescent patient has included Poswillo,[10] who thought that such surgery in the growing child would interfere with the functional matrix[11] and impede subsequent craniofacial growth and development. Obwegeser[12] also advocated deferring osteotomies until skeletal and dental maturity and popularized reconstruction of the temporomandibular joint and zygomatic arch with rib grafts as well as the rotation of the lower half of the craniofacial skeleton inferiorly and medially by the combination of a Le Fort I osteotomy, bilateral sagittal split osteotomy of the mandibular rami, and three-dimensional genioplasty (see Fig 103-15).

Advocates of osteotomies in children included Dingman and Grabb,[13] who recommended a metatarsal bone graft reconstruction of the affected mandibular ramus. Converse and Rushton[14] described a 12-year-old with unilateral craniofacial microsomia who also underwent a horizontal osteotomy of the ramus with insertion of an iliac bone graft in the resulting defect; a bite block was constructed to open the occlusion on the affected side. Delaire[15] recommended elongation of the affected ramus between the ages of 4 and 6 years by an inverted-L osteotomy with insertion of rib grafts in the horizontal component of the resulting defect. Converse et al[16] advocated a two-stage procedure during the period of mixed dentition to correct the maxillomandibular asymmetry. Other proponents of childhood osteotomies and bone grafts included Murray et al[17] and Munro and Lauritzen,[5] who also reported subsequent elongation and growth of the rib-grafted mandibular segment.

The development of distraction techniques[18,19] represented a true paradigm shift in the treatment of patients with either unilateral or bilateral craniofacial microsomia (see Figs. 103-2 and 103-3). The techniques are simpler and associated with less morbidity and infection; they obviate the need for intermaxillary fixation, autogenous bone graft harvesting, or blood transfusion. In addition, advocates of distraction recommend the technique even in infancy if there is a severe mandibular deformity with clinical evidence of sleep apnea.

Soft tissue hypoplasia is a prominent feature of craniofacial microsomia, especially in the cheeks (parotidmasseteric) and auriculomastoid areas. The results of nonvascularized transfers of fat and dermis-fat[20] are unpredictable, including a residual contour irregularity or even loss of the entire graft. Vascularized flap transfers are preferred because of long-term survival and the ability to deliver large volumes of fat. This concept was first established by the insertion of a tube flap in the preauricular area[21] and the use of a de-epithelialized pedicle flap.[22] These flap techniques have been superseded, however, by the introduction of de-epithelialized microvascular free flaps of dermis and fat (see Fig. 103-21).[23-25] Upton et al[26] restored soft tissue contour with microvascular transfers of omentum, but this technique has fallen out of favor because of the requisite need for a laparotomy and a secondary procedure to resuspend the omentum.

RECONSTRUCTIVE MODALITIES

Tracheostomy or Gastrostomy

In the neonatal period, tracheostomy is a lifesaving maneuver in patients with severe respiratory distress, but the need for this treatment modality has been lessened in recent years with the introduction of mandibular distraction in the infant patient.[27] Some children who require perinatal endotracheal intubation can successfully tolerate extubation several days later. If extubation is not possible, tracheostomy has traditionally been recommended.

As mentioned, the need for tracheostomy has been reduced since the introduction of mandibular distraction. For infants with severe eating problems, a gastrostomy is indicated to improve the nutritional status of the child and to provide the calories essential for growth and development. The nutritional problem is often aggravated by the increased energy requirements associated with respiratory insufficiency and is often corrected by mandibular distraction.

Mandibular Distraction

Mandibular distraction[18] can be employed at any age from the neonate to the adult. The technique involves an osteotomy on one or both sides of the mandible with the application of either an extraoral (Fig. 103-2) or intraoral (Fig. 103-3) distraction device.[18,19,28] The intraoral device is reserved for those patients with an adequate bone stock in the ramus and body of the mandible (Pruzansky type I or IIA). After a latency period of approximately 5 days, the device can be activated at the rate of 1 mm/day. In children younger than 3 years, it is appropriate to employ a rate of 1.5 mm/day to avoid premature consolidation.

In patients with unilateral craniofacial microsomia, activation of the distraction device is continued until there is leveling of the occlusal plane, inferior displacement of the ipsilateral oral commissure, and movement of the chin point to the midline

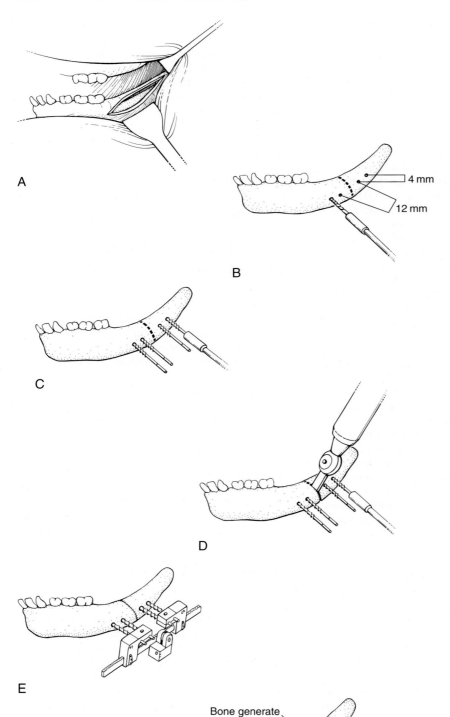

FIGURE 103-2. Technique of extraoral distraction. *A,* Intraoral incision. *B,* Line of osteotomy and sites of insertion of self-drilling pins. *C,* Partial osteotomy and insertion of fourth pin. *D,* Completion of osteotomy. *E,* The device has been attached. *F,* Generation of bone after activation of the device.

A

B

4 mm

12 mm

C

D

E

F

Bone generate

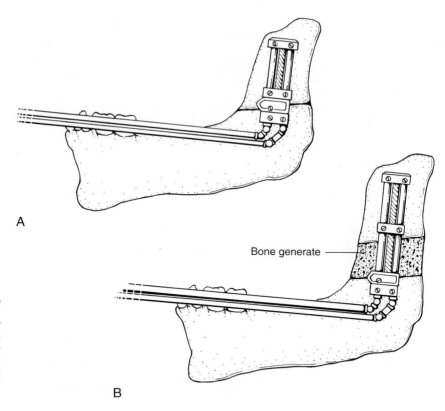

FIGURE 103-3. Technique of intraoral distraction. *A,* Device attached and osteotomy completed. *B,* Laying down of bone generate with activation of the device. Intraoral distraction requires a relatively large ramus for device application.

Bone generate

A

B

(Fig. 103-4). Such parameters may also be overcorrected in the growing child. In the younger patient with bilateral mandibular deficiency, the technique is employed bilaterally, and activation is continued until the mandibular anterior teeth are either edge to edge with or anterior to the maxillary anterior teeth. The technique is applicable in patients of all ages with either unilateral (Figs. 103-5 and 103-6) or bilateral (Fig. 103-7) craniofacial microsomia.

In preoperative planning, computed tomographic scans (axial and three-dimensional) are essential in defining the skeletal pathologic process and determining whether there is adequate bone stock for the osteotomy and pin placement. A curved reformat of the computed tomographic data yields a DentaScan (see Chapter 91) that is helpful in documenting the position of unerupted tooth follicles.[29]

The vectors of distraction are important and are determined by the placement of the pins and distraction device in reference to the maxillary occlusal plan (Fig. 103-8).[30] In the patient with unilateral craniofacial microsomia, the surgical goal is to increase the vertical or superoinferior dimension of the ramus (vertical vector). In bilateral distraction, the horizontal vector is employed. An oblique vector represents an intermediate orientation. With the introduction of multiplanar distraction devices and the development

of the concept of molding of the regenerate,[31] the clinician has the capability of achieving optimal mandibular morphologic features and occlusion.

With the accumulation of clinical experience, it has been demonstrated that mandibular distraction can be repeated (secondary distraction), that previously inserted rib grafts can also be distracted, and that the temporomandibular joint can be reconstructed by the technique of transport distraction.[32] In transport distraction (Fig. 103-9), a reverse L-shaped osteotomy is made in the ramal segment. A distraction device is placed across the osteotomy, and the leading edge of the transport segment is driven in the direction of the pseudo-glenoid fossa. The leading edge of the transport segment has a fibrous-cartilage surface that simulates the articular surface of the condyle.

Maxillomandibular Distraction

Maxillomandibular distraction[33] is also possible by performing a concomitant Le Fort I osteotomy (incomplete) at the time of the mandibular osteotomy (Fig. 103-10). The patient is placed in intermaxillary fixation, and as mandibular distraction proceeds, the maxillary segment is moved in an inferior and anterior direction. Thus, the occlusal cant is corrected, the

Text continued on p. 533

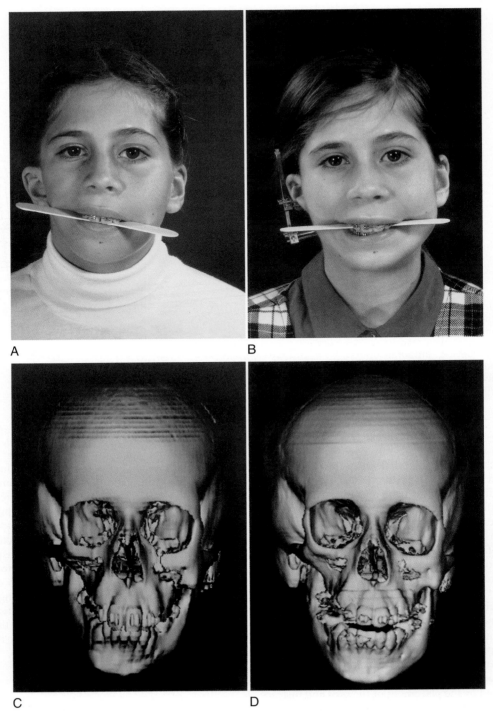

FIGURE 103-4. The treatment endpoints for unilateral distraction (illustrated with an extra-oral device). *A,* A young girl with right-sided craniofacial microsomia. Note that the chin is deviated to the affected side, the ipsilateral oral commissure is elevated, and there is an occlusal cant (documented by tongue blade). *B,* At the completion of device activation. Note the change in position of the tongue blade (occlusal plane) and chin point. *C,* Pre-distraction three-dimensional computed tomographic scan documenting the mandibular deficiency on the affected side, the occlusal cant, and the chin deviation. *D,* Post-distraction three-dimensional computed tomographic scan showing augmentation of the affected mandibular ramus and body, leveling of the occlusal plane, and translocation of the chin point to the midline.

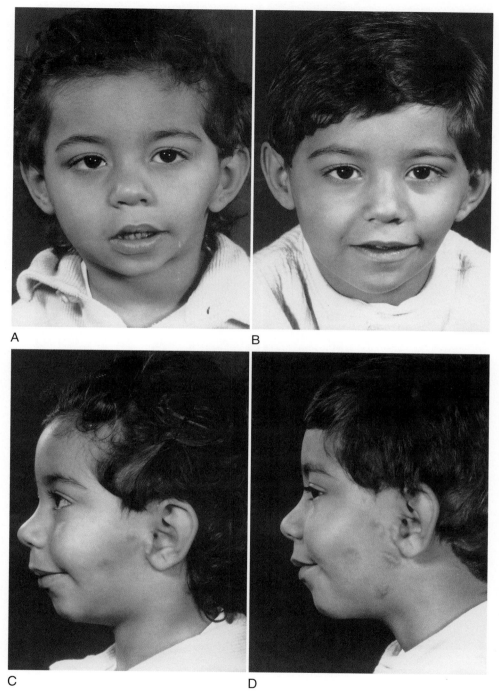

FIGURE 103-5. Unilateral mandibular distraction. *A,* Pre-distraction frontal view of a 2-year-old boy with left-sided craniofacial microsomia (type I). Note the deviation of the chin, occlusal cant, and hypoplasia of the affected cheek. *B,* Post-distraction frontal view with improvement in the position of the chin, oral commissure, and alar base. The occlusal plane has been leveled. *C,* Pre-distraction profile (affected side). *D,* Post-distraction profile. Note the increased sagittal thrust of the mandible. Some of the scars result from excision of preauricular skin tags.   *Continued*

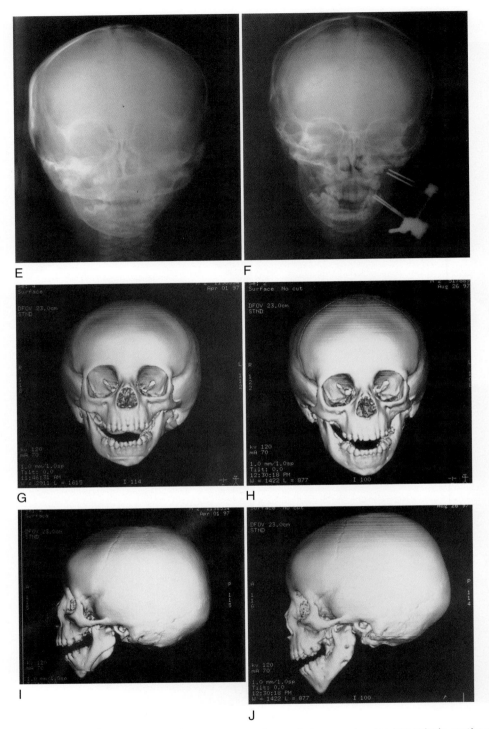

FIGURE 103-5, cont'd. *E,* Pre-distraction posteroanterior cephalogram showing hypoplasia on the affected side of the mandible and deviation of the chin. *F,* At the completion of device activation. Note the improvement in chin position and mandibular contour. The angle of the mandible has been reconstituted on the affected side. *G,* Pre-distraction frontal three-dimensional computed tomographic scan. Note the occlusal cant and chin position. *H,* Post-distraction frontal three-dimensional computed tomographic scan. Note the improvement in chin position, occlusal plane, and mandibular symmetry. *I,* Pre-distraction lateral three-dimensional computed tomographic scan. The hypoplasia of the affected mandibular body and ramus is apparent. *J,* Post-distraction lateral three-dimensional computed tomographic scan. Note the improvement in the shape and volume of the affected mandible. The bone generate is between the pin holes. (Partially reproduced from McCarthy JG, ed: Distraction of the Craniofacial Skeleton. New York, Springer-Verlag, 1999.)

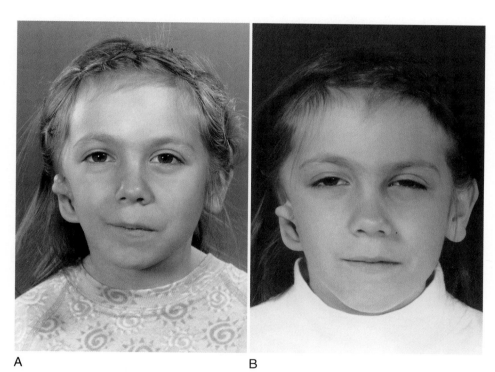

A   B

FIGURE 103-6. Unilateral mandibular distraction. *A,* Pre-distraction frontal view of a 7-year-old girl with right-sided craniofacial microsomia (Pruzansky type I). Note the chin deviation, elevation of the ipsilateral oral commissure, and hypoplasia of the cheek. There is a keloid of the auricular helix. *B,* Post-distraction frontal view. Note the improvement in chin and oral commissure position as well as in cheek contour. There is less alar base asymmetry.

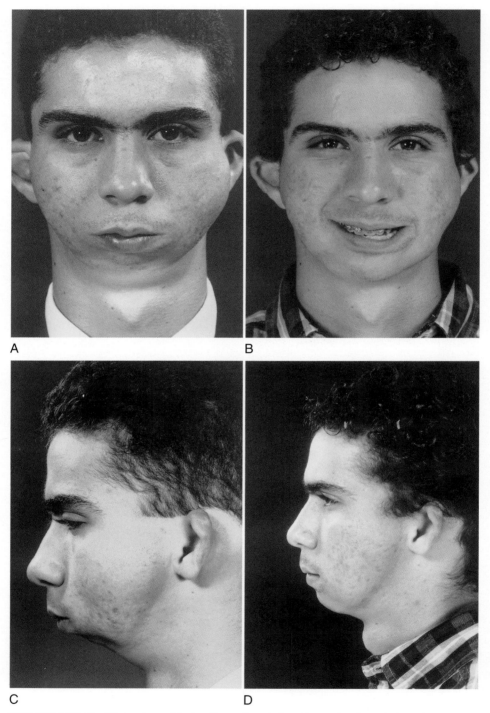

FIGURE 103-7. Bilateral mandibular distraction. *A,* Pre-distraction frontal view of a 21-year-old man with bilateral craniofacial microsomia (bilateral Pruzansky type IIA). Note the ear anomalies and severe hypoplasia of the chin and lower third of the face. *B,* Post-distraction frontal view showing restoration of the lower third of the face. He also underwent a genioplasty. *C,* Pre-distraction profile. *D,* Post-distraction profile. Note the increased sagittal thrust of the chin and mandible.

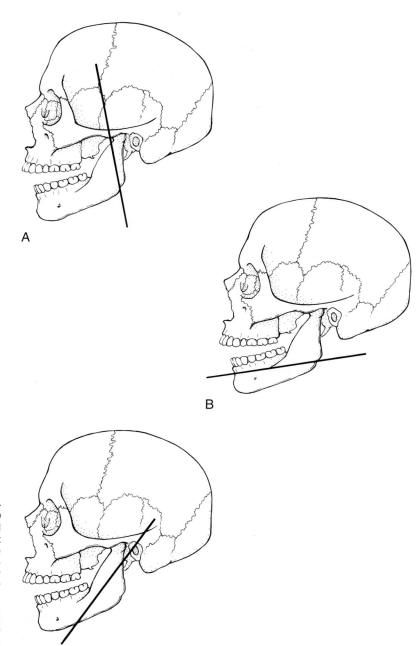

FIGURE 103-8. Vectors of distraction. *A*, The vertical vector is 90 degrees to the maxillary occlusal plane and is indicated for the patient with deficiency localized to the mandibular ramus. *B*, The horizontal vector is parallel to the maxillary occlusal plane and is indicated for deficiency of the mandibular body. *C*, The oblique vector is between the vertical and the horizontal vectors and is indicated for correction of combined mandibular ramus-body deficiency.

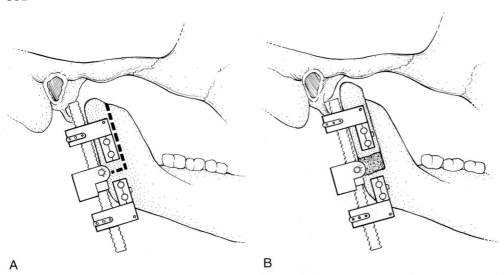

FIGURE 103-9. Technique of transport distraction. *A,* L-shaped osteotomy *(interrupted lines)* and application of the distraction device. *B,* With activation of the device, bone is generated in the ramus, and a condyle (with a fibrocartilage cap) is advanced into a pseudo-glenoid fossa.

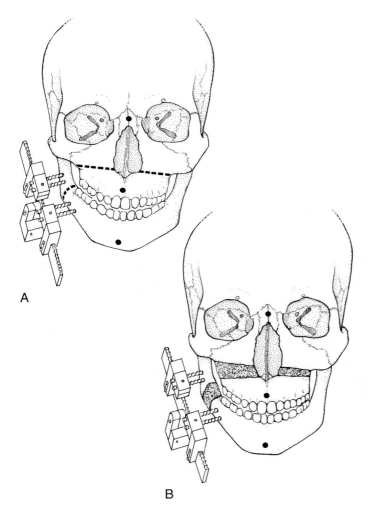

FIGURE 103-10. Technique of maxillomandibular distraction. *A,* The dots designate the asymmetry of the craniofacial midline. Note the Le Fort I and mandibular lines of osteotomy. The mandibular distraction device (four pins) has been applied. *B,* After activation of the device. The intermaxillary wires (or elastics) are not illustrated. Note the restoration of the craniofacial midline, improvement in the occlusal plane and chin position, and rotation-augmentation of the maxilla and mandible.

oral commissure is lowered, and the chin is moved to the midline.

The technique is especially indicated in the older child in whom spontaneous or orthodontically guided descent of the maxillary dentoalveolus is not possible. The Le Fort I corticotomy can also be performed on the younger patient without fear of injury to the unerupted maxillary teeth.

Bone Grafts

Rib or iliac bone grafting[5] has been the traditional method of reconstructing the Pruzansky type III skeletal defect (absence of the ramus and condyle) (Fig. 103-11). Through a bicoronal incision, complemented by a submandibular Risdon incision, the mandibular remnant is exposed in a subperiosteal plane. The projected location of the glenoid fossa is determined through the bicoronal incision. If the zygomatic arch is missing, this becomes part of the bone graft reconstruction. The cartilaginous end of the costochondral rib graft is placed in a groove of the reconstructed zygomatic arch, and the cartilaginous portion, simulating a condyle, prevents ankylosis. Rigid skeletal fixation is achieved at the mandibular remnant, and the patient is placed in intermaxillary fixation, which is removed at approximately 8 weeks (Fig. 103-12). Subsequent growth of the mandible is unpredictable, but such patients can undergo distraction of the bone graft–reconstructed mandibular site at a later date (Figs. 103-13 and 103-14).[34]

MANAGEMENT OF THE ABSENT RAMUS AND CONDYLE

The most challenging reconstructive problem is the patient with a Pruzansky type III mandibular deformity, that is, absence of the ramus and temporomandibular joint. The reconstructive goal is obvious: construct a ramus, condyle, and temporomandibular joint that simulate the contralateral side. Achievement of this goal, in turn, levels the occlusal plane, lowers the ipsilateral commissure, and centers the pogonion or chin point. It also provides a better skeletal foundation for the overlying soft tissues.

The traditional technique has been to reconstruct the glenoid fossa with a rib graft and the condyle-ramus with a costochondral rib graft (see Fig. 103-11). If the resulting ramus is inadequate in the vertical dimension, one could consider distraction of the bone graft, provided there is adequate bone stock.[34]

With the development of the distraction technique, one could also consider enucleation of tooth follicles in the body-ramus remnant after a curved three-dimensional computed tomographic reformat (DentaScan) documents the dental-skeletal status of the mandible. An interval of at least 4 months should elapse before transport distraction is performed to generate a ramus and neocondyle-glenoid fossa.[35]

Another recently developed technique, especially in bilateral craniofacial microsomia with a Pruzansky type III mandibular deformity, is the application of a rigid external distraction device. Distraction of the hypoplastic mandible (distraction histogenesis) is followed by reconstruction of the ramus with a microvascular free fibula flap (E. Stelnicki, personal communication, 2001).

Maxillomandibular Orthognathic Surgery

In the skeletally mature patient, traditional maxillomandibular orthognathic surgery is indicated. The mandibular osteotomies include the bilateral sagittal split of the ramus and the vertical or oblique osteotomy of the ramus (see Chapter 58). Obwegeser[12] combined the Le Fort I maxillary osteotomy with bilateral sagittal split of the mandibular ramus and genioplasty (Fig. 103-15) to ensure leveling of the occlusal plane and establishment of the optimal occlusal relationships. The sagittal split and vertical or oblique osteotomies allow repositioning of the tooth-bearing mandibular segments. Fixation, especially in the sagittal split procedure, is achieved with lag screws. The Le Fort I osteotomy is repositioned, according to preoperative plans, and rigid skeletal fixation is achieved with plates and screws. Genioplasty, usually in three planes, completes the procedure (Fig. 103-16).

PREOPERATIVE PLANNING

Careful preoperative planning is essential. The occlusal cant observed in unilateral craniofacial microsomia results from a reduction in the vertical dimension of the maxilla and mandible on the affected side. Some patients may also show, superimposed on this growth abnormality, facial findings characteristic of the long-face or short-face syndrome, as manifested by excessive or deficient maxillary gingival exposure at rest or on smiling. Thus, there exist several clinical variations for which the appropriate surgical plan must be chosen.

The objectives of surgery are to correct the occlusal cant while at the same time optimizing the lip-incisor relationship and correcting abnormal gingival exposure on smiling. There are three potential movements of the Le Fort I segment for correction of the defect (Fig. 103-17). In the first example (Fig. 103-17A), the left side is affected but the skeletal and soft tissue relationship is normal on this side. In this example, when the patient smiles, an excessive amount of teeth and gingivae show on the less affected (right) side. The Le Fort I segment is illustrated as elevated or impacted

Text continued on p. 540

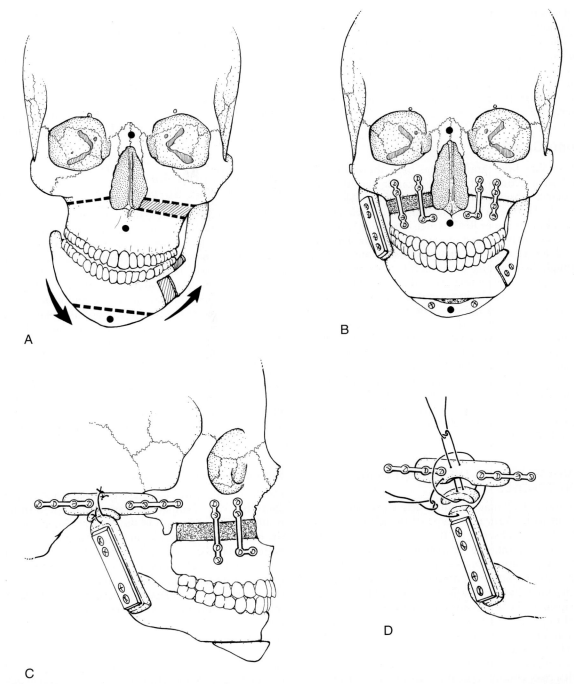

FIGURE 103-11. Technique of bone graft reconstruction of the mandibular ramus, condyle, and glenoid fossa in unilateral craniofacial microsomia. *A,* The dots designate the asymmetry of the craniofacial midline, and the arrows show the projected movement of the mandible. Note the Le Fort I line of osteotomy and the area of ostectomy on the nonaffected side of the maxilla. In the mandible, the genioplasty and sagittal split osteotomies are illustrated. *B,* After osteotomy and movement of the maxillary and mandibular segments and double-tier bone graft reconstruction of the ramus, condyle, and glenoid fossa. A bone graft has been placed in the maxillary defect. Rigid skeletal fixation has been established across the Le Fort I, sagittal split, and genioplasty osteotomies. *C* and *D,* Lateral views illustrating the details of the ramus, condyle, and glenoid fossa (bone graft) reconstruction. Note that a cartilage cap is interposed between the bone grafts, reconstructing the ramus, condyle, and glenoid fossa (undersurface of the zygomatic arch). A resorbable suture approximates these.

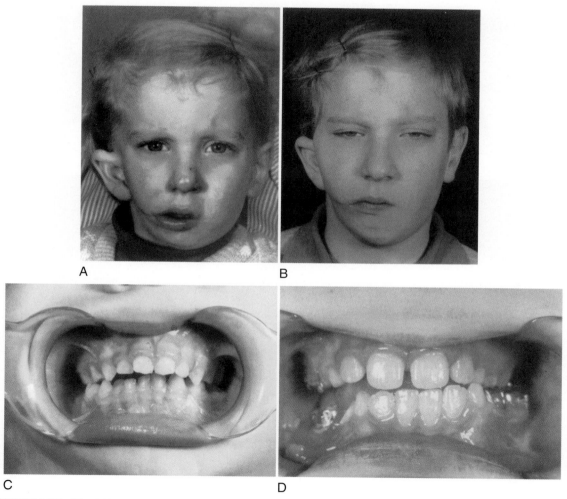

FIGURE 103-12. A 7-year-old boy who presented with sleep apnea and right-sided craniofacial microsomia. *A*, Preoperative appearance. *B*, Postoperative appearance (see Fig. 103-11). Note the improvement in the chin and oral commissure position. The sleep apnea was relieved. *C*, Preoperative occlusion. Note the disparity in the midincisor lines. *D*, Postoperative occlusion. Note the surgically created open bite and the shift of the mandibular midincisor line.

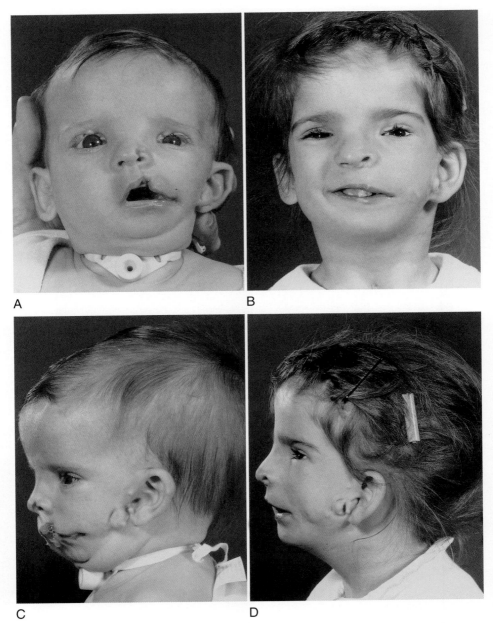

FIGURE 103-13. Technique of bone graft reconstruction of the mandibular ramus and condyle followed by distraction of the graft site at a second stage. *A,* A 6-month-old with left-sided craniofacial microsomia, multiple facial clefts, severe micrognathia, and tracheostomy. *B,* Appearance after first-stage costochondral bone graft reconstruction of the left ramus and condyle, followed by second-stage distraction of the double-tier rib graft. She also underwent repair of her multiple clefts. The tracheostomy has been removed. *C,* Preoperative profile. *D,* Postoperative profile.

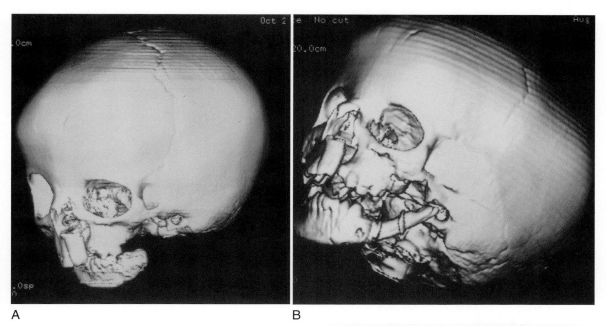

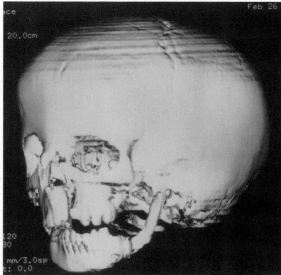

FIGURE 103-14. Three-dimensional computed tomographic scans of the patient illustrated in Figure 103-13. *A*, Preoperative image. Note the absent ramus and condyle (Pruzansky type III). *B*, Appearance after two-tier costochondral rib grafting (see Fig. 103-11). *C*, After second-stage distraction. Note the neo-gonial angle, lengthening of the bone grafts, and anterior projection of the mandible.

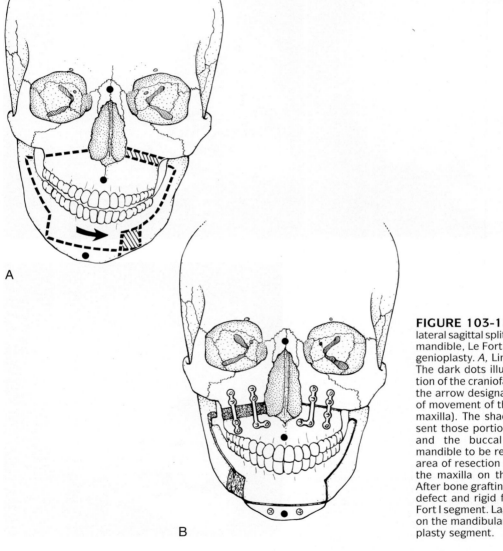

A

B

FIGURE 103-15. Combined bilateral sagittal split osteotomy of the mandible, Le Fort I osteotomy, and genioplasty. *A,* Lines of osteotomy. The dark dots illustrate the deviation of the craniofacial midline, and the arrow designates the direction of movement of the mandible (and maxilla). The shaded areas represent those portions of the maxilla and the buccal cortex of the mandible to be resected. Note the area of resection and impaction of the maxilla on the same side. *B,* After bone grafting of the maxillary defect and rigid fixation of the Le Fort I segment. Lag screws are used on the mandibular rami and genioplasty segment.

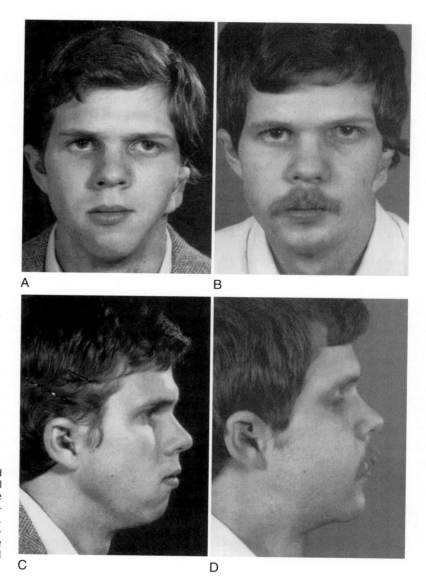

FIGURE 103-16. A 17-year-old with left-sided unilateral craniofacial microsomia reconstructed by the technique illustrated in Figure 103-15. *A* and *C,* Preoperative views. *B* and *D,* Postoperative appearance. Note the improvement in the chin-oral commissure position and contour.

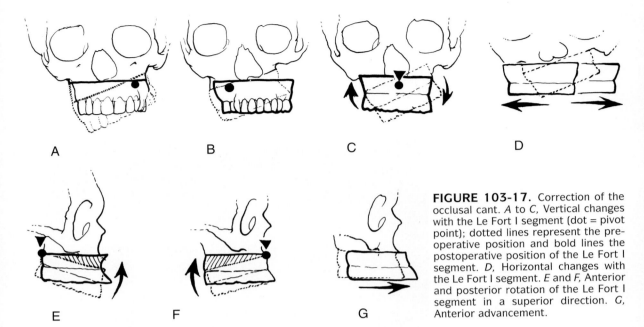

A   B   C   D

E   F   G

FIGURE 103-17. Correction of the occlusal cant. *A* to *C*, Vertical changes with the Le Fort I segment (dot = pivot point); dotted lines represent the preoperative position and bold lines the postoperative position of the Le Fort I segment. *D*, Horizontal changes with the Le Fort I segment. *E* and *F*, Anterior and posterior rotation of the Le Fort I segment in a superior direction. *G*, Anterior advancement.

on the right side only, correcting the cant of the occlusal plane. In the second example (Fig. 103-17*B*), the left side is affected and the Le Fort I segment is displaced inferiorly on this side. The patient, on smiling, shows a normal amount of gingivae and dental structures on the less affected (right) side and a deficient amount of these structures on the affected (left) side. For the skeletal and soft tissue relationship to be improved on the affected side, the Le Fort I segment is displaced inferiorly on the left side only. Note that the center of rotation is on the right as the occlusal plane is leveled. In the third example (Fig. 103-17*C*), the patient's left side is affected and the teeth appear slightly above the drape of the lips. The right side shows an excessive amount of gingiva on smiling. Correction of the occlusal cant is achieved by rotating the Le Fort I segment around a point at the midline (i.e., impaction on the right, lowering on the left). The skeletal deformity may also require other types of correction by movement of the Le Fort I segment to the left or right in the horizontal dimension (Fig. 103-17*D*). On evaluation of the lateral cephalogram, correction of the deformity may require that the segment be rotated superiorly or inferiorly either anteriorly or posteriorly (Fig. 103-17*E* and *F*) in combination with advancement or setback of the osteotomized segment (Fig. 103-17*G*). It is important to understand the secondary impact of these changes on the position of the mandible, its occlusion, and the soft tissue profile.

TWO-SPLINT TECHNIQUE. In the correction of an asymmetric skeletal deformity (unilateral craniofacial microsomia) when simultaneous surgery of both jaws is planned, two carefully constructed interocclusal splints are employed. The first or intermediate splint is used to establish the position of the osteotomized maxillary segment by referencing it to this splint that is wired to the nonosteotomized mandible. The mandible and splinted maxillary segment are rotated around the condyles and mobilized superiorly, ensuring accurate condylar "seating." The maxilla is fixed into position with plates and screws. The intermediate splint is removed, and a second splint is wired to the maxilla. The mandibular osteotomies are completed, after which the mandible is guided into its planned position as it is wired into the second splint.

The two-splint procedure functions only when both condyles and rami are of normal shape and size—usually not the case in unilateral craniofacial microsomia. The unequal ramal heights and condylar pathologic anatomy result in an asymmetric path of closure for the affected mandible. The mandibular body follows a path of opening and closing that is oblique rather than parallel to the craniofacial midsagittal plane. This complex three-dimensional motion cannot be accurately reproduced on conventional dental articulators. Thus, the intermediate splint does not accurately position the Le Fort I segment when the mandible is rotated upward toward the maxilla. Establishing the position of the Le Fort I segment is therefore dependent on calculations of the planned change derived from results of mock surgery on articulated study models, mock surgery on the cephalograms, and three-dimensional cephalometric or computed tomographic images.

UNILATERAL VERSUS BILATERAL RAMUS OSTEOTOMIES TO REPOSITION MANDIBLE. The mandible and maxilla in unilateral craniofacial microsomia demonstrate a true bilateral deformity. The primary deformity, by virtue of its effect on altering jaw position and function, induces compensatory shape and size changes on the unaffected or "less affected" side.[36] This is seen as a bowing out and elongation of the mandibular body and ramus on the less affected side. When the mandible is repositioned only by osteotomizing or bone grafting the affected ramus and rotation around the less affected condyle, the deformity of the less affected side becomes more apparent (Fig. 103-18). When the mandibular midline is centered in this fashion, the contour of the less affected side appears abnormally full and thrust laterally, whereas the affected side continues to appear deficient. The asymmetric bony mandibular anatomy and the associated asymmetric overlying soft tissue contribute to this effect. However, a ramal osteotomy on the contralateral side permits repositioning of the mandibular body in a manner that reduces, rather than emphasizes, the asymmetry. The optimally repositioned mandible results in minimal lateral displacement of the less affected mandibular body while maximal inferior and lateral displacement of the affected side is obtained.

Fronto-orbital Advancement and Cranial Vault Remodeling

Fronto-orbital advancement and cranial vault remodeling are occasionally indicated in the child with retrusion of the ipsilateral supraorbital rim and frontal bone.[37] A combined craniofacial route is required to provide surgical access to the frontal bone, orbits, and nasal radix. After an anterior craniotomy, a fronto-orbital advancement is performed. The frontal bone (forehead) can be reconstructed by remodeling the native frontal bone or replacing it with a harvested cranial bone graft (see Chapter 101).

Commissuroplasty

Commissuroplasty or closure of the lateral facial cleft[38] is indicated in patients with a macrostomia or a true lateral facial cleft. Vermilion and oral mucosal flaps are designed after the site of the projected oral commissure is determined (Fig. 103-19). The flaps are approximated and sutured with resorbable sutures. The orbicularis muscle stumps are skeletonized and closed in a vest-over-pants fashion with resorbable sutures. The cutaneous closure is incorporated in a Z-plasty to simulate the nasolabial fold. Closure is accomplished with nylon sutures (Fig. 103-20).

Microvascular Free Flap

The microvascular free flap has become the surgical workhorse in augmenting the deficient soft tissue of the cheek and preauricular and neck regions (Fig. 103-21). The preferred donor site is the parascapular area,[25] and different components of the flap can be used to restore the contour of the temporal, cheek, and upper lip regions. It is wise to defer the free flap until the underlying skeletal deficiencies have been corrected. Soft tissue restoration with a microvascular free flap can camouflage any underlying postsurgical skeletal irregularities (Fig. 103-22). Although autogenous dermis-fat grafts and fat injections have been recommended, long-term survival is less predictable, and there can be residual contour irregularities.

Text continued on p. 546

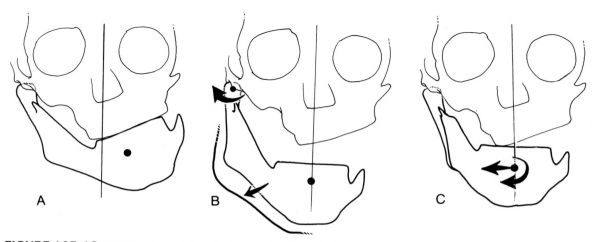

FIGURE 103-18. Unilateral craniofacial microsomia with underdevelopment of the mandibular ramus and absence of the condyle (left side). *A,* Preoperative appearance. *B,* Direction of the skeletal segment movement without associated osteotomy. *C,* Bilateral ramus osteotomies and direction of the skeletal segment movement.

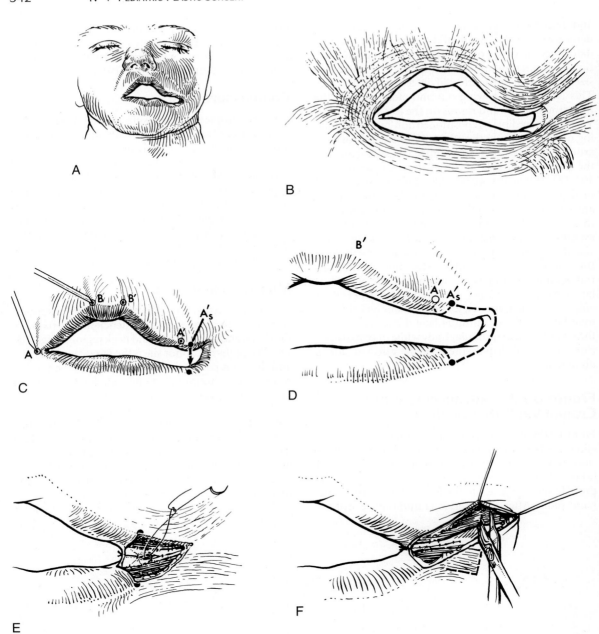

FIGURE 103-19. Correction of lateral facial cleft. *A*, Preoperative appearance, left-sided lateral facial cleft. *B*, Disruption of the orbicularis sphincter at the commissure. *C*, Markings are made on the white line with ink: A, oral commissure on unaffected side; B, philtral column on affected side; A', proposed oral commissure (distance = AB). A's is made the (overcorrected) surgical oral commissure because of expected postoperative contraction. A dot is placed opposite on the lower lip. *D*, Proposed vermilion turnover flap (outlined by the interrupted line). *E*, Closure of the oral mucosa. *F*, The upper and lower orbicularis muscle bundles are skeletonized and divided.

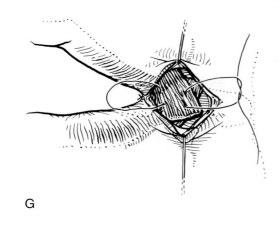

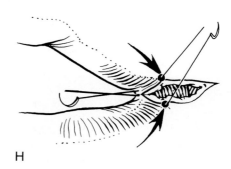

G

H

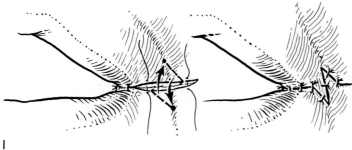

I

FIGURE 103-19, cont'd. *G,* Vest-over-pants closure of upper and lower divided ends of orbicularis muscle bundles. *H,* A simple suture is placed at the white lines at A's (see *C*). *I,* Proposed Z-plasty closure. The central limb must lie in the direction of the nasolabial fold.

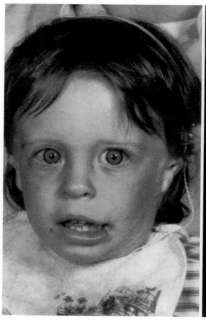

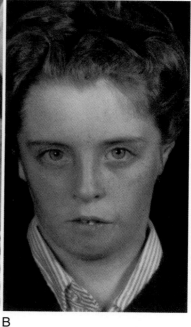

A

B

FIGURE 103-20. A 2-year-old boy with left-sided lateral facial cleft and bilateral microtia. *A,* Preoperative appearance. *B,* After correction by the technique illustrated in Figure 103-19.

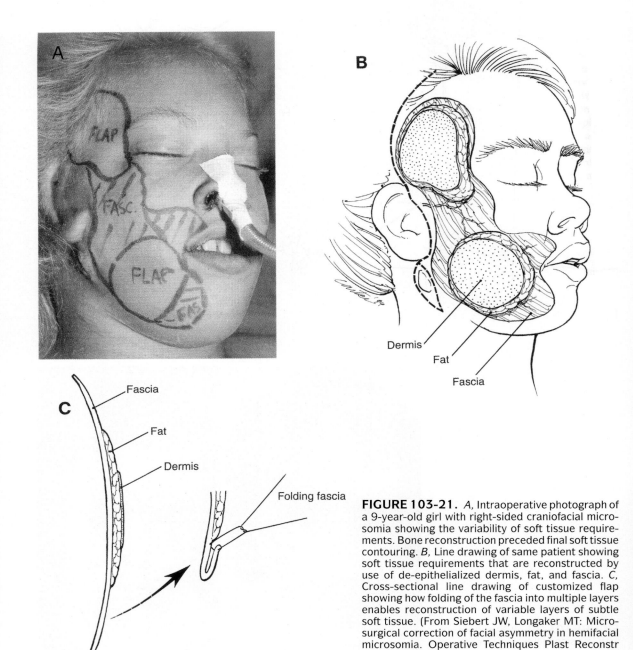

FIGURE 103-21. *A,* Intraoperative photograph of a 9-year-old girl with right-sided craniofacial microsomia showing the variability of soft tissue requirements. Bone reconstruction preceded final soft tissue contouring. *B,* Line drawing of same patient showing soft tissue requirements that are reconstructed by use of de-epithelialized dermis, fat, and fascia. *C,* Cross-sectional line drawing of customized flap showing how folding of the fascia into multiple layers enables reconstruction of variable layers of subtle soft tissue. (From Siebert JW, Longaker MT: Microsurgical correction of facial asymmetry in hemifacial microsomia. Operative Techniques Plast Reconstr Surg 1994;1:94.)

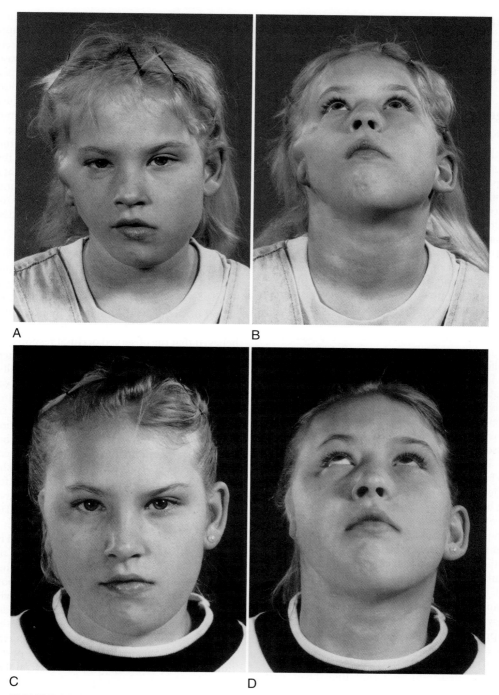

FIGURE 103-22. A 9-year-old girl with unilateral craniofacial microsomia after costochondral rib graft reconstruction of the right side of the mandible. *A,* Before microvascular free flap reconstruction of cheek and temporal areas (see Fig. 103-21). *B,* Preoperative basilar view. *C,* Postoperative frontal view. *D,* Postoperative basilar view. (From Siebert JW, Longaker MT: Microsurgical correction of facial asymmetry in hemifacial microsomia. Operative Techniques Plast Reconstr Surg 1994;1:93.)

Auricular Reconstruction

Auricular reconstruction is required in patients with microtia. The multistaged reconstruction is usually deferred until the child is at least 8 years of age (see Chapter 74).

Management of the Occlusion

EARLY INTERVENTION

Because the deciduous dentition is often used in the early interceptive orthodontic and surgical phases of care, the patient is referred for a pedodontic oral health evaluation between the ages of 12 and 18 months. This is intended to provide the parents with guidelines for their child's dental care and to begin preparing the child behaviorally to cooperate with oral examination and treatment.

The objectives of orthodontic treatment, in the deciduous dentition, are aimed at preventing or intercepting the development of severe malocclusion, an example of which is to provide adequate space for the eruption of the adult dentition by expansion and enlargement of the maxillary arch. In the mandibular dental arch, prevention of space loss due to premature shedding of a deciduous tooth may be achieved with a lingual arch space maintainer. On occasion, a mandibular first or second molar tooth bud may be present lying in the path of the anticipated distraction osteotomy or in the site of a planned bone graft. In some circumstances, the orthodontist may presurgically use orthodontic forces to erupt the tooth and to guide it out of the surgical site, sparing its early demise (Fig. 103-23).

A review of the orthodontic literature[39] shows that attempts have been made to use functional orthodontic appliance therapy to correct "mild" mandibular asymmetry in patients with craniofacial microsomia. The orthodontic literature is replete with papers debating the ability of functional appliance therapy to improve mandibular growth in children found among the "normal" population. It is doubtful that children born with mandibular anomalies of moderate to severe deficiency will achieve lasting benefit, if any, from functional appliance therapies. The authors are of the opinion that the therapeutic benefits or results of functional therapy in this population would be extremely limited, and therefore they favor early mandibular distraction osteogenesis or bone graft reconstruction.

TREATMENT PLANNING AND BIOMECHANICS OF MANDIBULAR DISTRACTION

Pre-Distraction Orthodontic Management

As in the preparation of a patient for orthognathic surgery, pre-distraction orthodontics may include removal of dental compensations, coordination of dental arch widths, and correction of occlusal plane disharmony and crowding. After these objectives are achieved with fixed orthodontic appliances, passive rectangular arch wires and surgical hooks are placed for the use of intermaxillary guiding elastics during the active stage of distraction. It appears that during this stage, before consolidation of the newly formed bone (regenerate), it is possible to mold the regenerate with intermaxillary elastics and to adjust the vector of distraction to achieve the planned occlusion. In the young child, an occlusal splint might be required at the end of device activation to maintain the leveled mandibular occlusal plane while room is left for the post-distraction correction of the maxillary occlusal plane.

Intermaxillary Elastics During Active Distraction

The vectors of distraction may be further modified by the use of intermaxillary elastics during the activation phase. After a bone regenerate is formed by linear activation of the distraction device, intermaxillary elastics can alter the skeletal and dental relationships. It is believed that the observed occlusal response to elastic forces is secondary to molding of the regenerate and dentoalveolar remodeling. Thus, intermaxillary elastics can be employed to modify the direction of skeletal change and to fine-tune the occlusal result. Intermaxillary elastics may be worn in class II, class III, vertical, or transverse directions during the activation phase. Anterior vertical intermaxillary elastics may be helpful in reducing an anterior open bite and may be employed transversely to correct or to prevent lateral shifting of the mandible (Fig. 103-24). In some patients for whom an open bite has been closed, intermaxillary elastics may be worn during the consolidation period for skeletal and dental retention (Fig. 103-25).[40]

The progress of distraction is monitored by documenting changes in the relationships of the maxillary and mandibular dentition and changes in the level of the occlusal plane, oral commissure, and position of the chin. In general, and especially in the growing child, activation of the device continues until the deformity is overcorrected (e.g., anterior crossbite in a micrognathic patient). The amount of overcorrection is influenced by the amount of expected post-distraction growth remaining in the craniofacial skeleton. A young child with much growth ahead would be overcorrected more than a child who is approaching completion of growth.[40] With the expectation that post-distraction growth will be "syndromic" and inadequate to keep up with the "normal side," there is a need for overcorrection of the ramus in the *very young* child.

Post-Distraction Orthodontic Management

In the unilateral distraction cases, the orthodontist is often confronted with a posterior open bite on the

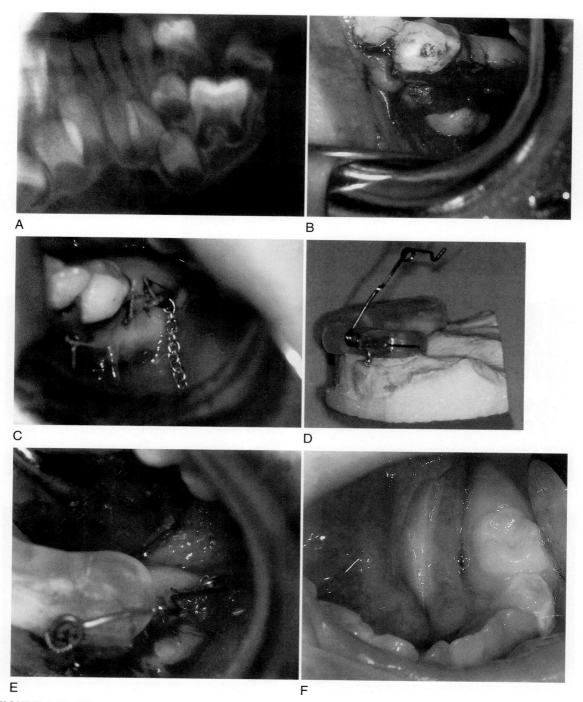

FIGURE 103-23. Orthodontic eruption of tooth at the osteotomy site. *A*, Radiograph demonstrating deciduous molars and permanent first molar. *B*, Surgical exposure of crown of first adult molar after extraction of deciduous molars. *C*, Chain attached to first adult molar at time of surgery. *D*, Bonded occlusal appliance with active spring used to elevate first adult molar. *E*, Activation of spring, engaging chain. *F*, Exposure of first adult molar resulting in an osteotomy site free of dentition.

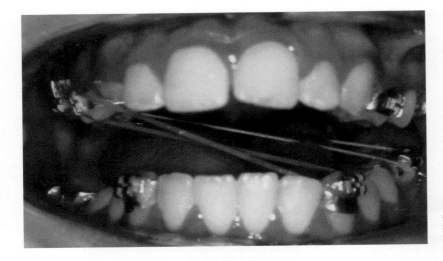

FIGURE 103-24. Translingual elastics preventing laterognathism during activation of a unilateral distraction device.

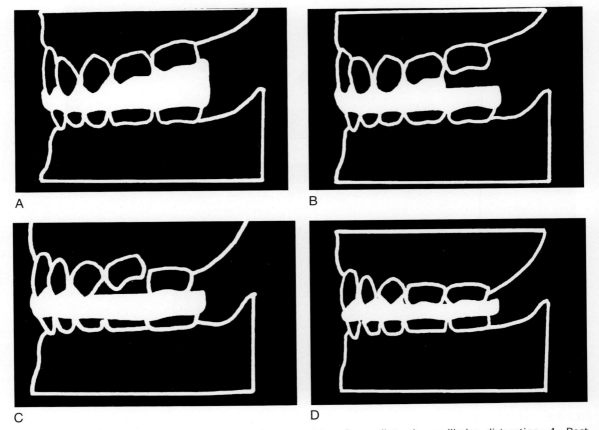

A

B

C

D

FIGURE 103-25. Management of the posterior open bite after unilateral mandibular distraction. *A,* Post-distraction open bite with occlusal bite plate. *B,* Reduction of bite plate occlusal to the posterior maxillary molar. *C,* Eruption of the posterior maxillary molar to the bite plate followed by anterior reduction of the bite plate. *D,* After occlusal eruption of the maxillary dentition to the reduced surface of the bite plate.

distracted side and crossbite on the contralateral side (see Figs. 103-24 and 103-25). The open bite may be managed with gradual adjustment of a bite plate (see Fig. 103-25B to D). The crossbite resulting from mandibular shift across the midsagittal plane may be corrected by a combination of transpalatal arches, lingual arches, intermaxillary cross elastics, and palatal expansion devices.

The posterior open bite that is often observed after unilateral distraction results from lowering of the mandibular occlusal plane on the affected side while the untreated maxilla still has its upward occlusal cant. It is important to prevent relapse of the mandibular occlusal plane correction resulting from uncontrolled occlusal overeruption of the mandibular teeth and alveolus. The posterior open bite plate is adjusted gradually to achieve eruption of the maxillary teeth and dentoalveolar process down to the level of the mandibular occlusal plane. During several months, the posterior-superior surface of the appliance is serially reduced under pairs of maxillary teeth to allow their gradual eruption and inferior descent.

After vertical unilateral distraction of the mandibular ramus, the mandibular body shifts toward the contralateral side, often resulting in posterior crossbites. The crossbite on the expanded side shows the maxillary teeth buccal to the lower teeth. On the contralateral side, the maxillary teeth are palatal to the mandibular teeth (palatal crossbite). The palate may be expanded to correct the crossbite with a classic palatal expansion device. Maxillary palatal expansion is typically a bilateral phenomenon: as the palatal crossbite is corrected, the buccal crossbite may worsen. To prevent this, intermaxillary cross elastics may be worn on the side of the buccal crossbite. The lower molars may be supported by a lingual arch to minimize the tendency for the cross elastic to tip the lower molars out toward the buccal aspect while the maxillary molars are tipped to the palatal aspect and into improved occlusal relationship with the lower dental arch.[40]

TREATMENT ALGORITHM
Neonatal Period and Infancy

In the evaluation of the newborn or infant, the surgeon must assess the respiratory function of the child. With a severe mandibular deficiency and associated glossoptosis, the nasal and oral pharyngeal spaces are severely constricted. A pediatric otolaryngologist is invaluable in documenting the respiratory status of the patient by physical and endoscopic examination. Pulse oximetry and sleep studies complement this evaluation.

Endotracheal intubation is occasionally indicated after delivery. If it appears that the need for endotracheal intubation will be prolonged, tracheostomy has traditionally been the technique employed. With the development of mandibular distraction, it has been demonstrated that distraction of the mandible can obviate the need for a tracheostomy.[27] Whichever modality is selected, the clinician must be aware that by one method or another, the airway must be secured.

Infants with sleep apnea often have associated feeding problems. Gavage feeding can be provided initially, but if the feeding problem continues, gastrostomy should be considered to ensure adequate calorie intake for the child. The nutritional requirements of the infant are accentuated by the energy demands associated with respiratory distress.

Fronto-orbital advancement and cranial vault remodeling may also be indicated in a small percentage of patients with a fronto-orbital deformity. Such surgery should be delayed until the child is at least 12 months of age.

A few patients may also require repair of an associated cleft of the hard or soft palate, and this should be done at approximately 12 months to facilitate speech development. It is also the optimal time to repair a macrostomia or lateral facial cleft.

Removal of ear tags or cartilaginous remnants in the cheeks is always satisfying for the parents, and this can also be done in the first year.

Early Childhood

During the period of early childhood (18 months through 3 years), reconstruction can be undertaken in the child with respiratory insufficiency or a moderate or severe example of skeletal deficiency.

For the child with a Pruzansky type III mandible (absent ramus and condyle), autogenous rib or iliac bone grafting of the hypoplastic mandible should be undertaken. As mentioned previously, such bone is amenable to a distraction procedure at a later stage (see Fig. 103-13). The procedure would result in an improved airway and facial appearance. It would also facilitate orthodontic work in establishing a functional occlusion.

For the patient with a type IIA or type IIB mandibular deformity, mandible distraction could be undertaken. In the unilateral case, activation of the distraction device should continue until the occlusal plane has been leveled, the oral commissure lowered, and sufficient anterior thrust of the mandible achieved.

Soft tissue augmentation is not undertaken at this stage. In like fashion, the child is not a suitable candidate for orthodontic therapy or auricular reconstruction.

Childhood

Childhood is defined as the period from 4 through 13 years when there is active growth. For much of this time, the child is in the period of mixed dentition. Primary mandibular distraction could be undertaken during this period if there is evidence of a significant occlusal cant, disparity of the oral commissure, and chin asymmetry and retrusion.

Experience has shown that in the patient undergoing mandibular distraction before 3 years of age, there is usually a spontaneous descent of the associated maxillary dentoalveolus with mandibular distraction.[41] Beyond that age, there are two choices for managing the tilt or cant of the maxillary dentoalveolus. In the first program, mandibular distraction can be accomplished and an orthodontic bite block constructed at the time of device removal to fill the resulting posterior void between the maxillary and mandibular dentition (see Fig. 103-25). During the subsequent year, the orthodontist can gradually reduce the bite block to allow serial descent of the maxillary dentoalveolus.[40] In the alternative method, combined maxillomandibular distraction (see Fig. 103-10) is performed with a combined Le Fort I corticotomy, sparing the unerupted maxillary dentition, and mandibular osteotomy with distraction device application.[33] With activation of the device and intermaxillary fixation, there is associated distraction of the maxilla with leveling of the occlusal plane.

It is during the childhood years that auricular reconstruction is undertaken and microvascular free flap augmentation of the cheek soft tissues can be considered.

Orthodontic therapy can be instituted as early as 4 years of age, depending on the level of the patient's cooperation. The following treatment options must be considered by the orthodontist:

1. Early intervention by a pediatric dentist to prepare the teeth for any orthodontic therapy.
2. Early orthodontic intervention:
   • Maxillary arch expansion to provide space for the adult dentition.
   • Mandibular lingual arch space maintenance for the adult dentition.
   • Forced eruption of a molar tooth bud out of the proposed path of the mandibular osteotomy to prevent extraction of a molar (see Fig. 103-23).
3. Distraction stabilization appliance for unilateral ramal vertical lengthening.[42]
4. Bite block therapy for controlled dentoalveolar elongation of the ipsilateral maxillary posterior segment.[40]

Adolescence and Adulthood

Adolescence/adulthood is defined as that period when craniofacial growth and development are completed, usually at a minimum of 15 years for girls and 17 years for boys. Treatment planning at this stage does not have to take into consideration the variable of subsequent growth and development. The role of the orthodontist involves preoperative planning as well as presurgical and postsurgical orthodontic therapy.

Orthognathic surgery plays a role at this point because in a single surgical maneuver, the craniofacial skeletal structure can be restored and optimal occlusion achieved as part of a combined orthodontic and surgical rehabilitation program. The surgical procedure described by Obwegeser[12] (Le Fort I osteotomy, bilateral sagittal split osteotomy of the mandible, and genioplasty) has proved to be the therapeutic workhorse in this situation (see Fig. 103-15).

In recent years, with the development of refined distraction devices and techniques, the role of maxillomandibular distraction in the mature patient has increased. For example, a Le Fort I osteotomy can be performed with three-dimensional repositioning of the maxilla and rigid skeletal fixation. Intraoral mandibular distraction can then be performed, and the mandible and its occlusion can be "docked" into the repositioned maxilla. The distraction technique also improves soft tissue contour and is associated with a lower rate of relapse. The development of the concept of molding of the regenerate by a combination of multiplanar distraction devices and skeletally and dentally anchored intermaxillary elastics ensures the achievement of optimal occlusion and skeletal structure.[31]

Genioplasty alone is the only skeletal reconstruction required in patients with a mild deformity characterized only by chin retrusion and asymmetry. A three-dimensional genioplasty can provide anterior advancement of the chin and three-dimensional repositioning to correct asymmetry (Figs. 103-26 and 103-27).[12]

GROWTH STUDIES

Mandibular Growth in Unilateral Craniofacial Microsomia: A Controversy

Polley et al[43] described the skeletal growth from early childhood to maturity of patients with unilateral craniofacial microsomia who did not undergo surgery. They reported that mandibular asymmetry is not progressive in nature. The authors of this chapter also agree that the "mandibular asymmetry is not progressive in nature"; however, a controversy exists around describing the ramal growth rates that are responsible for maintaining a constant ratio of size difference between the left and right mandibular rami during the years of mandibular growth. Polley et al[43] stated that "growth of the affected side in these patients parallels that of the nonaffected side." The authors take the contrary position that growth of the affected side occurs at a rate that is less than that of the unaffected side, a finding that in itself is responsible for the gradual return to

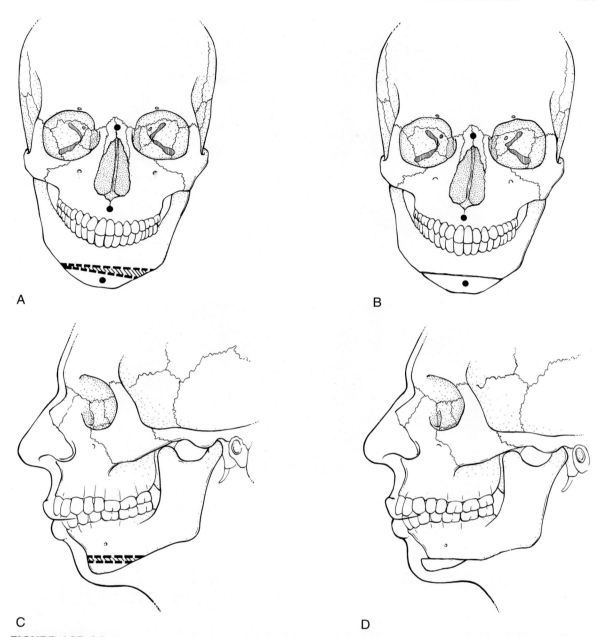

FIGURE 103-26. Asymmetric genioplasty. *A,* Preoperative frontal views showing area of resection *(shaded)* and lines of osteotomy. Dots designate the asymmetry of the craniofacial midline. *B,* Postoperative frontal view. *C,* Preoperative profile with line of osteotomy and area of resection *(shaded)*. *D,* Postoperative profile. Fixation is obtained with either lag screws or plate and screws.

asymmetry after early unilateral mandibular distraction in growing children with unilateral craniofacial microsomia. Close examination of the data published by Polley et al[43] shows that the ratio of affected ramus length to unaffected ramus length remains the same over time because of, rather than in spite of, different rates of growth on each side of the mandible.

Long-term Change and Growth After Distraction

In a longitudinal study of 10 patients with unilateral craniofacial microsomia and bilateral micrognathia who underwent correction of their mandibular deformities by distraction osteogenesis, clinical and

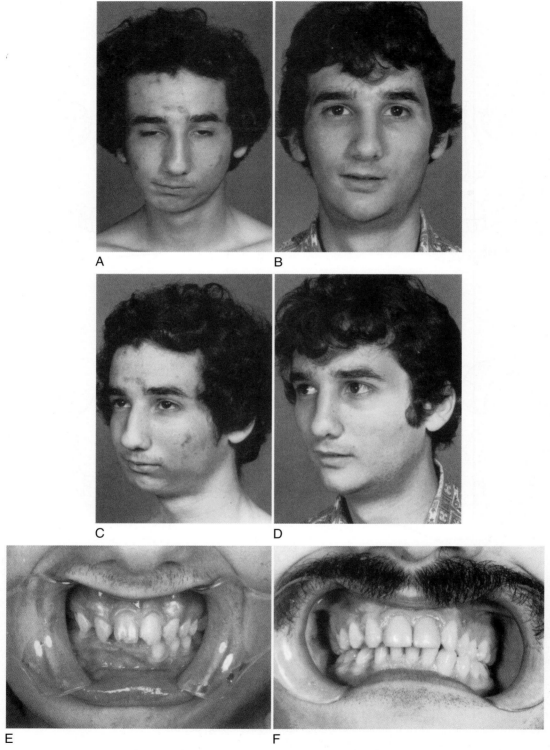

FIGURE 103-27. Adolescent man with right-sided craniofacial microsomia. *A* and *C,* Preoperative appearance. *B* and *D,* Postoperative views after rhinoplasty, onlay bone grafting, and genioplasty or horizontal osteotomy of the anteroinferior border of the mandible. *E,* Preoperative occlusion. *F,* After orthodontic and prosthodontic therapy.

cephalometric examinations were performed for a follow-up period ranging from 12 to 70 months.[44] Five patients underwent unilateral mandibular distraction, and five patients underwent bilateral distraction with an extraoral device. The average age at the time of distraction was 31 months (range, 19 to 43 months). In the period of observation after distraction, the 10 mandibles showed cephalometric and clinical evidence of growth. In the five unilateral cases, the side not operated on grew in a pattern that would be expected for the unaffected side of a mandible with unilateral craniofacial microsomia. The distracted side, however, grew with a variable response. Growth occurred at the site of the bone regenerate as well as in the adjacent body, ramus, and condylar head. No evidence of relapse was noted in any patient. The growth response of the side operated on was variable and appeared to be dependent on the genetic program of the native bone and the surrounding soft tissue matrix. Morphologic and volumetric improvements previously reported for the condyle were maintained long term, with continued growth of the condyle without evidence of deformational changes.

In the five patients who underwent bilateral distraction, the neomandible grew during the period of observation. Both sides of the mandible grew at comparable rates. The sites not operated on, including the body and condyle, also showed evidence of growth throughout the study period.

Comparison of lateral cephalograms revealed that a clockwise rotation of the mandible occurred with the passage of time. Clockwise mandibular rotation occurred secondary to the expected vertical growth of the maxillary dentoalveolus as the children passed from the primary to the mixed and finally the permanent dentition. Tooth development and eruption occurred with no evidence of developmental delay.[40]

REFERENCES

1. Pruzansky S: Not all dwarfed mandibles are alike. Birth Defects 1969;1:120.
2. Kaban LB, Moses MH, Mulliken JB: Surgical correction of hemifacial microsomia in the growing child. Plast Reconstr Surg 1998;82:9.
3. Gosain AK, McCarthy JG, Pinto RS: Cervico-vertebral anomalies and basilar impression in Goldenhar syndrome. Plast Reconstr Surg 1994;93:498.
4. Longacre JJ, DeStefano GA, Holmstrand KE: Surgical management of first and second branchial arch syndromes. Plast Reconstr Surg 1963;31:507.
5. Munro IR, Lauritzen CG: Classification and treatment of hemifacial microsomia. In Caronni EP, ed: Craniofacial Surgery. Boston, Little, Brown, 1985:391-400.
6. Converse JM, Shapiro HH: Treatment of developmental malformations of the jaws. Plast Reconstr Surg 1954;10:473.
7. Gorski M, Tarczynska IH: Surgical treatment of mandibular asymmetry. Br J Plast Surg 1969;22:370.
8. Stark RB, Saunders DE: The first branchial syndrome: the oral-mandibular auricular syndrome. Plast Reconstr Surg 1962;29:229.
9. Brown JB, Fryer MP, Ohlwiler DA: Study and use of synthetic material, such as silicones and Teflon, as subcutaneous prosthesis. Plast Reconstr Surg 1960;26:264.
10. Poswillo DE: Otomandibular deformity: pathogenesis as a guide to reconstruction. J Maxillofac Surg 1974;2:64.
11. Moss ML: The primacy of functional matrices in orofacial growth. Dent Pract Dent Rec 1968;19:65.
12. Obwegeser HL: Correction of the skeletal anomalies of otomandibular dysostosis. J Maxillofac Surg 1974;2:73.
13. Dingman RO, Grabb WC: Reconstruction of both mandibular condyles with metatarsal bone grafts. Plast Reconstr Surg 1964;34:441 [follow-up clinic, Plast Reconstr Surg 1971;47:594].
14. Converse JM, Rushton AM. In Gillies H, Millard DR Jr, eds: The Principles and Art of Plastic Surgery, vol I. Boston, Little, Brown, 1957:314.
15. Delaire J: De l'interet des osteotomies sagittales dans la correction des infragnathies mandibulaires. Ann Chir Plast 1970;15:104.
16. Converse JM, Horowitz SL, Coccaro PJ, Wood-Smith D: Corrective treatment of the skeletal asymmetry in hemifacial microsomia. Plast Reconstr Surg 1973;52:221.
17. Murray JE, Kaban LB, Mulliken JB: Analysis and treatment of hemifacial microsomia. Plast Reconstr Surg 1984;74:186.
18. McCarthy JG, Schreiber JS, Karp NS, et al: Lengthening of the human mandible by gradual distraction. Plast Reconstr Surg 1992;89:1.
19. Molina F, Ortiz-Monasterio F: Mandibular elongation and remodeling by distraction: a farewell to major osteotomies. Plast Reconstr Surg 1995;96:825.
20. Davis WB: Reconstruction of hemiatrophy of face. Plast Reconstr Surg 1968;42:489.
21. Gillies H, Millard DR Jr: The Principles and Art of Plastic Surgery. Boston, Little, Brown, 1957.
22. Brown JB, McDowell F: Skin Grafting, 3rd ed. Philadelphia, JB Lippincott, 1958:114.
23. Fujino T, Rytinzaburo T, Sugimoto C: Microvascular transfer of free deltopectoral dermal-flat flap. Plast Reconstr Surg 1975;55:428.
24. Wells JH, Edgerton MT: Correction of severe hemifacial atrophy with a free dermis-fat flap from the lower abdomen. Plast Reconstr Surg 1977;59:223.
25. Siebert JW, Longaker MT: Microsurgical correction of facial asymmetry in hemifacial microsomia. Operative Techniques Plast Reconstr Surg 1994;1:93.
26. Upton J, Mulliken JB, Hicks PD, Murray JE: Restoration of facial contour using free vascularized omental transfer. Plast Reconstr Surg 1980;66:560.
27. Denny AD, Talisman R, Hansen PR, Recinos RF: Mandibular distraction in very young patients to correct airway obstruction. Plast Reconstr Surg 2001;108:302.
28. Diner PA, Kollar EM, Martinez H, Vasquez MP: Intraoral distraction for mandibular lengthening: a technical innovation. J Craniomaxillofac Surg 1996;24:92.
29. Katzen JT, Holliday RA, McCarthy JG: Imaging the neonatal mandible for accurate distraction osteogenesis. J Craniofac Surg 2001;12:26.
30. Grayson BH, McCormick S, Santiago PE, McCarthy JG: Vector of device placement and trajectory of mandibular distraction. J Craniofac Surg 1997;8:473.
31. McCarthy JG, Hopper RA, Hollier LH, et al: Molding of the regenerate in mandibular distraction. Part II. Clinical experience. Plast Reconstr Surg 2003;112:1239.
32. Stucki-McCormick S, Winich R, Winich A: Distraction osteogenesis for the reconstruction of the temporomandibular joint. N Y State Dent J 1998;64:36.
33. Ortiz-Monasterio F, Molina F, Andrade L, et al: Simultaneous mandibular and maxillary distraction in hemifacial microsomia in adults: avoiding occlusal disasters. Plast Reconstr Surg 1997;100:852.

34. Stelnicki EJ, Hollier L, Lee C, et al: Distraction osteogenesis of costochondral bone grafts in the mandible. Plast Reconstr Surg 2002;109:925.

35. McCarthy JG: Reconstruction of the Pruzansky III mandible by tooth enucleation and subsequent transport distraction. Presented at the Biannual Meeting of the International Society of Craniofacial Surgeons, Visby, Sweden, June 2001.

36. Grayson B, Boral S, Eisig S, et al: Unilateral craniofacial microsomia. Part I—mandibular analysis. Am J Orthod 1983;84:225.

37. McCarthy JG, Grayson B, Coccaro PG, Wood-Smith D: Craniofacial microsomia. In McCarthy JG, ed: Plastic Surgery. Philadelphia, WB Saunders, 1990:3054.

38. McCarthy JG, Fuleihan NS: Commissuroplasty in lateral facial clefts. In Stark RB, ed: Plastic Surgery of the Head and Neck. Boston, Little, Brown, 1986.

39. Harvold EP, Vargervik K, Chierici G: Treatment of Hemifacial Microsomia. New York, AR Liss, 1983.

40. Grayson BH, Santiago PE: Treatment planning and biomechanics of distraction osteogenesis from an orthodontic perspective. Semin Orthod 1999;5:9.

41. McCarthy JG, ed: Distraction of the Craniofacial Skeleton. New York, Springer-Verlag, 1999.

42. Hanson P, Melugin MB: Orthodontic management of the patient undergoing mandibular distraction osteogenesis. Semin Orthod 1999;5:25.

43. Polley JW, Figueroa AA, Liou EJ, Cohen MN: Longitudinal analysis of mandibular asymmetry in hemifacial microsomia. Plast Reconstr Surg 1997;99:328.

44. Hollier LH, Kim JH, Grayson B, McCarthy JG: Mandibular growth after distraction in patients after 48 months of age. Plast Reconstr Surg 1999;103:1361.

45. Kaban LB, Mulliken JB, Murray JE: Three-dimensional approach to analysis and treatment of hemifacial microsomia. Cleft Palate Craniofac J 1981;18:90.

Hemifacial Atrophy

JOHN W. SIEBERT, MD ✦ HOOMAN SOLTANIAN, MD
✦ ALEXES HAZEN, MD

Restoration of a harmonious and symmetric appearance is a crucial aspect of surgical treatment for many congenital and acquired deformities of the face. Facial contour deformities can result from a variety of causes, be unilateral or bilateral, and range in severity from mild to severe. Progressive facial atrophy (or Romberg disease) is the most frequently seen cause of facial contour deformity indicating surgical correction. Other causes include connective tissue disorders, nerve palsy, burns, trauma, hemifacial microsomia, and other congenital abnormalities. For the purposes of this chapter, we focus on facial atrophy, although the same basic principles and surgical technique can be applied to the entire range of deformities.

Whereas there are many well-described methods to accomplish restoration of facial contour and facial "harmony," microsurgical techniques have become the "gold standard." It has been the authors' experience during the past 15 years that free tissue transfer yields the best and most predictable results. Fasciocutaneous flaps specifically have demonstrated the most superior aesthetic results; they can be sculpted and shaped with more precision, allowing the return of facial symmetry and harmony.

BACKGROUND

Romberg Disease

Romberg disease is a progressive hemifacial atrophy of unknown etiology. Parry first described this clinical phenomenon in 1825, and it was then detailed by Romberg in 1846.[1,2] Romberg disease usually begins in the first 2 decades of life. Females are affected 1.5 times more than are males. Romberg disease is unilateral in 95% of patients, with both sides of the face affected equally. The atrophy is progressive and usually affects the skin and subcutaneous tissue. In patients with severe disease (usually with onset in childhood), the muscles and bones may also be affected.

The etiology of Romberg disease is not well understood. Although it is distinct from scleroderma, it may represent a localized form of this disease. Atrophic tissue in Romberg disease histologically shows chronic inflammation and scarring. The pathogenesis of Romberg disease has been proposed by four different theories: infection resulting in a degenerative effect on the sympathetic nervous system, trigeminal neuritis, an increased sympathetic condition triggering the initiation of facial atrophy, and chronic neurovasculitis.[3-5] The progression of the atrophy may last 2 to 10 years. After this, the disease process seems to enter a stable or "burnout" phase.

Connective Tissue Disorders

Systemic lupus erythematosus and scleroderma are the most common connective tissue disorders resulting in soft tissue atrophy with facial involvement. Lupus erythematosus is an inflammatory connective tissue disorder of unknown cause occurring predominantly in women (90% of patients). It can have a variable course. Patients often have antinuclear antibodies including anti-DNA antibodies (more specific for systemic lupus) in their serum. Various forms of lupus can result in telangiectasia and skin atrophy.[6-8]

Scleroderma, seen four times more often in women, causes diffuse fibrosis of the skin, blood vessels, synovia, and vital organs such as the kidneys. The pathogenesis is not fully clear. A combination of vascular abnormalities, excess collagen, and deposition of matrix substance are being discussed as possible causes of this disorder. The skin is involved in more than 95% of patients.[9-12]

INDICATIONS AND OPTIONS FOR SURGERY

Patients who have suffered from Romberg disease or other connective tissue disorders resulting in facial atrophy may have a deformity that is often composed of all components of the facial form, from skin and subcutaneous tissues to muscle and bone. The options for correction of facial deformities caused by facial atrophy include synthetic materials such as liquid silicone[13-16] and implants, bone and cartilage grafts, fat and dermal grafts, and free tissue transplantation. The results of facial contouring with silicone injections have generally been unsatisfactory with the possibility of delayed scar and contracture formation as well as occasional skin breakdown. Removal of free silicone is at times a difficult task and can make future reconstructive efforts more challenging. The use of injectable materials seems appealing at first glance. For mild defects, injection of synthetic materials appears to be a "quick fix" and is of little cost to the patient and little time to the surgeon. However, contrary to the initial promise of injectable and prosthetic materials, the clinical results have been disappointing. Whereas these materials are easy to use, with low risk to the patient, the results are often dissatisfying to patient and surgeon alike.

Autologous fat injections have the obvious advantage of being cost-efficient and relatively simple to perform with no risk of "rejection" or allergic reaction. Large defects are less suitable for fat injections.[17,18] However, injectable materials such as fat, collagen, and Cymetra have the difficulty of being resorbed over time. More permanent materials, on the other hand, are susceptible to infection, seroma, and capsule formation and have unpredictable results.

Who is a candidate for facial contour correction with a free flap? Whereas other authors have claimed that not all patients are candidates for free flap surgery, the following approach is applicable to patients with both severe and mild abnormalities.[3] Muscle or musculocutaneous flaps are often too bulky for facial contouring and have thus been largely discarded. Omentum has been used for facial recontouring,[19,20] but it has many disadvantages, including intraabdominal harvest and difficulty in long-term flap fixation (with no dermal or facial attachments to fix the tissue to the desired location). The groin flap and superficial inferior epigastric flap are other options for fasciocutaneous free tissue transplantation. The superficial inferior epigastric flap is useful when large amounts of skin coverage are required (Fig. 104-1). However, this flap limits the possibility of incorpo-

rating thin, pliable fascia beyond the width of the skin paddle design. Therefore, this flap would not allow optimal management of subtle, midline-associated deformities often seen with hemifacial atrophy. The authors have found that flaps based on the circumflex scapular pedicle are the most versatile flaps for restoration of facial contour. The following sections focus primarily on the techniques of harvesting and use of those flaps.

TIMING OF THE OPERATION

Many of the underlying causes of facial atrophy have a progressive nature. It is important to ensure that the deformity has reached a stable stage before embarking on surgical correction. It is preferable to wait a minimum of 18 to 24 months after the atrophy stops progressing. The authors have performed free tissue transplantation for facial contouring in patients varying in age from 5 to 67 years. The superficial temporal vessels are of adequate size for microvascular anastomoses, even in the younger patients.

In patients with severe defects, when the subcutaneous tissue is almost completely atrophic, earlier intervention with free tissue transplantation can improve or prevent further atrophy of the overlying skin and may prevent or lessen subsequent skeletal wasting. If there are correctable skeletal abnormalities present, these should be addressed before the attempt to improve the soft tissue coverage. In patients with bilateral defects, free tissue transplantations are scheduled at least a month apart. The revision is performed bilaterally 6 months after the second free flap.

SURGICAL TECHNIQUE
Parascapular and Inframammary Extended Circumflex Scapular Flaps[21-28]

The areas of facial deformity are marked with the patient in the upright position. Attention is given to the three-dimensional nature of the asymmetry. A two-dimensional template can be used with special markings for the areas in need of thicker soft tissue augmentation (dermis, fat, and fascia) and the areas where the edges of the flap will be tapered and interdigitated with the normal tissue to avoid unsightly step-offs (Fig. 104-2).

The ipsilateral donor site is preferably used. This allows a two-team approach to the recipient area on the face and the donor site on the back. The horizontal and vertical branches of the circumflex scapular artery can be outlined on the skin with use of a hand-held Doppler probe. The required soft tissue flap is marked on the skin in a vertical to oblique

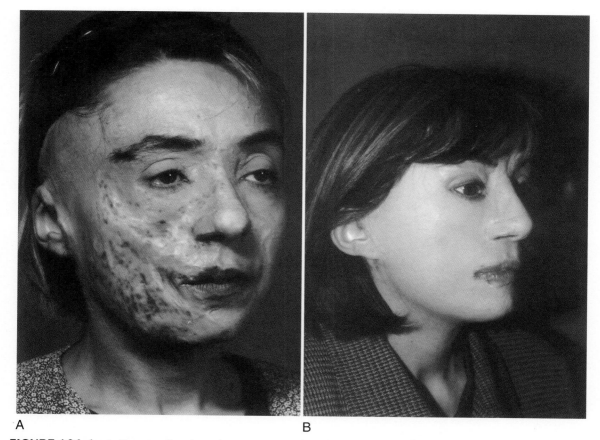

FIGURE 104-1. *A,* Preoperative view of a 41-year-old woman with a history of giant hairy nevus involving the right half of the face and nose. *B,* Postoperative view.

orientation, depending on the length needed. An inframammary extended circumflex scapular flap can be based on the anterior branches of the circumflex scapular artery (Fig. 104-3).[22]

The patient is placed in the supine position with padding behind the ipsilateral shoulder. This allows simultaneous exposure of the scapular and the facial areas. After closure of the donor site, the padding is removed so the face can be assessed more easily for symmetry. The ipsilateral upper extremity is prepared and draped along with the remaining operative areas. The upper arm and shoulder can be easily positioned during the harvest for a better visualization of the circumflex scapular vessels.

The table is positioned in the operating room in a fashion allowing the surgeon access to both sides of the head and the ipsilateral side of the patient. The anesthesia equipment is located along the contralateral side of the table. A crossbar is placed at the level of the shoulders and draped into the field so it can be used to stabilize the ipsilateral upper extremity during the harvest.

The recipient site on the face is injected with a diluted epinephrine solution. The face is dissected through a limited preauricular incision extending just to the earlobe. The facial dissection is performed in a subcutaneous plane to completely release all the soft tissue tethering. This is carried out beyond the borders of atrophy for adequate placement of the flap during the later phase of the operation. It may be required to dissect deep to the alar base at the piriform aperture to allow repositioning of the alar base to a more symmetric position with reconstruction of the deficient alar support. Frequently, the dissection is continued into the upper lip and adjacent oral commissure to lengthen the ipsilateral upper lip. Malposition and tethering of the ear can be addressed in a similar fashion.

The superficial temporal artery and vein are most commonly used as recipient vessels and are visualized through the preauricular incision. Exposure of the

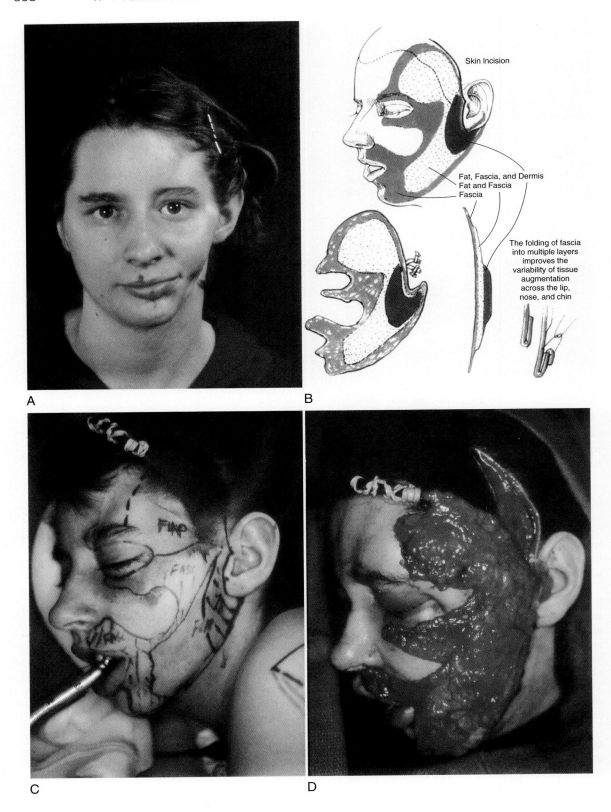

Skin Incision

Fat, Fascia, and Dermis
Fat and Fascia
Fascia

The folding of fascia
into multiple layers
improves the
variability of tissue
augmentation
across the lip,
nose, and chin

A

B

C

D

FIGURE 104-2. *A,* An 18-year-old woman with left-sided hemifacial atrophy. *B,* Diagrammatic representation of flap inset and composite tissue needed and used. *C,* Preoperative markings representing tissue deficits and soft tissue irregularities. *D,* Flap vascularized to superficial temporal vessels by microvascular technique. Variable tissue requirements are addressed with a single flap. Flap contour and bulk are then customized to desired shape and size. Areas of fascia and overlying fat can be trimmed and folded as necessary and placed in areas with greater soft tissue requirements.

superficial temporal vessels can require dissection well into the parotid gland.[21] Rarely, there is a need for an extension of the incision into the neck or a separate Risdon incision. Once an adequate skin envelope is developed, meticulous hemostasis is obtained and surgical sponges are placed within the pocket.

The parascapular flap can be harvested simultaneously. The flap commonly has an ellipsoid design that

simplifies the primary closure of the donor site. The circumflex scapular pedicle is located within the triangular space bordered by the teres major muscle inferiorly, the teres minor muscle superiorly, and the long head of the triceps muscle laterally. The flap is designed in a fashion to capture the vascular pedicle. An important point in the flap design is the location of the tissue requirements on the face in relation to the proposed location of the anastomosis to the superficial temporal vessels. If tissue augmentation is necessary both superior and inferior to the future anastomosis below the zygomatic arch, the donor flap will extend onto the shoulder as well as down into the inframammary fold. The amount of skin can be limited to the areas of the face with the most severe degree of atrophy and those that need the thickest flap. This approach has resulted in few instances in which full-thickness flap tissue (skin, fat, and fascia) requirements exceeded more than 8 to 9 cm in width. Therefore, tension-free closure of the donor site is the norm. Distinct blood supply of the fascia allows the harvest of extensions of the dorsal thoracic fascia, which can be used for

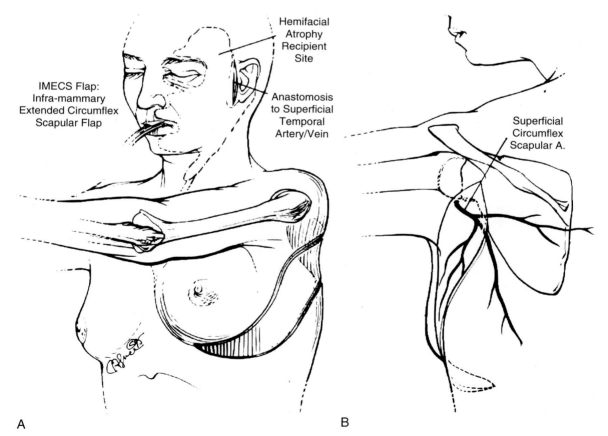

A   B

FIGURE 104-3. *A* and *B,* Diagram of inframammary extended circumflex scapular (IMECS) flap and corresponding vascular pedicle.

precise contouring of those areas with a lesser degree of atrophy. Fascial extensions can be folded into two or more layers to allow correction of variable deficits with the same flap.

The skin and subcutaneous tissue are incised, and the flap is elevated in a subfascial plane in a retrograde fashion. The vascular pedicle can be followed to the level of the thoracodorsal vessels. If there is need for additional bulk, portions of regional muscles, such as the teres major muscle, can be harvested. After adequate hemostasis, the wound is closed in layers over a closed suction drain.

Anastomoses to the superficial temporal vessels are performed in an end-to-end fashion, the vein followed by the artery. The flap is draped in its final orientation on the face. The skin is de-epithelialized, and the flap's thickness is tailored to meet the requirements of various regions. The transition between thicker and thinner areas is tapered to achieve a more natural facial contour. The facial structures and the transferred flap are edematous at this point. It is almost impossible to overresect or overthin the flap during the first operation. In the majority of patients, the optimal aesthetic reconstruction is achieved with a second procedure to revise the flap and to finalize the facial contouring.

At this point, the facial pocket is checked for hemostasis. The flap is secured in the area close to the anastomoses and also sutured to the periosteum of the infraorbital rim and zygoma with nonabsorbable material to prevent downward shift. The head of the bed is raised to help with natural contouring of the flap. The fascial extensions of the flap are secured in adequate positions with nylon sutures brought out through the skin and tied over petrolatum gauze (Fig. 104-4). It is important to stretch the flap out to its optimal dimensions to avoid sagging or redundancy of the flap. A skin island for monitoring purposes does not need to be saved unless there would be undue pressure on the flap with direct closure of the facial incision (this may be found in patients with a deformity due to sequelae of irradiation). A closed suction drain is placed superficial to the flap before skin closure.

POSTOPERATIVE CARE

No dressing is used on the face. Patients should receive one aspirin per day starting in the recovery room

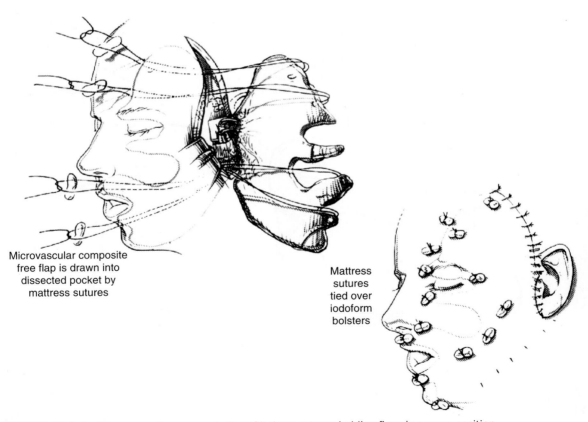

Microvascular composite free flap is drawn into dissected pocket by mattress sutures

Mattress sutures tied over iodoform bolsters

FIGURE 104-4. Diagrammatic representation of bolster sutures holding flaps in proper position.

(rectally). This continues orally for 1 month. The Doppler signals are monitored in the artery and vein postoperatively for 2 days. Intravenous hydration continues until oral intake is adequate. Patients leave the hospital between 3 and 5 days postoperatively. The facial drain is usually removed before discharge. The donor site drain and preauricular and facial sutures are removed on postoperative day 7.

The authors have not experienced a single instance of flap loss in more than 200 free tissue transplantations for correction of facial asymmetry. The rate of unplanned re-exploration has been less than 5% for hematoma or suspected vascular thrombosis. The final aesthetic result was not compromised in these patients.

Revisions are planned beginning approximately 5 months after free tissue transplantation to allow complete resolution of edema. Ancillary aesthetic procedures can be performed at the time of the revisional surgery.

REVISIONS

Most patients who undergo this operation will require revision, if only to debulk the flap. Revisions are best timed from 5 months after initial surgery. This will allow swelling to be reduced to normal and the flap to become well vascularized. If debulking is all that is required, the initial preauricular incision may be used, and either liposuction or direct excision with scissors may be performed (Fig. 104-5). Some patients may require other procedures with the overall goal of total facial harmony. With increasing aesthetic demands of patients with facial contour deformities, it has become necessary to include some of the standard aesthetic procedures into the overall plan. Procedures such as face lift, blepharoplasty, lateral canthoplasty, genioplasty, and rhinoplasty can be performed at the time of revisional surgery to enhance the final results (Figs. 104-6 to 104-8).[21]

SUMMARY

Optimization of facial aesthetic results for the challenging problem of restoration of facial contour has been achieved with free tissue transplantation. With increasing experience, the authors' indications for free tissue transplantation have been extended to the presence of any subtle contour deformity not amenable to correction with local or regional tissue rearrangements. The authors' technique has become more refined, and careful attention is paid to both the recipient and donor site scars. The limited preauricular incision minimizes the stigmata of facial surgery, or more specifically, it eliminates an unsightly neck incision. If recipient vessels in the neck are needed, the access should be provided through an incision parallel to the skin creases in the neck separate from the preauricular incision. The attempt to connect these two incisions often results in a prominent scar. An attempt should be made to eliminate even subtle contour abnormalities in the face, including the forehead, lips, chin, periorbita, nose, and ears. The donor site can be minimized and hidden by careful preoperative planning (Fig. 104-9). When the inframammary extended circumflex scapular flap is used, the scar will be largely under the arm. With further experience, one may also be able to harvest large fasciocutaneous flaps with smaller and smaller incisions. The authors' operative times, initially approximately $6^{1}/_{2}$ hours, have been reduced to approximately 5 hours. The overall goal is one of facial harmony, which may include, as previously stated, ancillary procedures and revisions. It is more difficult to achieve symmetry in patients with a unilateral defect. The reconstructed side can never duplicate the normal contralateral side in all aspects, including form and texture. Optimal results are more easily achieved with bilateral contour problems; it is less challenging to match one reconstruction to another than to match the uninvolved contralateral side of the face.

Text continued on p. 568

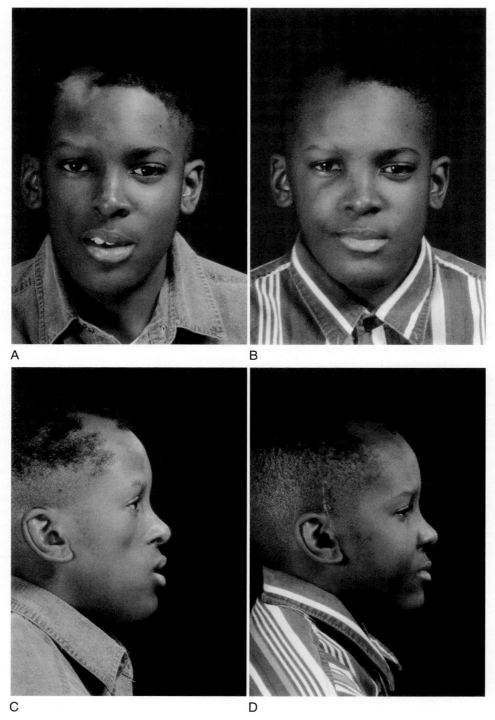

FIGURE 104-5. *A, C,* and *E,* Preoperative views of a 12-year-old boy with linear scleroderma. *B, D,* and *F,* Postoperative appearance (2¹/₂ years later) after parascapular free flap. Note lip lengthening, nasal lengthening, and facial contouring on postoperative views.

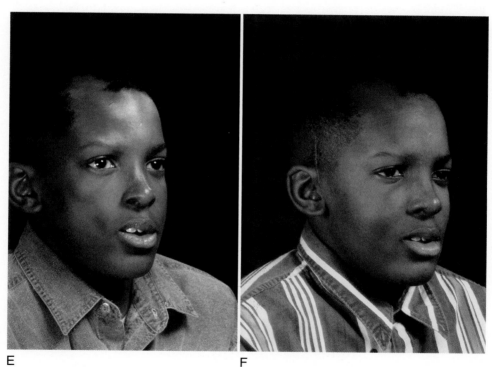

E   F

FIGURE 104-5, cont'd.

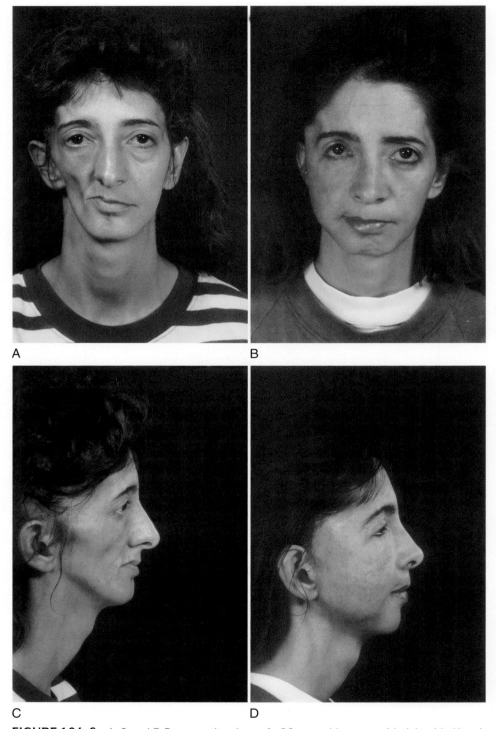

FIGURE 104-6. *A, C,* and *E,* Preoperative views of a 26-year-old woman with right-sided hemifacial atrophy. *B, D,* and *F,* Postoperative views 2¹/₂ years later. The patient underwent a parascapular free flap and, at the time of revision, rhinoplasty, blepharoplasty, and a lip-switch procedure for vermilion atrophy.

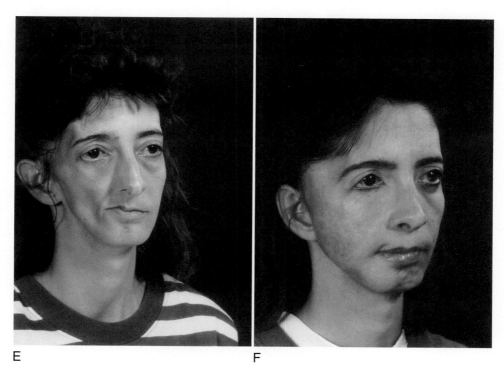

E

F

FIGURE 104-6, cont'd.

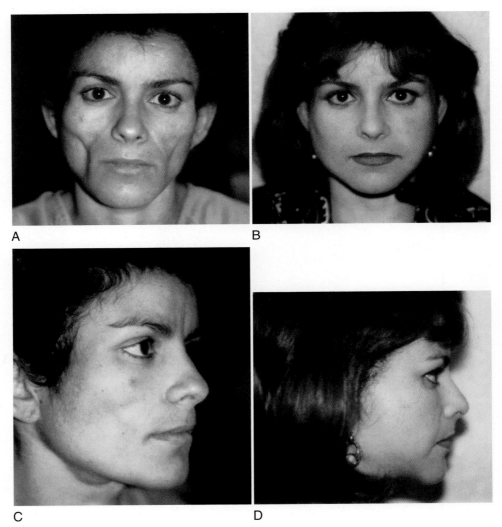

FIGURE 104-7. *A, C,* and *E,* A 27-year-old woman with bilateral facial atrophy associated with systemic lupus erythematosus. *B, D,* and *F,* Postoperative appearance after bilateral free tissue transplantation with superficial inferior gastric flaps. The patient underwent a revision at 6 months. Note symmetry and restoration of youthful appearance.

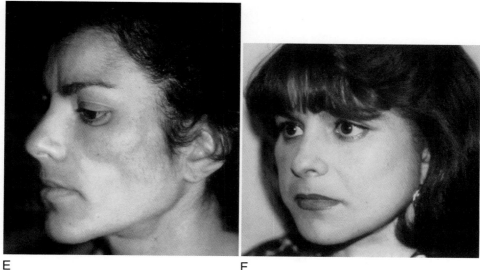

E   F

FIGURE 104-7, cont'd.

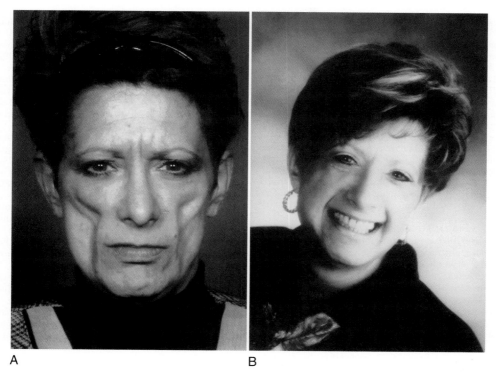

A   B

FIGURE 104-8. *A,* Preoperative view of a 42-year-old woman with nonspecific collagen vascular disorder and bilateral wasting. *B,* View 2 years postoperatively with appearance demonstrating facial animation and excellent symmetry.

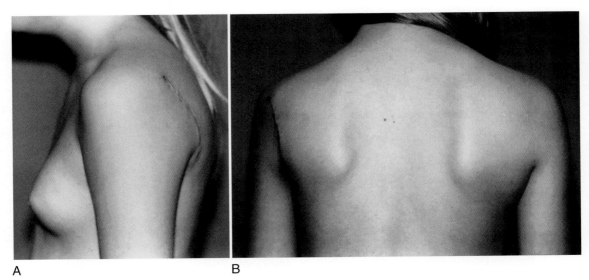

FIGURE 104-9. *A* and *B,* Typical early donor site in a 12-year-old girl after parascapular free flap (current incisions are more limited).

REFERENCES

1. Romberg HM: Trophoneurosen. Klinische Ergebnisse. Berlin, Forstner, 1846:75-81.
2. Parry CH: Collections from the Unpublished Medical Writings of the Late C. H. Parry. London, Underwoods, 1825:478.
3. Wells JH, Edgerton MT: Correction of severe hemifacial atrophy with a free dermis-flat from the lower abdomen. Plast Reconstr Surg 1977;59:223-230.
4. Converse JM: Reconstructive Plastic Surgery. Philadelphia, WB Saunders, 1968:1271-1286.
5. Pensler JM, Murphy GF, Mulliken JB: Clinical and ultrastructural studies of Romberg's hemifacial atrophy. Plast Reconstr Surg 1990;85:669-674, discussion 675-676.
6. Callen JP, Klein J: Subacute cutaneous lupus erythematosus. Clinical, serologic, immunogenetic, and therapeutic considerations in seventy-two patients. Arthritis Rheum 1988;31:1007-1013.
7. Chlebus E, Wolska H, Blaszczyk M, Jablonska S: Subacute cutaneous lupus erythematosus versus systemic lupus erythematosus: diagnostic criteria and therapeutic implications. J Am Acad Dermatol 1998;38:405-412.
8. Tan EM, Cohen AS, Fries JF, et al: The 1982 revised criteria for the classification of systemic lupus erythematosus. Arthritis Rheum 1982;25:1271-1277.
9. Falanga V, Tiegs SL, Alstadt SP, et al: Transforming growth factor-beta: selective increase in glycosaminoglycan synthesis by cultures of fibroblasts from patients with progressive systemic sclerosis. J Invest Dermatol 1987;89:100-104.
10. Ho-Asjoe M, Khan J, Frame JD: Dermal grafting for a patient with scleroderma. Case report. Scand J Plast Reconstr Surg Hand Surg 1996;30:325-327.
11. LeRoy EC: Increased collagen synthesis by scleroderma skin fibroblasts in vitro: a possible defect in the regulation or activation of the scleroderma fibroblast. J Clin Invest 1974;54:880-889.
12. Norton WL, Hurd ER, Lewis DC, Ziff M: Evidence of microvascular injury in scleroderma and systemic lupus erythematosus: quantitative study of the microvascular bed. J Lab Clin Med 1968;71:919-933.
13. Rees TD, Ashley FL: Treatment of facial atrophy with liquid silicone. Am J Surg 1966;111:531-535.
14. Rees TD, Ashley FL, Delgado JP: Silicone fluid injections for facial atrophy. A ten-year study. Plast Reconstr Surg 1973;52:118-127.
15. Maas CS, Denton AB: Synthetic soft tissue substitutes: 2001. Facial Plast Surg Clin North Am 2001;9:219-227, viii.
16. Franz FP, Blocksma R, Brundage SR, Ringler SL: Massive injection of liquid silicone for hemifacial atrophy. Ann Plast Surg 1988;20:140-145.
17. Mordick TG 2nd, Larossa D, Whitaker L: Soft-tissue reconstruction of the face: a comparison of dermal-fat grafting and vascularized tissue transfer. Ann Plast Surg 1992;29:390-396.
18. Ersek RA, Chang P, Salisbury MA: Lipo layering of autologous fat: an improved technique with promising results. Plast Reconstr Surg 1998;101:820-826.
19. Losken A, Carlson GW, Culbertson JH, et al: Omental free flap reconstruction in complex head and neck deformities. Head Neck 2002;24:326-331.
20. Wallace JG, Schneider WJ, Brown RG, Nahai FM: Reconstruction of hemifacial atrophy with a free flap of omentum. Br J Plast Surg 1979;32:15-18.
21. Siebert JW, Longaker MT: Aesthetic facial contour reconstruction with microvascular free flaps. Clin Plast Surg 2001;28:361-366, ix.
22. Siebert JW, Longaker MT, Angrigiani C: The inframammary extended circumflex scapular flap: an aesthetic improvement of the parascapular flap. Plast Reconstr Surg 1997;99:70-77.
23. Siebert JW, Longaker MT: Secondary craniofacial management following skeletal correction in facial asymmetry. Application of microsurgical techniques. Clin Plast Surg 1997;24:447-458.
24. Siebert JW, Anson G, Longaker MT: Microsurgical correction of facial asymmetry in 60 consecutive cases. Plast Reconstr Surg 1996;97:354-363.
25. Longaker MT, Siebert JW: Microsurgical correction of facial contour in congenital craniofacial malformations: the marriage of hard and soft tissue. Plast Reconstr Surg 1996;98:942-950.

26. Longaker MT, Flynn A, Siebert JW: Microsurgical correction of bilateral facial contour deformities. Plast Reconstr Surg 1996;98:951-957.

27. Longaker MT, Siebert JW: Microvascular free-flap correction of severe hemifacial atrophy. Plast Reconstr Surg 1995;96:800-809.

28. Upton J, Albin RE, Mulliken JB, Murray JE: The use of scapular and parascapular flaps for cheek reconstruction. Plast Reconstr Surg 1992;90:959-971.

Index

Note: **Boldface** *roman numerals indicate volume. Page numbers followed by f refer to figures; page numbers followed by t refer to tables.*